Classification of nursing diagnoses

PROCEEDINGS OF THE SIXTH CONFERENCE

Classification of nursing diagnoses

PROCEEDINGS OF THE SIXTH CONFERENCE

North American Nursing Diagnosis Association

Edited by

Mary E. Hurley, R.N., M.A., CCRN

Assistant Director of Nursing,
Mount Sinai Medical Center,
New York, New York

with 38 illustrations

The C. V. Mosby Company
St. Louis • Toronto • Princeton   1986

MOSBY

A TRADITION OF PUBLISHING EXCELLENCE

Editor: Barbara Ellen Norwitz
Developmental editor: Sally Adkisson
Manuscript editor: Patricia J. Milstein
Production: Gayle May, Barbara Merritt

Printed in the United States of America

The C.V. Mosby Company
11830 Westline Industrial Drive, St. Louis, Missouri 63146

Library of Congress Cataloging-in-Publication Data

Main entry under title:

Classification of nursing diagnoses.

   Proceedings of the Sixth Conference for the
Classification of Nursing Diagnoses, held in Saint
Louis, Mo., Apr. 4-6, 1984.
      Includes bibliographies and index.
      1. Diagnosis—Congresses.   2. Nursing—Congresses.
I. Hurley, Mary E.   II. North American Nursing
Diagnosis Association.   III. Conference for the
Classification of Nursing Diagnoses (6th : 1984 :
Saint Louis, Mo.) [DNLM: 1.   Nursing Process—
congresses. WY 100   C614   1984]
RT48.C554   1986   616.07′5   85-31046
ISBN 0-8016-3766-X

GW/VH/VH   9   8   7   6   5   4   3   2   1   03/D/302

Contributors

Gordon A. Allen, Ph.D.
Miami University, Oxford, Ohio

Linda S. Baas, R.N., M.S.N., CCRN
University Hospital, Cincinnati, Ohio

Kathleen A. Baldwin, R.N., M.S.N.
Peoria City County Health Department,
Peoria, Illinois

Ann M. Becker, R.N., M.S.N.
St. Louis University School of Nursing,
St. Louis, Missouri

Andrea U. Bircher, R.N., Ph.D.
University of Oklahoma, College of
Nursing, Oklahoma City, Oklahoma

Kathleen A. Breunig, R.N., M.N.
Veterans Administration, Medical
Center, Milwaukee, Wisconsin

Genee Brukwitzki, R.N., M.S.N.
Division of Nursing, Alverno College,
Milwaukee, Wisconsin

Lynne Cheatwood, R.N., B.S.N.
Miami Valley Hospital, Dayton, Ohio

Rene Clark, R.N., M.N., Ed.D
University of Kansas, College of Health
Sciences, Department of Pediatric
Nursing, School of Nursing, Kansas City,
Kansas

Jacqueline Clinton, R.N., Ph.D., F.A.A.N.
University of Wisconsin-Milwaukee,
School of Nursing, Milwaukee, Wisconsin

Luna Collado, R.N., B.S.N.
Veterans Administration, Westside
Medical Center, Chicago, Illinois

Jennifer L. Craig, R.N., Ph.D.
University of British Columbia,
Vancouver, B.C., Canada

Laraine Crane, R.N., M.S.N.
St. Luke's Samaritan Health Care, Inc.,
Milwaukee, Wisconsin

Joan Marie Crosley, R.N., M.S.
Long Island Jewish Medical Center, New
Hyde Park, New York

Kathryn T. Hubalik Czurylo, R.N., M.S.
Veterans Administration, Westside
Medical Center, Chicago, Illinois

Joan M. Duslak, R.N., M.S.N.
Veterans Administration, Westside
Medical Center, Chicago, Illinois

Suzanne Falco, R.N., Ph.D.
St. Luke's Hospital and University of
Wisconsin-Milwaukee, Milwaukee,
Wisconsin

Richard J. Fehring, R.N., D.N.Sc.
Marquette University College of Nursing,
Milwaukee, Wisconsin

Marilyn Frenn, R.N., M.S.N.
Marquette University College of Nursing,
Milwaukee, Wisconsin

Grammatice Garofallou, R.N., M.S.
The Hospital of the Albert Einstein
College of Medicine, Bronx, New York

Marjory Gordon, R.N., Ph.D., F.A.A.N.
Boston College School of Nursing,
Chestnut Hill, Massachusetts

Pamela Gotch, R.N., M.S.N.
Medical College of Wisconsin and St.
Luke's Hospital, Milwaukee, Wisconsin

Margaret R. Grier, R.N., Ph.D.
College of Nursing, University of Illinois
at Chicago, Chicago, Illinois

Edward J. Halloran, R.N., Ph.D., F.A.A.N.
University Hospitals of Cleveland and
Frances Payne Bolton School of Nursing,
Case Western Reserve University,
Cleveland, Ohio

Nancy Hnat, R.N., B.S.N.
The Hospital of the Albert Einstein
College of Medicine, Bronx, New York

Lois M. Hoskins, R.N., Ph.D.
The Catholic University of America,
Washington, D.C.

Dorothea Fox Jakob, R.N., M.A.
City of Toronto, Department of Public
Health, Western Health Area, Parkdale
District, Toronto, Ontario, Canada

Jean L. Jenny, R.N., M.Ed., M.S.
School of Nursing, University of Ottawa,
Ottawa, Ontario, Canada

Lucille A. Joel, R.N., Ed.D., F.A.A.N.
Rutgers University College of Nursing,
Newark, New Jersey

Phyllis E. Jones, R.N., M.Sc.
University of Toronto, Faculty of
Nursing, Toronto, Ontario, Canada

MaryLou Kiley, R.N., Ph.D.
University Hospitals of Cleveland and
Frances Payne Bolton School of Nursing,
Case Western Reserve University,
Cleveland, Ohio

Mi Ja Kim, R.N., Ph.D., F.A.A.N.
College of Nursing, University of Illinois
at Chicago, Chicago, Illinois

Lark W. Kirk, R.N., M.S.N.
The Washington Hospital Center,
Washington, D.C.

Phyllis B. Kritek, R.N., Ph.D., F.A.A.N.
University of Wisconsin-Milwaukee,
School of Nursing, Milwaukee, Wisconsin

Nancy R. Lackey, R.N., Ph.D.
The University of Kansas School of
Nursing, Kansas City, Kansas

Jane Lancour, R.N., M.S.N.
Lancour and Lancour L.T.D. and Medical College of Wisconsin, School of Nursing, Milwaukee, Wisconsin

Norma M. Lang, R.N., Ph.D., F.A.A.N.
School of Nursing, University of Wisconsin-Milwaukee, Milwaukee, Wisconsin

Karen S. Lawson, R.N., M.N.
Department of Nursing, Northeastern Oklahoma, A & M College, Miami, Oklahoma

Chi Hui Kao Lo, R.N., M.S.
Ph.D. Candidate, College of Nursing, University of Illinois at Chicago, Chicago, Illinois

Annette G. Lueckenotte, R.N., M.S.
Illinois Wesleyan University School of Nursing, Bloomington, Illinois

Margaret Lunney, R.N., M.S.N.
Hunter Bellevue School of Nursing, New York, New York

Janet Lutze, R.N., B.S.N.
Health Concepts, Milwaukee, Wisconsin

Patricia A. Martin, R.N., M.S.
Miami Valley Hospital, Division of Nursing, Dayton, Ohio

Ann E. McCourt, R.N., M.S.
New England Sinai Hospital, Stoughton, Massachusetts

Gertrude K. McFarland, R.N., D.N.Sc.
U.S. Department of Health and Human Services, Health Resources and Services Administration, Division of Nursing, Rockville, Maryland

Elizabeth A. McFarlane, R.N., D.N.Sc.
The Catholic University of America, Washington, D.C.

Audrey M. McLane, R.N., Ph.D.
Marquette University College of Nursing, Milwaukee, Wisconsin

Ruth E. McShane, R.N., M.S.N.
University of Wisconsin-Milwaukee, Milwaukee, Wisconsin

Norma M. Metheny, R.N., Ph.D.
St. Louis University, St. Louis, Missouri

Christine A. Miaskowski, R.N., M.S.
The Hospital of the Albert Einstein College of Medicine, Bronx, New York

Judith Fitzgerald Miller, R.N., M.S.N.
Marquette University College of Nursing, Milwaukee, Wisconsin

Carol A. Morris, R.N., M.S., M.N.
Department of Nursing, Northeastern Oklahoma, A & M College, Miami, Oklahoma

Judith L. Myers, R.N., M.S.N.
St. Louis University, St. Louis, Missouri

Deborah M. Nadzam, R.N., M.S.
University Hospital of Cleveland, Cleveland, Ohio

Charlotte Naschinski, R.N., M.S.
Saint Elizabeth's Hospital, National Institute of Mental Health, U.S. Department of Health and Human Services, Washington, D.C.

Syble M. Oldaker, R.N., Ph.D.
Clemson University, College of Nursing, Clemson, South Carolina

Anne G. Perry, R.N., M.S.N.
St. Louis University, St. Louis, Missouri

Barbara E. Pokorny, R.N., M.S.N.
United Community Services, Public
Health Nursing Department, Norwich,
Connecticut

Marion M. Resler, R.N., M.S.N.
St. Louis University, St. Louis, Missouri

Laura Rossi, R.N., M.S.
Brigham and Women's Hospital, Boston,
Massachusetts

M. Gaie Rubenfeld, R.N., M.S.
The Catholic University of America,
Washington, D.C.

Polly Ryan, R.N., M.S.N.
St. Luke's Hospital, Milwaukee,
Wisconsin

Ann M. Schreier, R.N., Ph.D.
The Catholic University of America,
Washington, D.C.

Pamela M. Schroeder, R.N., M.S.N.
St. Luke's Samaritan Health Care, Inc.,
Milwaukee, Wisconsin

Judeen Schulte, R.N., M.S.N.
Division of Nursing, Alverno College,
Milwaukee, Wisconsin

Franklin A. Shaffer, R.N., Ed.D.
National League for Nursing, New York,
New York

DeLanne A. Simmons, R.N., M.P.H.
Visiting Nurse Association of Omaha,
Omaha, Nebraska

Deborah Ann Smith, R.N., B.S.N.
Columbia Hospital, Milwaukee,
Wisconsin

Martha A. Spies, R.N., M.S.N., CCRN
Deaconess College of Nursing, St. Louis,
Missouri

Rosemarie Suhayda, R.N., M.S.N.
University of Illinois at Chicago Health
Sciences Center, Chicago, Illinois

Marita G. Titler, R.N., M.A.
Coe College, Cedar Rapids, Iowa

Karen G. Vincent, R.N., M.S.
Coastal Community Counseling Center,
Braintree, Massachusetts

Ann Marie Voith, R.N., B.S.N.
Columbia Hospital, Milwaukee,
Wisconsin

Mary B. Walsh, R.N., M.S.N.
The Catholic University of America,
Washington, D.C.

Ramona M. Wessler, R.N., Ph.D.
St. Louis University, St. Louis, Missouri

Una E. Westfall, R.N., M.S.N.
Oregon Health Sciences University,
School of Nursing, Portland, Oregon

Ellen G. Wilson, R.N., M.S.N.
North Chicago Veterans Administration
Medical Center, Chicago, Illinois

Karen A. York, R.N., M.S.N.
Miami Valley Hospital, Dayton, Ohio

Preface

The Sixth Conference on the Classification of Nursing Diagnoses was held in St. Louis, Missouri, April 4 to 6, 1984. The meeting differed from past conferences in several ways. This was the first conference to convene under the recently formed North American Nursing Diagnosis Association (NANDA). In order to recognize the international scope of membership in the association, the word "national" was dropped from the program title but it was decided to continue the sequential numbering.

Since the more formal structuring of the Association 2 years earlier, a state of transition had existed. The Association leaders had been diligently working to make the new bylaws operational. Previously, the review and refinement of nursing diagnoses had been the major focus of the conferences' small-group work sessions. The new bylaws called for the development of a criteria-based review process for all nursing diagnoses and the coordination of the review by a Diagnosis Review Committee. Small-group work sessions were deleted at the Sixth Conference, pending the development and implementation of the review process.

The program consisted of thirteen invited papers presented at general sessions. Six additional sessions contained 21 submitted papers that had been selected for presentation by a review panel. Additionally, eighteen poster exhibits were displayed.

In addition to these formal sessions, certain other events made the meeting noteworthy. This conference saw the first business meeting of the new association convened under Marjory Gordon, President. Preceding the meeting was an awards ceremony recognizing the contributions of five of the original leaders in nursing diagnosis. Special interest groups and regional groups also met and discussed issues of concern related to nursing diagnosis and the Association.

In view of the recent establishment of NANDA and the rich history of the nursing diagnosis movement, the theme of the conference, Nursing Diagnosis—A Janus View, was particularly appropriate. The events of the meeting offered several opportunities for participants to look at nursing diagnosis from a past and future perspective and encouraged both reflection and strategic planning.

The editor of the proceedings has tried to organize the material in a way that will provide continuity and clarity as well as highlight the many perspectives from which nursing diagnosis was reviewed.

Section I begins with the keynote address by Dr. Mi Ja Kim and continues with the general sessions papers divided by category. Section II contains the papers presented at simultaneous sessions. These are also grouped according to category as much as possible. The poster presentations are listed alphabetically by the author's last name in Section III, and Section IV contains the currently accepted nursing diagnoses. The Chairperson of the Program Committee, Audrey McLane, provides an excellent overview of some of the major conference papers in Section V. Also included in this section are the minutes of the business meeting. Several appendices contain reference data that should prove informative and useful.

The three day meeting gave credence to the belief that nursing diagnosis was and is steadily gaining support and momentum within the nursing profession. This meeting had the largest attendance in the history of the conferences. Equally significant was the quality of the papers and posters presented. Much work remains to be done in the area of nursing diagnosis. The conference aided this endeavor by providing an opportunity for sharing ideas, gaining information, and setting direction and priorities, all of which are needed to identify and meet the many challenges that still remain before us.

I wish to express my gratitude to Karen Murphy, Executive Director, NANDA, Dr. Phyllis Kritek, Vice President, NANDA, and Sallyanne Castro, Secretarial Assistant, for their help and support during the preparation of these proceedings.

Mary E. Hurley
Editor

Contents

xi

Section III

Poster presentations, 380

CHAPTER 1

Nursing diagnosis: a Janus view

MI JA KIM, Ph.D., R.N., F.A.A.N.

It is a great honor and privilege to deliver the keynote address at this historical conference in which the language of the nursing profession is being shaped and discussed. As the title denotes, I shall follow the characteristics of the Roman God, Janus. That is, I will look back on the footprints of the National Conference Group on Classification of Nursing Diagnoses and the North American Nursing Diagnosis Association (NANDA) for the past 11 years and will look forward to the future work of nursing diagnosis and NANDA.

Looking back, I am reminded of the editorial by Edith Lewis in *Nursing Outlook* (1975) entitled, "The stuff of which nursing is made." In this editorial, Lewis stated that "we must admit the idea (of the First National Conference on Classification of Nursing Diagnoses)* struck us as a bit pretentious. . . . As we listened to the formal and informal presentation at that meeting [the Nursing Diagnosis session of the 1974 ANA Convention*], we soon discovered that there is much more to a nursing diagnostic classification system than first meets the eye" (Lewis, 1975). Indeed the skepticism and criticism about the words "nursing diagnosis" abounded when the National Conference Group on Classification of Nursing Diagnosis embarked on its voyage in 1973. However, as was pointed out by Lewis, there was, there is, and there will be much more substance to a Nursing Diagnosis Classification system than the mere words may indicate. I believe the work of NANDA has far-reaching impact to every facet of the nursing profession, particularly to nursing practice, where increasing numbers of nurses are expected to use nursing diagnoses in everyday practice.

One of the major reasons why I believe nursing diagnosis is so important to the nursing profession is that it provides the language that is *uniquely* nursing—by which we describe nursing and with which nursing can identify. It expresses the phenomena of nursing science and art in nursing language and provides a means by which the nursing science base can expand. Abdellah

---

*Added to clarify the meaning of the quotations.

(1969) defined nursing science as "a body of cumulative scientific knowledge, drawn from the physical, biological, and behavioral sciences that is uniquely nursing." Furthermore, Crawford, Default, and Rudy (1979) stated that concepts and theories that are borrowed from other sciences must be redefined and synthesized according to the perspective of nursing. A similar thought was echoed by McMurrey (1982), who said that "knowledge becomes unique because of the unique perspective of the discipline in which that knowledge is incorporated."

I believe nursing diagnoses bring this unique perspective of the nursing discipline to the theories, principles, and concepts of other sciences and expresses them in the nomenclature which nurses can use in their practice, research, and teaching. When nursing diagnoses have established validity and reliability and are found clinically relevant and useful, they can become the building blocks of the nursing science knowledge base and of the nursing diagnosis taxonomical system. However, developing a nursing diagnosis taxonomy that is theoretically sound and clinically useful is one of the most complex and difficult tasks that the nursing profession has ever faced.

The development of nursing diagnosis taxonomy is a difficult and complex endeavor. The *New York Times* carried an article by Webster on February 14, 1982, with the title, "Classification is more than a matter of fish or fowl." The article began with the question, "If it flies, has two legs, yellow feathers and sings, it's a canary. Right?" The author answered by saying, "Well, yes, if you're satisfied with simple answers." However, if the same question was posed to a taxonomist, he or she would ask whether or not the canary was "a pure-bred Hartz Mountain finch or an American hybrid, where it fits on the evolutionary scale, or what species it's most closely related to" (Webster, 1982). In addition, the taxonomist would have to choose one of three major systems of taxonomical research which are currently used by scientists. I quickly discovered that these taxonomist scientists are not any different from nurse scientists and that they, too, have a lot of controversy among themselves as to the methods of developing a taxonomy. Time and space do not permit a lengthy discussion about this controversy; only a brief description of their approaches will be made here.

There are three taxonomical branches. The first is the evolutionary taxonomy, which stresses relationships of organisms based on their evolutionary history. The second is phenetics, a Greek word meaning *appearance*, which focuses on observable similarities. The third is cladistics, a Greek word meaning *branch*, which attempts to establish the temporal sequence of "branching" within an order or family of species on its evolutionary tree.

Gould, a Harvard evolutionary biologist (Webster, 1982), offered the following comments regarding these three classification theories. He described the *cladist* as a scientist who rejects overall similarity and works with branching order alone; the *phenetist* as one who works with overall similarity alone and tries to measure it in the vain pursuit of objectivity; and the *traditional* taxonomist as one who tries to balance both kinds of information. This is a legitimate act but disparate and often falls into hopeless subjectivity because they conflict with each other. Depicting the situation, he said that "trying to change a cladist's mind is like trying to deprogram a Moonie" (cited in Webster, 1982). In view of the strengths and weaknesses of these taxonomical branches, I suggest that nursing could benefit by using all three systems when possible, to arrive at a classification system.

The difficulty of developing a taxonomy system was also well described by Cattel and Shierer (1961) in their book entitled, *The Meaning and Measurement of Neuroticism and Anxiety.* On the other hand, the reasons for the difficulty of developing a taxonomy were listed as "theoretical orientation; relative emphasis on etiology, complaint, and behavior; and the differences between adults and children" (Chandler and Lundahl, 1983). In every instance, however, all disciplines recognized the need and importance of having a taxonomy. Dreger (1977), for instance, listed the major benefits of having a taxonomy as the following: having a taxonomy would bring clarity to the problem, improve communication among professionals, facilitate research, and provide the necessary conceptual understanding from which the most appropriate and effective intervention choices can be made.

I will now review the historical growth and development of nursing diagnosis and NANDA. The Task Force Group reports of the Third, Fourth, and Fifth National Conferences that were presented by Gordon (1982, 1984) describe detailed accounts of the progress of the National Conference Group. Tables 1, 2, and 3 highlight some of the salient features of the past five national conferences. As can be seen in Table 1, all five National Conferences were held in St. Louis, with the number attending ranging from 119 to 199, except this sixth conference in which more than 450 nurses are in attendance. The major reason why the number attending stayed below the 200 line during the first five National Conferences was that the Conference was by and large by invitation based on expertise and experience. This method was appropriate for the purpose of the conference, that of developing, refining, and approving nursing diagnoses during the initial growing period. Nurses with different functional areas, namely teaching, practice, administration, research, and theory, were present at every Conference. The large number attending this Conference reflects the open invitation to all nurses and the different purpose of the Conference, that is, dissemination of information.

Table 2 shows the methods used to generate and approve nursing diagnoses, and the theorists' involvement. The first four National Conferences used an inductive approach by small groups to generate nursing diagnoses. A hand vote by all attending at the end of the Conferences was used to approve nursing

TABLE 1   The profile of national conferences

Year	Place	No. at-tending	Functional area of attendants	Type of conference
1973	St. Louis	119	Teacher, clinician, administrator, researcher, theorist	Invitation by expertise
1975	St. Louis	156	Teacher, clinician, administrator, researcher, theorist	Invitation by expertise
1978	St. Louis	350	Teacher, clinician, administrator, researcher, theorist	Invitation by expertise/experience
1980	St. Louis		Teacher, clinician, administrator, researcher, theorist	Invitation by expertise/experience
1982	St. Louis	199	Teacher, clinician, administrator, researcher, theorist	Invitation by expertise/experience
1984	St. Louis	>450	—	Open

TABLE 2   Methods of developing approved list and theoretical framework

Year	Method of generating nursing diagnoses	Method of approval of nursing diagnoses	Theorists' involvement
1973	Inductive approach by small groups	Hand vote by all attending	0
1975	Inductive approach by small groups	Hand vote by all attending	0
1978	Inductive approach by small groups	Hand vote by all attending	Theoretical framework by 14 nurse theorists
1980	Inductive approach by small groups	Hand vote by all attending	Theoretical framework Refinement with clinical specialists' input
1982	Inductive approach by small groups and approval by the task force	Written vote by all attending	Theoretical framework Refinement by small group work Nursing diagnosis taxonomy begun
1984	None	None	None

TABLE 3   **Activities of national conferences**

Year	No. of papers presented invited/peer reviewed		ANA convention nursing diagnosis session	Proceedings editors	Administrative structure
1973	3	0		Gebbie and Lavin	Task force
			1974 Gordon and Roy		
1975	1	0	—	Gebbie	Task force
1978	6	4	—	Kim and Moritz (one volume for 1978 and 1980)	Task force
1980	8	6	Kim and McLane		Task force and Steering Committee
1982	9	45	Gordon, Kim, and McLane	Kim, McFarland, and McLane	NANDA organized

diagnoses. At the Fifth National Conference, the outcome of the small groups which still used an inductive approach was subjected to and approved by the Task Force Group. Another important difference at the Fifth Conference was that the diagnoses had to be submitted with research or clinical data prior to the Conference for consideration by the National Conference Group.

The historical account of the development of the theorist group is found in the reports given by Sr. C. Roy (1982, 1984) at the Third, Fourth, and Fifth National Conferences, published in the Proceedings. I simply want to point out that the theorists participated in the development of a conceptual framework to organize the nursing diagnoses that were generated by the inductive approach. It was thought that both inductive and deductive approaches would facilitate the process of developing a nursing diagnosis taxonomy. Under the leadership of Sr. C. Roy, 14 nurse theorists met at the Third National Conference and developed a conceptual framework which was refined with input from clinical specialists at the Fourth National Conference. At the Fifth National Conference two small groups worked with the conceptual framework. One group examined the relationship of the Unitary Man framework to defining characteristics of nursing diagnoses. The other group developed a taxonomy using the framework. For example, the first small group, led by K. Gebbie (1984), categorized defining characteristics of *Airway Clearance, Ineffective* as follows: abnormal breath sounds and cyanotic were assigned to the category: exchanging. The work of the second small group, led by P. Kritek (1984), demonstrates the beginning effort of relating nursing diagnoses to the Unitary Man framework and building a taxonomic tree. Her report shows many missing elements in the taxonomy which indicate urgent need for more intense work in these areas.

Table 3 shows the activities of the National Conference Group. Most notably, the number of peer-reviewed papers increased drastically at the Fifth National Conference and the trend continued in the Sixth National Conference. Sessions on Nursing Diagnosis were presented at the ANA Conventions in 1974 by Gordon and Roy; 1980 by Kim and McLane; and 1982 by Gordon, Kim, and McLane. These facts reflect the giant steps, taken in the area of nursing diagnosis in recent years. The work of the National Conferences has been captured in the form of Proceedings. The First proceedings was edited by Gebbie and Lavin (1973), the second by Gebbie (1976), the third and fourth together by Kim and Moritz (1982), and the fifth by Kim, McFarland, and McLane (1984). For 7 years, the organization existed in a very loose form operated by the Task Force Group and the Clearinghouse located at the School of Nursing, St. Louis University. This loose and flexible organization served a purpose in the initial phase. However, increasing demands and complexity of the work necessitated the election of a Steering Committee at the Fourth National Conference. Finally, a formal organization, the North American Nursing Diagnosis Association (NANDA), was established at the Fifth National Conference in 1982.

The major issues related to nursing diagnosis have changed over time. From 1973 to about 1978, attention appeared to focus on the word, "diagnosis." Questions such as "Can nurses diagnose?" were asked. As this issue gradually subsided, a new issue emerged concerning the concept and definition of nursing diagnosis. Nurses debated what the criteria for nursing diagnosis were and, more specifically, how the nursing diagnosis should be defined in terms of nursing interventions. Under the rubric of these questions the following two subquestions can be posed for our consideration. Should nursing interventions be 100% independent in solving the patient's problem all the time? Could nursing interventions be independent most of the time (e.g., >70%) and interdependent some of the time (e.g., <30%) in solving the patient's problem?

In order to provide answers to these questions, 87 nurses who attended a recent workshop on nursing diagnosis were asked to rate each nursing diagnosis by the percent level of independence, interdependence, and dependence of their nursing interventions (Kim, 1984). *Independent* was defined as nursing interventions which can be carried out without a physician's order and which can solve the patient's problems without consultation or collaboration with physicians or other health professionals. *Interdependent* was defined as nursing interventions which can be carried out with a physician's order and which provide the solution of the patient's problem in a collaborative manner. *Dependent* was defined as nursing interventions which were carried out with a physician's order and without nursing judgment or decision-making.

Table 4 shows the results of this survey. Only selected nursing diagnoses are shown here. The grand average of independent, interdependent, and de-

TABLE 4   **Degree of independence of nursing interventions for nursing diagnoses**

Nursing Diagnosis	Nursing intervention (%)					
	Independent		Interde-pendent		Dependent	
	Mean	SD*	Mean	SD	Mean	SD
Airway clearance, ineffective	57	36	36	34	7	14
Activity intolerance	57	37	34	36	9	18
Anxiety	59	34	30	32	11	21
Bowel elimination, constipation	60	32	31	30	9	19
Breathing patterns, ineffective	39	33	44	34	17	26
Cardiac output, decreased	31	30	44	33	25	32
Comfort, alt. in, pain	59	32	30	30	11	21
Coping, ineffective, individual	61	33	33	31	6	11
Fluid volume deficit	40	35	47	35	13	21
Grieving, anticipatory	70	32	23	29	7	15
Injury, potential for	68	36	27	36	4	8
Knowledge deficit	70	33	25	31	6	14
Mobility, impaired physical	56	35	34	9	9	18
Noncompliance	66	35	28	33	6	11
Nutrition, alt. in, less than body requirements	48	35	44	34	8	13
Self-care deficit	74	31	20	28	6	16
Skin integrity, impairment actual	71	32	22	30	6	14
Sleep pattern disturbance	69	32	23	29	8	18

*SD = standard deviation

pendent nursing interventions for all of these nursing diagnoses were as follows: independent 59%, interdependent 32%, and dependent 9%. The nursing diagnoses with higher than 70% independent nursing interventions were: grieving, anticipatory (70%); knowledge deficit (70%); self-care deficit (74%); and skin integrity (71%). On the other hand, nursing diagnoses that were perceived to have less than 50% independent nursing interventions were: breathing patterns, ineffective (39%); cardiac output, decreased (31%); fluid volume deficit (40%); and nutrition, alteration in, less than body requirements (48%).

It is discomforting to note that no one nursing diagnosis was perceived to have 100% independent nursing interventions and that the highest mean for percent independent intervention was only 74% (self-care deficit). Further-more, it is disappointing to note that this group of nurses perceived all nursing diagnosis interventions collectively as only 59% independent. Judging from the wide standard deviations, the percent of independent nursing interventions varied a great deal, which could be a reflection of the reality of practice or the respondent's point of view. A randomized study would be necessary to gen-eralize beyond this sample; however, the result of this survey suggests that the definition of nursing diagnosis cannot be limited, implicitly or explicitly, to independent nursing interventions only.

The history of nursing functions can be divided roughly into four blocks of time. From the beginning of nursing to the 1960s, nursing functions were perhaps more dependent than interdependent. From the early 1960s up to the 1970s the reverse might have been true, in that nursing functions were more interdependent than dependent. Between 1970 and the 1980s, the notion of dependent function diminished considerably and nursing functions were de-scribed primarily in terms of interdependent and independent. However, the proportion of interdependent nursing functions was perhaps still higher than independent nursing functions. From 1980 on into the future, I predict that independent nursing functions will be higher than the interdependent nursing functions and the so-called "fuzzy" diagnoses will become clear and focused in the nursing domain.

The issue of the boundary of nursing discipline is inseparably linked to the topic of independent versus interdependent (collaborative) nursing functions. This issue can be addressed in light of the recent decision and the reasoning for the decision by the judge of the Missouri Supreme Court. In making the decision in favor of two certified nurse practitioners, the judge expressed the difficulty of defining and drawing the "thin line that separates the practice of medicine and the practice of professional nursing in modern day delivery of health services" (Selby, 1984). Furthermore, the comments made by a physician regarding nursing diagnosis indicate a distinct possibility that nursing and medicine could successfully collaborate for patient care and that interdepen-dence on each other is a natural course of practice in today's health care setting. Marion E. Alberts, the Scientific Editor of the *Journal of the Iowa Medical Society*, wrote an article on "Commenting editorially: nursing diagnosis," in which he urged all physicians to learn about nursing diagnosis and recom-mended that physicians meet with nursing staff and have a meaningful dialogue about this "very useful and exciting concept" (nursing diagnosis). He further noted that "the legal responsibilities of the nurse are broadening, and the wise physician will soon realize the nurse of the future will work with and not for the medical profession" (Alberts, 1983).

Now looking forward from the Janus view, two broad categories will be considered. One deals with the concept and use of nursing diagnosis and the other relates to the key roles that NANDA could play in determining the success of nursing diagnosis taxonomy. First, the concept and use of nursing diagnosis will be addressed in terms of practice, education, and research. Second, the key roles will be suggested in terms of nomenclature/taxonomy development, research funding, regional networking, communication channels, and dissemination of information.

In regard to the practice setting, the concept and definition of nursing diagnosis with respect to the level of nursing functions, independent versus interdependent, need to be clarified and put to rest. This would eliminate unnecessary polarization among nurses on the issue and allow us to move forward with more important tasks, such as developing a nursing diagnosis taxonomy and diagnosis-specific nursing interventions. Among the three functional areas of nursing, practice has made the most impressive progress in the use of nursing diagnosis. Another important issue that faces nurses in the practice setting is the concept and use of etiology. Discussions with clinical experts in various specialty fields indicate that not every nursing diagnosis can have an etiology. I am told that in psychiatric nursing, for instance, identifying the etiology or etiologies is as difficult as identifying the nursing diagnosis itself and that psychiatric nurses frequently operate with contributing or associated factors. I further learned from the practice setting that a nursing diagnosis often serves as the etiology for another nursing diagnosis. This brings up the complexity of the concept of etiology which was presented by Forsyth at the Fifth National Conference (Forsyth, 1984). Box 1 illustrates the possi-

---

BOX 1   **Complexity of etiology***

	Z ← (N.Dx.†)	Y ← (N.Dx.)	X ← Presumed cause (N.Dx.?)	W Cause of the cause
Example: Practice setting: Critical care unit		Decreased cardiac output	Tachy- or bradyarrhythmia	Myocardial ischemia and/or hypokalemia
Ambulatory or commu- nity setting	Activity intolerance	Decreased cardiac output		

---

*Modified from Forsyth, G.: In Kim, M.J., McFarland, G.K., and McLane, A.M., editors: Classification of nursing diagnosis—proceedings of the Fifth National Conference, St. Louis, 1984, The C.V. Mosby Co.
†N.Dx., Nursing diagnosis.

bility of endless "cause of the cause" relationships depending upon one's level of sophistication, expertise, specialty, and practice setting. For instance, in the critical care unit, decreased cardiac output may be a nursing diagnosis with the etiology of tachy- or- bradyarrhythmia, which in turn could be caused by myocardial ischemia and/or hypokalemia. On the other hand, in the ambulatory or community setting, activity intolerance may be an appropriate nursing diagnosis with the etiology of decreased cardiac output which, in turn, could be caused by two other levels of etiologies as stated above. Hence, one is compelled to ask which one of these is the nursing diagnosis, or are all three of them the nursing diagnoses? It seems that understanding the level and the type of expertise in different practice settings is the key factor for developing a reality-based nursing diagnosis taxonomy, and I often wonder whether much of the controversy surrounding so-called "fuzzy" nursing diagnosis categories can largely be explained on this basis.

The concept and the use of nursing diagnosis in the educational setting have been quite limited compared to the practice setting. A curriculum could be developed incorporating nursing diagnosis for baccalaureate, masters, and doctoral programs. In order for nursing diagnosis to be taught properly, courses such as logic and mathematics should be taught in the freshman or sophomore year before entering the nursing process course. Following this, nursing diagnoses that are more concrete could be taught in the beginning year and nursing diagnoses with increasing complexity and abstractness could be taught in the advanced years, such as junior and senior levels. Master's programs could build on the BSN curriculum, with a major research emphasis on selected nursing diagnoses to develop and test construct validity and reliability. Doctoral programs could be developed using a nursing diagnosis specialty as a focus for the doctoral study option. Students could conduct research to establish internal and external validity of nursing diagnoses so that scientifically valid diagnosis-specific nursing interventions could be generated for clinical use.

Educational needs of staff nurses regarding the diagnostic process and the concept of nursing diagnosis have been met fairly well by continuing education workshops at local and regional levels. Indeed, the number of continuing education workshops on nursing diagnosis have increased impressively in recent years. However, well-coordinated comprehensive educational programs at regional levels by well-trained teachers would be more efficient and economical in reaching staff nurses with expert knowledge.

As noted earlier, research studies on the concept and the use of nursing diagnosis have definitely increased during the past 4 years. I shall address the following questions about future research endeavors. What kind of studies are needed in the future, and which ones should have priority? How should research activities interface with nursing theories and nursing practice?

First, what kind of studies are needed? Before I present the types of studies, I would like to point out that the numerous research questions which were generated for each diagnosis at the Fifth National Conference can serve as the beginning points of inquiry and that these are listed in the Proceedings (Kim, McFarland, and McLane, 1984). Three general categories of studies are suggested for the future: (1) descriptive, (2) empirical or statistical, and (3) experimental.

The descriptive study is usually guided by some theoretical framework which provides an understanding of the phenomenon of nursing. The major purposes of the descriptive study would be: (1) to identify and synthesize available data (knowledge) to establish construct validity of nursing diagnoses and (2) to identify etiologies and nursing interventions for nursing diagnoses. Both of these objectives can be largely accomplished by a comprehensive literature review of primary sources, with the understanding that nursing perspectives should be brought to bear on the theories, principles, and concepts of other sciences. When data are not available in the literature, survey and clinical study are suggested. Since the priority is to establish validity and reliability of nursing diagnoses, the qualifications of the nurse sample are extremely important. In keeping with the idea that nursing diagnosis should be made by professional nurses, preferred educational criterion for the sample of nurses is BSN degree and certainly not undergraduate students or non-RN's. Whenever possible, nurse experts such as clinical specialists should be consulted for validation of nursing diagnoses, either in survey or clinical studies.

Empirical or statistical approaches often rely on observed behaviors such as clusters of signs and symptoms and inferences made from the clusters by the researcher. However, Edelbrock (1979) stated that the results of this approach are of questionable clinical relevance since they generally lack a conceptual framework. This could be remedied with Chandler and Lundahl's (1983) recommendation that as a priority, researchers develop a conceptual framework which proposes diagnostic categories so that diagnoses can be tested by empirical methods.

The major purposes of experimental studies are: (1) to develop outcome criteria and test nursing interventions for nursing diagnoses and (2) to develop a conceptual framework and/or test nursing theories in conjunction with nursing diagnoses. However, experimental studies cannot be carried out until clinically valid and reliable nursing diagnoses are available. Nursing interventions that are directed by nursing diagnoses should bring forth results that can be evaluated by outcome criteria.

In regard to the relationship between theory and research, Fawcett (1978) described it as "a double helix" whose core has theory directing research and research findings shaping the development of theory. Likewise, research related to nursing diagnosis should be guided by a theory, and the research findings of nursing diagnoses in turn should contribute to the enhancement of nursing theory. The relationship of theories and research to practice can be described as shown below:

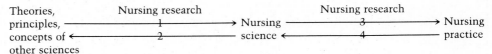

Step 1 shows that the theories, principles, and concepts of other sciences become nursing science through nursing research, and step 2 shows the role and the responsibility of nursing science feeding back into other sciences. Step 3 shows the role of nursing science to nursing practice via nursing research, and step 4, vice versa. It is important to point out that nursing practice is guided by nursing science, which is developed by research, and that nursing practice is the source of research.

Still with futuristic eyes, I will present my wish list to officers of NANDA. First and foremost, generation and refinement of nursing diagnosis nomenclature and further development of a nursing diagnosis taxonomy are of prime importance. To fulfill the leadership role of NANDA in these areas I suggest the following:

1. Develop a process by which incoming data such as diagnostic labels, etiologies, references, etc., can be systematically examined and recommended for approval to be included on the list.
2. Examine nursing diagnoses, etiologies, and defining characteristics which are already published in the Proceedings and elsewhere so that they can become part of the approved list.
3. Develop criteria by which nursing diagnosis can be evaluated in terms of problem, etiology, and signs and symptoms so that standardized nomenclature can be developed.
4. Clarify the concept and usefulness of "etiology."
5. Consult a taxonomist for development of a nursing diagnosis taxonomy.

Next, active research support for nursing diagnosis studies should be instituted, particularly in relation to the Diagnostic Related Group system. NANDA could provide seed money for research projects or engage in fundraising endeavors so that a nationwide study could be instituted.

Third, develop a highly organized and functional regional network with regional directors and state coordinators who will assess needs, coordinate activities, and serve as liaisons to NANDA.

Fourth, develop a mechanism by which nurses at large can communicate with and participate in the activities of NANDA. Dialogue on issues concerning nursing diagnosis and ideas about the operation of NANDA from nurses at large would be helpful for the growth of the organization.

Fifth, NANDA could enlarge the scope of information dissemination. The current nursing diagnosis newsletter could be expanded and could follow the format of a peer-reviewed journal.

I realize that the magnitude of these suggestions is overwhelming, but my confidence in the ability of the current leaders leaves me no doubt that they will give attentive ears to these suggestions.

In closing, I wish to reemphasize the key point made by Alberts (1983): nurses of today and certainly the future work *with* and *not for* physicians. I believe nursing diagnosis can serve as the key element that will promote such a relationship.

REFERENCES

Abdellah, F.: The nature of nursing science, Nursing Research **18**:390-393, 1969.

Alberts, M.E.: Commenting editorially—nursing diagnosis, J. Iowa Med. Soc. **73**:273-276, 1983.

Cattel, R., and Schierer, I.: The meaning and measurement of neuroticism and anxiety, New York, 1961, Ronald Press.

Chandler, L.A., and Lundahl, W.T.: Empirical classification of emotional adjustment reactions, Amer. J. Orthopsych. **53**:460-467, 1983.

Crawford, G., Default, K., and Rudy, C.: Evolving issues in theory development, Nurs. Outlook **27**:346-351, 1979.

Dreger, R.: The children's behavioral classification project: an interim report, J. Ab. Child Psychol. **5**:289-297, 1977.

Edelbrock, C.: Empirical classification of childen's behavior disorders: progress based on parent and teacher ratings, School Psychol. Dig. **8**:355-369, 1979.

Fawcett, J.: The relationship between theory and research: a double helix, Adv. Nurs. Sci. **1**:49-62, 1978.

Forsyth, G.L.: Etiology: in what sense and of what value. In Kim, M.J., McFarland, G.K., and McLane, A.M., editors: Classification of nursing diagnoses—Proceedings of the Fifth National Conference, St. Louis, 1984, The C.V. Mosby Co.

Gebbie, K.M., editor: Summary of the Second National Conference—Classification of nursing diagnoses, St. Louis, 1976, Clearinghouse, National Group for Classification of Nursing Diagnoses.

Gebbie, K.: Small group work on diagnostic labels. In Kim, M.J., McFarland, G.K., and McLane, A.M., editors: Classification of nursing diagnoses—Proceedings of the Fifth National Conference, St. Louis, 1984, The C.V. Mosby Co.

Gebbie, K.M., and Lavin, M.A., editors: Proceedings of the First National Conference—Classification of nursing diagnoses, St. Louis, 1975, The C.V. Mosby Co.

Gordon, M.: Historical perspective: the National Conference Group for Classification of Nursing Diagnoses (1978, 1980). In Kim, M.J., and Moritz, D.A., editors: Classification of nursing diagnoses—Proceedings of the Third and Fourth National Conferences, New York, 1982, McGraw-Hill Book Co.

Gordon, M.: Report of the Task Force Conference Group for Classification of Nursing Diagnoses. In Kim, M.J., McFarland, G.K., and McLane, A.M., editors: Classification of nursing diagnoses—Proceedings of the Fifth National Conference, St. Louis, 1984, The C.V. Mosby Co.

Kim, M.J.: Level of nursing functions associated with nursing diagnoses. (Unpublished data.)

Kim, M.J., McFarland, G.K., and McLane, A.M., editors: (1984). Classification of nursing diagnoses—Proceedings of the Fifth National Conference, St. Louis, 1984, The C.V. Mosby Co.

Kim, M.J., and Moritz, D.A., editors: Classification of nursing diagnoses—Proceedings of the Third and Fourth National Conferences, New York, 1982, McGraw-Hill Book Co.

Kritek, P.: Report of the group work on taxonomies. In Kim, M.J., McFarland, G.K., and McLane, A.M., editors: Classification of nursing diagnoses—Proceedings of the Fifth National Conference, St. Louis, 1984, The C.V. Mosby Co.

Lewis, E.P.: The stuff of which nursing is made, Nurs. Outlook **23:**89, 1975.

McMurrey, P.H.: Toward a unique knowledge base in nursing. Image **14:**12-15, 1982.

Roy, C.: Framework for classification systems development: progress and issues. In Kim, M.J., McFarland, G.K., and McLane, A.M., editors: Classification of nursing diagnoses—Proceedings of the Fifth National Conference, St. Louis, 1984, The C.V. Mosby Co.

Roy, C.: Historical perspective of the theoretical framework for the classification of nursing diagnosis (1980). In Kim, M.J., and Moritz, D.A., editors: Classification of nursing diagnoses—Proceedings of Third and Fourth National Conferences, New York, 1982, McGraw-Hill Book Co.

Selby, T.L.: Court overturns ruling restricting NPs practice, Amer. Nurse **3:**20, 1984.

Webster, B.: Classification is more than a matter of fish or fowl, *New York Times,* February 14, 1982.

CHAPTER 2

Classification, taxonomy, structure

ANA Steering Committee on Classifications of Nursing Practice Phenomena: current and future directions

NORMA M. LANG, Ph.D., R.N., F.A.A.N.

It is with great pleasure that I bring you greetings from the American Nurses' Association. I am very pleased to be here to discuss the current and future Directions of the ANA Committee on Classifications of Nursing Practice Phenomena.

The American Nurses' Association has consistently had a representative present at each of the Nursing Diagnoses conferences. I am pleased that this meeting provides us with an opportunity to discuss mutual goals and processes of the American Nurses' Association (ANA) and the North American Nursing Diagnosis Association (NANDA). Although I am the invited spokesperson this morning, I think it is important that you know that Marjory Gordon and Roberta Thiry, present at this conference, are also members of the Steering Committee. Marjory Gordon, well known as a leader of NANDA, serves as the official liaison person between ANA and NANDA. Other ANA Steering Committee members are: Ada Sue Hinshaw, Kathryn Barnard, Virginia Saba, Marlene Ventura, Jean Steel, and Roberta Conti.

Let me begin my remarks by clarifying the title of the committee. The current group is called the ANA Steering Committee on Classifications of Nursing Practice Phenomena. I think it is significant that the group did not continue to be labeled, as it was at the time of appointment and as were others in the past, a Task Force on a Taxonomy for Nursing.

Historically, several groups within ANA were assigned the task of developing *a* taxonomy. Several approaches were examined, including a taxonomical structure for nurses as well as for nursing. Although outlines for proposals were developed, no specific products were forthcoming.

In 1982, the Steering Committee on Classifications of Nursing Practice Phenomena was established. The Steering Committee is responsible to the Cabinet on Nursing Practice in cooperation with the Cabinet on Nursing Research and recently the Cabinet on Nursing Services.

Early in its deliberations, the current ANA Steering Committee invited consultant philosophers of science to discuss alternatives for taxonomic structures. One was Glenn Webster, whom NANDA subsequently invited to its conference. After hours of discussion with these consultants, the group recommended that the ANA not pursue the development of *a* taxonomy but rather to encourage and monitor groups who are attempting such a task. The consultants warned that nursing is a discipline that is "too rich in data" to try to limit it to a single taxonomy at this time. A single taxonomy, established by the professional association at this time, would or could severely limit the development of the professional practice of nursing.

The ANA group recommended that it be titled the Steering Committee on Classifications of Nursing Practice Phenomena. The plural form of classifications is significant to note.

The group further recommended and is in the process of implementing the following committee goals.

1. To recommend ANA policy regarding classification systems.
2. To develop a blueprint for the work toward the identification of classifications for nursing practice phenomena of concern.
3. To maintain a collaborative relationship with the North American Nursing Diagnosis Association (NANDA).
4. To monitor the "state of the art" of classification systems.
5. To promote an understanding of the "state of the art" of classification systems.

The origins of the Steering Committee were rooted in the ANA Social Policy Statement. After the statement was published in 1980, an implementation committee was established. One of the major developments the committee thought to be needed was further elaboration of the definition of nursing.

Nursing is the diagnosis and treatment of human responses to actual and potential health problems. (ANA, 1980.)

Only broad categories of human responses were offered as examples in the statement. These were such categories as:

Self-care limitations

Pain and discomfort

Impaired functioning in such areas as rest, sleep, ventilation, circulation, activity, nutrition, elimination, skin, and sexuality

Emotional problems related to illness and treatment, life-threatening events, or daily experiences, such as anxiety, loss, loneliness, and grief

Self-image changes required by health status

These broad categories were not intended to be nursing diagnoses, but were to serve as examples of broadly stated phenomena of concerns. The publication was to serve as a beginning point, with the aim of encouraging nurses to continue to develop theory-based diagnosis, treatment, and evaluation of human responses to actual and potential problems.

I will highlight a few of the activities under each goal to give you a sense of the scope of the committee's work.

Goal number one is to suggest ANA policy regarding classification systems. The committee has agreed on the following statements.

The professional association should:

1. Support diversity in the development and testing of classification systems to describe nursing phenomena until stable systems evolve
2. Collaborate with multiple inter/intradisciplinary groups in identifying and developing classification systems for health care, as well as monitoring and studying the interrelationships of these systems to nursing classification systems
3. Promote or facilitate the classification of human responses which nurses diagnose and treat and for which they assume accountability

In addition:

4. Classification systems developed or used by the nursing profession will be adaptable to the various client/health care delivery situations (i.e., hospitals, nursing homes, primary care).
5. When an existing classification is selected for use, promote consistent application of the classification scheme whether used for reimbursement, peer review, standards development, structuring practice, certification, or other purposes.

Goal number two is to develop a blueprint for the identification of and classifications for nursing practice phenomena by ANA structural units. Part of this goal is being met by requesting that the Council of Nurse Researchers work with NANDA in developing strategies for the empirical testing and validation of the current nursing diagnoses. Tomorrow, Dr. Jacqueline Clinton, ANA Council of Nurse Researchers, will be presenting a paper on Nursing Diagnoses Research Methodologies. Tonight and tomorrow Dr. Clinton and Dr. McFarland and others will be meeting to discuss strategies to further this goal.

Another part of this goal is being met by working with the ANA Divisions and Councils on Practice. This activity is labeled a collaborative effort to identify phenomena of concern. Several approaches are under consideration, including the selection of the ten most common NANDA nursing diagnoses utilized by each Division on Practice. A third part of this goal is to develop a research prospectus on identification of phenomena by practicing nurses. A fourth part of this goal is the development of a paper further elaborating on the definitions contained in Nursing: A Social Policy Statement; with a special focus on the intersections between medicine and nursing. *Goal number three* relates specifically to the relationship between the American Nurses' Association and the North American Nursing Diagnosis Group.

Both Roberta Thiry and Marjory Gordon provided leadership for the Steering Committee in the establishment, implementation, and monitoring of these activities with the aim of furthering the goals of each organization.

The activities of NANDA to facilitate the ANA steering committee's goal were proposed as follows:

1. Continue current objectives and related responsibilities of (a) developing, defining, and classifying nursing diagnosis; (b) providing a clearinghouse for information; and (c) promoting the identification and classification of nursing diagnosis
2. Disseminate to ANA Cabinet on Nursing Practice a bibliography of publications, newsletters, list of experts, and notice of national conferences and other relevant materials
3. Serve as a resource as ANA develops policy statements that are relevant to nursing diagnosis and classification systems
4. NANDA members are available to serve as a resource to ANA
5. During NANDA diagnostic category review, consider utilizing ANA clinical experts as panelists
6. Continue to encourage members to identify and clinically validate nursing diagnoses
7. Promote the definition of nursing (Social Policy Statement) and other relevant ANA activities through information dissemination activities
8. Continue to identify ongoing practice and research activities in nursing diagnosis
9. Help identify experts to assist in the dissemination of information at state and regional levels

In turn, activities of the American Nurses' Association in identifying and investigating nursing practice phenomena that could facilitate diagnostic classification activities of NANDA include the following:

1. Collaborate with NANDA to implement the definition of nursing (Social Policy Statement) (papers presented at NANDA conferences, etc.)
2. Focus on specifying interventions and outcomes for currently identified nursing diagnoses (clinical units)
3. Recognize NANDA's leadership in the development of classification and coordination of classification activities and thus share information with NANDA on ANA activities related to nursing diagnosis
4. Use NANDA members as consultants in the area of nursing diagnosis and diagnostic classification

5. Disseminate news items through *The American Nurse* on the progress of NANDA and other groups in classification on nursing diagnoses
6. Facilitate obtaining research funds to clinically validate current diagnoses as well as identify new diagnoses
7. Cooperate with NANDA to develop conferences that identify the state of current knowledge relative to each diagnosis; continue to collaborate in joint ANA-NANDA programs at the ANA conventions
8. When feasible, hold regional conferences on the Standards of Practice and *Nursing: A Social Policy Statement,* which include how to implement the definition of nursing (diagnosis and treatment). Consider using NANDA members to assist in these conferences. Encourage implementation of nursing diagnosis as stated in the Standards of Practice.
9. Continue to appoint a liaison person from the Cabinet on Nursing Practice to NANDA
10. Collaborate with NANDA to provide a forum for groups developing classification systems at NANDA meetings
11. Facilitate communication among experts in classification at the state level through constituent state nurses' associations

The steering committee also designated Marjory Gordon as the liaison person to facilitate communication between the North American Nursing Diagnosis Association and the American Nurses' Association for at least the period in which the ANA Steering Committee is active. Thereafter, the liaison activity would continue through the Cabinet on Nursing Practice.

In response to the proposed activities from the ANA Steering Committee, NANDA's president, Marjory Gordon, responded regarding the collaborative efforts of the ANA and NANDA. She wrote that the outline of collaborative activities should promote the development and classification of nursing diagnoses, the implementation of this concept within the nursing process and permit nursing to realize the social commitments of the profession described in the Social Policy Statement.

Dr. Gordon also sent a packet of information from the Clearinghouse. Information about the NANDA conference in April, 1984, and a call for papers was sent to ANA Cabinets and Divisions. When policies for reviewing diagnoses are developed by this organization, a copy will be sent to the Steering Committee. A NANDA committee has been charged with identifying experts on state and regional levels. When their listing is complete, a copy will be sent to ANA. A short column for *The American Nurse* about the conference, 1984, and a summary after the conference is to be prepared by the NANDA Public Relations Committee.

Dr. Gordon encouraged the Steering Committee to submit a paper on their work on the HCFA grant involving nursing diagnosis for the conference. She concurred with the suggestion of state of the art conferences on each diagnosis, stating that NANDA would be pleased to collaborate on this project. Further plans for collaboration based on the items identified in the ANA letter were to be discussed at the next NANDA Board of Directors meeting. Dr. Gordon experssed her pleasure to be the liaison from the Steering Committee to NANDA. Finally, Dr. Gordon wrote that the special interest group session at the Council of Nurse Researchers meeting was well received and that NANDA looked forward to the further assistance from this Council.

The *fourth goal* of the Steering Committee is to monitor the state of the art of classification systems. The Steering Committee requested that the ANA Center for Nursing Research staff prepare a monograph on the current classification systems and their relationships with reimbursement. Dr. Susan Hartly and Dr. Richard McKibbon prepared such a monograph, entitled "Hospital Payment Mechanisms, Patient Classification Systems and Nursing Relationships and Implications," published by ANA in the 1983 series of monographs. The monograph has been well received and utilized by many groups of people. The Steering Committee has requested that the staff continue to monitor the state of the art and to prepare periodic written reports.

The Steering Committee also receives reports of projects dealing with reimbursement of nursing such as the ANA-CHAMPUS project in which a system of peer review is being established for nursing services receiving direct reimbursement. This project will help meet the need for a list of phenomena to be added to those of medicine and other disciplines for the purpose of reimbursement.

The Steering Committee continues to monitor the effect of diagnostic related groups on nursing. Future reports form the ANA project on Refinement of Nursing within the diagnostic related groups should yield useful data for nursing classification systems.

The Steering Committee, in its *goal number five,* aims to promote an understanding of the state of the art of classifications for nursing practice phenomena. Let me share one of the successes with you. The Committee assisted in focusing the ANA Clinical Sessions held in November of 1983 in Denver around the Social Policy Statement definition of nursing practice. Specifically the Committee wanted the conference structured around the phenomenological concerns of nursing practice, with the diagnosis and treatment of human responses to actual and potential problems.

I had the task of summarizing the conferences and providing a challenge for the future. I would like to share a little of the analysis of the abstracts and presentations in terms of the social policy statement.

I attempted to synthesize the conference by coding each of the abstracts from the verbal presentations and written abstracts according to the characteristics identified in the "centerfold" (Fig. 1) of the Social Policy Statement (ANA, 1980).

Each presentation/abstract was coded according to:
1. Was a phenomenon of concern/nursing diagnosis identified?
2. Was a nursing intervention/action tested?
3. Were effects/outcomes/evaluation measures tested?
4. Was there an identified theoretical framework or theory?
5. Was the focus on an overall classification scheme?

My coding of each abstract was then verified by several other persons, including Dr. Roberta Thiry and ANA staff who attended the specific verbal presentations.

Keeping the severe limitations in mind (this was not a highly controlled study), I will share the summary of findings with you.

Fifty-two abstracts and verbal presentations were reviewed. The identification of phenomena of concern or nursing diagnosis received the most attention at the conference. Over twenty presentors focused on phenomena. A theoretical framework could be identified in eight of those studies.

Fourteen authors related a diagnosis to an action or intervention. In seven studies diagnosis, intervention, and effects were related. In two studies the focus was solely on an intervention. Two authors focused solely on outcomes or effects. Only one author focused on all of the characteristics identified in the social policy statement. Those characteristics are theory, nursing diagnosis, treatment, and effects. Four authors focused on classification development as a whole; ten on population descriptions; eight on nurses or organization of nursing practice; and one on the computerization of data.

The goal, as outlined in the Social Policy Statement, is to strongly encourage studies that will focus on each part of the grid; that would include a nursing phenomenon, action, and effect within a theoretical framework.

Another action under the Steering Committee's goal five is the possible development of consensus conferences. A consensus process is the development of a structure and strategies for identifying known information and applying and evaluating such information in nursing practice, administration, and education. The overall purpose of the conference would be to develop and evaluate a consensus process for the identification of known information (defining characteristics, theory application, nursing action, and effects) about selected nursing phenomena and strategies for the utilization and evaluation of such knowledge in nursing practice and the delivery of health care.

In summary, the Steering Committee on Classifications of Nursing Practice Phenomena is a committee of the ANA Cabinet on Nursing Practice in collaboration with the Cabinets on Nursing Research and Nursing Service. The focus of the committee is to prepare a blueprint for the profession to work toward classifying phenomena of concerns to nurses. Specific activities to date relate to recommending policies regarding classification systems; maintaining a collaborative relationship with the North American Nursing Diagnosis Association; monitoring the state of the art of classification systems; and facilitating state of the art conferences.

I believe that NANDA and the ANA Steering Committee have a good beginning for their collaborative work. I look forward to many products/outcomes from this collaboration.

REFERENCE

American Nurses' Association: Nursing: A social policy statement, Kansas City, MO, 1980, The Association.

Development of a taxonomic structure for nursing diagnoses: a review and an update

PHYLLIS B. KRITEK, Ph. D., R.N., F.A.A.N.

As your program indicated, it is my intent today to speak to the general topic of "Taxonomic Issues." I have broadened that concept somewhat to provide both a review and an update of the development of a taxonomic structure for nursing diagnoses. In this sense my comments receive a context from the theme of the Conference: A Janus View, focused on past activities, current issues, and future developments of nursing diagnoses.

Gebbie and Lavin (1975), reporting the proceedings of the First National Conference on the Classification of Nursing Diagnoses, gave emphasis to two basic activities of this body, then called the National Group for the Generation and Classification of Nursing Diagnoses. One involved the generation of labels or names of nursing diagnoses, the other involved creation of some system of classification. The latter task, at our 1973 inception, was a central focus of concern. Two major outcomes of this emphasis emerged: an explanation of the principles of classification for nursing diagnoses and a delineation of several possible classification systems for nursing diagnoses.

Eleven years after the fact, it may be useful to briefly review these outcomes. In exploring principles of classification for nursing diagnoses, two key considerations were emphasized (Gebbie and Lavin, 1975). The first was the critical need for a principle of order for such a system, the second was the recognition that such a principle of order "can be one of many possibilities, and depends very much on the purposes of the classification system, its users, and its workability." It was noted, in this context, that one seeks to create some balance between complexity and simplicity. Extant taxonomies for other sets of phenomena were explored. This exploration, particularly of the work of Bloom (1956) and that of Krathwohl, Bloom, and Masia (1964), clarified key characteristics of a taxonomy. A summary of this view of the nature of a taxonomy is as follows:

1. In a true taxonomy, ordering and arrangement are based on a single principle or consistent set of principles.
2. Principles must be consistent with sound theory in the discipline.
3. Taxonomic ordering must be testable against empirical evidence about real phenomena.
4. Taxonomic ordering should point to phenomena yet to be discovered.
5. Taxonomic ordering should reveal relationships among phenomena.
6. Taxonomic ordering should reveal the essential properties of phenomena.

23

    7. Taxonomic ordering should be logically developed and internally consistent.

This overview of taxonomies evoked some general guides to action in nursing's pursuit of a taxonomic structure, summarized as follows:

    1. Be logical, concise, and consistent.
    2. Incorporate current knowledge of nursing phenomena.
    3. Be descriptive, objective, detached, and neutral.
    4. Incorporate all possible nursing world views.
    5. Identify central themes and concepts.
    6. Identify potential limitations.
    7. Accommodate future developments and changes.
    8. Assure practical workability.
    9. Be comprehensive.
   10. Be communicable.
   11. Avoid overlap.

Given this generalized overview of the task at hand, participants at the First Conference concurrently addressed two activities: naming phenomena and ordering it within a framework. Several frameworks emerged, including one based on Maslow's 1954 hierarchy (Gebbie and Lavin, 1975), one based on Abdellah's 1960 problem list (Gebbie and Lavin, 1975), and other group-generated models. In the end labels were reported in terms of four levels of duration (intermittent, chronic, acute, or potential) and four etiologies (anatomical, physiological, psychological, and environmental). They were ordered according to the alphabet.

I have given considerable time to the review of the First Conference Proceedings with some sense of purpose. Looking back to our roots provides grounding in understanding our present and anticipating our future. The proceedings of subsequent national conferences carry the themes created in the first: a commitment to classification, a sense of frustration with the difficulty of the task, a desire to follow one's own rules, and the recognition of the absence of easy answers. But efforts were made. Most "popular knowledge" views of NANDA's efforts tend to emphasize the generation of an alphabetical list of named phenomena. The struggle toward classification is simply less understood, and less overt. But it persists.

Sr. Callista Roy's leadership in creating the theorist group was in part a response to the problems encountered in creating a classification schema for nursing diagnosis. Our First Conference guidelines argued that we should incorporate all possible world views. What better way than to bring together key proponents of various world views and ask them to create a composite world view, which they did quite ably.

But we, collectively, were not quite content with, or grateful for, the message. It overwhelmed us. The chasm between the practical world of impaired gas exchange and the conceptual world of a pattern of unitary man called exchanging seemed difficult to bridge at best. It was at this point of impasse that a group of participants in the Fifth National Conference publicly and systematically emerged to reactivate the question: can we create a taxonomic structure for nursing diagnoses beyond the alphabet? The question had always been there as background noise. It simply required a conscious focus.

As chairperson of that group, I can summarize our answer to the question quite briefly: maybe. A study of the Fifth Conference Proceedings (Kim, McFarland, and McLane, 1984) will provide you with more detail and the time to scrutinize outcomes of this group. The effort itself can be briefly described. A group of twenty conference participants generated an initial taxonomic structure for nursing diagnoses using the patterns of unitary persons as a basis for their classification schema. Both taxonomic trees and a nomenclature emerged from this classification.

While some of you have some knowledge of both this process and its outcome, the vast majority do not, so some review is in order. The Fifth Conference Taxonomy Group used decision making by consensus to create an initial taxonomy of nursing diagnoses. After a discussion of options available, the group decided to focus on the existing NANDA diagnosis list, to use the theorists' "patterns of unitary persons" as a classification schema, and to sort the list vertically by levels of abstraction and horizontally by unitary patterns. Cues, interventions, and qualifiers were largely ignored during sorting but were viewed as germane to further classification tasks. Labels themselves were occasionally modified for clarity, and category names created when needed and appropriate. Several blank spaces were "built in" to accentuate the tree's incompleteness. No attempt was made to formally relate these trees to the Theorist Group's distinctions of empirical data, summary concept, or dimension as described by Roy (1984).

The finished products of the Taxonomy Group follow; in their entirety they serve to highlight some of the insights the group gained in doing this task.

Box 1 demonstrates the four levels of abstraction identified by the group, going from I (most abstract) to IV (most concrete). The group hypothesized that the lower the level, the closer to practice phenomena. Indeed, this exercise speaks to one of the most persistent complaints made by practicing nurses who attempt to use the NANDA list. The level I and II concepts doubtless serve not as diagnostic labels but as category name sets: they are probably, therefore, relatively dysfunctional for precision in rendering clinical judgements.

Table 1 sketches the parallelism constructed by the group between Patterns of Unitary Persons and Level I concepts, those considered most abstract. Parentheses indicate those terms introduced by the group. This list, and the marked number of parenthetical inclusions, demonstrate a second major in-

BOX 1   **Classification by levels of abstraction**

Level I

Comfort	Fear	Nutrition
Communication	Knowledge	Self-concept
Coping	Mobility	Thought processes
	Spiritual	

Level II

Bowel elimination	Deficit diversional activity
Cardiac output, alterations	Fluid volume deficit, actual
Pain	Fluid volume deficit, potential
Verbal communication, impaired	Impaired gas exchange
Coping, ineffective family	Injury
Coping, ineffective individual	Knowledge deficit
Impaired physical mobility	Alteration in nutrition
Parenting	Body image
Self-care deficit	Self-esteem
Role performance	Personal identity
Sensory perception	Sexual dysfunction
Sleep pattern disturbance	Alterations in thought processes
Spiritual distress	Tissue perfusion
Noncompliance	Urinary elimination
Airway clearance	Grieving
Violence	Ineffective breathing
Skin integrity, actual	Skin integrity, potential

Level III

Constipation
Diarrhea
Incontinence
Cardiac output, decreased

Alteration in nutrition
  -More
  -Less
  -Potential for more than required

Sensory perceptual alteration
  -Visual
  -Auditory
  -Kinesthetic
  -Gustatory
  -Tactile
  -Olfactory
Tissue perfusion, alteration
  -Cerebral
  -Cardiopulmonary

Self-care deficit
  -Feeding
  -Bathing/hygiene
  -Dressing/grooming
  -Toileting
Potential for
  -Injury
  -Poisoning
  -Suffocation
  -Trauma
Alteration in parenting
  -Actual
  -Potential

Coping, family
  -Potential for growth

Grieving
  -Anticipatory
  -Dysfunctional

BOX 1   **Classification by levels of abstraction—cont'd**

Level III—cont'd

Tissue perfusion, alteration—cont'd
  -Gastrointestinal
  -Peripheral
  -Renal

Urinary elimination,
  Alteration in patterns
Home maintenance management,
  impaired
Rape trauma syndrome

Level IV

Rape trauma syndrome
  -Rape trauma
  -Compound reaction
  -Silent reaction

TABLE 1   **Parallels of patterns and level I content**

Patterns of unitary persons	Alterations in human responses (normless)
Exchanging	Nutrition, elimination (oxygenation), (circulation), (physical integrity)
Communicating	(Communication)
Relating	(Role)
Valuing	Spiritual (state)
Choosing	Coping (participating)
Moving	Activity, rest, (recreation), (activities of daily living), (self-care)
Perceiving	Self-concept, sensory/perceptual
Knowing	Knowledge (learning), thought processes
Feeling	Comfort (emotional integrity)

---

sight discovered by the Taxonomy Group. The NANDA list may further frustrate users because of marked incompleteness. It is virtually impossible to trace most concepts through all levels of abstraction with the labels currently identified.

Figs. 1 through 9 are the actual trees created by the group. It is noteworthy that the pattern labeled exchanging is clearly more well developed than any other. Many are remarkably underdeveloped.

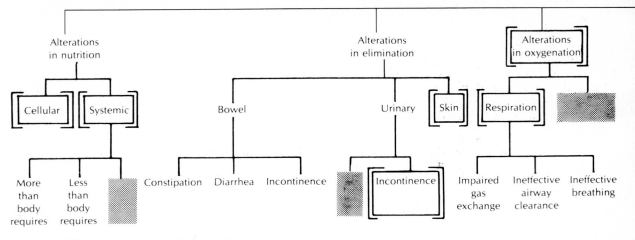

FIGURE 1   Pattern 1: Exchanging.

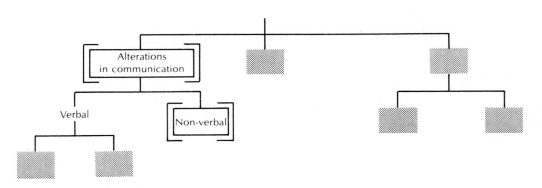

FIGURE 2   Pattern 2: Communicating.

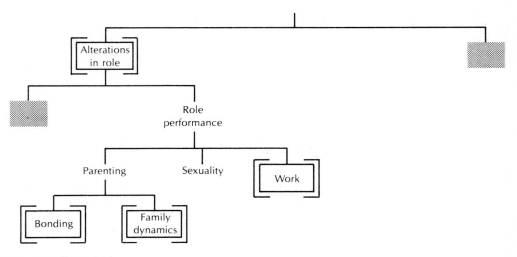

FIGURE 3   Pattern 3: Relating.

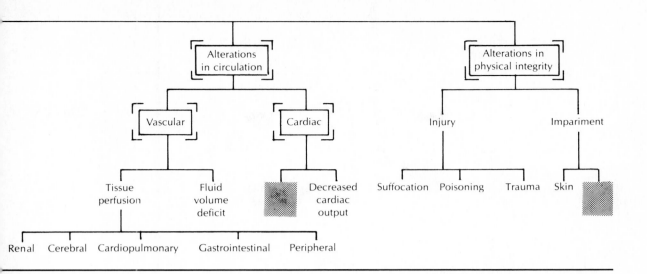

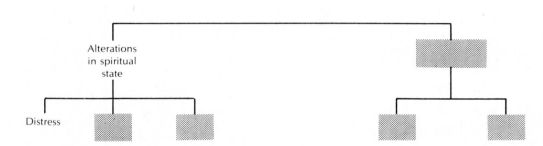

FIGURE 4 Pattern 4: Valuing.

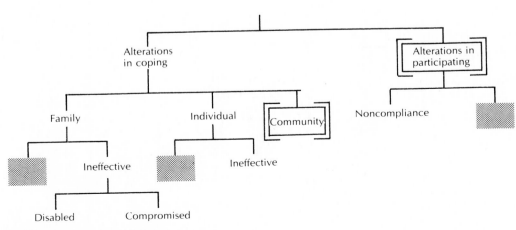

FIGURE 5 Pattern 5: Choosing.

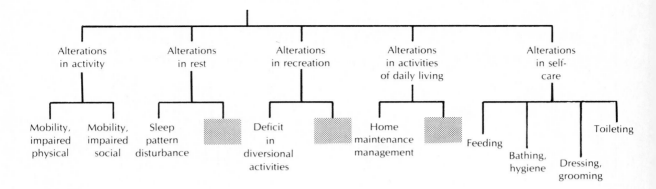

FIGURE 6   Pattern 6: Moving.

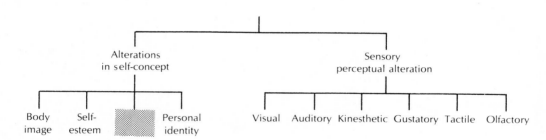

FIGURE 7   Pattern 7: Perceiving.

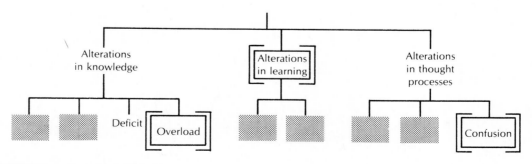

FIGURE 8   Pattern 8: Knowing.

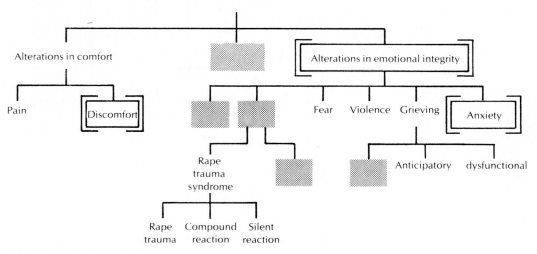

FIGURE 9   Pattern 9: Feeling.

Finally, in Box 2 a possible nomenclature, based on this classification schema, is developed. As Glenn Webster (1984) noted at the last conference, one of the key reasons for standardization is computer storage and access of information. Box 2 demonstrates a possible system of numerically coding the proposed taxonomy.

BOX 2   **Taxonomy structure**

1. *Exchanging*
    1.1. *Alterations in nutrition*
        1.1.1. (Cellular)
        1.1.2. (Systemic)
            1.1.2.1. More than body requires
            1.1.2.2. Less than body requires
            1.1.2.3. _____
    1.2. *Alterations in elimination*
        1.2.1. Bowel
            1.2.1.1. Constipation
            1.2.1.2. Diarrhea
            1.2.1.3. Incontinence
        1.2.2. Urinary
            1.2.2.1. (Incontinence)
            1.2.2.2. _____
        1.2.3. Skin

1.3. *(Alterations in oxygenation)*
    1.3.1. (Respiration)
        1.3.1.1. Impaired gas exchange
        1.3.1.2. Ineffective airway clearance
        1.3.1.3. Ineffective breathing
    1.3.2. _____
1.4. *(Alterations in circulation)*
    1.4.1. (Vascular)
        1.4.1.1. Tissue perfusion
            1.4.1.1.1. Renal
            1.4.1.1.2. Cerebral
            1.4.1.1.3. Cardiopulmonary
            1.4.1.1.4. Gastrointestinal
            1.4.1.1.5. Peripheral
    1.4.2. (Cardiac)
        1.4.2.1. Decreased cardiac output
        1.4.2.2. _____
1.5. *(Alterations in physical integrity)*
    1.5.1. Injury
        1.5.1.1. Suffocation
        1.5.1.2. Poisoning
        1.5.1.3. Trauma
    1.5.2. Impairment
        1.5.2.1. Skin
        1.5.2.2. _____
2. *Communicating*
    2.1. *(Alterations in communication)*
        2.1.1. Verbal
            2.1.1.1. _____
            2.1.1.2. _____
        2.1.2. (Nonverbal)
    2.2. _____
    2.3. _____
        2.3.1. _____
        2.3.2. _____
3. Relating
    3.1. (Alterations in role)
        3.1.1. Role performance
            3.1.1.1. Parenting
                3.1.1.1.1. (Bonding)
                3.1.1.1.2. (Family dynamics)
            3.1.1.2. Sexuality
            3.1.1.3. (Work)
        3.1.2. _____
    3.2. _____
4. Valuing
    4.1. (Alterations in spiritual state)
        4.1.1. Distress

        4.1.2. _____

        4.1.3. _____

     4.2. _____

        4.2.1. _____

        4.2.2. _____

5. Choosing
   - 5.1. Alterations in coping
     - 5.1.1. Family
       - 5.1.1.1. Ineffective
         - 5.1.1.1.1. Disabled
         - 5.1.1.1.2. Compromised
       - 5.1.1.2 _____
     - 5.1.2. Individual
       - 5.1.2.1. Ineffective
       - 5.1.2.2. _____
     - 5.1.3. Community
   - 5.2. (Alterations in participating)
     - 5.2.1. _____
     - 5.2.2. _____
6. Moving
   - 6.1. (Alterations in activity)
     - 6.1.1. Mobility, impaired physical
     - 6.1.2. Mobility, impaired social
   - 6.2. (Alterations in rest)
     - 6.2.1. Sleep pattern disturbance
     - 6.2.2. _____
   - 6.3. (Alterations in recreation)
     - 6.3.1. Deficit in diversional activities
     - 6.3.2. _____
   - 6.4. (Alterations in activities of daily living)
     - 6.4.1. Home maintenance management
     - 6.4.2. _____
   - 6.5. (Alterations in self-care)
     - 6.5.1. Feeding
     - 6.5.2. Bathing, hygiene
     - 6.5.3. Dressing, grooming
     - 6.5.4. Toileting
7. Perceiving
   - 7.1. Alterations in self-concept
     - 7.1.1. Body image
     - 7.1.2. Self-esteem
     - 7.1.3. Personal identity
     - 7.1.4. _____
   - 7.2. Sensory/perceptual alteration
     - 7.2.1. Visual
     - 7.2.2. Auditory
     - 7.2.3. Kinesthetic
     - 7.2.4. Gustatory

      7.2.5. Tactile
      7.2.6. Olfactory
8. Knowing
  8.1. Alterations in knowledge
      8.1.1. Deficit
      8.1.2. (Overload)
      8.1.3. _____
      8.1.4. _____
  8.2. (Alterations in learning)
      8.2.1. _____
      8.2.2. _____
  8.3. Alterations in thought processes
      8.3.1. (Confusion)
      8.3.2. _____
      8.3.3. _____
9. Feeling
  9.1. Alterations in comfort
      9.1.1. Pain
      9.1.2. (Discomfort)
  9.2. (Alterations in emotional integrity)
      9.2.1. (Anxiety)
      9.2.2. Grieving
          9.2.2.1. Dysfunctional
          9.2.2.2. Anticipatory
          9.2.2.3. _____
      9.2.3. Violence
      9.2.4. Fear
      9.2.5. _____
          9.2.5.1. Rape trauma syndrome
              9.2.5.1.1. Rape trauma
              9.2.5.2.2. Compound reaction
              9.2.5.3.3. Silent reaction
          9.2.5.2 _____
      9.2.6. _____
  9.3. _____

The process of generating this classification schema somewhat serendipitously unearthed several useful insights into the implicit principles of classification embedded in the existing NANDA alphabetical list. In reviewing the group's product over time, it appears to me that the four levels of abstraction each involves a specific principle of classification:

Level I: Patterns of unitary persons
               Human response patterns
               Human response pattern categories

Level II: Alterations in human responses
            Normless category labels
            Assessment categories
Level III: (Unnamed)
            Phenomena of concern categories
            (not phenomena themselves)
Level IV: (Unnamed)
            Phenomena of concern

In addition, the process unearthed several principles that have not yet been effectively addressed.

   I. Probable principle:
     Actual vs. potential
     (Dichotomous Trees)
  II. Possible principles:
     Intensity
     (More/less, deficit/excess, etc.)
     Risk
     (Dysfunction, impaired, disabling, etc.)
     Acuity
     (intensity + risk = potentiality ?)
     Developmental level
     (range)
 III. Unexamined principles:
     Relationship to norms
     Change over time
     Weighting
     Interactions
     Health maximization

This list implicitly identifies the next set of hard questions which the NANDA Taxonomy Committee and other concerned nurses must explore.

Having briefly reviewed the past and the present, what remains to be stated is some view of the future. What has been said is a backdrop, and guides our future directions. The process of creating a functional taxonomy of nursing phenomena seems to me a process that will, in my lifetime, involve a high commitment to tentativeness, ambiguity, and provisional outcomes. Yet, equally, it seems to me that the creation of this tentative, ambiguous, provisional taxonomy should begin, that we would collectively benefit from the effort. The process itself may be the most important outcome, uncovering, as it did for the Taxonomy Group, some key quandaries, summarized as follows:

  1. Distinguishing among
    A. Category set labels
    B. Diagnostic labels
    C. Empirical indicators

2. Identifying omissions in
   A. Principles of classification
   B. Levels of abstraction
   C. Diagnostic labels
3. Balance between
   A. Change
   B. Stability
4. Generalized imprecision

I would like then, facing the future, to make some commitments. Rollo May (1975), in discussing the courage necessary to exercise creativity, states that "commitment is healthiest when it is not *without* doubt, but *in spite* of doubt." I am, thus, making this commitment in spite of my personal doubt. But May's observation is made as a preface to a discussion of creative courage which involves the discovery of the new patterns, symbols, and form needed to build new societies. Discussing professions, he observes that "the need for creative courage is in direct proportion to the degree of change the profession is undergoing."

I believe we need to take this proposed taxonomy and, returning to our guidelines of 1973, tenaciously pursue its development. I believe the *generation* and *classification* of nursing diagnoses (both now imperfect processes) should occur in tandem. Each process enhances, and challenges, the other. To continue to develop, test, and approve labels in a conceptual vacuum makes little sense. The Theorist Group has offered us much that can guide us in our struggle to develop and describe a conceptual framework for classifying nursing diagnoses. Literally thousands of nurses have contributed their time and energy to the careful description and naming of various nursing phenomena. The bridge that I believe is necessary to span these two important activities is the further development and testing of a classificatory schema, utilizing NANDA's list and framework.

Janus-like, we need to look backward and forward. Recently Brown, Tanner, and Padrick (1984) again demonstrated a persisting weakness in nursing research, one they call its "major limitation." This is nursing research's noncumulative nature. They observe, "Research was not linked clearly enough to prior work, nor did it appear to refine, extend, or refute theoretical formulations." This is the work we need next. We need to look at NANDA's prior work. We need to test, refine, extend, and refute. And we need to do so systematically.

Returning to the general guides to action in nursing's pursuit of a taxonomic structure, we find the scope of the task clearly outlined. I believe some first steps are obvious. We need, as an organization, to formally review and accept the proposed taxonomy. We need to encourage and support research which tests, refines, extends, and refutes the taxonomy as it currently exists. We need to begin to "fill in the blanks," especially at the category level where devel-

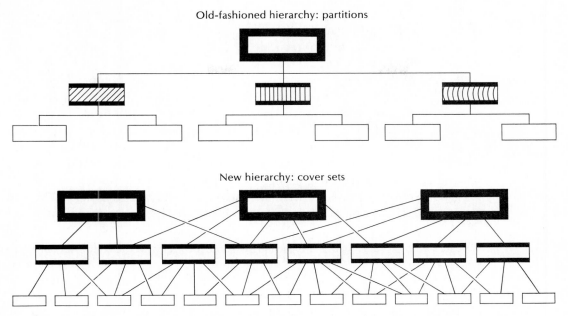

Old-fashioned hierarchy: partitions

New hierarchy: cover sets

FIGURE 10 *Top,* Old fashioned hierarchy (partitions). *Bottom,* New hierarchy (cover sets). (Adapted from Atkin, 1981. Multidimensional man.)

opment may primarily involve identifying functional umbrella concepts. We need to identify the solutions nurses have already created for the omissions in our current taxonomy, and test their feasibility for inclusion. We need to systematically incorporate new diagnoses into our taxonomy.

All of which begins to sound firm, final, fixed, and permanent, which is clearly not my intent. I believe I am arguing for the next step, taken gingerly, but bravely, balancing the demands for progress with the desire for provisional solutions.

It may be useful, in that spirit, to conclude with what I perceive as the next hard challenge on the horizon. John Naisbitt (1983), in his analysis of major futuristic trends on the United States, identifies one as a move away from hierarchies and toward networks. Since the late 1930s and with the introduction of electronic computation, statistical classification techniques have increased at an exponential rate. We have the technology to manipulate data sets in multidimensional space, to systematically and mathematically create and investigate networks. The proposed NANDA taxonomy exists in a narrow, two-dimensional space. It is a classic hierarchy, partitioning reality into theoretical, mutually exclusive categories. Ron Atkin (1981), a mathematician with a passion for the human, has worked extensively with social scientists eager to protect their intuitive need to have things connected to each other, to recognize relationships and networks. To respond to that need,

Atkin proposes a new kind of hierarchy, with categories which are actually cover sets. He argues that since we live in a multidimensional world, we must adapt our conceptual systems to reflect that world reality, and adapt our technology accordingly.

Fig. 10 illustrates the contrasting imagery of these two types of hierarchies and demonstrates the network effect of the latter. This multidimensional network of concepts and relationships goes well beyond the linear, two-dimensional taxonomy we now have. Atkin sketches the challenge before us and renews my faith in the tentativeness of knowledge. If indeed we are now generating a descriptive theory of nursing at the level of factor-isolation, imagine the challenge of factor-relating!

I would like to conclude with a thought from Arthur Koestler (1970), the essayist who has had a pervasive impact on twentieth-century intellectual life.

The scientist's discoveries impose his own order on chaos, as the composer or painter imposes his; an order that always refers to limited aspects of reality, and is based on the observer's frame of reference, which differs from period to period as a Rembrandt nude differs from a nude by Manet."

REFERENCES

Atkin, R.: Multidimensional man: Can man live in 3-dimensional space? New York, 1981, Penguin Books.

Brown, J. J., Tanner, C.A., and Padrick, K. P.: Nursing's search for scientific knowledge, Nurs. Res. **33,** 26-32, 1984.

Gebbie, K. M., and Lavin, M. A., editors: Classification of nursing diagnoses—Proceedings of the First National Conference, St. Louis, 1975, The C. V. Mosby Co.

Kim, M. J., McFarland, G., and McLane, A., editors: Classification of nursing diagnoses—Proceedings of the Fifth National Conference, St. Louis, 1984, The C. V. Mosby Co.

Koestler, A.: The act of creation, London, 1970, PAN Books.

Kritek, P. B.: Report of the group work on taxonomies. In Kim, M. J., McFarland, G., and McLane, A., editors: Classification of nursing diagnoses—Proceedings of the Fifth National Conference, St. Louis, 1984, The C. V. Mosby Co.

May, R.: The courage to create, New York, 1975, Bantam Books.

Naisbitt, J.: Megatrends, New York, 1982, Warner Books, Inc.

Roy, S.C.: Framework for classification systems development; progress and issues. In Kim, M. J., McFarland, G., and McLane, A., editors: Classification of nursing diagnoses—Proceedings of the Fifth National Conference, St. Louis, 1984, The C. V. Mosby Co.

Webster, G. A. (1984). Nomenclature and classification system development. In Kim, M.J., McFarland, G., and McLane, A., editors: Classification of Nursing Diagnoses: Proceedings of the Fifth National Conference (pp. 14-25). St. Louis: Mosby.

Structure of diagnostic categories

MARJORY GORDON, Ph.D., R.N., F.A.A.N.

Currently, 62 diagnostic categories describing phenomena of therapeutic concern to nurses have been accepted for clinical testing by the North American Nursing Diagnosis Association (Kim, McFarland, and McLean, 1984). Some authors have criticized the complexity (Lunney, 1982), esoteric language (Shamansky and Yanni, 1983), lack of specificity (Gordon, 1982; Tanner and Hughes, 1984), and the diversity in level of abstraction (Ray, 1984). Notwithstanding these problems, the diagnostic categories are being used and tested in clinical practice and new diagnoses are being identified.

A *diagnostic category* represents a group of equivalent phenomena that are labeled and classified. The categories used in clinical practices describe either (1) a health condition and its etiology or probable cause(s) or (2) a potential problem (high-risk state) that does not have a cause per se. Defining characteristics are the observable referents of a problem or etiology (Carpenito, 1983; Jones and Jakob, 1982; Gordon, 1976; Mundinger and Jauron, 1975; Purushotham, 1981).

A diagnostic category refers to a cluster of behaviors that are recognizable as a pattern that occurs repeatedly in many person-environment situations. Etiologic labels have the same characteristics. Whereas problem labels are used descriptively to represent the state of the client, etiologic labels are used as explanatory concepts. At some level of probability, etiologic factors are recognized as contributing to or maintaining the health problem.

As Mundinger and Jauron (1975) have clearly pointed out, definitive treatment (as opposed to palliative symptom relief) is not possible without understanding the probable cause of a problem. Clinicians use both descriptive concepts (problem labels) and explanatory concepts (etiologic labels) to describe phenomena. Theoretically, treatment is directed toward eliminating or modifying factors producing the problem. It is important to note that a clinician's concept of a client's problem and the concept of etiology are inferred from clinical data. The *relationship* between a specific problem and etiologic factors is a second inferential conclusion, twice divorced from reality-based observation.

At this point in classification system development, there is a need to examine the state of development and refinement of diagnostic categories used in clinical practice. Because diagnosis is an integral part of nursing process, consideration of the cognitive processes in which categories are used is necessary during refinement. Poorly developed diagnostic and etiologic categories can increase the risk of errors in diagnosis and treatment, deprive patients of quality care, and place the clinician in jeopardy for malpractice. The purpose of this paper is to examine current diagnostic categories from a structural perspective and relate structural factors to the diagnostic reasoning process and treatment decisions.

INTERACTION OF CATEGORY AND PROCESS

A brief overview of the interaction between categories and the diagnostic judgment process will serve to clarify the importance of structural characteristics. Human beings, faced with the need to identify something not immediately perceptible, use a process of inference and cue search (Carnevali, 1984; Gordon, 1982; Tanner, 1983). They generate tentative diagnostic hypotheses to guide the search for further information. When sufficient information is collected to support a particular diagnostic hypothesis, a judgment is made. The level of confidence in a diagnostic judgment is related to the assessment of highly valid and reliable indicators.

Diagnostic categories are used as hypotheses. For example, when restlessness is observed in a 55-year-old construction worker who is awaiting cardiac surgery, clinicians generate tentative diagnostic hypotheses about the meaning of restlessness. We hear a nurse say: "Well, it could be fear (death, surgical outcome), or anxiety, or even a cardiac problem with alteration in comfort: anginal pain." The defining characteristics of fear, anxiety, and pain direct the search for further information. Experts would focus further assessment on highly valid and reliable diagnostic criteria (defining characteristics) of these conditions. Not only is this an efficient procedure, but it prevents information overload. The few diagnostic cues that are specific and reliable indicators convey maximum information. This is evident in clinicians' deductive reasoning and the conditional proposition: "Well, if it's anxiety then . . . (cues) . . . but if it is fear then I'll see . . . (cues) . . ." The more quickly the pool of relevant hypotheses can be reduced, the less the inferential and memory strain incurred by the diagnostician. Human cognitive processes are limited; for example, short-term, working memory is said to have a capacity for 7 ± 2 separate bits of information (Miller, 1956).

Level of generality

Generality refers to the inclusiveness of a category; the more general a category, the more inclusive. Abstraction refers to the conceptual distance from perception; an abstract category is remote from real-world, perceptual data. Currently identified diagnostic categories are at various levels of abstraction and generality (Roy, 1984). The use of abstract categories to label a patient's health problem can be problematic when treatment decisions have to be made. Definitive treatment and outcome projection require definitive diagnosis.

We categorize our experience of the world into namable chunks at a useful level of abstraction. These are stored in memory, presumably, as prototypes or representations and used for identifying phenomena and determining an action-response. In practice the rule of "best fit" to the stored "textbook picture" is both cognitively efficient and usually sufficiently accurate. The idea of a prototype-category or "best example" is useful in refining and constructing diagnostic categories. The prototype is the mean representation. It is defined by a cluster of highly valid and reliable signs and symptoms (Rosch, 1978).

Irrespective of the conceptual focus for nursing diagnosis ultimately decided upon, prototype-categories must be at a sufficiently useful level of abstraction to conserve cognitive resources. Categories are useful when they permit going beyond the information given to actions and consequences. For example, if something is a bird (category), we also infer that it must have feathers and wings (Bruner, Goodnow, and Austin, 1956). Rosch and co-workers (1976) have identified a level of abstraction "that is appropriate for using, thinking about, or naming" a phenomenon in most situations where the phenomenon occurs. They call these *generic* or *basic level categories.* In the vertical dimension of a taxonomy other categories are subordinate or superordinate to the prototype-category.

Basic level, or generic, categories form the level of generality where discontinuities are readily perceived, such as the discontinuity between eggs and apples. As Berlin (1978) stated, "Psychologically, generic taxa are highly salient . . . they refer to the most commonly used, everyday categories." Usefulness of categories is a function of their (1) distinctiveness or contrast with other categories and (2) total cue validity or within-category, family resemblance (Rosch, 1978). Basic level categories have attributes common to all or most members of the category and are more distinct from other categories. Both distinctiveness and high cue validity contribute to cognitive efficiency and usefulness. In contrast to the basic level, members of more general superordinate categories (furniture is an example) have more distinctive than common characteristics. Members of categories subordinate to the basic level, such as white plastic kitchen chairs, have many common features and less distinctive features. One could suppose that alterations in skin integrity would be less useful (as defined above) than decubitus ulcer, stage one, or sacral decubitus, stage one. The methodology used by Rosch (1978) or Tversky (1978) in studying language categories suggests a way of determining the most useful level of abstraction for diagnostic categories used in clinical practice. Their research also suggests the possibility that action-responses (treatments) related to basic level categories are more numerous than the action-responses to abstract, superordinate categories (Rosch and associates, 1976). If this finding holds true for diagnostic categories, treatment planning may be profoundly affected by the level of generality. Do fewer treatments "come to mind" with the diagnosis, alteration in parenting, than the more specific diagnosis, low parent-infant attachment? Problematic diagnostic categories could be identified by studies of clinicians' errors in problem identification and treatment.

A cluster of defining signs and symptoms for a diagnosis may be most useful if structured by highly valid, distinctive (differentiating) diagnostic criteria—in other words, the prototype of a category. This should provide the "mean" representation to which atypical or boundary cases can be related. Although the term *prototype* is not commonly used in health science catergorizations, the Jones Criteria are an example often quoted in medicine (Feinstein, 1982). These are a set of criteria for diagnosing acute rheumatic fever (American Heart Association, 1965) first introduced in 1944 to improve the quality of clinical diagnosis. Since that time, many revisions have been made.

Cognitive economy dictates that distinctiveness and clarity of diagnostic categories are important variables in information processing. Yet, as Sokal (1974) argues; "There are birds that lack wings, vertebrates that lack red blood cells and mammals that do not bear their young." In the classification of health problems, the same diversity is encountered. To overcome real-world classification difficulties, Beckner (1959) suggested (1) that empirical concepts can be defined by multiple attributes which form a loose cluster, and (2) although many characteristics can be identified, only a proportion of the defining characteristics may be required to *assign* an observed phenomenon to the category. (Sneath and Sokal [1973] suggested the name *polythetic* to describe concepts with a dysjunctive arrangement of class attributes, such as A, B, *and* C.) The criteria required for *identifying* a member of a category would be included in the prototype suggested by Rosch (1978). The problem of fuzzy boundaries between diagnostic categories cannot be totally eliminated. Clinical judgment skills have to be exercised.

Naming

The limited capacity of human memory provides an argument for concise category-labels. "Alterations in nutrition: potential for more than body requirements" has nine linguistic symbols. These nine symbols need to be held in short-term memory stores while characteristics of the condition are being tested. This may strain memory capacities. Potential obesity would be a more concise designation. Potential skin breakdown, nutritional deficit, exogenous obesity, and self-concept disturbance would be examples of concise labels for the concepts currently described by lengthy names. Most labels with extraneous words contain the broad term *alteration*. They are either general classifications (alteration in parenting) or contain both the general classification and specific diagnosis (alteration in bowel elimination: constipation). The specific diagnosis would probably suffice for terms used clinically. Clear concise labeling is important; for the most part, the current category-labels meet this criterion and contain terms familiar to nurses and other professionals.

Bircher called attention to the fact that category-names should be consistently developed within a system of nomenclature. Labeling of phenomena can be arbitrary (the Bircher syndrome), descriptive (unresolved role conflict), or dynamic (ineffective coping) as well as causal or an analog (Bircher, 1982). The Association has used the preferred, descriptive method of labeling. In general a category-name reflects the operational definition of the concept being categorized and is consistent with other concepts categorized in the system.

Operational definitions and defining characteristics

Presence of defining characteristics or diagnostic indicators increases the support for a diagnostic hypothesis; absence suggests the hypothesis should be rejected. Diagnostic categories and their defining characteristics provide structure for the cognitive processes involved in diagnosis and provide labels for the final, diagnostic judgment.

Although some diagnoses have been listed for over 10 years, operational definitions of *critical* defining characteristics are absent. As may be seen in Table 1, 42 diagnoses lack a definition, and the critical defining characteristics (diagnostic criteria) of 47 are not specified. In general, few prototype categories have been developed. The number of characteristics specified for accepted diagnostic categories varies. Examination of the current listing of 62 diagnoses (Kim, McFarland, and McLane, 1984) revealed approximately 789 defining characteristics with a mean of 13.6. The range was 0 (Personal Identity Disturbance) to 64 (Potential for Trauma). Questions arose. Do all of the listed characteristics need to be present for the diagnosis to be made? If so, then for fear, anxiety, and pain 40 characteristics would need to be assessed. The recall, assessment, and transformation of information that would be required produce high cognitive strain and increase the risk of errors. Which characteristics should be required learning in educational programs? Careful examination of currently identified characteristics by three clinicians and this author suggested that, for most diagnostic categories, there may be only one or two characteristics that *must be present* for the condition to be diagnosed. The remaining characteristics may provide supporting or redundant cues which influence confidence levels in uncertainty-geared judgments. If operational definitions were available, critical characteristics could be identified and subjected to clinical testing.

Qualitative examination of categories suggested that the concepts at a high level of abstraction (the more inclusive concepts that are categorized) have a greater than average number (13.6) of characteristics. Examples include alter-

TABLE 1   Diagnostic categories lacking definitions or critical defining characteristics*

Categories lacking definitions (N = 42)	Categories lacking critical defining characteristics (N = 47)
Activity intolerance	Activity intolerance, potential
Activity intolerance, potential	Airway clearance, ineffective
Airway clearance	Bowel elimination, alterations in: constipation
Anxiety	Bowel elimination, alterations in: diarrhea
Bowel elimination, alteration in: constipation	Bowel elimination, alterations in: incontinence
Bowel elimination, alteration in: diarrhea	Breathing pattern ineffective
Bowel elimination, alteration in: incontinence	Cardiac output, alteration in: decreased
Breathing pattern, ineffective	Comfort, alteration in: pain
Cardiac output, alteration in: decreased	Coping, ineffective family: compromised
Comfort, alteration in: pain	Coping, ineffective family: disabling
Communication, impaired verbal	Coping, ineffective family: potential for growth
Diversional activity deficit	Diversional activity deficit
Family process, alterations in	Family process, alteration in:
Fluid volume deficit, actual (1)	Fear
Fluid volume deficit, actual (2)	Fluid volume deficit, actual (1)
Fluid volume, alterations in: excess	Fluid volume deficit, actual (2)
Fluid volume deficit: Potential	Fluid volume deficit, alterations in: excess
Gas exchange, impaired	
Grieving, dysfunctional	Fluid volume deficit, potential
Mobility, impaired physical	Gas exchange, impaired
Nutrition, alteration in: less than body requirements	Grieving, anticipatory
Nutrition, alteration in: more than body requirements	Grieving, dysfunctional
Nutrition, alteration in: potential for more than body requirements	Health maintenance alteration
Oral mucous membranes, alteration in	Injury, potential for; poisoning, potential for; suffocation, potential for; trauma, potential for
Rape trauma syndrome: compound reaction	Knowledge deficit
Rape trauma syndrome: silent reaction	Mobility, impaired physical
Self-care deficit: feeding, bathing/hygiene, dressing/grooming, toileting	Nutrition, alteration in: less than body requirements
Self-feeding deficit (specify level)	Oral mucous membranes, alteration in
Self-bathing/hygiene deficit (specify level)	Powerlessness (severe, moderate, low)
Self-dressing/grooming deficit (specify level)	Rape trauma syndrome
Self-toileting deficit (specify level)	Rape trauma syndrome: compound reaction
Body image disturbance	Rape trauma syndrome: silent reaction

TABLE 1   **Diagnostic categories lacking definitions or critical defining characteristics—cont'd**

Categories lacking definitions (N = 42)	Categories lacking critical defining characteristics (N = 47)
Self-esteem, disturbance in	Self-feeding deficit (specify level)

Role performance, disturbance in	Self-concept, disturbance in
	  Self-esteem, disturbance in
	  Role performance, disturbance in
	  Personal identity, disturbance in

Sensory perceptual alterations (6 specified)	Sensory perceptual alterations (6 specified)
Sexual dysfunction	Sexual dysfunction
Skin integrity, impairment of: actual	Skin integrity, impairment of: actual
Skin integrity, impairment of: potential	Skin integrity, impairment of: potential
Thought processes, alteration in	Social isolation
Tissue perfusion, alteration in (5 specified)	Thought processes, alteration in
Urinary elimination, alteration in pattern	Urinary elimination, alteration in patterns
Violence, potential for (self, others)	Violence, potential for (self-directed or directed at others)

*Analysis based on: Kim, M.J., McFarland, G., and McLane, A. Classification of nursing diagnoses—Proceedings of the Fifth National Conference, St. Louis, 1984, The C.V. Mosby Co.

ation in parenting, alteration in nutrition: less than body requirements, sensory perceptual alterations, impairment of skin integrity, sleep pattern disturbance, and alteration in mucous membranes. To use an analogy, the observable characteristics of furniture (an abstract concept) would be greater in number than the observable characteristics of a less inclusive concept (kitchen chairs). Most clinicians would agree that abstract diagnostic concepts require further discrimination. At least four types of sleep pattern disturbances and multiple nutritional deficits are encountered in practice. Are all sleep pattern disturbances treated in the same manner? In fact, three critical defining characteristics specified for this category are probably separate diagnostic entities that are *treated differently* (sleep onset disturbance, interrupted sleep pattern, and the early awakening pattern which may be a sign of another health problem). Sleep pattern reversal, a fairly common problem in some clinical settings, is not listed. Broad, general diagnostic categories are of limited usefulness in treatment planning. On the other hand, if further discriminations do not alter intervention, or are not associated with different outcomes (prognosis), they are only of academic interest. An example of very fine discriminations is the 56 categories of pain suggested by Campbell (1978). Is such fine discrimination of the pain category required for treatment planning?

Further qualitative examination of current diagnoses revealed many imprecise defining characteristics. Yet these characteristics are used (1) as the behaviors which are assessed through questions and observations during diagnostic hypothesis testing, (2) as criteria to differentiate between diagnostic categories, (3) as criteria for diagnostic judgment, and (4) as measurable signs or symptoms to evaluate the resolution of a problem and, consequently, as a basis for decisions to continue or discontinue treatment. Structurally, categories for classifying patients' health problems should provide the diagnostician with the power to discriminate between presence and absence of a problem and to differentiate among problems. Distinctive criteria provide this. Defining characteristics which are listed for more than one diagnosis, such as restlessness, do not aid in discriminations between or among categories. One example of a useful category that has discriminatory power is self-feeding deficit, level 0-1. The diagnostic criterion is distinctive and measurable: inability to bring food from a receptacle to the mouth. The level of the health problem is quantified by a 1-4 designation. In contrast, two defining characteristics of potential fluid volume deficit, increased output and altered intake, are ambiguous and nonprecise for evaluating the presence or absence of this condition.

We construct categories for cognitive efficiency, but human behavior is not necessarily presented in discrete packages; fuzzy categories will always be with us. Yet, our professional responsibility to patients requires the highest level of precision and accuracy in diagnosis and treatment that can be attained. Distinctive and measurable characteristics have to be of prime concern in category construction; otherwise, errors in usage will result. Jones and Jacob (1982) noted that there is a considerable difference in the *treatment* of anxiety and fear, yet a high rate of errors was found in the diagnosis of these conditions. Why? It is interesting to note that fear is listed as a defining characteristic of anxiety, although anxiety is defined as "often nonspecific in focus"; the definition of fear includes a focus on "an identifiable source" (Kim, McFarland, and McLane, 1984). In some cases the ability to discriminate among levels of a problem is also important for definitive diagnosis and treatment planning. For example, activity intolerance is a category where specification of the level of tolerance is critical for continuing care decisions. Currently, no levels are designated.

Not all diagnostic concepts can be quantified numerically. Yet, methods exist for scaling subjective signs, symptoms, and categorical data, such as fatigue, discomfort, degrees of activity tolerance, or skin breakdown (New York Heart Association, 1964; CURN Project, 1981; Sisson, 1978; Feinstein, 1982). Our diagnostic judgments are sufficiently important for quantification or qualification to be considered in refinement and construction of categories. Research of Amborn (1976), Cranley (1981), Norbeck and associates (1981), Gould (1983), and Guzzetta and Forsythe (1979) represents efforts to specify criteria or levels. McCourt (1981) has further developed the functional level classification for self-care deficits. Atwood (1980), Diers (1979), Evaneshko and Kay (1982), Oiler (1982), and Schatzman and Strauss (1973) offer ideas about methods for refinement.

Etiological factors. Clinicians experience difficulty in specifying etiological factors for a problem; in many instances they record the medical diagnosis. Although this may be attributed to the higher level processes involved in causal thinking or not appreciating multicausal relations, it could also be attributed to the clarity and specificity of our etiological categories. Examination of etiologies for the current diagnostic categories reveals (1) ambiguity of terms, such as "psychological injuring agents" or "health beliefs" (non-specified), (2) lack of operational definitions, and (3) absence of diagnostic criteria for etiological concepts. In some instances both diagnostic and etiological categories contain the same characteristics, varying only in specificity. At present, clinicians find it may be useful to use the list of 62 diagnostic categories and their defining characteristics as a set of concepts for describing individual patients' problems and etiological or contributing factors. This is supported by data obtained in the Jones and Jakob project (1982). The largest number (49%) of contributing factors in their sample of 2,772 diagnoses were from the list of diagnostic categories.

Potential problems. During refinement and construction of concepts categorized as potential problems, the concepts of risk and cause have to be considered. A cause cannot exist for a problem that has not occurred. Thus, etiology in the usual sense of probable cause is not applicable. The phrase "not applicable" is stated under etiology for one potential problem, potential impairment of skin integrity. Examination of the remaining seven potential problems currently categorized reveals that four have etiological factors specified and three note that etiologies are to be developed. There are contributing factors for a potential or high risk state; these are referred to as risk factors. Thus for a potential problem, defining characteristics (risk factors) and etiological factors are the same. It is not necessary or logical to specify etiological factors for a potential problem. Carpenito (1983) suggested that actual problems can be used as potential problems with the designation *potential.* This is true but it needs to be clear that it is the transformed etiological factors that guide problem identification. It would be more precise to define risk factors for each potential problem.

It is predicted that diagnostic criteria for actual or potential health problems will be (1) small in number, (2) highly valid indicators related to the operational definition of the diagnostic concept, and (3) reliable indicators that nearly always occur when the condition is present. Establishing validity and reliability of diagnostic criteria requires research. Yet, a great deal of logical analysis needs to be done prior to testing criteria. Let us consider some of the logical assumptions that influence the refinement and construction of diagnostic criteria used in nursing diagnosis.

To accurately and confidently diagnose a subjective state of feeling, knowing, perceiving, or valuing requires subjective data, such as verbal reports. Examples of categories describing subjective states are powerlessness, spiritual distress, anxiety, and grieving. In contrast, diagnosis of states or processes, such as airway clearance or skin integrity, relies more heavily on observational data. Second, when diagnosing a process, such as ineffective coping or grieving, both historical and current (patient, family) information is required. Diagnostic criteria should reflect this. Any diagnosis of an alteration or disturbance, such as sleep pattern disturbance or alteration in parenting, implies change or deviation. Criteria for diagnosing an alteration or disturbance must include the degree of change from individual baselines (historical data) or from normative baselines. The diagnoses of deficits such as knowledge or diversional activity implies there is a needed amount determined either by present or future needs (knowledge deficit) or by subjective report of need.

Diagnosing an actual problem on the basis of historical or contextual data is stereotyping. Current, state-of-the-patient data is required. An example frequently seen is the diagnosis of self-concept disturbance based on the prior occurrence of hysterectomy. Hysterectomy is a historical, contextual cue. Self-concept is a subjective state and disturbance implies change. Diagnosis is made by comparing the historical and current self-concept pattern. If cues to self-concept disturbance are present, "hysterectomy" may serve to increase the confidence level. Refinement and construction of diagnostic criteria should take into account typologies of clinical information (Gordon, 1982) and the type of phenomenon being described.

The work required for refinement of diagnostic categories used in practice most closely approximates concept analysis. The activities involved in explication of concepts are discussed by Chinn and Jacobs (1983), Walker and Avant (1983), and Wilson (1963). Concept development is a cyclic process involving repeated conceptual and research activities. As knowledge accumulates, concepts undergo further revision. The plea at this time is that (1) we consider knowledge of the diagnostic process in refinement of diagnoses currently categorized, and (2) always remember that diagnoses are concepts constructed by the intellect. Because of this they can be modified or discarded when not useful. Hardening of our categories, like hardening of the arteries, is dangerous.

REFERENCES

Amborn, S.A.: Clinical signs associated with the amount of tracheobronchial secretions, Nurs. Res. **25**:121-126, 1976.
American Heart Association: Jones criteria revised for guidance in the diagnosis of rheumatic fever, Circulation **32**:664, 1965.
Atwood, J.: Developing instruments for measurement of criteria, Nurs. Res. **29**:104-108, 1980.
Avant, K.: Nursing diagnosis: Maternal attachment, Adv. Nurs. Sci. **2**:45-55, 1979.

Beckner, M.: The biological way of thought, New York, 1959, Columbia University Press.

Berlin, E.: Ethnobiological classification. In Rosch, E., and Lloyd, E., editors: Cognition and categorization, Hillside, NJ, 1978, Lawrence Erlbaum Associates.

Bircher, A.: On the development and classification of diagnoses, Nursing Forum, **14:**11-29, 1975.

Bruner, J.S., Goodnow, J.J., and Austin, G.A.: A study of thinking, New York, 1956, John Wiley & Sons, Inc.

Campbell, C.: Nursing diagnosis and intervention in nursing practice, New York, 1978, John Wiley & Sons, Inc.

Carpenito, L.J.: Nursing diagnosis: Application to clinical practice, Philadelphia, 1983, J.B. Lippincott Co.

Cranley, M.S.: Development of a tool for measurement of maternal attachment during pregnancy, Nurs. Res. **30:**281-282, 1981.

Diers, D.: Research in nursing practice, Philadelphia, 1979, J.B. Lippincott Co.

Evanshenko, V., and Kay, M.: Ethnoscience research technique, West. J. Nurs. Res. **4:**49-64, 1982.

Feinstein, A.R.: The Jones Criteria and the challenge of clinimetrics, Circulation **66:**1-5, 1982.

Gordon, M.: Nursing diagnosis and the diagnostic process, Amer. J. Nurs. **76:**129-130, 1976.

Gordon, M.: Nursing diagnosis: Process and application, New York, 1982, McGraw-Hill Book Co.

Guzzetta, C.E., and Forsythe, G.L.: Nursing diagnostic pilot study: Psychophysiological stress, Adv. Nurs. Sci. **2:**27-44, 1979.

Jones, P., and Jakob, D.: Nursing diagnosis: Differenting fear and anxiety, Nursing Papers **14:**20-29, 1982.

Jones, P., and Jakob, D.: The definition of nursing diagnosis (Unpublished manuscript. University of Toronto, Faculty of Nursing.)

Kim, M.J., McFarland, G., and McLane, A., editors: Classification of nursing diagnosis—Proceedings of the Fifth National Conference, St. Louis, 1984, The C.V. Mosby Co.

McCourt, A.: Measurement of functional deficit in quality assurance, American Nurses' Association Quality Assurance Update **5:**1-3, 1981.

Miller, G.A.: The magical number seven, plus or minus two: some comments on our capacity for processing information, Psychol. Rev. **63:**81-97, 1956.

Mundinger, M., and Jauron, G.: Developing a nursing diagnosis, Nurs. Outlook **23:**94-98, 1975.

Norbeck, J.S., Lindsey, A.M., and Carrieri, V.L.: The development of an instrument to measure social support, Nurs. Res. **30:**264-269, 1981.

Oiler, C.: Phenomenological approach in nursing research, Nurs. Res. **31:**178-181, 1982.

Purushotham, D.: Nursing diagnosis, Canad. Nurse **81:**46-48, 1981.

Rosch, E.: Principles of categorization. In Rosch, E., and Lloyd, B., editors: Cognition and categorization, Hillside, NJ, 1978, Lawrence Erlbaum Associates.

Rosch, E., and others: Basic objects in natural categories, Cognitive Psychol. **8:**382-439, 1976.

Roy, C.: Framework for classification system development: Process and issues. In Kim, M.J., McFarland, G., and McLane, A., editors: Classification of nursing diagnoses—Proceedings of the Fifth National Conference, St. Louis, 1984, The C.V. Mosby Co.

Schatzman, L., and Strauss, A.L.: Field research: strategies for a natural sociology, Englewood Cliffs, NJ, 1973, Prentice-Hall, Inc.

Shamansky, S.L., and Yanni, C.R.: In opposition to nursing diagnosis: a minority opinion, Image **15:**47-50, 1983.

Sisson, J.C.: Quantifying clinical information, South. Med J. **71:**1416-1418, 1978.

Sneath, P.H.A., and Sokal, R.R.: Numerical taxonomy, San Francisco, 1973, W.H. Freeman Co.

Tanner, C.A.: Research on clinical judgment. In Holzemer, W.L.: Review of research in nursing education, Thorofare, NJ, 1983, Slack.

Tanner, C.A., and Hughes, A.G.: Nursing diagnosis: issues in clinical practice research, Top. Clin. Nurs. **5:**30-38, 1984.

Tversky, A.: Studies of similarity. In Rosch, E., and Lloyd, B., editors: Cognition and categorization, New York, 1978, Lawrence Erlbaum.

Walker, L.O., and Avant, K.C.: Strategies for theory construction in nursing, Norwalk, CT, 1983, Appleton-Century-Crofts.

Wilson, J.: Thinking with concepts, Cambridge, England, 1963, Cambridge University Press.

CHAPTER 3

Framework

The design for relevance, revisited: an elaboration of the conceptual framework for nursing diagnosis

LARK W. KIRK, M.S.N., R.N.

As the title suggests, the focus of this paper is primarily conceptual in character. What is presented is a distillation of selected thoughts related to both the formulation and the use of nursing diagnoses within the context of providing nursing care. The conceptual material bears more than a little resemblance to the original conceptual framework for nursing diagnosis authored by the Nurse Theorists' Group and explained by Roy (1978, 1980, 1982). Yet this work also represents another origin; it is an attempt to coax out an as-yet vague and ill-appreciated clinical utility from the conceptual system for nursing posed by Rogers (1970, 1980, 1983, 1984). Additionally, several writings of Gordon and colleagues (Gordon, 1976, 1978, 1982; Gordon and Sweeney, 1979; Gordon and associates, 1980) have played a prominent part in shaping this thinking. The impetus for organizing these thoughts has come from the twin beliefs that nursing diagnosis is a productive, meaningful tool for contemporary nursing and that Rogers' system, though not fully explicated by Rogers with respect to practice concerns, harbors an unrealized and perhaps important utility for shaping nursing care activities.

We have called this new derivative view "the design for relevance, revisited," for it was originally inspired, in part, by the following passage from Rogers' 1970 book:

> The resolution of health problems and the setting of goals directed toward achieving a healthy people require a new concept of the unity of man and a recognition of man's capacity to feel and to reason. Man possesses major resources within himself for determining the direction in the developmental process.... **A design for relevance requires the seeing of a pattern.** (Emphasis added.)

Upon reading this passage, one is led immediately to question what is meant by "the seeing of a pattern." Indeed, we might need to start by asking what the term "pattern" means and considering how it has been represented within the nursing literature. For example, it is useful to consider at least three different definitions which have appeared in the writings of nursing authors.

Gordon (1982) has defined pattern as a "sequence of behavior across time." Rogers (1970, 1983), however, has said that pattern is both a human and an environmental characteristic. And Crawford (1982), in an insightful analysis of the various uses in nursing of the word "pattern," has offered yet a third definition: "the configuration of relationships between elements of a particular phenomenon."

All three definitions are useful and important. Those by Gordon and by Crawford are operationally useful; Rogers' definition is abstract and general. None of the definitions should be taken to exclude the others; none appears to give a final answer, once and for all, regarding what "pattern" means. Therefore, to achieve some closure on the matter for the aims of practice, what may be useful is to consider what, from a nurse's viewpoint, *characterizes* patterns. On this point, Gordon has provided a highly valuable set of four pattern characteristics.

According to Gordon (1982), patterns are descriptive units with the potential to enhance or sharpen the nurse's understanding of the client and are focused on (1) client and environment, (2) developmental content, and (3) function. In addition, they meet a fourth vital characteristic: utility for practice.

Given these leading criteria and some knowledge of Rogers' system—both its strengths and its shortcomings—an attempt was made to formulate a transitional sort of framework for practice. It was intended that this framework would approximate an understanding of Rogers' system, as originally written and revised over the past 14 years, as well as make use of the similarity in terms and assumptions which exists between Rogers' work and that of the Nurse Theorists' Group (NTG). This framework, it was recognized, would not achieve a complete elaboration of Rogers' system, nor would it be exactly the same as that produced by the Nurse Theorists' Group. Further, no claim would be made that this was a fully specified model. Instead, ten assumptions were framed, as the basis for this speculative new scheme or design. These assumptions were:

1. "Pattern" describes the fundamental flux of energy between the human and the environment.
2. The unit of analysis in nursing care is a client's life as a whole, and this "whole" is a singular pattern of experience.
3. Assessing a client consists of "glimpsing" this pattern.
4. Diagnosis, an activity concluding assessment and which is done *with* a client, consists of forming value-based statements about the pattern.
5. "Client" may mean one or more persons.

6. The client's awareness of pattern is both innate and beneficial, but his or her pattern recognition abilities can be sharpened.

7. Ability to affect one's own pattern is the basis of the process that is commonly called "coping" and is a critical life skill. This ability too can be improved.

8. Successful nursing care results in enhancing the development of a client. That is, nursing care influences or supports the natural process and direction of change toward new situations of increased complexity and diversity within the client's singular life pattern. Such new situations reflect an arrangement both more ordered and more satisfying to the client.

9. One key measure in nursing practice, though very general in nature, is the client's perception that a beneficial change has occurred.

10. The primary activities of nursing practice are goal seeking and setting. These are performed jointly by the nurse and client and experienced as a "creative journey."

The point of emphasis in this design is that there is a singular pattern of experience to one's life. Pattern is considered here an experienced phenomenon. Further, and associated with the coherence of this pattern, are increasing order and a trend toward ever more complexity. And along with these changes is a perceived satisfaction on the part of the client.

At this writing some preliminary efforts have been made to apply this view in the clinical setting. These efforts have included the pilot testing of early versions of the ideas in several practice realms. Though we will not detail this history here, it may be worthwhile to explain how the idea of a *singular pattern* has been interpreted as meaningful within the care process, in terms of our current and latest version of this design.

Within the practice of nursing and the design presented, pattern is considered as something to be recognized, judged by client and nurse, and influenced from time to time. To enhance pattern recognition, on the part of both client and nurse, themes for pattern recognition may be used. This occurs primarily during the assessment/diagnosis of the client's problems and within the evaluative phases of care.

At present, nine themes are suggested for use:
Perceiving
Knowing
Energy substrate—intake/utilization/excretion
Elemental exchange—fluid and gases
Physically expressed energy—kinetics and repair
Energetics of the sleep/wake index
Relating
Feeling and communicating
Valuing

These nine were chosen after reviewing (1) the general conceptual framework described by the Nurse Theorists' Group, (2) the typology that Gordon has been evolving in the literature since 1980, and (3) responses from "small group sessions" at the Fourth National Conference (Rossi and Krekeler, 1980). In particular, there was an attempt when identifying these pattern recognition themes to maintain as much similarity as justified between this design and that of the earlier influencing works. Yet responding to and incorporating several concerns identified by the small groups at the conference was also a goal. These matters, it should be emphasized, did not concern Gordon's scheme but that of the Nurse Theorists' Group. The assumption was made that "small group reactions" represented the voice of the more clinically active nursing diagnosis contingency at that time. Therefore, by tailoring the theorist-generated framework to their comments and suggestions, a new hybrid view could be offered which could be expected to speak more effectively to contemporary practice concerns.

The first matter addressed was the great importance group members ascribed to the pattern called "exchanging." One group cross-listed the existing diagnoses and showed that the great majority of them fell under this heading (Rossi and Krekeler, 1980). A second and apparently independent group identified that "the human experience is interaction" and proposed that "material and nonmaterial exchange" could be used to organize or reorganize a conceptual basis (Rossi and Krekeler, 1980). Also, it was noted that there was a general concern expressed among conference attendees that the biophysical dimension of the human was not well addressed by the theorist group (Feild, 1980). On these bases, we were encouraged to go forward with our design and, specifically, to state that (1) the focus of concern for nursing should be a singular pattern of experience and (2) the fundamental characteristic of this pattern was client-environment exchange.

The three operationalizations of pattern mentioned here in the context of nursing diagnosis are (1) the patterns of unitary man named by the Nurse Theorists' Group (Roy, 1978, 1980), (2) Gordon's (1980, 1982) well-known functional pattern typology, and (3) the pattern recognition themes presented here. These three are shown side by side for comparison in Table 1.

In general, the view corresponding to the new design and naming "pattern recognition themes" includes six of the original nine patterns of unitary man identified by the Nurse Theorists' Group. In addition, this new design has themes which correspond generally to Gordon's typology elements called "elimination, nutritional/metabolic, activity/exercise, and sleep/rest."

To promote understanding regarding how these pattern recognition themes are incorporated in the process of care, a care guide has been prepared (Kirk, 1983, 1984). An outline is shown in Box 1.

This guide is an emergent product, preceded by three progressively more thoughtful versions of assessment tools for determining nursing diagnoses

TABLE 1   Three views for nursing diagnosis and nursing care

Patterns of unitary man (NTG*)	Functional pattern typology (Gordon)	Pattern recognition themes (Kirk)
Exchanging	Self-perception/self-concept	Perceiving
Communicating	Sexuality/reproductive	Knowing
Relating	Value/belief	Energy substrate—intake excretion utilization
Valuing	Coping/stress tolerance	Elemental exchange—fluid and gases
Choosing	Cognitive/perceptual	Physically expressed energy—kinetics and repair
Moving	Role/relationship	Energetics of sleep/wake index
Perceiving	Elimination	Relating
Knowing	Health perception/health management	Feeling and communicating
Feeling	Activity/exercise	Valuing
	Sleep/rest Nutritional/metabolic	

*Nurse Theorist Group.

BOX 1   Care guideline, "The design for relevance, revisited"—MINC Project*

Discovery-oriented portion
   Introduction—to client
   Client's perception of own field—focusing questions
   Vital signs
   Evidence of past pattern aberrancy
   Overt pattern readjustment routines
   Pattern-recognition themes (9)
   Experience-modulating patterns
   Physical examination component
   Summaries of assessment
      Closure items
      General observations
      Supplementary data
      Summary of impressions, including evidence of both pattern coherence and pattern disruption
Nursing diagnoses
Planning materials
   Idea words list
   Formatted care plan
Result-oriented portion
   Review of each diagnosis, each outcome
   Restatement of nursing diagnoses, back to framing, if needed
Appended
   Idea words list
   Physical examination guideline
   Formulas for energy/protein/and water requirements

*Models In Nursing Care (Kirk, 1983, 1984).

(Kirk and Choy, 1982; Kirk, 1982a, 1982b). Presently, the guide incorporates a structured yet open-ended tool for data collection and summarization, plus elements that address the role of the client as a source of strategies for problem solution. The data collection and summarization portions are directed toward both (1) assessment/diagnosis and (2) evaluation phases in the care process. Materials appended to the care guide include (a) a supplemental guide for physical examination, (b) formulas for calculating selected nutritional requirements and corrections to these for sleep, activity, and specific bodily alterations (that is, alterations such as stress in various degrees, amputations of body parts, and time and degree of exertion versus periods of sleep), and (c) an "idea words" list. This list contains two dozen change-oriented, choice-oriented verbs which can be given to a patient to enable him or her to better speculate with the care-providing nurse about possible solutions to problems which have been described in the newly defined nursing diagnoses.

Having introduced this new design for the reader's consideration, we are not done. A few other thoughts, also on a conceptual plane but more general, are offered next. These subsequent thoughts may be viewed as completely separate from the "design for relevance" just described, although they did arise during the formulation of that design and they have influenced the direction in which that nursing care tool has evolved.

REFLECTIONS ON THE PROCESS OF NURSING CARE

Nursing practice as problem solving, a view generally credited to Yura and Walsh (1967), is widely used as a basis for organizing thoughts about care. Relatedly, one interesting matter at which we might look more closely is a vital but little-discussed precursor: *problem finding.*

Within materials in the field of education, specifically some remarks on creativity theory (Dillon, 1982), a thought-provoking discussion was noted regarding how problems are found. A summary of key points in this article is shown in Table 2.

The thesis advanced by Dillon was that problems exist at three levels of actuality and that at each of these levels one is called upon to engage in a

TABLE 2   A conceptual scheme for comparing levels of problem finding and solving

Problem level (existential/psychological)	Problem	Activity	Solution
I. Existing/evident	As problematic	Perceiving the situation (**recognition**)	As resolved
II. Emergent/implicit	For elements of a problem	Probing the data (**discovery**)	For elements of a solution
III. Potential/inchoate	A defined problem	Producing the problem-event (**invention**)	A defined solution

specific type of thought and activity in order to locate or "find" the problem. The scheme suggests a special meaningfulness for nursing practice and particularly nursing diagnosis, since the latter is largely a problem-specifying or problem-locating activity. Implicit in Dillon's view is the idea that the less evident a problem is, the more effort is called for on the part of person (or persons) serving as the problem locator. Yet regardless of problem "level," some effort must be expended in problem finding prior to problem solution.

Dillon asked four leading questions at the close of his paper, presumably to promote further thought on the matter of problem location as an activity in its own right. These questions, deeply puzzling, were as follows:

What steps are involved in problem finding and how do they relate to one another?

How are problem *finding* and *solving* related?

What is the relationship between problem solving and other variables of interest (such as "creativity" or "cognitive style")?

To what extent can people be identified as either "finders" or "solvers" of problems and what might distinguish them as such?

We will not attempt to fully elaborate answers to these questions but instead will add a few more of our own from a nursing perspective.

Within the context of nursing practice activity, who is responsible, nurse or client, for problem finding?

Similarly, who is responsible, nurse or client, for problem solution?

Further, if these responsibilities are shared, what process is entailed?

Such matters represent difficult issues. They have been addressed in part within writings which discuss the self-help and self-care movements in health care.* They are knotty matters to address: it would be an error to suggest otherwise. It may be worthwhile simply to clarify our own ideas and commitments regarding the type of "helping" beliefs and approaches which we as nurses adopt with our clients.

An important paper published recently in the nursing literature (Cronenwett, 1983) has addressed this, shedding a much-needed light on the helping content implicit in major nursing frameworks. That paper provides a synopsis of four types of helping models proposed by social psychologist Brickman and co-workers. As Cronenwett explains, the names of the four helping models are "moral, enlightenment, compensatory, and medical." These four are distinguished on the basis of two parameters of implied or accepted client responsibility: (1) responsibility for the origin of a problem and (2) responsibility for its solution. The "moral" model is characterized by viewing the client as highly responsible for both. The "enlightenment" helping model describes high

---

*For reviews of these trends and discussion of associated conceptual problems see King, 1980; Zola, 1979.

responsibility for problem origin yet low responsibility for problem solution. The "compensatory" model places low responsibility for problem origin with the client but gives him or her a high degree of responsibility for problem solution. And, finally, the "medical" model of helping gives little responsibility to clients for either aspect of their problem(s), origin or solution. Three conclusions within Cronenwett's paper may be of particular relevance to our struggle to understand and elaborate nursing from a problem-diagnostic and problem-solution stance. First, she noted that the medical model was identified by Brickman and colleagues to be the manner of helping most broadly adopted by our physician colleagues. Second, her analysis demonstrated that nursing practice–related descriptions tend to favor the compensatory model. And third, nursing authors also show allegiance to forms of "blended models" of helping.

Clearly, then, a critical question for us to address is what model or models of helping correspond most closely to our current modes of caring in nursing practice. Since the first nursing diagnosis conference was convened, the stated intent has been to incorporate the views of the client in the diagnostic process. From the proceedings of the first conference held in 1973 we note, "nursing diagnosis should be seen as a process that involves the interaction of the nurse with the patient or client. This interaction leads to a consensually validated statement of the problem" (Gebbie and Lavin, 1975). With respect to nursing considered most generally, the involvement of clients and concern for the client's opinions, hopes, and wishes is clearly the dominant ethic. This is so much so, in fact, that no reference is needed on this point. Therefore, it is proposed that the model of helping which is most consistent with the stated views of NANDA, and contemporary nursing in general, is the compensatory model. Additionally, we extend this model of helping somewhat to include client participation in *all* phases of the care process.

Not a radical position, we believe that client participation is consistent with the growing trend toward increasing levels of consumer involvement in the design and use of health care. Indeed, we suspect that in many cases the increased involvement of clients when nursed with the compensatory type of helping model will be well received. Such an approach may even come to be routinely expected by informed consumers of nursing services.

But how will nurses mediate this new arrangement and secure maximum client involvement in care? And, as suggested by the previous discussion, how can this involvement effectively extend to include the client actively in both the *finding* of the problems (or nursing diagnoses as they are currently conceptualized) and the *solving* of them? Attempting to remain consistent with Rogers' views and those stated by the Nurse Theorists' Group, we present a reconceptualization, of sorts, of the nursig process. Based on the idea that nursing practice is creative in both procedure and product, we suggest that a potentially useful way to view nursing is as a "creative journey" (one of the original 10 assumptions listed earlier in this paper).

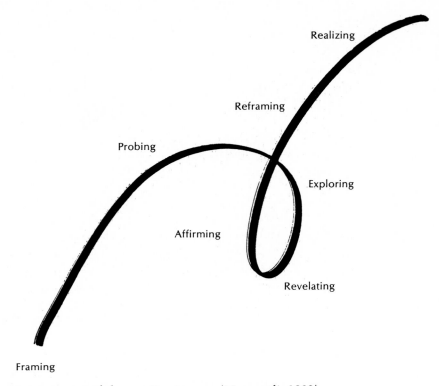

Realizing

Reframing

Probing

Exploring

Affirming

Revelating

Framing

FIGURE 1   The seven passages of the creative journey (Motamedi, 1982).

Motamedi (1982), writing outside the nursing literature, proposed a model of creative productivity. This is a view laden with meaning for nursing. He termed this process "the creative journey," naming seven passages, and he diagrammed the journey as shown in Fig. 1.

There is potential to use this model as a guide for organizing shared work toward creative ends. We propose the idea of shared work toward creative ends as a new way of naming nursing practice. Such naming incorporates the finding of the problem, the diagnosis of the patient, the glimpsing of the pattern, and the involvement of the client or patient as referred to in the "compensatory" model of helping.

Motamedi's seven passages, as shown, were framing, probing, exploring, revelating, affirming, reframing, and realizing. For clarification, we have proceeded to draw analogies, such as they exist, between the familiar nursing process (including the step of diagnosis) and a creative journey (see Table 3).

Steps of the nursing process are compared with their corresponding "passages." In the very last lines of this listing, on the left, reference is made to "Loop 2." The reason for this, as the reader surely has surmised, is that a description of nursing care as a creative journey requires the consideration of more than just a single "cycle" of Motamedi's original model. In terms of generalizing Motamedi's model to nursing practice, Fig. 2 depicts what may, in fact, be more relevant for us to consider as nurses. As a point of clarification, the terms bracketed and appearing to the right of the diagram are to suggest that continuing to those passages is discretionary. That is, the decision to proceed beyond the second instance of "exploring"—or the evaluation phase, in the vernacular of nursing—is discretionary depending upon the mutual judgment of the client and nurse.

Of course, whenever such a large dose of new terminology is introduced there is need for sufficient definitions. In recognition of this, descriptions of the seven passages and what we see as their possible relevance to nursing care are presented here. These elaborations, except for the nursing or care references, appear largely as abstracted from Motamedi's paper.

Framing is understood to contain the initial experience in which a phenomenon appears in context and is recognized. At this time both "meaning" and "involvement" are first organized. Labeling or naming of the phenomenon begins. **Probing** is described as broad scanning for more information about the phenomenon. Quizzing and resensing help assess potential risks and rewards of further pursuit. **Exploring** consists of forming and reviewing working hypotheses and tentative strategies. Knowledge of the phenomenon gradually shifts from noticing to knowing. Inductive, intuitive, and janusian thinking* predominate. Courage may be needed at this time to pursue the journey further. **Revelating** is the passage during which new insights, continually applied, yield discovery. Here, the gap between the pursuer(s) and the phenomenon is narrowest. **Affirming** is the passage which includes the first effort that confirms the revelation. More objective than the passage just preceding, affirming ends with perceived credibility, confidence, and certainty regarding the revelation. **Reframing** is the period in which the content of the revelation and affirmation becomes more ordinary. It is characterized by an increasing objectivity. *New meaning* is organized. We speculate that it is here that a nursing care plan can be first formalized. **Realizing** is the sharing of the new information or knowledge, the product that has been derived. We interpret that this passage corresponds to implementation of the new plan.

As indicated in Fig. 2, a second loop (or more) may be conceptually useful for the nursing application of the creative journey model. *Framing, Probing,* and *Exploring* in the second loop correspond to the activities and understandings which nurses usually discuss as the evaluation of outcomes from the care

---

*"Janusian thinking" refers to the simultaneous consideration of two opposites and has been identified as a basic way of thinking associated with creative output. For additional information about this and a related entity, "homospatial thinking," the reader is referred to the original writings on these topics (Rothenberg, 1971, 1976, 1979).

TABLE 3   The nursing process and the creative journey

Passages	Steps
Framing Probing Exploring	Assessment
Revealing Affirming	Diagnosis
Reframing	Planning
Realizing	Implementing
Framing (Loop 2) through exploring, and further if needed	Evaluation

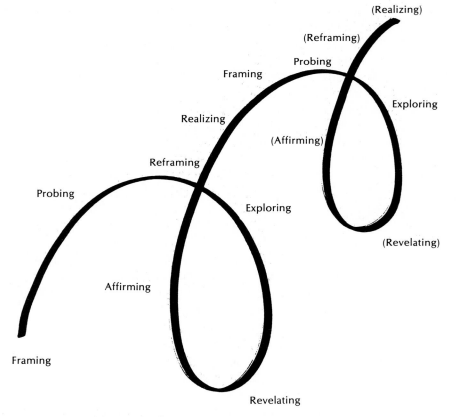

FIGURE 2   Nursing care process expressed as a "creative journey."

plan. During these latter instances of Framing, the phenomenon is renoted. Investment of the parties is continued. Probing then corresponds to a refocusing to achieve an understanding of the new, present situation. And Exploring, in this later time, refers to generation of new hypotheses for understanding the new situation. Value decisions are applied regarding the need for further examination of the situation. It may be useful to say that this point is where nurses, along with their clients, decide whether new interventions are needed, whether new problems have come into existence, and what their next activities and goals will be.

Highlights of the creative journey model are that it has both objective and subjective phases. Also, persons may proceed "backward" along the sequence of passages, if needed, before forward progress toward realization is made. In the nursing application of this model, the realization which is achieved as an outcome is a blend of both new health (or a satisfying, coherent, and complex pattern which has an empirical referent or set of referents) and a new understanding of the self, in health terms. Thus, both a new health or patterning and knowledge of the self are the results or products of nursing care.*

In summary, several collections of thought on a conceptual plane have been provided which may be of interest to nurses attempting to understand their patients and implement nursing diagnosis in a meaningful fashion. The "design for relevance, revisited," was represented as an attempt to better explicate Rogers' conceptual system in terms of its meaning for contemporary nursing care practices. An attempt was made to maintain linkage between that design and the conceptual framework of the theorist group and to demonstrate the contributions to this thinking derived from the work of Gordon and colleagues. Ten assumptions about pattern and nursing and human beings were proposed.

It was pointed out that problem finding is a necessary precursor to problem solving. The embedded nature of problem finding was discussed, while describing a scheme that identifies three existential levels of "problems." Also included was a discussion of attitudinal sets about helping, and four models of helping based upon these attitudes were briefly mentioned. It was stated that the "compensatory model of helping," featuring client involvement, was most consistent with contemporary nursing practice, in general, and most congruent with the intent of NANDA. This participatory mode was then elaborated as a process of shared work and called the "creative journey."

In closure, this material clearly must be viewed as a speculative, open-ended approach to understanding and conducting one's nursing practice. Plans are underway to test this scheme, this "design for relevance," in terms of its

---

*The author is indebted to Professor Rosemary Ellis, thinker in nursing, for sensitizing her to the oft-seen conceptual fuzziness beween empirically evident problems and knowledge problems.

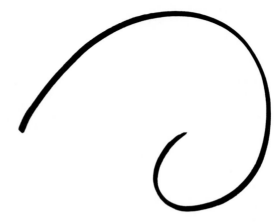

FIGURE 3   Mired in initial assessment, journey thwarted.

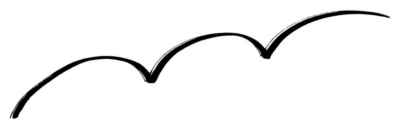

FIGURE 4   One or both parties reluctant or unable to participate.

capacity to usefully guide nursing care. There will be a simultaneous testing of frameworks for practice of both Orem (1971, 1980) and Roy (1970, 1971, 1976, 1984).

To reinforce our tentativeness about the utility of these ideas, a few final ideas and diagrams are offered depicting possible outcomes which may occur.

One possible result, to be avoided, is that a nonending or unfocused data collection period could take place. Should this occur, we might expect the unhappy, unfruitful situation of becoming mired in data analysis.

Alternatively, we could find a lack of investment on the part of one or both parties, a situation which would not support the shared work process. Instead, a superficiality could characterize this situation.

Similarly, though for a different reason, a partial participation such as that due to a "proxy" participant may lead to a somewhat less accurate or less complete "journey" experience. This would perhaps occur, of necessity, in

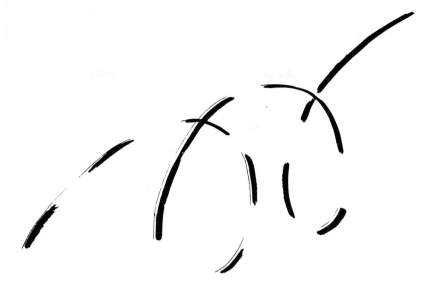

FIGURE 5   Significant other as " proxy" participant, information sketchy.

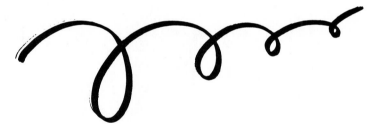

FIGURE 6   Decreasing shared work.

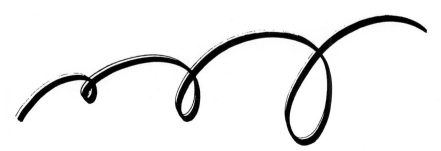

FIGURE 7   Increasing shared work.

circumstances when the goals, ideas, or wishes of the patient himself or herself cannot be known but are instead represented by a loved one or some other advocate within the process of care.

Trends over time may show a decrease in the shared work, either in the amount and/or depth or complexity, *or* an increase in same. The former situation could be exemplified by a large and difficult set of nursing diagnoses slowly being resolved to the client's satisfaction. The latter might be seen when there is some initial reluctance to participate followed by a trend toward more investment, the result being an increasingly more complex and detailed scheme of nursing care.

And for your final consideration, we represent the generalization of nursing care as an iterative creative process. In diagrammatic form, this is perhaps the ideal with respect to the potential of nursing practice to contribute meaningfully and in an ongoing fashion to the general social good.

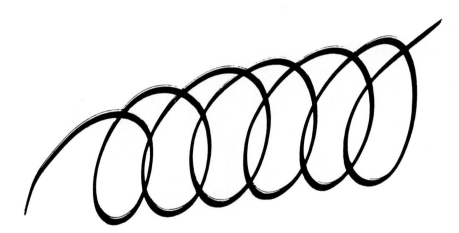

FIGURE 8   Iterations of nursing care as a "creative journey."

REFERENCES

Crawford, G.: The concept of pattern in nursing: conceptual development and measurement, Adv. Nurs. Sci. **5:**1-6, 1982.

Cronenwett, L.R.: Helping and nursing models, Nurs. Res. **32:**342-346, 1983.

Dillon, J.T.: Problem finding and solving, J. Creative Behav. **16:**97-111, 1982.

Feild, L.: Comments included in Responses of clinical specialists to the unitary man framework. In Kim, M.J., and Moritz, D.A., editors: Classification of nursing diagnoses—Proceedings of the Third and Fourth National Conferences, New York, 1982, McGraw-Hill Book Co.

Gebbie, K.M., and Lavin, M.A., editors: Classification of nursing diagnoses—Proceedings of the First National Conference, St. Louis, 1975, The C.V. Mosby Co.

Gordon, M.: Nursing diagnosis and the diagnostic process, Am. J. Nurs. **76:**1298-1300, 1976.

Gordon, M.: The diagnostic process. In Kim, M.J., and Moritz, D.A., editors: Classification of nursing diagnoses—Proceedings of the Third and Fourth National Conferences, New York, 1982, McGraw-Hill Book Co.

Gordon, M.: Nursing diagnosis: process and application, New York, 1982, McGraw-Hill Book Co.

Gordon, M., and Sweeney, M.A.: Methodological problems and issues in identifying and standardizing nursing diagnoses, Adv. Nurs. Sci. **2**:1-16, 1979.

Gordon, M., Sweeney, M.A., and McKeehan, K.: Nursing diagnosis: looking at its use in the clinical area, Am. J. Nurs. **80**:672-674, 1980.

Kim, M.J., and Moritz, D.A., editors: Classification of nursing diagnoses—Proceedings of the Third and Fourth National Conferences, New York, 1982, McGraw-Hill Book Co.

King, C.: The self-help/self-care concept, Nurse Pract. **5**(3):34-35, 39, 46, 1980.

Kirk, L.W.: Tool for determining the nursing diagnoses of the hospitalized adult (preliminary version). Unpublished document, 1982a.

Kirk, L.W.: Tool for determining the nursing diagnoses of the hospitalized adult. Unpublished document, 1982b.

Kirk, L.W.: The design for relevance, revisited: a guide for the delivery of nursing care based on Rogers' conceptual system. Unpublished document, 1983-1984. Produced in conjunction with the Models in Nursing Care Project (Director, Sr. C. Roy; Co-Directors, R. Wu and L.W. Kirk).

Kirk, L.W., and Choy, S.: Health assessment tool for the adult client in ambulatory settings. Unpublished document, 1982.

Motamedi, K.: Extending the concept of creativity, J. Creative Behav. **16**:75-88, 1982.

Orem, D.E.: Nursing: concepts of practice, New York, 1971, McGraw-Hill Book Co.

Orem, D.E.: Nursing: concepts of practice, ed. 2, New York, 1980, McGraw-Hill Book Co.

Rogers, M.E.: An introduction to the theoretical basis of nursing, Philadelphia, 1970, F.A. Davis Co.

Rogers, M.E.: Nursing: a science of unitary man. In Riehl, J.P., and Roy, C., editors: Conceptual models for nursing practices, ed. 2, New York, 1980, Appleton-Century-Crofts.

Rogers, M.E.: Science of unitary human beings: a paradigm for nursing. In Clements, W.I., and Roberts, F.B., editors: Family health: a theoretical approach to nursing care, New York, 1983, John Wiley & Sons, Inc.

Rogers, M.E.: Instructional materials on the science of unitary human beings. (Personal communication, 1984.)

Rossi, L., and Krekeler, K.: Small group reactions to the theoretical framework, "unitary man." In Kim, M.J., and Moritz, D.A., editors: Classification of nursing diagnoses—Proceedings of the Third and Fourth National Conferences, New York, 1982, McGraw-Hill Book Co.

Rothenberg, A.: The process of janusian thinking in creativity, Arch. Gen. Psychiatry **24**:195-205, 1971.

Rothenberg, A.: Homospatial thinking in creativity, Arch. Gen. Psychiatr. **33**:17-26, 1976.

Rothenberg, A.: The emerging goddess: the creative process in art, science, and other fields, Chicago, 1979, University of Chicago Press.

Roy, C.: Adaptation: a conceptual framework for nursing, Nurs. Outlook **18**:42-45, 1970.

Roy, C.: Adaptation: a basis for nursing practice, Nurs. Outlook **19**:254-257, 1971.

Roy, C.: Theoretical framework for classification of nursing diagnosis. In Kim, M.J., and Moritz, D.A., editors: Classification of nursing diagnoses—Proceedings of the Third and Fourth National Conferences, New York, 1982, McGraw-Hill Book Co.

Roy, C.: Historical perspective of the theoretical framework for the classification of nursing diagnosis. In Kim, M.J., and Moritz, D.A., editors: Classification of nursing diagnoses—Proceedings of the Third and Fourth National Conferences, New York, 1982, McGraw-Hill Book Co.

Roy, C.: Framework for classification systems development: progress and issues. In Kim, M.J., McFarland, G.K., and McLane, A., editors: Classification of nursing diagnoses—Proceedings of the Fifth National Conference, St. Louis, 1984, The C.V. Mosby Co.

Roy, C.: Introduction of nursing: an adaptation model, ed. 2, Englewood Cliffs, N.J., 1984, Prentice-Hall, Inc.

Yura, H., and Walsh, M.B.: The nursing process: assessing, planning, implementing, and evaluating, Washington, D.C., 1967, Catholic University of America Press.

Zola, I.K.: Helping one another: a speculative history of the self-help movement, Arch. Phys. Med. Rehabil. **60**:452-456, 1979.

Nursing diagnosis: where does the conceptual framework fit?

ANDREA U. BIRCHER, Ph.D., R.N.

This progress report of experiences and results in the pursuit of the question "Nursing Diagnosis: Where does the conceptual framework fit?" presents neither final conclusions nor right answers. It is a sharing of findings, given the current state of the art. I hope that the ideas expressed are interesting and challenging and will lead to further exploration, thought, dialogue, debate, and discourse.

In order to arrive at a meaningful answer to the question asking "where the conceptual framework fits into the realm of nursing diagnosis," this paper looks at two major areas: nursing diagnosis and conceptual frameworks.

NURSING DIAGNOSIS

The answer to the question "What is a nursing diagnosis?" is not clear. Carnevali and associates (1984) state that there is "not yet widespread acceptance of one approach, nor one overall conceptual framework." Griffith and Christensen (1982) suggest that nursing diagnosis is the least understood and most controversial of, and as such the weakest link in, the nursing process (Aspinall, 1976).

Reviews of literature on nursing diagnosis and related topics result in similar impressions. The frequent arrival of new papers and books concerned with some aspect of nursing diagnosis seems staggering. This difficulty is augmented when one tries to maintain a focus of critical inquiry and to pursue the opening avenues in relevant topics of related fields: medical diagnosis, research methodology, concepts and theories, and others.

In light of the question of the fit of nursing diagnosis and conceptual framework, much of the reading I reviewed was irrelevant or inconclusive. The pursuit of the basic question of fit between nursing diagnosis and conceptual framework was sustained, however, by a strong conviction of the importance of the topic of nursing diagnosis to the advancement of nursing as a profession. After 5 years the confusion in nursing diagnosis literature continues unabated, even grows in volume and complexity and indicates recurring and continuing difficulties. But bitter reality is better than defended, avoided, or distorted reality. There is also the realization that the plethora of comments and definitions of nursing diagnosis found in the literature can be ordered.

The many comments can be grouped into five bunches, each corresponding to one of the five critical attributes of the concept of nursing diagnosis which emerged from the concept analysis presented at the Third National Conference for the Classification of Nursing Diagnoses (Bircher, 1982):

1. Nomenclature, name/label/symbol: some definitions and descriptions of nursing diagnosis, its nature and its purpose (for example: "a clear, concise, definitive statement, name, or phrase of a client's health status or concern" [Griffith and Christensen, 1982] or a "concise phrase or term summarizing a cluster of empirical indicators representing a pattern of unitary man" [Nursing Diagnosis Approved List; Roy, 1982; many others])

2. Signs and symptoms defining characteristics: discussions referring to observables of behavior or appearances which constitute the defining characteristics of a given nursing diagnosis (Gordon, 1982; Nursing Diagnosis Approved List; Nursing Diagnosis Theorists, 1980)

3. Taxonomy/natural history/Level I theory: comments including the excellent North American Nursing Diagnosis (NANDA) Taxonomy Committee Association Report by Kritek (1984) (Carnevali and associates, 1984)

4. Taxa/content: discussions focusing on the area of taxa and the specific knowledge/content relevant to each diagnostic label, client condition, or concern (Bircher, 1975b, 1977; Gordon, 1982; Kim, 1984)

5. Clinical judgment/diagnosing: conclusions, judgments, opinions, or decisions made as a result of nursing assessment activities (Bircher, 1975a; Gebbie and Lavin, 1975; Carnevali and associates, 1984; Chambers, 1962; Griffith and Christensen, 1982)

6. Other: clear definition of nursing problems, guides to nursing actions, and the like

At least some comments of what a nursing diagnosis is, or ought to be, fall into each of the five areas of the critical attributes of nursing diagnosis: nomenclature, defining characteristics, taxonomy, taxa/content, and judgment. This analysis or classification confirms and validates the framework of five critical attributes of the concept of nursing diagnosis as presented at the Third National Conference for the Classification of Nursing Diagnoses (Bircher, 1982).

Before the issues of nursing diagnosis and conceptual framework can be discussed meaningfully in greater detail, a few accepted, basic assumptions about nursing have to be reviewed. These assumptions form a background of knowledge which influences the approaches taken to the topic, the selection of focus, and the line of inquiry and reasoning pursued.

BASIC ASSUMPTIONS

Nursing is scientific humanism. As such, nursing uses science, its products of knowledge, and its methods and technology as tools to develop a science of nursing. This science produces the knowledge, methods, and technology which provide the art of nursing with the tools it needs to accomplish its goals: effective and mature coping by people with their activities and the demands of daily living, continuing growth and development, and their responses to illness and life-cycle experiences.

Nursing is a learned professional discipline, even though all nurses do not always act professionally or in accord with standards of a learned profession. The focus of professional nursing is on current human experience, level of functioning, coping ability, strengths and capabilities in problem solving and goal achievement, identification and attainment of the next developmental learning tasks, firm commitment, and constructive contribution to realistic life goals and purposes.

Nursing, as a profession, recognizes that human beings are unfathomably mysterious and unique ends in themselves. Human beings are not reducible to something else. They are not energy systems, though they may be characterized by some such attributes. Nor are human beings organisms, although they obviously share in the nature and characteristics held by all organisms. Human beings are human beings. Simultaneously, they are objects with potential for action and subjects with felt states (Sullivan, 1953). Thus nursing, to live up to its claim of holistic care and concern for the whole person, has to gain and use expertise in both the subjective and the objective realms of human experience and being. Langer (1967) points out that neither empirical positivist methods of scientific research nor phenomenological methods or other ethnoscientific approaches are appropriate to the study of the phenomena of the whole person. This is because the characteristics and phenomena of symbols, language, mind, self, personality, culture, religion, and the like, which set apart human beings from other animals, arise in the interaction of the objective and subjective aspects of experience. The question is not which of the two methods should be used in nursing. Aspects of both have to be combined and new methods which will do justice to the study of human phenomena must be found. To be true to its aims and purposes, nursing has to go beyond finding knowledge and methods in other fields and importing them in toto. Nursing, in order to progress and assume its potential stature as a full-fledged helping profession, has to begin to develop its own knowledge and methods, that are adequate and appropriate to the complex phenomena of concern to nursing: holistic human experience and coping with the full range of human responses to them.

Nurses are fortunate to have the nursing process to help them deal effectively with this overwhelming complexity of demand. The nursing process accounts for the interpersonal interactions and relationships between client and nurse as well as the nurse's thought processes and resulting clinical judgments. Both aspects of the nursing process are essential to effective nursing. It is the critical thinking aspect, however, which helps nurses to manage complexity (Bircher, 1973), and there are as many versions of this aspect as there are nurses discussing it. The version presented here is used because the six aspects given are analytically distinct, identifiable entities which require development of special competencies paralleling each aspect of the nursing process and different actions for successful use.

1. Assessment: observing, ordering, and presenting information about the clients, their condition, and their life situations
2. Acquisition, presentation, and use of the formal body of knowledge relevant to the presenting client situation
3. Nursing diagnosis: the conjunction of observations and knowledge (more about this later)
4. Planning care: setting goals and priorities, prescribing intervention regimens, and carrying out nursing actions
5. Implementation of the plan: giving deliberate, purposive nursing care and therapy
6. Evaluation: appraising the extent of goal achievement, the meeting of standards, and the quality of performance of the implementor(s)

The remainder of this paper focuses on selected areas of nursing diagnosis, the nature of conceptual frameworks, and their relationship.

WHAT IS A NURSING DIAGNOSIS?

For the purpose of this discussion, Bircher's (1982) exposition of nursing diagnosis as a complex concept, a tripartite relationship, is accepted.

The first of the three aspects is the **referents.** The referents of nursing diagnosis involve five critical attributes:

The *first* is called name or nomenclature. It is concerned with all matters of naming. This area involves decisions and a consensus about what to call a given thing, phenomenon, idea, experience, or response pattern. The first critical attribute of nursing diagnosis essentially involves the development and use of the profession's technical language.

The *second* is called defining characteristics. This involves the area of symptomatology, the study and making of decisions about observable cues, the presence or absence of which determines assignment of a given nursing diagnosis to a client condition.

The *third* is called taxonomy. This area deals with the issues of conceptualization—categories, concepts, symptoms, clustering, principles, conceptual frameworks, theories, and models. Concepts and frameworks form the foundation of and make possible cognition. Taxonomies are also called level one theory, or the natural history phase of science (Denzin, 1970; Dickoff and James, 1968; Kerlinger, 1965; Northrop, 1947). A taxonomy forms a sound scientific basis for a profession to the extent to which it meets the rules of categorization.

The *fourth* concerns the area of taxa, or units, and the related subject matter content of the categories and concepts that make up the taxonomy or framework used. The framework used may be a loose aggregate of concepts or a logical hierarchical system such as a formal theory. A framework or theory is useful in guiding action to the extent it emerges from and forms a superstructure for a sound taxonomy.

The *fifth* critical attribute is clinical judgment, the thought processes which are undertaken by the clinician. These thought processes allow the clinician to recognize a client condition as an example of a known entity and therefore to have understanding of its genesis, progression, and predictable events as well as its consequences for human health, effective functioning, and coping with responses to life cycle experiences. These thought processes and judgments allow the clinician to select the most effective intervention from those known to influence or control the progression of the event or condition.

The second part of the tripartite relationship is the **idea.** The idea is a central nervous system organization of the patterns of facts which constitute the critical attributes of the concept, and at the same time serve as recognitional capacity. Recognitional capacity allows a person to bring knowledge and logical reasoning to bear on his decisions and action in a given situation. In the case of nursing diagnosis it is this recognitional capacity or transfer learning which allows warranted and correct application of professional and scientific knowledge, procedures, and skills. Such application enhances the likelihood that actions result in effective and efficient attainment of desired goals.

The third aspect of the tripartite relationship is the **name** assigned to symbolize the complex of referents, idea and symbol. The symbol is one aspect, but it stands for the entire, complex notion of nursing diagnosis.

As such, nursing diagnosis is not a thing, not a label, not a statement, not a procedure of activity which nurses do, such as CPR. It does not solve problems or clarify client conditions, health problems, or nursing care issues. Nursing diagnosis does not assure a successful intervention outcome or clarity of communication. It is an idea available to and used by a nurse. A nursing diagnosis is a concept, an intellectual tool for abstract thought. The essence of this abstract thought is a clinical judgment made by the nurse. It is a judgment which involves the uniting of clinical observations about a new never before seen specific client condition or situation with the formal body of knowledge of a class of characteristics or conditions which are similar and therefore relevant to the specific case. Nursing diagnosis is a bridge over the knowledge-practice gap. This is so because the matching of clinical observations with the formal class knowledge allows the clinician to identify the new case as an illustrative example of a general known category or class. Since all members of that class share known characteristics and proclivities toward given developments and consequences, such matching allows the clinician to go beyond the information given in the specific case. Knowledge gained from the other cases in the class may be applied to the new case with high likelihood of correct interpretation of meaning and anticipation of future developments and consequences. The clinician can then select interventions which are known to be successful in obtaining desired goals in these kinds of client situations. The correct matching of individual case characteristics with a group or class of known similar cases is the very essence of clinical judgment, the fifth critical attribute of nursing diagnosis (Bruner, 1973; Kant, 1959; London and associates, 1963).

Since nursing diagnosis is the third analytically distinguishable aspect of the nursing process, the accuracy and validity of the nursing diagnosis determine the value and effectiveness of the three aspects of the nursing process which follow it. Inaccuracy of nursing diagnoses results in nursing care which is at best haphazard, at worst deleterious to clients. This occurs by either omission of necessary, or commission of inappropriate or harmful interventions. Nursing diagnosis is the hub of effective and efficient nursing interventions and quality care.

How to make a correct, valid nursing diagnosis is essentially a question of how individual clinicians convert the raw materials of their sense impressions into knowledge. It is also a question of why, because of that conversion, a nurse is able to act more efficiently and effectively. Kant, the famous German philosopher, addressed this question in his *Critique of Pure Reason*. The following discussion is excerpted and adapted from Kant and complemented with more recent work as indicated by other references cited:

As persons go about their daily business in the world, they are sensitive and receptive. They are affected by experiences with things, phenomena, and people. As persons undergo such experiences, they have sensations. Those aspects of sensations and experiences which correspond to the things or phenomena apprehended are called intuitions. The essence of such intuitions is a synthesis of space and time with external and internal responsiveness and with those sensations which correspond to the noted things or phenomena. Intuitions are the mental representations of the appearance of things or phenomena encountered in experience. Intuitions enable persons to note things and to develop object constancy. Intuitions form the essential foundations of all but are themselves not cognitions.

Cognition means to know. A person cannot know anything except by intuition. Cognitions are at once empirical, a matter of sensuous intuition and conception, a matter of abstract principle. They may be objective, subjective, or a combination of both.

Cognition always has a systematic unity, a logical completeness which serves a desired end. It may be experiential. This means that knowledge is based on past experiences with things or phenomena and related sensations. On the other hand, cognition may be rational. This kind of knowledge is based on abstract logical principles. Full understanding of a thing, a person, or a phenomenon requires an interaction of both kinds of knowledge.

Kant goes on to explicate the nature of cognition and suggests that it consists of three major aspects: (1) understanding, the process and product of developing and using representation and conceptions—namely categories and concepts; (2) judgment, the process and product of comparison and decision whether or not an item noted in experience is a specific example of a conception and consequently may properly be subsumed under the rules and laws of that conception, and (3) reason, the process and product of developing and using a hierarchical system of abstract, logical, and universal principles in order to draw inferences and conclusions—singularly or serially—from facts, premises, and available evidence.

The principles of reason are not the same as the categories and concepts of understanding or intuitions, nor are they the same as the principles of esthetics, ethics, or mathematics. Principles of reason are ideal patterns of things or phenomena. These patterns are not derived from sensation or from experience. Instead they are derived by logical and dialectic processes, by positing a thesis and an antithesis, and by resolving the contradiction of the two at a higher level of abstraction and universality. The aim of reason is comprehension, the complete unity of known truths. In order to attain this aim, reason cannot permit knowledge about things to remain in an unconnected, haphazard, chaotic state. Instead, reason continually strives toward a state where the sum of knowledge forms a logically unified, hierarchical system of conceptions and abstract universal principles.

Reason supplies the principles through which all subsumed particular items can be known in accord with a logical system. Reason is able to bring order to the varied manifold of conceptions and representations of understanding. Because of the logical unity of the system of universal principles, reason makes possible the extension of cognition beyond the limits of experience. Reason also enables a person to remember the past and to anticipate future events and experiences. Once a person realizes the power of reason in speculating about things met in experience, it becomes easy to see the application of reason in pure speculation and fantasy. However, such speculative thought, whether haphazard or systematized in formal theory, is sheer fantasy. For realistic use of reason, and for effective action, the empirical validation of speculative thought is necessary. The means for such validation is empirical research. The aim of such research is validation of fantasy or theoretical statements and subordination of particular facts or items to general conceptions or principles. The aim of science is to arrive at new conceptions which differ from old ones in kind, have greater logical rigor, are more general and more universal, have wider application in human experience, and have more predictive and greater explanatory powers.

Repeated observations and searches for reliable recurrently observable or inferable elements eventually yield a mass of items. Such items are then clustered, ordered, and organized into increasingly more systematic groups. From such groups commonalities are abstracted. Logical explanations (theories) are constructed and tested. Such theories are revised into ever more logically and hierarchically ordered systems which eventually allow deduction and thereby lead to the generation of predictions and explanations of, as yet, never observed phenomena.

In summary, nursing diagnosis is an abstract concept, an intellectual tool which is neutral. It is as powerful and constructive, or as weak and destructive, as the extent to which it is used appropriately and effectively toward the achievement of an end. Neglect of any one of the five critical attributes of the concept of diagnosis, such as only labeling or listing indicators, destroys the validity, power, and usefulness of the idea of nursing diagnosis. The essence and value of the concept of nursing diagnosis lie in the thought processes, clinical judgments, and ethical standards of the clinician. In order to execute sound clinical judgment, a knowledge of labels, manifest characteristics (signs and symptoms), taxonomy and related higher-level theories, and subject matter content for each taxon are needed. In short, the more logically rigorous and empirically validated the theoretical knowledge is, and the more appropriately it is applied, the more effective and therefore the more powerful the idea of nursing diagnosis becomes.

CONCEPTUAL FRAMEWORKS

All knowledge is a conceptual framework. Knowledge is a linguistic or other symbolic system which represents an ideational phenomenon rather than a concrete thing (Burr, 1973). A conceptual framework describes and symbolizes known and surmised aspects, phenomena, and human experiences of the world. By so doing it allows them to be thought about and communicated (Burr, 1973).

Price (1980) suggests that the most important issue facing the mental health field is conceptual. The same thing can be said for nursing. Rychlack (1981) suggests, and Langer (1967) concurs, that avoiding serious examination of concepts, meanings, assumptions, and principles of theory development has led to naive realism in some fields, especially in behavioristic psychology, and has actually served to hold back psychology in its development as a scientific discipline.

In literature much is said about conceptual frameworks. The term is often used as a synonym for other terms such as theory, theoretical framework, practice model, value system, belief system, and the like (Argysis and Schoen, 1978; Fawcett, 1984; King, 1971; Mullen, 1983; Newman, 1979). The following discussion focuses on the nature of conceptual frameworks as it emerges from a selective concept-focused literature review about concepts, conceptual frameworks, theories, philosophy of science, epistemology, research, psychiatry, psychology, and psychopathology. For purposes of this paper the terms concepts, conceptual frameworks, theory and model are used to refer to four analytically distinguishable ideas, four different conceptual entities.

The following questions emerge to guide the inquiry:

1. What is a concept?
2. What is a framework?
3. What is a conceptual framework?
4. What is a theory?
5. What is a model?
6. What is the relation of conceptual frameworks, theories, and paradigm models?
7. Nursing diagnosis: where does the conceptual framework fit?

What is a concept?

Human experience has many facets: sense experience, perception, emotion, feeling, imagination, thinking, valuing, willing, judging, planning, deciding, behaving, relating, coping, problem solving, goal achieving, and the like. Language cannot possibly do justice to the fullness of such an ever-flowing stream of human experience, yet language is the only tool available with which human beings can hope to master and control such experiences. Language is a vast system, a pattern of interrelated, intellectual tools, with which a person dissects, constructs, and analyzes experiences, notices or neglects phenomena and their relationships to his or her own experiences (as well as channels of reasoning or avenues of action) (Sartori citing Whorf, 1984). By use of language human beings divide the stream of their experiences into basic groupings of reliably recurring elements. These patterns achieve a cohesive unity and thus become ideas. Such ideas (concepts) are the basic units of thought. Certain words are assigned to these ideas and serve as names for these ideas. The ideas and the words assigned to them can be organized into networks of ideas called conceptual frameworks. Such network construction is done in accord with the rules provided by the language of which they are a part. Languages provide three different kinds of rules: (1) rules of semantics, which deal with the meaning of words—(a) the intensional or connotative meaning and (b) the extensional or denotative meaning; (2) rules of syntactics, which are concerned with the relationship among signs or words and with grammar and sentence structure; and (3) rules of pragmatics, which focus on the relationship of words or signs to human behavior (Sartori citing Whorf, 1984).

Language is monitored by thought in accord with the logical system of reasoning used by the thinker. Language molds thought through its vocabulary, which embodies an overall approach to perceiving and conceiving the world and human experiences within it (Sartori citing Whorf, 1984). Language, thought, and culture greatly interpenetrate, influence, enhance, and determine each other. All three evolve in a mutual feedback fashion (Sartori citing Whorf, 1984).

Human beings can use language in two ways to control the stream of their experiences.

The first is an *affective* way. It is a way of using language to control subjective experiences to feel, to will, to be, to intend, to enjoy living, well-being and beauty, or to endure and suffer discomforts and miseries of fate. In this mode, the goal is to experience self fully and authentically, to actualize self, and to realize one's own human potential. It should be noted that the control of experience by language is a reciprocal matter. Language controls experience to some extent, yet experience also exerts some control on language (Sartori citing Whorf, 1984).

The second is a *reciprocal* way of controlling experiences. The goal of this approach is to know, to order information and facts in such a way that they can be used for gaining greater understanding. This use of language enables a person to predict, explain, control, and produce things (Sartori citing Whorf, 1984).

The goals of using language in this way are description, prediction, explanation, and control. These, however, are the very goals of science. They also include the goals of practice professions, namely, the control and production of given things, phenomena, human experiences, and action patterns. All sciences depend on concepts. Much of the work of theorizing is taken up with clarification of concepts (Blumer, 1931; Sartori citing Merton, 1984). A look at the state of concepts of a science is one quick and telling way of evaluating that science.

Concepts are the building blocks of theories. They are more fundamental than theories (Greenwood, 1962; Sartori, 1984). Concepts are the tools with which professionals perform their work (Sartori, 1984). Whatever is known to anyone is mediated by concepts, which in turn are represented by language. Vague or ambiguous language leads to double-talk, and double-talk leads to fuzzy if not confused thinking. In turn, bad thinking leads to poor work (Langer,

1967; Macnamara, 1977; Northrop and Morgenau, 1950; Sartori, 1984; Vermulapalli, 1984).

It is interesting to note comments in the literature about the paucity of work and progress made in the understanding of the nature and the methodology of concept development and concept clarification (Bellak, 1973; Blalock, 1982, 1984; Blumer, 1931, 1970; Sartori, 1984; Wagner, 1984).

Definition of concept. The meaning of the term concept is a combination of taking in and putting together. To conceive is to take into the mind sensory experiences and to put them together into a picture. This process of conceiving mentally involves apprehension by imagination or by reason, and forms an idea in the mind (American Heritage Dictionary, 1970; Webster's New Collegiate Dictionary, 1973).

A concept is more than just a word or empty label. A concept is a significant symbol, a word that has been given special meaning in the course of human interactions (Mead, 1934; Northrop and Morgenau, 1950). Thus a concept is a matter of both a word and a special meaning idea attached to that word.

A concept is a clear-cut verbal and logical operation in which a person uses a series of logically selected ideas in order to arrive at a conclusion. The person automatically disregards all extralogical considerations (Luria, 1976). A concept is a process of classification, of placing a number of items into a category. This is accomplished by isolating one or more essential qualities that pertain to a generic category and by disregarding all individualistic peculiarities. For example, an apple tree is classified as a tree; a spider monkey is classified as an animal. A concept represents attributes shared by a group. A concept is a stereotype.

A concept has also been defined as a statement of the structure, of the critical attributes in the description of a group or category to which it applies (Hunt, 1962). A concept is a decision rule about things, their critical attributes, nature, appearance, structure, function, underlying dynamics, and causes. Use of such decision rules allows determination of whether a thing possesses the critical attributes which allow its subsumption under a category or concept (Hunt and Hoveland, 1963). Delineation of fit of an item within a given class allows the assigning of the name of the class to a specific matching item. With correct identification and naming, all knowledge pertaining to the class as a whole is applicable to that specific item (Hunt, 1962; Hunt and Hoveland, 1963).

Such identification of items as members of known classes is of crucial value, for it helps orient a person to a situation. It allows the person to determine that the never encountered item is, for example, a dog. Dogs have given properties and ways of behavior which are associated with likely experiences to be had in contact with all dogs, while other experiences are not likely to be had in the presence of dogs. In this manner the individual can anticipate the future, plan action to achieve pleasant anticipated happenings, and avoid unpleasant, dangerous, and harmful ones. Such subsuming of items of experience under concepts, then, is one crucial element of timebinding, of relating present experiences to past experiences and knowledge derived from them, as well as relating them to the future. Bruner (1973) calls this "going beyond the information given." A person, provided he or she has the necessary information and knowledge, can anticipate the future, plan and execute actions which intervene in the course of events, influence the outcomes, bring about alternative outcomes, enhance or prevent occurrences, and work effectively toward the attainment of desired goals. Thus, through the subsumption of discrete items under categories or concepts, a person may gain a certain measure of control over experiences encountered (Bircher, 1966; Hook, 1959, 1971; Mead, 1934). Langer (1942) calls this process of gaining control over events the bringing of experience under the control of concepts. This process of subsuming items under a category or concept is called categorical thinking (Luria, 1976).

Concepts are the tools essential for mastery of human experiences (Blumer, 1931; Greenwood, 1962; Peterson, 1977; Pope and Singer, 1980). Without the development and use of concepts, human experience would forever remain a never ending unpredictable flux of discrete, kaleidoscopically changing, and incomprehensible prototaxic experiences (Blumer, 1931; Bruner, 1973; Greenwood, 1962; Piaget, 1958; Rychlak, 1981; Sullivan, 1953).

Concepts are something presumed and inferred but never actually present in things or experiences. They are not directly observable; they do not arise in, are not derived from, and cannot be determined by facts. Concepts begin and end in perceptions. They are continuations and elaborations of sense perceptions. Concepts are abstractions and generalizations—generic ideas which are constructed by human beings about their own experiences. Thus, concepts are free creations of thought, inventions of the mind (Blumer, 1931; Dickoff and James, 1968; Morgenau citing Einstein, 1975).

Langer (1942) points out that, though concepts are creations of the mind, a person is successful not because of the number of kinds of experiences he or she encounters but because of the number of formulating notions, the number of concepts with which he or she meets the world. Langer (1967) states that a science develops and thrives to the extent that more and more powerful concepts are introduced. New concepts lead to new ways of thinking, and the effect is revolutionary. New ways of thinking transform questions asked, experiences observed, and criteria used. In so doing, the appearance, patterns, values, and meanings of facts are changed.

In summary, the term "concept" refers to an entity constructed by human beings. This entity at once encompasses a word or name, a meaning or idea, a pattern of facts or properties observable or inferred, a complex mental process of abstract thought, a central nervous system organization, a specific intrapsychic structure which serves a recognitional capacity, a decision rule for classification and labeling of items of experience, and a summary of past experiences for the subsumption of current experiences and the anticipation of future experiences likely to occur under given circumstances. Thus concepts are substantively developed guides to expectations and evaluation of what a thing, situation, event, phenomenon, person, experience, or response ought to be. As such, concepts are intellectual tools for abstracting, simplifying, generalizing, symbolizing, integrating and interpreting experiences, and for guiding action.

The following broad range of functions of concepts has been identified in the literature:

1. Organizing: central nervous system, intrapsychic structure, sensation, perceptions, information, data, evidence, facts, values, expectations
2. Categorizing: ordering, summarizing, simplifying
3. Abstracting
4. Generalizing
5. Modifying/symbolizing
6. Symbolic/representational
7. Language
8. Alerting
9. Recognitional
10. Orienting
11. Timebinding
12. Interpretive
13. Attention-focusing
14. Thought
15. Problem-solving
16. Experience mastery
17. Action-guiding
18. Theory development
19. Scientific
20. Clinical practice
21. Activities of daily, personal living

Discussion in detail of these functions, and of the development of concepts, lies beyond the scope of this paper.

What is a framework?

The term framework implies the work of framing. To frame, according to the dictionary, means to construct, to put together, to arrange, and to adjust the various parts of something in a way that ensures a desired outcome, or the attainment of a given purpose or goal. A framework is a structure for supporting, enclosing, or defining something. A structure is a complex entity, an intricate configuration or arrangement of elements, parts, or constituents. The interrelations of these constituents provide the basic principle and organization of the complex entity. The parts and their synergistic interrelationships determine the nature and objective meanings of the entity, regulate its functions, and limit its possible action (American Heritage Dictionary, 1970; Bonham, 1980). A framework provides the current, official, and consensual definition of a situation (Goffman, 1963, 1964). In the case of developing or verbalizing ideas, a framework serves as a point of reference, as a set of coordinate axes in terms of which propositions and actions may be specified and in reference to which physical laws or rules of conduct may be stated and used to guide action (American Hertiage Dictionary, 1970; Durkheim, 1938, 1962).

What is a conceptual framework?

Conceptual frameworks are tools of thought. Like all tools, they are constructed for given purposes. For a complete job of carpentry, more than one tool is needed. So it is with conceptual frameworks. They consist of sets or networks of concepts and provide a more or less integrated view or perspective of a thing, phenomenon, experience, or other aspect of the world. The use of more than one conceptual framework provides greater depth of meaning and understanding in a way similar to sight, where binocular vision provides for depth perception.

Conceptual frameworks are word pictures, intellectual road maps of the territory of things, phenomena, human experiences, response patterns and their respective structures, functions, antecedents, consequences, relationships, underlying dynamics, and causes. They are not theories. They are broad pretheoretical bases from which theories may be derived (Fawcett, 1978, 1984).

Conceptual frameworks are the broad background of ideas which make possible reasoning and thinking and which form the context for perception, study, report writing, decision making, and action (Newman, 1979). Conceptual frameworks are also ways to integrate and synthesize knowledge from one or more fields, sciences, or disciplines. It is said that conceptual frameworks are logically interrelated sets of ideas, concepts, feelings, subjective biases, perspective world views, or visions in terms of which other ideas, experiences, and things are interpreted and assigned meaning (Mullen, 1983; Schafer, 1983). Thus, conceptual frameworks provide sets of statements which delineate salient aspects such as characteristics, components, functions, developmental phases, and underlying, orienting, organizing, and explanatory principles. But it is said that conceptual frameworks are insufficient to be theories. They lack the rigorous logic of a formal system of causal relationships. This deprives them of certainty of description, explanation, and predictability, which are characteristic of formal theories (Denzin quoting Homan, 1970).

The structure of a conceptual framework consists of the following components: (1) concepts, (2) broad generalizations or statements of relationships, (3) criteria entering into concept formation, and (4) rules of inclusion or exclusion in the concepts or categories of the conceptual framework (Biddle and Thomas, 1966; Fawcett, 1984; Peterson, 1977).

Conceptual frameworks are said to provide a network, a set of more or less well-related categories or concepts and relevant methods within which questions, facts, concepts, and theories fit together. Conceptual frameworks allow persons to order facts and observations and to integrate them into a coherent system. Conceptual frameworks can, but do not necessarily, integrate concepts in a way similar to that by which concepts integrate facts, sense perceptions, and intuitions (Fawcett, 1984; Kant, 1952). Conceptual frameworks are one link in a chain of a person's mental activities which turn sense perceptions of the outside world and related human experiences into knowledge of things, situations, events, and the like (Blumer, 1931; Denzin, 1978). Conceptual frameworks determine the meaning of concepts, and of items and experiences subsumed under them. They do so to the extent that they provide for connections among concepts and establish underlying themes, structures, functions, dynamics, and causal relationships. Conceptual frameworks encompass and allow a person to order given realms of experience and to identify the necessary conditions and essential determinants of reality (Frosch, 1983; Mullen, 1976). They identify areas where theory development is needed. Thus conceptual frameworks influence actions and direct the search for organization among facts and concepts, as well as the search for meaning (Northrop, 1947, 1967).

In nursing literature conceptual frameworks are delineated as a means to make explicit what is implicit in experience and in beliefs. As such conceptual frameworks are an approach to the study and management of problems or situations (Fawcett, 1978; Haber and associates, 1978; Newman, 1979; Peterson, 1977).

What is a theory?

Current usage suggests several meanings for the term theory: (1) original mental viewing or contemplation, (2) idea or plan of a way to do something, (3) systematic statement of principle involved, (4) formulation of apparent relationships or underlying principles of certain observed phenomena or human experience which may or may not have been verified to some extent (this is distinct from hypothesis), (5) that part of an art or science which consists of the knowledge of its principles and methods rather than its practice or procedures, and (6) popularly, a mere conjecture or guess (Webster's New Collegiate Dictionary, 1973).

A theory is a statement of a set of hierarchically interrelated, internally consistent, definitions and propositions which present a systematic view of a part of the world. It is a word picture, a symbolic snapshot of one aspect of the world (Braitwaith, 1953; Denzin, 1970; Kerlinger, 1974; Northrop, 1947, 1967). A theory orders abstracted and conceptualized observations and proposition to specify surmised relationships among concepts, their properties, their underlying principles and dynamics, and their causal influences related to or thought to be salient in one given aspect of the actual world. It is an attempt to present as clear, rounded, and systematic a picture of the principles and dynamics of a subject as is possible at a given time. It represents the current understanding and thinking surrounding that subject. This means that a theory is but a best guess, an estimate available at a given time. A theory is an abstraction and a generalization. It is always an oversimplification and therefore a distortion of the actual world represented. This also means that a theory about a significant aspect in the world will be continuously revised, refined, changed, or replaced with another one which is more able to account for the observations and new understanding gained in study, reasoning, and contemplation.*

Formal theory, also called theory proper or causal theory, is a statement not of fact observed or of logical relations of such facts to other facts but of formulated principles which are inferred from empirical manifestations of facts. Theory proper not only states but also organizes a set of principles underlying and summarizing diverse concepts into a rigorous hierarchy, a logical deductive system. Theory proper organizes information and thereby can indicate what empirical facts are likely to be encountered under given sets of circumstances. To do so successfully, a theory proper has to have two distinguishable aspects. First is a body of logically interrelated propositions which delineate the general principles of an empirical system. Second is a description of the actual empirical system, be that a thing, situation, event, phenomenon, human experience, or response pattern (Bershady, 1973). Given these two aspects, a theory proper imposes a rigorous, logical, hierarchical organization on words, or other representative symbols, and their overt or covert properties, facts, and manifestations. Theory proper makes possible the inferring and articulating of underlying dynamics, principles, and singular or multiple causal relations (Bruner, 1973; Burr, 1973; Chinn and Jacobs, 1983; Dickoff and James, 1968; Patterson, 1978).

Meaningful organization of information and human experience involves four aspects: description, explanation, prediction, and control. Theory proper makes possible these four aspects, since with an adequate description of the empirical aspect of the world and with a logically sound hierarchically rigorous statement of underlying dynamics and principles, prediction and control become possible. *Description* involves a factual statement and recording, a symbolic recreating, and a categorical identification (genus and species) of significant things, phenomena, human experiences, and response patterns. Descrip-

*Burr, 1973; Burton, 1974; Dickoff and James, 1968; Greenwood, 1962, 1963; Johnson, 1978; Kerlinger, 1965, 1973; King, 1978; Kuhn, 1962, 1970; Laszlo, 1972; Mills, 1959; Patterson, 1978; Rogers, 1970; Schafer, 1983; Stevens, 1979; Zderad, 1978.

tion is the process which identifies, judges, and subsumes noted items under the categories or concepts of a conceptual framework or theory. *Explanation* involves one or more statements of how and why two things are related, generated, influenced, destroyed, or otherwise affected. *Prediction* involves statements of conditions under which given things do occur. *Control* involves a statement of how description, prediction, and explanation can be used, and what has to be done in order to produce, manipulate, delimit, or prevent the occurrence of a thing (Dickoff and James, 1968; Kerlinger, 1973). A given theory may deal with one, several, or all four of these aspects of organization of experience.

It is possible that two or more theories account for the same patterns of facts, concepts, even laws—for example, Freud's three theories of anxiety. Furthermore, concepts of one theory may become basic terms of another theory or of another science (Denzin, 1970).

Theory—the substantive focus on the nature of things, phenomena, and human experience and response patterns—is one component of knowledge. It is one of four major aspects of the scientific enterprise, the purpose of which is the development and validation of knowledge. The second aspect is methodology, the development of procedure for observation, data collection, measurement, and analysis of evidence. The third is research activity, the implementation and use of such procedures. The fourth is a disciplinary imagination. It is a vision which in sociology is called the sociological imagination. It is a vision of and commitment to a purpose, to an idea of what is and what might be in the given discipline (Mills, 1959; Denzin, 1970).

All human beings are theory-building animals, but they pursue it in a less formal and less systematic way than do the sciences. Human life is an interpretive process in which people, singly or collectively, guide themselves by defining and determining the meaning of objects and experiences which they encounter (Denzin citing Becker, 1970). With the articulation and elaboration of these definitions and meanings, the human universe becomes a complex network of descriptions of and explanations about interconnected relationships between parts and principles of a unified whole (Capra, 1972; Hebb, 1965). In the construction of such descriptions and explanations (that is to say, in the invention of such theories) emerge the articulated vision of experience and the full-fledged nature of a field as a science (Denzin, 1970; Zderad citing Laing, 1978). A science, on the other hand, progresses only as fast as theories are developed, tested, and revised (Burr, 1973). Until a paradigm model, a consensually adopted theory, emerges in a field, one has to contend with many different, apparently equally plausible, theories of the things, phenomena, human experiences, and coping patterns under study (Burton, 1974 [preface]; Kuhn, 1962, 1970).

Human beings cannot understand or explain experiences or actual things and events in the world any more than they can construct reality by observing, seeing, hearing, and feeling (alone or in combination). What is needed to do so is a mental process that organizes actuality—what actually occurs in the world. Such organization develops explanations and predictions about what people experience. This includes statements of what those experiences and happenings mean: what kind of influences they will have on the welfare of people. The mental processes which accomplish this are contemplation combined with the use of symbols, namely thinking (Kaplan, 1964; Rychlak, 1981).

Theory, technology and action go hand in hand. They have reciprocal roles. Just as with ideas, tools, and action, they may be considered independently of each other, but mankind is best facilitated by their conjunction. If considered separately, a theory is of greater value than is research, technology, or action. A theory provides a coherent vision by articulating and ordering information and human experiences. It constructs reality and implies possible approaches or solutions to problems confronted. Yet, without research, technology, and action, theory becomes sterile, a figment of the imagination. On the other hand, research without a theory, and without application of its findings in practice or daily life, becomes noncumulative, even confused (Blumer, 1931; Burton, 1974; Denzin, 1970; Mills, 1959; Wagner, 1984). Theory and research, as well as conceptualization of ideas and action, interdigitate and, when so intertwined, produce a synergistic effect, both in science and in activities of daily human living.

What is a model?

In nursing, currently, the term model is used synonymously with the term conceptual framework. Nursing literature suggests that a model is a delineation of the nature of human beings, the state of health, the environment, and the services provided by nurses. Such beliefs, it is said, derive from the basic, biological, behavioral, and social sciences, from the humanities, and from professional experiences. As such, a model is seen as a more or less systematized set of ideas, both explicit and implicit, which practitioners actually use to direct their own actions in clinical nursing practice. Such models include a statement of the scientific and ethical reasoning and the personal motives which account for a nurse's behavior, or for the structure of a given curriculum (Beckstrand, 1980; Fawcett, 1984; Hardy, 1978; King, 1971; Paterson, 1977).

In nursing, models are said to require the following essential elements in order to be used for guiding nursing practice or curriculum development:

1. The nursing process. This is a statement of the services to the consumer and a description of nursing as a deliberative problem-solving process, which is the core of nursing services provided, including restorative, rehabilitative, preventive, health-maintaining, and health-promoting care.
2. The goal. This is a statement of the view of health and well-being, as well as the outcome health status expected from the service.

3. Rationale. This is a statement of why clients need the service, such as help in coping with illness, recovery, rehabilitation, and health maintenance or promotion.

4. Nursing practice. This is a statement or description of the level of services to be provided, advanced clinical specialty, professional, technical, or auxiliary roles.

5. Client description. This is a statement of description of basic assumptions about, and basic approaches to be taken toward, the client's needs.

6. Care setting. This is a statement or description of the care setting where the service will be rendered.

Continued development of concepts in each of the six areas is said to be needed for increasing clarification of the model and its implementation (Peterson, 1977).

In science a model is an ideational guideline and standard for practice, which is built upon a theory (Abdellah and Levine, 1965; Riehl and Roy, 1974). A model is an exemplary or paradigm theory, which delineates a consensually adopted mode of practice in a scientific or professional field (Kuhn, 1970). It includes a field's laws of practice, its theories, instrumentations, and methods, and their respective applications. Together these form, and from these spring, more or less coherent traditions of scientific research, for example, Newtonian physics and Freudian psychology.

In order to qualify as a paradigm theory, also called scientific model, a statement of practice has to demonstrate unprecedented achievements: attract a group (or groups) of persons who carry it on, open conditions that leave unsolved problems, be a component of existing laws and theories, and possess applications and instrumentations as well as rules and standards for scientific practice. In the early stages of development the users of a paradigm exhibit random fact gathering. In the second stage the group demonstrates taxonomic work. This phase is also known as the natural history phase of science, or Level I theory development (Dickoff and James, 1968; Northrop, 1947, 1967). In the third phase implied theories are explicated and developed. This occurs first at the descriptive, then at the explanatory and predictive, and finally at the prescriptive levels. These levels are also known as Level II, III, and IV theories, or de-facto and normative theories (Dickoff and James, 1968; Northrop, 1947, 1967). In the fourth phase new paradigms replace older ones and provide new and more rigorous definitions of the field (Kuhn, 1970).

What is the relation of conceptual frameworks, theories, and paradigm models?

It follows from the foregoing discussion that conceptual frameworks, theories, and paradigm models are systems of concepts. All three are figments of the imagination, which are constructed for specific purposes and which serve as

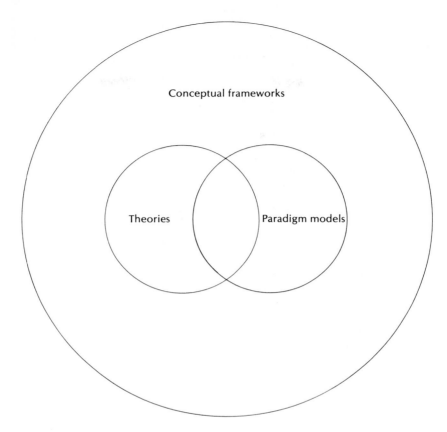

FIGURE 1   Theories and paradigm models as subsets of conceptual frameworks.

intellectual tools. Conceptual frameworks are defined, on the one hand, as loose aggregates of broad concepts. Theories, on the other hand, are defined as rigorously logical hierarchical systems of precisely conceived underlying principles which account for and explain diverse surface manifestations, and therefore allow prediction and control of experience. Other discussions, both about conceptual frameworks and about theories, fall between these two extremes. At times it is impossible to distinguish comments about the nature of conceptual frameworks from those about theories. This suggests that all theories are conceptual frameworks but not all conceptual frameworks are theories. Theories are a subset of conceptual frameworks (see Fig. 1). Furthermore, paradigm models have a similar relationship to conceptual frameworks. Paradigm models are also a subset of conceptual frameworks. Thus all paradigm models are conceptual frameworks but not all conceptual frameworks are paradigm models. In addition, some paradigm models are theories, and some theories are paradigm models. Thus theories and paradigm models are two different but overlapping subsets of conceptual frameworks (Fig. 1).

Three major dimensions of significant variation for conceptual frameworks emerge from this rational inquiry into the nature of concepts, conceptual frameworks, and theories. The three dimensions are (1) logical rigor—loose aggregation or deductive-hierarchical interrelations of component conceptions, (2) articulateness—implicitness or explicitness of ideas and assumptions, (3) empirical validity—accepted on faith or hearsay or supported by fact and evidence.

The first of the three dimensions is a continuum, a dimension which ranges from loose aggregation to tight logical coherence; from jumbled mixed-up individual jigsaw puzzle pieces to an interlocking fit of each piece with all others in such a way that the puzzle is solved and the picture completed.

In general, literature suggests that, compared to theories, conceptual frameworks lack rigorous statements of postulates about the interrelations of their components, beliefs, and assumptions and do not confine themselves to punctilious conceptualization, verbal description, and denotatively defined terms of one or more identified things, phenomena, or human experiences as do theories (Kuhn, 1970).

Progress and success in science are achieved in direct proportion to which logical rigor contributes to and moves forward the development of hierarchical deductive systems of symbolic representation, namely, theories relevant to and accounting for the things of concern in a given field or discipline. Without precisely delineated and rigorously logical hierarchical theories, scientific action is not considered to be possible (Blumer, 1931, 1970; Denzin, 1970; Gale, 1979).

The second dimension of variation between conceptual frameworks and theories emerges from the conceptual framework literature. On the one hand, that literature speaks to implicitness of ideas, beliefs, and other aspects of conceptual frameworks. On the other hand, theory literature comments on the importance of articulation and explicit postulation of assumptions, relations, and the like. This suggests a dimension which moves from one extreme, of implicitness and intuition, to the other extreme, of explicit articulation or complete symbolic representation of the salient aspects of whatever is under study (Polanyi, 1966).

Whether conceptual framework or theory, it is not a matter of dealing with actual facts or things, nor is it a matter of dealing with written or spoken statements. Conceptual frameworks and theories essentially constitute a central nervous system organization. They are symbolic pictures in the head of a person and represent those aspects of the world which the person has experienced as meaningful in the past. Lippman (1960) called these symbolic representations "... Pictures in the head ... (of) ... the world outside. ..." Human beings, Lippman states, develop effective action plans on the basis of the expectations, the pictures they have in their heads. People use ideas and conceptions they hold in mind to anticipate events and to plan their course of action. But, Lippman goes on to point out, people act in the actual world. People are likely to be successful, effective, and efficient in their action to the extent that their expectations are congruent with the actuality of the world outside.

Unconscious intrapsychic structure, personality organization, intuitive ideas, expectations, and beliefs lie at one end of this second dimension of articulateness. At the other extreme lie fully articulated and explicated formal scientific theories.

Expectations, ideas, beliefs, even aspects of the unconscious can be symbolized and articulated in language. Freud's "Where there was Id there shall be Ego" and the continuing thriving of psychoanalysis and its derivatives are but one kind of evidence supporting this view (Kaplan, 1980). In turn, verbalized ideas can be conceptualized, rearranged, and developed into a formal scientific theory by imposing the rigorous logical structure of a hierarchical system of principles appropriate to the phenomenon under consideration.

Still other comments, primarily in the literature about theories and science, focus on the need for empirical validation of ideas and theories. However, sterile fantasy is mentioned. Thus a third continuum emerges on which conceptual framework and theories vary, the dimension of empirical validity. Scientific progress is achieved by conceptualization, by reassessing and reformulating problems, no less than by exploring facts (Korzbski, 1933, 1954; Northrop, 1947, 1967; Shye, 1978). Whether in personal life or in science, whether loose aggregate or a logically rigorous hierarchical system, it is the conceptual framework that provides for order and coherence of information and for translation of facts into meaningful knowledge. Such translation of facts into knowledge is required for the anticipation of future events, for prediction, and for planning and guiding effective action. The greater the empirical validity of a person's ideas or a scientific theory, the more effective will be the actions which are planned and guided by them.

At the other extreme, emotional disturbances are the consequence of cognitive insufficiency, of lack of accurate and complete pictures in the head about the world outside and experiences to be had in it (Bircher, 1981; Lippman, 1960). Furthermore, psychoses and other acute mental illnesses can be viewed as the collapse of a belief system, a collapse of the cognitive structure of a person without the integration of a new conceptual framework which is adequate to the subjective experience and the objective actualities of that person's life at that point in time. Such a view is consistent with Korzybski's (1933, 1954) views, which suggest that science and sanity go hand in hand.

Empirical validation and reality testing are two different versions of the same process. Both serve the same purpose, to check out whether the surmised is actually so. This view of cognitive insufficiency is also congruent with Langer's (1942) comment that success in life does not depend as much on the wealth of experiences an individual has had as it does on the notions formulated, the concepts with which he or she meets the world of experiences. It is the wealth, quantity, and quality of concepts and their interrelations, the conceptual frameworks, which allow a person to bring his or her experiences under control, to attain purpose and meaning, to anticipate events, and to plan and guide action toward successful goal achievement. Experience has to be brought under the control and guidance of concepts and their related knowledge to achieve such success (Kant, 1952, Langer, 1942).

One important point is the fact that, short of acute psychosis, there is no such thing as not having a conceptual framework. There are only questions of how explicit, logically rigorous, hierarchical, empirically valid, and appropriate to given purposes a conceptual framework used is. Perhaps in the future other dimensions will be identified which influence the power and usefulness of conceptual frameworks for human action. Two that might be considered are the dimensions of internalization and appropriateness. Based on the discussion in this paper, it may be said that the dimensions of logical rigor, empirical validation, and the extent of articulateness determine the power and usefulness of a conceptual framework for achieving desired goals. This is true for ordinary persons in the pursuit of daily living and for scientific inquiry, as well as for professional and clinical practice.

Nursing diagnosis, where does the conceptual framework fit?

The foregoing discussion on concepts and conceptual frameworks suggests that their quality and use make a difference. How does this apply in the area of nursing diagnosis?

Nursing diagnosis is a concept, a complex tripartite relationship of (1) a name or a matter of nomenclature, namely, the symbol "nursing diagnosis"; (2) a pattern of referents, namely, the five critical attributes of name, referents taxonomy, taxa, and clinical judgment; and (3) the idea, the recognitional capacity. The clinician's ability to recognize a new client condition, experience, or response as one illustrative example of a general class of the same will determine how effective the clinician will be in assisting the client to reach health goals. As such the idea of nursing diagnosis is one specific example of the general class of concepts. Therefore, what has been said of concepts and conceptual frameworks is also true of nursing diagnosis. Since the notion of nursing diagnosis encompasses a broad field, conceptual frameworks can be useful to help order the ever growing mass and diversity of information accumulating in libraries. Conceptual frameworks can also be expected to help highlight important areas and cues, to focus attention, and to keep issues in mind during planning and guiding client care.

The following example of a nursing diagnosis label was written with no discernible guidance of a conceptual framework. The only constraint is that Mundinger and Jauron's (1975) format of two linked phrases is used.

Nursing diagnosis I

> Unproductive group discussion related to overuse of
> allocentric focus
> concrete narrative description
> illustrative examples
> nominal definitions
> magical thinking
> hypothetical thinking/could-ism
> imperative thinking/should-ism
> circular reasoning
> intuitive decision making

Clearly the writer of this first nursing diagnostic label had to have some concept and framework, but short of the focus on mental phenomena a specific conceptual framework is not discernible.

The second example is also taken from actual clinical work. Two nursing diagnoses were written for the same patient.

Nursing diagnosis II

> Unmet belonging needs related to
> communication deficit
> death of mother 3 months ago
> abandonment by sister
> exploitation by brother
> history of battery and incest
> marital conflict
> mistrust of others
> loneliness
> self isolation/withdrawal
> lack of friends
> lack of support systems

Nursing diagnosis III

> Unmet self-esteem needs related to
> ambivalence
> anxiety, anger, rage, guilt
> despair, helplessness, hopelessness
> denial, projection, rationalization
> delusions of persecution
> overgeneralizing, overinclusiveness
> autistic thinking, bipolar thinking
> maladaptive coping/blaming
> pleasure principle domination
> short attention span

Again, psychiatric conceptions clearly are used, but no systematic use is made of a psychoanalytic framework. On the other hand, two concepts from Maslow's (1954) hierarchy of needs are recognizable: belonging needs and self-esteem needs. These are a higher level of abstraction and help to separate a large number of important problems into two groups, one regarding problems of interpersonal relations, the other psychological/psychopathological matters. It should be noted that there were no remarkable conditions or concerns in the other three realms or they would have been given as other nursing diagnoses. The value of this use of five realms derived from Maslow's principle of a hierarchy of needs, is that it allows a holistic focus—all five realms have to be accounted for; yet, unless there are remarkable items at hand, they need not be spelled out. Furthermore, concepts, problem formulations, and statements can be included in any language or level of sophistication and from any school of thought. Thus in the pressure of reality practice, with incomplete information gathering or for a number of other reasons, this is a practical, interim approach to nursing diagnostic labeling. It is also an excellent way of helping students learn to grasp the idea of ordering information in accord with a category set. Furthermore, the category set formed by the five realms of needs is most appropriate to the purposes of holistic nursing care.

Problems, however, can be seen. The two nursing diagnosis labels are unwieldy. Could the same process be used to develop subcategories? Or could several of the problem items mentioned be combined at a higher level of abstraction? Using the framework of ego functions, as developed by Bellak, Hervich, and Gediman (1973), the following nursing diagnostic labels emerge for the same clinical information:

Nursing diagnosis IIa
Unmet belonging needs related to
  impaired object relations
  lack of individuation-separation
  passive dependency
  passive aggression
  mistrust

There are advantages and disadvantages of this nursing diagnostic label, as opposed to the previous one on unmet belonging needs. Descriptive detail has been lost. On the other hand, ego function deficit has been identified. The clinician would have to be knowledgeable about ego functions in order to be able to use this kind of a diagnostic statement.

Nursing diagnosis IIIa
Unmet self-esteem needs related to
  impaired regulation and control of drives, affect, and impulses
  impaired thought processes
  impaired mastery competence

Again, descriptive and specific details have been lost, as will occur in abstraction and summarization. On the other hand, simplicity of statement has been gained. It has to be emphasized here that most of the ego functions as defined by Bellak, Hervich, and Gediman (1973) fall into the self-esteem realm. Under a broad umbrella category system such as the five realms, one can mix several different frameworks such as family theory in the belonging realm, and ego functions in the self-esteem realm, and other theories into these two or other realms. The purist scholar would be aghast, but the practitioner would appreciate the realism and practicality of this kind of an approach. One can only hope that someday nursing will have a taxonomy and related taxa knowledge which will permit the use of that system. In so doing the client will be better served than by use of a strange mixture of conceptual frameworks from other disciplines or haphazard and intuitive approaches.

Another way to use the ego function framework for writing nursing diagnostic labels follows:

Nursing diagnosis IIb
> Impaired regulation and control of drives, affects, and impulses related to
>> rage breaking through into consciousness

Nursing diagnosis IIIb
> Impaired thought processes related to
>> magical thinking
>> nominal thinking
>> overgeneralization
>> condensation
>> autistic logic

Here the ego functions are used as major framework without use of the five realms. The advantage is that this focuses more on the psychological area of concern. However, other areas are deleted from mention. There are other advantages to this approach, provided that ego function disturbances are the major concerns in client care. Those advantages concern the plan for interventions. Long-term goal no. 1 would logically be "effective ego functions of regulation and control of impulse, affect, and drives." Long-term goal no. 2 would be "effective phase specifically mature thought processes." The short-term goals would state each subsumed area in terms of positive achievement, i.e., legitimate, own, and master anger experiences; distinguishing facts from desires; generic thinking; drawing warranted generalizations and conclusions.

Again, this is not to present the right way of labeling diagnoses but to show the function of conceptual frameworks in ordering, grouping, and simplifying the vast amount of relevant information gathered by nurse clinicians. The focusing of attention which occurs through the use of a conceptual framework should be noted. Another way the use of a conceptual framework makes a difference is in the analysis of information gleaned from the literature. A grouping and ordering function, is foremost, but an analysis of scope is possible. For example, a realm analysis, using the five exhaustively and mutually exclusively defined realms derived from Maslow's hierarchy of needs, provides insight into the otherwise not so apparent focus of emphasis in Gordon's (1982) *Typology of Functional Health Patterns* (Bircher, 1983).

Gordon postulates eleven functional health patterns. These fall into the five realms as follows:

1. Biological/physiological realm	Sleep/rest pattern (no. 6)
	Exercise pattern (no. 4)
	Nutritional metabolic pattern (no. 2)
	Elimination pattern (no. 3)
	Sexual reproductive pattern (no. 9)
	Health care perceptual pattern (no. 1)
2. Safety/environmental realm	None
3. Belonging/sociocultural realm	Role relationship pattern (no. 8)
4. Self-esteem/psychological realm	Cognitive perceptual pattern (no. 5)
	Self-perception/self-concept pattern (no. 7)
	Value belief pattern (no. 11)
5. Self-actualizing/spiritual realm	None

It is left to the reader to decide how holistic is the distribution of functional health patterns. However, a warning is in order. This distribution is much more holistic than many, if not most, found in nursing practice. The point is not to make judgment of quality or correctness. It is to stress that this is a vast improvement from those computer programs which only allow for physiological, laboratory, medication, and custodial care entries into nursing records. The realm analysis demonstrates the influences of a conceptual framework. Instead of eleven patterns, the attention is drawn to five realms; one realm with six patterns, one realm with three patterns, one realm with one pattern, and two realms without any patterns. The potential to stimulate thought and possible work lies in the question: Are there other client conditions, experiences, and response patterns that, if identified and articulated, would be fruitful in giving holistic nursing care?

There are many other ways to illustrate the influence of the use of a conceptual framework. For example, in nursing it is generally accepted that a nursing conceptual framework should include at least four areas, namely, health, human being, environment, and nursing. Table 1 shows, with simple + for yes, s for some, and − for no, how a number of nursing models mention these areas. Again, the point is not to find fault or to evaluate, but to show the function of conceptual frameworks applied to information available.

This approach to the nursing models might also be taken by using the five critical attributes of the concept of nursing diagnosis, and to identify where and to what extent these models meet the critical attributes necessary to have a viable diagnostic system (see Table 2).

CONCLUSION

In conclusion, it is stressed that all theories are conceptual frameworks, but not all conceptual frameworks are theories. All conceptual frameworks, how-

TABLE 1   Conceptual frameworks in nursing and the nursing model

	Approved nursing diagnosis	Unitary man	Human health competency system	Gordon's patterns	Quality nursing care	Orem, D.	King, I.	Rogers, M.	Orlando, I.
Health	−	s	+	−	+	s	s	+	+
Human beings	−	s	+	s	+	s	+	+	s
Environment	−	s	+	s	+	s	+	+	s
Nursing	−	s	+	s	+	s	+	+	+

Key: +, yes; s, some; −, no.

TABLE 2   The nursing diagnosis concepts and nursing models

Critical attributes of nursing diagnosis concept	Selected nursing models							
	Approved nursing diagnosis	Unitary man	Human health competency system	Gordon's patterns	Quality nursing care	Orem, D.	King, I.	Rogers, M.
	1.	2.	3.	4.	5.	6.	7.	8.
Nomenclature labels		s	+					
Signs and symptoms	s	s	s					
Taxonomy/category system	s	s	+	+	s	s		
Taxa/content	s		+			s	+	s
Clinical judgment			+		s	+		+

Key: see Table 1.

ever, allow access, direct attention, sensitize, highlight cues and areas, inable the making of finer distinctions, and identify areas of relevant knowledge. If based on a sound taxonomy, conceptual frameworks do reduce complexity and allow for diagnosing, that is to say, allow a nurse to identify a new, never before seen instance of client condition, experience, or response as a member of a known class or category of conditions, experiences, or responses. That recognition is the essence of nursing diagnosis. In so diagnosing, use of a conceptual framework allows the nurse to go beyond the information given in the current situation and apply knowledge (scientific or professional) gained from past similar experiences. Going beyond the information given in the present case makes possible prediction, anticipation, preparation for events to come, and control of events, experiences, and responses to them. If backed up by sound Level II, III, and IV theories, taxonomies serve as intellectual road maps to the territories of life experiences and professional practice. Theories make the difference between groping in the dark and enlightened, planned, purposive action. Theories allow the derivation of meaning, of consequences to be anticipated. In the coincidence of immediate experience and the conceptual framework, which serves as integral central nervous system organization, the person experiences reality. Thus, mind is a framework of expectations, a conceptual framework more or less explicit, logically rigorous, hierarchical, and empirically valid. Such a mental conceptual framework may be more or less psychological, or it may reflect the structure of subject matter, or the accumulated knowledge in a field. Whichever it may be, a person's theory in action, as Argyris and Schoen (1978) call it, is the actual framework which guides their actions, regardless of what framework may be espoused verbally.

Nursing diagnosis: a Janus view. In terms of conceptual frameworks, nursing has come from a past with loose aggregates of concepts and carapaces. Currently, nursing is contemplating the value of struggling with nursing diagnosis and conceptual frameworks. Some nurses are considering taxonomic work. Will nurses avail themselves of the powerful intellectual tool of conceptual frameworks, of logically rigorous, heirarchic deductive systems? Will nursing work on, and actually manage to put together many pieces of the puzzle called effective functioning, mastery of human experiences, and coping with related responses? The task is large but the benefits could be great. Only time will tell.

REFERENCES

Abdellah, F., and Levine, E.: Better patient care through nursing research, New York, 1965, The Macmillan Co.

Argyris, C., and Schoen, D.: Theory in practice, San Francisco, 1978, Jossey-Bass, Inc., Publishers.

Aspinall, M.: Nursing diagnosis—the weak link, Nurs. Outlook 24(7):433-437, 1976.

Beckstrand, J.: A critique of several conceptions of practice theory in nursing, Res. Nurs. Health 3(2):69-79, 1980.

Bellak, L., Hervich, M., and Gediman, H.: Ego function in schizophrenics, neurotics and normals, New York, 1973, John Wiley & Sons, Inc.

Bershady, H.: Ideology and social knowledge, New York, 1973, John Wiley & Sons, Inc.

Biddle, B., and Thomas, E., editors: Role theory, New York, 1966, John Wiley & Sons, Inc.

Bircher, A.: Thinking patterns. Language as experience and guide to action. Unpublished Ph.D. dissertation, 1966, University of California, Berkeley.

Bircher, A.: Quality nursing care. Paper presented at the Oklahoma District Nurses' Association Mini-Convention, 1973.

Bircher, A.: On the development and classification of nursing diagnoses, Nurs. Forum **14**(1):10-29, 1975.

Bircher, A.: More on the development and classification of nursing diagnoses. Paper presented to the Special Interest Group on Nursing Diagnosis. American Nurses' Association, Council of Nurse Researchers' annual meeting, Hollywood, Fla., 1975.

Bircher, A.: Reflections on nursing research, OUCN Res. News **1**(2):2-10, 1977.

Bircher, A.: Nursing diagnosis, psychiatric mental health nursing, and the DSM III. Paper presented at the Second Annual Perspectives of Psychiatric Nursing Conference, New York, 1981.

Bircher, A.: The concept of nursing diagnosis. In Kim, M., and Moritz, D., editors: Classification of nursing diagnoses—Proceedings of the Third and Fourth National Conferences, New York, 1982, McGraw-Hill Book Co.

Bircher, A.: A realm analysis of Gordon's typology of functional health patterns. Oklahoma City, 1983, University of Oklahoma College of Nursing.

Bircher, A.: Process definitions of concepts: prototype of research method development for nursing. Keynote address at the Fourth Annual Nursing Research Conference, University of South Florida College of Nursing, Tampa, 1985.

Blalock, H.: Conceptualization and measurement in the social sciences, Beverly Hills, Calif., 1982, Sage Publications, Inc.

Blalock, H.: Basic dilemmas in the social sciences, Beverly Hills, Calif., 1984, Sage Publications, Inc.

Blumer, H.: Science without concepts, Am. J. Sociol. **36**(4):515-533, 1931.

Blumer, H.: What is wrong with social science theory? In Filstead, W., editor: Qualitative methodology, Chicago, 1970, Markham.

Bonham, G.: Demystifying the humanities, Change **12**(7):16-17, 1980.

Braitwaith, R.: Scientific explanation, London, 1953, Cambridge University Press.

Bruner, J.: Beyond the information given (J. Anglin, editor), New York, 1975, W.W. Norton & Co., Inc.

Burr, W.: Theory construction and the sociology of family, New York, 1973, John Wiley & Sons, Inc.

Burton, A.: Operational theories of personality, New York, 1974, Brunner/Mazel, Inc.

Capra, F.: The new physics as a model for a new medicine, J. Sociol. Biol. Struct. **1**(1):71-77, 1978.

Carnevali, D., Mitcheli, P., Woods, N., and Tanner, C.: Diagnostic reasoning in nursing, Philadelphia, 1984, J.B. Lippincott Co.

Chambers, W.: Nursing diagnosis, Am. J. Nurs. **62**(11):102-104, 1962.

Chinn, P., and Jacobs, M.: Theory and nursing: a systematic approach, St. Louis, 1983, The C.V. Mosby Co.

Denzin, N.: The research act, Chicago, 1970, Aldine Publishing Co.

Dickoff, J., and James, P.: A theory of theories: a position paper, Nurs. Res. **17**(3):197-203, 1968.

Durkheim, E.: The rules of sociological method, Glencoe, Ill., 1938, Free Press of Glencoe.

Fawcett, J.: The what of theory development. In theory development: what, why, how? New York, 1978, National League for Nursing.

Fawcett, J.: Analysis and evaluation of conceptual models of nursing, Philadelphia, 1984, F.A. Davis Co.

Frosch, J.: The psychotic process, New York, 1983, International University Press.

Gagne, R.: Memory structures and learning outcomes, Rev. Ed. Res. **48**(2):187-222, 1978.

Gale, G.: The theory of science: an introduction to the history, logic and philosophy of science, New York, 1979, McGraw-Hill Book Co.

Gebbie, K., and Lavin, M., editors: Classification of nursing diagnoses, St. Louis, 1975, The C.V. Mosby Co.

Goffman, E.: Behavior in public places, Glencoe, Ill., 1963, Free Press of Glencoe.

Goffman, E.: Sociology 204: "Frames," (lecture notes), University of California, Berkeley, 1963, 1964.

Gordon, M.: Nursing diagnosis: Process and application, New York, 1982, McGraw-Hill Book Co.

Greenwood, E.: Relationship of sciences to the practice professions, J. Am. Inst. Plan. **24**(2):223-231, 1954.

Greenwood, E.: Research methods in social work (lecture notes), University of California, Berkeley, 1962, 1963.

Griffith, J., and Christensen, P.: Nursing process. Application of theories, frameworks and models, St. Louis, 1982, The C.V. Mosby Co.

Haber, J., Lich, A., Shudy, S., and Sidelau, B.: Comprehensive psychiatric nursing, New York, 1978, McGraw-Hill Book Co.

Hardy, M.: Evaluating nursing theories. In theory development: what, why, how? New York, 1978, National League for Nursing.

Hebb, O.: The need of theory. In Severin, F., editor: Humanistic view points in psychology, New York, 1965, McGraw-Hill Book Co.

Hook, S.: Psychoanalysis, scientific method, and philosophy, New York, 1971, University Press.

Hunt, E.: Concept learning, New York, 1962, John Wiley & Sons, Inc.

Hunt, E., and Hoveland, C.: Programming a model of human concept formation. In Feigenbaum, E., and Feldman, J., editors: Computers and thought, New York, 1963, McGraw-Hill Book Co.

Johnson, D.: State of the art of theory development in nursing. In Theory development: what, why, how? New York, 1978, National League for Nursing.

Kant, I.: Critique of pure reason, New York, 1959, Encyclopaedia Britannica.

Kaplan, A.: The conduct of inquiry, New York, 1964, Harper & Row, Publishers.

Kaplan, H., Freedman, A., and Sadock, B., editors: Comprehensive textbook of psychiatry, ed. 3, Baltimore, 1980, The Williams & Wilkins Co.

Kerlinger, F.: Foundations of behavioral research, ed. 2, New York, 1973, Holt, Rinehart & Winston.

King, I.: Toward a theory for nursing, New York, 1971, John Wiley & Sons, Inc.

Korzybski, A.: Science and sanity, Lakeville, New York, 1933, International Non-Aristotlian Library.

Kritek, P.: Taxonomy committee report. Presented at the Sixth Conference on Nursing Diagnosis, April, 1984.

Kuhn, T.: The structure of scientific revolutions, ed. 2, Chicago, 1970, The University of Chicago Press.

Langer, S.: Philosophy in a new key, Cambridge, Mass., 1942, Harvard University Press.

Langer, S.: Mind: an essay on human feeling. Vol. I, Baltimore, 1967, John Hopkins Press.

Lazlo, S.: The systems view of the world, New York, 1972, George Braziller, Inc.

Lippman, W.: The pictures in our heads and the world outside. In Mills, C.W., editor: Images of man: the classical tradition in sociological thinking, New York, 1960, George Braziller, Inc.

London, J., Wenkert, R., and Hagstrom, W.: Adult education and social class. Cooperative research report #1017, Berkeley, 1963, Survey Research Center, University of California.

Luria, A.: The making of mind, Cambridge, 1979, Harvard University Press.

Luria, A.: Cognitive development: its cultural and social foundations, Cambridge, 1976, Harvard University Press.

Macnamara, J.: On the relation between language and thought. In Macnamara, J., editor: Language, learning, and thought, New York, 1977, Academic Press, Inc.

Maslow, A.: Motivation and personality, ed. 2, New York, 1954, Harper & Row, Publishers.

Mead, G.: Mind, self, and society, Chicago, 1934, University of Chicago Press.

Mills, C.: The sociological imagination, New York, 1959, Oxford University Press, Inc.

Morgenau, H.: The method of science and the meaning of reality, Main Currents of Modern Thought (retrospective issue) **32**(225):7-15, 1975.

Mullen, E.: Personal practice models. In Rosenblatt, A., and Waldfogel, D., editors: Handbook of clinical social work, San Francisco, 1983, Jossey-Bass, Inc., Publishers.

Mundinger, M., and Jauron, E.: Developing a nursing diagnosis, Nurs. Outlook **23**(2):94-98, 1975.

Newman, M.: Theory development in nursing, Philadelphia, 1979, F.A. Davis Co.

Northrop, F.: The logic of the sciences and the humanities, New York, 1967, The World Publishing Press.

Northrop, F., and Morgenau, H.: The nature of concepts. Their interrelation and role in social structure—Proceedings of the Tenth Stillwater Conference, Stillwater, Okla., June, 1950.

Patterson, J.: The tortuous way towards nursing theory. In theory development: what, why, how? New York, 1975, National League for Nursing.

Peterson, C.: Questions frequently asked about development of a conceptual framework, J. Nurs. Ed. **16**(4):22-32, 1977.

Piaget, J.: The construction of reality in the child, New York, 1958, Basic Books, Inc., Publishers.

Polanyi, M.: The tacit dimension, New York, 1966, Doubleday & Co., Inc.

Pope, K., and Singer, J.: The stream of consciousness, New York, 1978, Plenum Publishing Corp.

Price, R., Katterer, R., Bader, B., and Monahan, J.: Prevention in mental health, Beverly Hills, 1980, Sage Publications, Inc.

Riehl, J., and Roy, C.: Conceptual models in nursing practice, New York, 1980, Appleton-Century-Crofts.

Rogers, M.: An introduction to the theoretical basis of nursing, Philadelphia, 1970, F.A. Davis Co.

Roy, C.: Theoretical framework for classification of nursing diagnoses. In Kim, M.J., and Moritz, D.A., editors: Classification of nursing diagnoses: Proceedings of the Third and Fourth National Conferences, New York, 1982, McGraw-Hill Book Co.

Rychlak, J.: Introduction to personality and psychotherapy: the theory construction approach, Boston, 1981, Houghton Mifflin Co.

Sartori, G.: Social science concepts: a systematic analysis, Beverly Hills, Calif., 1984, Sage Publications, Inc.

Shye, S., editor: Theory construction and data analysis in the behavioral sciences, San Francisco, 1978, Jossey-Bass, Inc., Publishers.

Schafer, R.: The analytic attitude, New York, 1983, Basic Books, Inc., Publishers.

Stevens, B.: Nursing theory: analyses, application, evaluation, Boston, 1979, Little, Brown & Co.

Sullivan, H.: The interpersonal theory of psychiatry, New York, 1953, W.W. Norton & Co., Inc.

Vermulapalli, G.: The unnecessary conflict between teaching and research, Chron. Higher Ed. **28**(22):25, 1984.

Wagner, D.: The growth of social science theories, Beverly Hills, Calif., 1984, Sage Publications, Inc.

Zderad, L.: From here and how to theory: Reflections on how. In theory development: what, why, how? New York, 1978, National League for Nursing.

Discussion

Question: Are there any plans for NANDA to take an official stand on the taxonomy you have proposed?

Phyllis Kritek: NANDA is in the process now of going from a loose-knit to a formal structure. Since we have a taxonomy committee it seems to me inappropriate until the committee has deliberated and sought advisement, including, I think, working with the ANA group, to bring anything forward for this conference. This is what I consider our transition conference. It is my hope, though, that the taxonomy committee could bring forward for a general assembly review and debate at the 7th Conference a taxonomy which NANDA would adopt as its own.

Richard Fehring: I am Richard Fehring, member of the planning Committee. I have a question for Dr. Kim. This morning when you were breaking down the percentage of independent and dependent nursing actions you said you had done a survey. I would be interested in the characteristics of the nurses utilized in that study and if they were primarily from hospital settings?

Mi Ja Kim: I knew some of the researchers would ask that question. Unfortunately, I do not have the data analyzed to that point, but by just looking at the raw data, first of all, the majority of them are from hospital settings and, secondly, a majority of them are B.S.N. and graduate prepared. I cannot say more at this time—the data has to be analyzed to make some relationships, and that is the plan.

Nancy Grayson: I am Nancy Grayson from the University of Illinois. I have a comment that I would like to hear some reaction to, especially from Phyllis. I think that taxonomic work is very important. One of the things that troubles me, however, is what I consider a little more elementary, and I consider myself brave getting up here and saying this. I need definitions. I think the taxonomic structures that you propose suggest there is a problem, because not everything is on the same plane. But still, even with the terminology that goes into the taxonomy I would be willing to bet if we all wrote out our definitions in this room today, we would have 450 definitions. And I would like to hear your comment about that.

Phyllis Kritek: Part of how I have tried to make sense out of whether we ought to do a taxonomy or not is to look at the history of science and what has happened in other disciplines. In the best of all worlds, I would prefer definitions for all of it. But I also would prefer a full list; by that I mean, I have several things I would like. At one point, soil was considered a chemical, and "chemists" spent an enormous amount of time studying it so they could get its properties, not knowing it was many, many, many chemicals and that soils varied across the surface of the earth. My feeling is that in the process of pushing at all of these parameters to bring something out, in particular what nurses already know and are practicing, we will drive ourselves to ask the right questions and grapple for better answers. So, for me the process of trying to create a taxonomy is really predicated on the assumption that by trying to find out if there is order out there, we will begin to ask that question. This group viewed these five things as falling under exchanging. Are they right or wrong? I do not know. Do we need to debate it? Yes, I think so. But, I know what you are saying about courage, and I do not think one ought to be anxious about it. It all should be criticized, because it is all pretty imperfect. But the criticisms unearth the next hard questions, I think, and let us do that a lot.

Mary Lou Kiley: This is for Dr. Kritek. I am Mary Lou Kiley from University Hospitals of Cleveland and the Frances Paine Bolton School of Nursing. I support your position that we should proceed with the taxonomy as it is and continue to try to refine it. I am also reminded of the development of the medical classifications, the ICD9s and the DSM3s. The DSM3s twenty-five years ago were in a state similar to our nursing diagnoses. Residents carried them around in a paper notebook in their pockets. I have a question which you might want to answer. I feel that we need to describe what we are seeing in patients and to continue to do that to a considerable extent before we can move into interventions. I feel, in the talks this morning, we are pushing for interventions, and I just wonder if that might not be somewhat premature. Again, I do not think we should put any limits. I think if people want to study interventions, they certainly should. But I do not think that we know enough yet about the full range of our diagnoses.

Phyllis Kritek: I agree. My conviction is that we have not described our phenomena yet, and therefore it is absolutely indefensible to say that we can fully explain our interventions or our outcomes. But I have held that position for ten years, and am beginning to hear myself in the background. By the same token, if folks are doing that, I do not go around saying "Quit doing that," "Do not play with interventions." One reason why I was interested in the taxonomy was I thought it was another way to ferret out incomplete lists and to start worrying about exactly your point. The other thing I was interested in was why are so many staff nurses frustrated with some of the diagnoses and in love with others? And the reason, I think, is because some are functional and some are not. We need to first say that out loud as a group and quit being defensive or worried about it and then say here are some ways we are going to try to solve it. How does it look to you? People also have this fantasy that NANDA has taken the position that you must use the list under the following conditions. I think we have to send a message of tentativeness and exploration to everyone and then ask them to feed us their information: please enrich our knowledge base.

Comment: One more word about the definitions. I think the defining characteristics that were published at one time but are not refined to the extent that one would like them to be do make very good definitions.

Phyllis Kritek: That is very helpful. Thank you. That is a good point, and I had not thought of that. You mentioned DSM. I have to mention one of my favorite disorders of childhood and adolescence, which is defined as "leaving home without permission."

Regina Maibusch: Regina Maibusch from Milwaukee, Wisconsin. I have a question and comment which hinges on the question the previous speaker at this microphone had, about definitions for those titles—not the diagnoses, now, but the titles in the theorists' framework. How do we develop in a practice setting, in an acute care setting, a data base? What kind of questions are we going to ask? We do not have definitions for those terms yet. And the variety of people that we get—some who stay forty-eight hours, twenty-four hours, same day surgery—how much of such a list can we use? I am working with a group now who is trying to revise their data base for admitting patients to the acute care setting. How do I do this? How do I use that?

Phyllis Kritek: You will definitely get Kritek's world view here. But it seems to me you solve that problem in the most realistic, appropriate, functional ways you can in your own environment and live with the tentativeness of the process. We are not there yet. There are hospitals and health care agencies that have developed very elaborate taxonomic structures with multiple diagnoses, many of which have never even seen the light of day in NANDA. I cannot get real upset with that at this point. It seems to me the more we can collectively try to utilize everything that is generated and approved by NANDA, the better, in terms of leading to some level of general consensus. But we are going to have to all create temporary solutions in our own real worlds. Remember until Einstein, physics had a temporary solution. They just did not know it.

Regina Maibusch: I would like to ask if anyone in this audience has tried to develop a data base using the theorists' framework rather than something else? If so, I would be interested in speaking to them.

Bill Windells: I am Bill Windells from Burlington, Vermont, Medical Center Hospital and University of Vermont School of Nursing. I was pretty confused and at the same time interested with the black holes that appeared on your classification diagrams and would like to know how they got there. Is there any preliminary thought on what they might be or are they just an expression of humility?

Phyllis Kritek: I think I will go with the last one. I like that. . . . They are part caprice and part deliberate. The one thing that the taxonomy group was very conscious of was how people deal with "the lists": if it is not on this list, you do not have a phenomenon. We were very apprehensive about that kind of response with the taxonomic trees. So what we wanted to do was build in an overt visual cue that said: "Look! It is incomplete!" That was our primary motive. In addition to that, sometimes just to structurally put the thing together, we had to put some blanks in, especially when there was a category label needed for a level two phenomenon and there were level three phenomena with names, but we did not know the group or level two name. So, part of it was necessity: part of it was this basic commitment to tentativeness. Then toward the end of the last conference, an effort by the group was made to just go through and see where else we could put blanks to create as unfinished an image as possible. So the third piece called caprice is also there.

Linda Carpenito: Linda Carpenito. Dr. Kim, do you think the percentage would be higher in independents if you used the two part statement with the category, because in reality the diagnosis seems to come alive related to specifying the interventions? I am thinking that you could probably look at one category, give two different diagnostic statements depending on your contributing factors, and probably the percentages would change greatly. What do you think?

Mi Ja Kim: I have to think very fast, because I did not consider that. I think that it is an excellent suggestion. In terms of operationalizing and structuring a study it might create a lot of problems. My original intent of the study was to just give us a sense of where we are at. I just wanted to have a really rough idea, and please do not take this study as something that was very well controlled and so forth. As you can tell, the data were analyzed last week, and that is how recent and how fast I cranked out the data. But I think in my next venture I would consider that. If I do that, then the complexity of ideology comes into the picture along with the problem that we do not have all identified ideologies for the diagnoses. So obviously we would have to look at selective nursing diagnoses which we think have some established ideologies. That is how I would look at it, but that is a good idea. Thanks, Linda.

Dottie Jones: Dottie Jones from Boston, Massachusetts. I would like to respond to what Phyllis talked about earlier in terms of this use of the whole framework that has been presented. I think as you listen to Phyllis you get the feeling that there are, in fact, levels of abstraction, and that abstraction in terms of how it translates to concrete practice conjures up a lot of things. When you get to level four, it would seem apparent that this is the level where we are really looking to assessing the more concrete things we see in practice. Things like functional assessment may become very apparent at several of those levels. And I think you translate that to the needs of the setting that you are involved in in terms of defining what the smaller pieces are and what the questions are. I think the other question it raises is, are there levels of diagnoses for each of these levels of phenomena that are being described? In fact, there may be different ways to assess different levels, where you go from the very concrete to the more abstract which may reflect the phenomenon of the individual or the concern of that total person. We have not gotten there yet. So I think that you cannot look at exchanging in its most abstract form and think about how to do that right now. You may need to go to the much more functional and work inductively rather than deductively, or maybe in both directions, to arrive at multiple levels of understanding of the phenomenon.

Phyllis Kritek: I just want to respond to Dottie. I think you have made several observations. And I think that one is the whole issue of what happened with exchanging during the group work, in contrast to some of the other, less physiological or less physical or less concrete patterns. I know none of the patterns are concrete, but the perception that the exchanging pattern seems to give, the sense that this is touchable, this is a see, hear, touch, taste kind of thing to me reflects some of what the philosophy of science is dealing with now in terms of questioning the whole view of reality as only a cause and effect kind of reality. This raises some rough questions for things like choosing and valuing, I think. So we may have to deal with many different kinds of parameters based on which pattern we are looking at.

Harriet Werley: I just want to say I am impressed with the progress that has been made, and I am impressed with the non-rigidity with which you are moving along. I appreciate that. I see encouragement to move along in this way and that way and the other way. I want to call something to your attention that I think shows another movement to help push this along, and that is a little flier on a book on nursing interventions. While the diagnosis business is being approached from several aspects, here is a group moving forward with interventions now. If you have not found the flier, do look it up. It would seem to me that there is a lot in there that would be another tack on the subject. If one group, for instance, has a way of defining what it is they are going to do in their research or their thinking of moving ahead, it will put some other pieces in place and probably help fill some of those vacant spots that are up there on your diagrams. In conjunction with the different things that are being done and the non-rigidity of feeling it has to go down all one path, any of you who are familiar with that circuitous path of research know how it backtracks. You will go this way, and you will go that way, and you will plug in this, and you will plug in that, and I think eventually the pieces will fall in place. Just to hear that physician saying what he said about nursing diagnosis shows the long way that nursing has come. I can remember the early years when Marge Gordon would try to get some research proposals in, and we used to always say well, it was because there were physicians on the review group, and the word diagnosis raised a red flag with them, so they were in opposition to giving a favorable review. Well, I think you have passed a lot of hurdles, and that is good. I am impressed, too, to see the scholarly volumes come out and because this is a movement in history, I would urge you to continue in the scholarly vein as this will be investigated by a lot of people. You can be proud of the scholarly way in which your volumes are coming out. So I commend you all.

Linda Carpenito: Just a comment on Marge's discussion of going from general to specific. I agree wholeheartedly, except in certain situations. We used to have a very general diagnostic category called Alteration in Respiratory Function. That was removed from the list and replaced by three very specific diagnoses. Now we find in clinical practice that when you have factors that may contribute to an alteration in respiratory function like ineffective diaphragmatic movement or post-anesthetic state, these three do not fit. I express that caution, not disagreement, because sometimes I think we need that broad category to refer to in certain clinical situations, when overall function, not parts, are affected.

Phyllis Kritek: My question is for Marge Gordon. I am always confused when you use the terms "diagnostic category," "diagnostic concepts," and "diagnostic labels." Do they all mean the same thing or three different things? Another term used is "name phenomena." Would you differentiate for us what you mean by those four specific terms or phrases?

Marjory Gordon: I think probably the general definition of a diagnostic category is a division in a classification system. The general definition in the literature of diagnostic category is a division in a classification system in a book. Something like potential skin breakdown or alteration in skin integrity can be in a book as a diagnostic category or in a categorization system or a class in a classification. But where did that come from? That probably is a concept or an idea that has observable reference signs and symptoms, and that concept is classified and then called a category. But you are right. The distinction between category and concept is probably not used clearly. Diagnostic label would be the label for a diagnosis which one might find in a classification system and one might use to label a patient's problem. We notice things in the clinical area, and then what emerges is like a cluster of signs and symptoms that we think hang together, have relationship. It is a phenomenon.

Cindy Dougherty: Cindy Dougherty, the University of Iowa, and my question is addressed to Marjory Gordon. I want to go back to the beginning of your discussion about etiology and making our nursing diagnostic labels very simple. This question came up, and we had some heated debate about it in our small group section a few days ago, whenever that was. In critical care, for the diagnosis of physiological nursing problems, the etiology most frequently goes back to a medical diagnosis. Let me give you the example. If someone has decreased cardiac output, the cause is usually a myocardial infarction. Now, we can call it all kinds of things, myocardial ischemia etc., but is it our aim, when we are naming the things that nurses diagnose and treat, to rename other phenomena that have already been identified by other groups? How can we name physiological problems or go about outlining our etiologies without renaming medical diagnoses?

Majory Gordon: I would have to go back and ask you your definition of etiology, but let me just throw this out. Etiology has a definite impact on the interventions.

Cindy Dougherty: Yes.

Marjory Gordon: Okay. So we agree on the definition. Okay, what are you going to do about myocardial infarct?

Cindy Dougherty: In my opinion, there are many things we can do about myocardial infarction. The nursing diagnosis is something that comes from the myocardial infarction. And in critical care we can do some things about that.

Marjory Gordon: Sure, but maybe the diagnosis comes from the person who has had a myocardial infarct, and maybe legally if you really diagnose a myocardial infarct, you might send that patient to the physician.

Cindy Dougherty: No, I am diagnosing decreased cardiac output.

Marjory Gordon: Okay, I know in critical care you do have the measurements because the physician has already placed lines, etc., and you can get those measurements. I guess I would argue usefulness. Mi Ja Kim and I have debated this over and over. My question is are we really going to re-label the 999 diagnoses? Maybe we need to get something that is useful for clinical practice. But I think the other thing to consider, is maybe nursing practice is both medical and nursing diagnoses-based. So, do we really have to change congestive failure into decreased cardiac output, or can we use that to write our disease-based interventions?

Cindy Dougherty: I hope we do not have to completely rename, but if we use your format, we are sort of lost a little bit.

Andrea Bircher: I appreciate your loss, but may I respond in part? The issue of etiology is a very problematic one. I am sorry I did not get all of my points made but the conceptual framework that you bring to the situation you see has bearing. What do you do with a patient who you see has a myocardial infarction but then you learn about his stress-related history and life experience? Or take the patient with stomach ulcers who ends up to really have a repression of anger? If you take a whole person systems view, your decreased cardiac output and the pathophysiology that are—may be secondary. It may be the result of a problem in another major area. It may be a sociological problem. It may result from a lack of meaning, lack of purpose in life. So, if you take a person approach, you may find that your decreased cardiac output is a symptom rather than an etiology for a nursing diagnosis.

Eileen Jones: I am Eileen Jones, University of Wisconsin, Oshkosh. I think you gave us a really good synopsis of the state of the art in relation to the diagnostic categories we have now and the various levels of abstraction and so on. It sounds like we need to do a lot of work on these. We need to refine them, etc. But yesterday in the NANDA business meeting, Phyllis seemed to emphasize that we need to develop new ones rather than work on the old ones. Did I misunderstand? Are you differentiating what should happen in practice versus what the Association is going to do in its formal process?

Marjory Gordon: Oh, I am sorry. I was not talking for the Association. I was talking about the profession. We probably do need to both refine and categorize what we have and construct new ones.

Phyllis Kritek: You did hear that correctly. I think the intent behind that position is that emphasis will be given in the diagnostic review process to creating mechanisms for accepting, reviewing, and acting on new diagnoses. I do not use the term, category, and that is probably why I raised the question. I tend to think of it as label. After we have implemented that mechanism we should have a useful process for reconsidering those we have. We would then have set norms and standards to which we would then subject old labels and/or categories. Hopefully, it will be a more expeditious process. I think Marge has helped us see that we have got to get it down to some useable set of labels. If I can get more and more of these useable practice labels in place with the indicators that we need, then it will quickly become clear how to clean up the existing list and turn it into a taxonomic tree.

Carol Tippey: Carol Tippey from Iowa, Mt. Mercy College. I am trying to teach the abstract concept of wellness to may students who are dealing with well, elderly clients. I am wondering if you have some thoughts on how to help students and other clinical people deal with naming something as abstract as the concept of wellness seems to be at this point. Also, do you think there is a different diagnostic process for dealing with problems of wellness? My perspective is we are not really looking at etiologies of problems if we are looking at defining characteristics of wellness in a person who is not either having a problem or potentially at risk for a problem. Does that make some sense? I would like Dr. Gordon to address this if possible.

Marjory Gordon: Let me ask, if a person by your health status evaluation process is well, are you going to charge for that? Are you going to make a diagnosis and charge for that? Also, there is discussion about growth and wellness, yet we do not have anything regarding that except one category, and that is potential for growth, ineffective family coping. No, I do not think the diagnostic process is different if it is identification.

Andrea Bircher: Let me quickly respond to that. I do not think it is a matter of a change of diagnostic process. I agree with Marjory. I think the difference is that you have different concepts and need different background knowledge. Background knowledge in wellness and health is not as clearly defined as pathology and pathophysiology in particular. Now, psychopathology already gets confused. I think we have an issue here of the null hypothesis in which you see that for which you have words. We all have a lot of words for psychopathology, problems, and being sick. We define nursing in terms of helping people cope with their actual and potential responses to health problems. I say to you that if we are what we say we are, and prevention and promotion of health is part of our uniqueness, we need to start coping with life experiences and growth and development. Now, I would like to make a comment concerning something that I think is adding some confusion. A colleague and I are proposing that there is another whole area of nurse decision-making, which is the monitoring of decisions that are a large part of nursing practice and cut across both nursing and medical diagnoses. There is a diagnostic process, a decision-making process, that goes along with that. I think if the independent nursing diagnoses are separated out from the decisions related to monitoring of care, I think it will cope with some of this confusion. And I think both the wellness concepts, where the nurse is monitoring the health of an individual as well as medical diagnosis, can be addressed through the area of a monitoring decision process.

CHAPTER 4

Cost and quality assurance

DRGs: impact on health management and health professions

FRANKLIN A. SHAFFER, Ed.D., R.N.

I have heard many questions concerning what a "DRG" is. Some say it's "D Rotten Government." Others are convinced it's "Docs Ruined by Government." Still others, more self-conscious about some kind of monitoring process that is going on, call it "Docs in a Box." While each of these approaches to DRG may provide a fascinating and descriptive insight into different responses that the new prospective payment system has drawn from the health care management community, none of them really tells us what DRG actually is. In fact, our greatest problem today as health care professionals may well be that we live in a changed and unfamiliar environment, and that it really bothers us that we do not really understand the ramifications of DRGs. Good at what we do, we are nonetheless suddenly encountering a new era in which every aspect of the system of rewards for what we do is changing. We inhabit a strange and seemingly hostile environment in which all of the rules—all of the criteria for organizational success or failure—have been turned upside down. And this is no wonder in a nationwide system in which the dominant value for reimbursement has shifted from "more is better" to "less is more" (Pointer and Ross, 1984). Management tactics that worked exceedingly well in the past are no longer effective; hospitals that do not "quickly acquire a different repertoire of strategies and tactics will become organizational mastodons" (Pointer and Ross, 1984).

In this context, nursing must rise to the challenge of the new environment and set as its goal: to acquire expertise at understanding exactly what DRG is and to use this knowledge to improve the quality of nursing care while maintaining or even reducing cost. Why is it always those who accept change as an *opportunity* rather than as a *setback* who advance? It is because they are the ones who have the presence of mind to explain the way to others and thus to assume new positions of leadership and responsibility. The choice is ours.

WHAT DRG IS AND WHERE IT IS GOING

Today we start by looking briefly at recent economic and legislative developments that have created and will continue to redefine the DRG (Diagnosis Related Group) prospective payment system.

On April 20, 1983, legislation was passed that will revolutionize the American health care delivery system. The impact of this legislation will be felt by health care management for years to come. On that date, President Reagan signed *Public Law* 98-21, the Social Security Amendment of 1983. This payment system began on October 1, 1983, and will take effect at every hospital in the country during the reporting period beginning on or after that date. The rapidity with which Congress passed the prospective payment policy, which is based on diagnosis related groups (DRGs) was remarkable: the process took approximately one month. Only three months earlier, former Health and Human Services Secretary Richard Schweiker first submitted the prospective payment proposal. This rapid passage contrasts sharply with three years of unsuccessful lobbying during the Carter administration. Why the sudden and dramatic change?

There are several major reasons that can explain why Congress acted in record time. While a factor that contributed to the fast Congressional action was concern over the looming federal deficit, the major reason was the danger of insolvency of the Medicare trust fund—the primary reimbursement source for health care in this country. When this fund begins to run out, it is predictable that whatever has to be done to contribute to its replenishment will be done. In fact, the Prospective Payment Assessment Commission (PROPAC) is mandated to recalibrate the DRGs in 1986, and it is speculated that the Medicare trust fund will become insolvent by 1990. I can assure you that if the fund *is* actually about to run out again at that time, we will be meeting again to discuss the new and sweeping changes. But the soaring cost of health care will continue to be the primary reason for this fund's depletion, and there are many factors contributing to this drain. Among these are population changes, the effects of supply and demand, new technology, and intensity of service.

Retrospective reimbursement

For the legislators who passed the DRG prospective payment system, the major reason for the excessive increases in hospital costs has been attributed to the system of reimbursement. This system is based on a network of public and private third-party payers, which includes Medicare, Blue Cross, Blue Shield, and various private insurers. Therefore, direct payments by patients toward national health costs have decreased, while private insurance payments have escalated steadily. With the advent of Medicare and Medicaid in 1965, public reimbursements rose precipitously and private, direct payments declined further. Thus, the true cost of health care was insulated by public funding.

Further, before the DRG implementation, third-party payers continued to reimburse providers on a retrospective or "cost" basis computed on the patient's length of stay in the hospital chargeable at a fixed amount per day—regardless of what treatment was rendered. Providers were paid for reasonable costs *after* the delivery of the service. This system, promising to pay for whatever services were rendered for each case, created incentives for overutilization. Therefore we can see that the cost-based, retrospective system stifled demand among both patients and providers for more prudent and efficient delivery of care.

PROSPECTIVE RATE SETTING

What, then, are the components of prospective, as opposed to retrospective, rate setting that are going to help to prevent the Medicare trust fund from running out? Dowling (1979) notes that, under a prospective rate setting system, "providers are paid at rates set in advance and are considered fixed for the pertinent period (typically a year)." Some external authority, such as the Health Care Financing Administration, must be empowered to supervise rate setting. Dowling summarized the general concept of prospective payment in four steps:

1. An external authority is empowered (by statute, market power, or voluntary compliance by providers) to set provider charges and/or third party payment rates.
2. Rates are set in advance of the prospective year during which they apply and are considered fixed for the year (except for major, uncontrollable occurrences).
3. Patients and/or third parties pay the prospective rates rather than the costs actually incurred by providers during the year (or charges adjusted to cover these costs).
4. Providers are at risk for losses or surpluses.

In short, prospective rates are both a means of exerting more external influence over hospital activities and a means of building cost containment constraints and/or incentives into hospital payment.

THE HCFA PROSPECTIVE PAYMENT PLAN

What does the Health Care Financing Administration (HCFA) plan have to do with the prospective payment system that we have just outlined? To answer this we have to look at the important considerations of the new federal legislation which were initiated in early HCFA demonstration contracts with New Jersey and other states. As I mentioned before, on or after October 1,

1983, Medicare payment for inpatient operating costs will be based on a fixed amount, determined in advance, for each case, according to one of 467 diagnosis related groups (DRGs) into which a case is classified. The prospective payment will be considered payment in full; hospitals are prohibited from charging beneficiaries more than the statutory deductible and coinsurance.

The HCFA plan replaces the retrospective cost reimbursement system and the cost-per-case limits and rate of increase ceiling created by the Tax Equity and Fiscal Responsibility Act of 1982 (TEFRA), P.L. 97-248, for most hospitals. In addition, through fiscal year 1985, payments for Medicare inpatient hospital costs under the prospective payment system will be no more or less than projected under the TEFRA provisions.

Cost data from previous years will be used by HCFA to develop a fixed rate per DRG. Medicare will pay a hospital a flat rate for each of 467 DRGs. If patient treatment in a DRG category costs a hospital less than this rate, the hospital keeps the surplus as profit. This is the first time that the government has endorsed such profit-taking by nonprofit hospitals. If, however, patient treatment in a DRG category costs a hospital more than the prespecified Medicare DRG rate, the hospital absorbs the loss. Because of the varying expertise of different hospitals in various diagnostic categories, there will be DRGs which will make money for some hospitals and which will lose money for others.

Overall, the HCFA Prospective Payment Policy incorporates those elements of the programs piloted in New Jersey and other states that can be easily administered on a national level. Discharged patients will be categorized into 467 groups based upon diagnosis, age, treatment procedure, discharge status, and sex. The program began nationwide on the hospitals' first accounting period on October 1, 1983. It will progress in a "stepped" or "layered" fashion, phasing in over a three-year period as follows:

- In the first year 25% of the payment will be based on regional DRG rates, and a 75% weighting will be based on the hospital's historic cost experience.
- In the second year 50% of the payment will be based on a combination of national and regional DRG rates (25% national, 75% regional); 50% of the payment will be based on each hospital's last experience.
- In the third year 75% of the payment will be based on a combination of national and regional DRG rates (50% national, 50% regional); 25% of the payment will be based on each hospital's cost experience.
- In the fourth year 100% of the payment will be based upon national DRG rates.

In contrast with New Jersey and other DRG prospective payment systems, the national system will apply only to Medicare, not to all third-party payers. The national DRG category rates will be adjusted for rural and urban hospitals within nine census regions. Further, in addition to hospitals' historical cost data, rates will be based on annual industry-wide increase in hospital costs. For example, rates will be updated in fiscal years 1984 and 1985, using an index of the costs of goods and services purchased by hospitals plus one percentage point. After fiscal year 1985, DRG rate increases will be set according to the opinion of a commission of experts.

Also, in contrast with New Jersey's and other states' implementations, under the HCFA Prospective Payment Policy, capital-related costs will be excluded from the prospective rate and will be progressively instituted as follows:

- For the first 3 years of implementation capital costs other than return on equity will be reimbursed on a reasonable basis.
- Return on equity will be reimbursed at the same rate as the average interest rate on the Medicare Hospital Insurance Trust Fund, which is down one and one-half times from the current rate.
- After October 1, 1986, all capital costs, including return on equity, will be prospectively reimbursed.

Direct and indirect teaching costs will be handled very similarly to the manner in which they have been treated in New Jersey.

- Direct teaching costs—including the costs of nursing education programs—will continue to be paid on a reasonable-cost basis. They will be excluded from the prospective payment determinations.
- Indirect teaching expenses will be reimbursed at twice the amount of the teaching adjustment under the Tax Equity Fiscal Responsibility Act (TEFRA).

New Jersey and other states have implemented an extensive appeals process by which hospitals who believe they have somehow been misclassified under one DRG category or another can appeal these decisions. HCFA's plan is rather limited and, if used, opens the hospital's record for in-depth scrutiny. While the HCFA plan requires hospitals to contract with professional review organizations to review the quality of care provided, the appropriateness of Medicare admissions, and the appropriateness of care to patients designated as outliers, the extensiveness of the appeals process seen in New Jersey has not been replicated by HCFA. It may well be that the administrative complexities of administering appeals processes compelled the legislators to leave their adoption to individual state discretion.

Concerning state options for bypassing the DRG system, the Secretary of Health and Human Services can permit alternative cost control systems so long as these do not result in Medicare expenditures above those under the DRG system. The criteria for these systems would be discretionarily set by the Secretary. A waiver for such exceptions would be submitted to the Secretary.

Excepted from the HCFA Prospective Payment Plan would be psychiatric, long-term care, children's hospitals, and rehabilitation hospitals. Also excepted would be hospitals in Puerto Rico and the territories.

Physicians will not be reimbursed according to medical diagnoses. The Secretary, however, will be required to collect data and to report to Congress concerning this issue by December 31, 1984, concerning the advisability and feasibility of including physician payments in DRG rates.

Quality control and system monitoring are to be implemented in relation to admission patterns and DRG categories. This kind of monitoring is already part of the total cost limit program required by the 1982 law. For prospective payment, the medical review mechanism will identify unusual changes in the volume of admissions, case mix, total reimbursement, and discharge status. The cause of any such fluctuations will be investigated. Additionally, a system of DRG verification will be implemented to assure that the DRGs assigned to individual cases are correct, focusing in particular on their tendency to creep into costlier classifications.

As Bisbee (1982) stated, "A change to DRG-based reimbursement would involve a major repositioning of the 'carrots and sticks' that influence hospital behavior." In this sense the new system has effectively plunged health care into the competitive world of business. The system's incentives for efficiency, along with the decreasing demand for inpatient hospital services, are the new forces driving health care toward a competitive marketplace. All of this requires health care professionals to acquire new kinds of managerial skills. From the perspective of expenditure and percentage of the gross national product, health care is the largest business in the United States. How nursing will adapt to the demand for professional restructuring to accommodate the requirements of this business will be considered below. What is important as a beginning is that we as nursing professionals immediately become informed of the implications of the new legislation that is quickly rendering obsolete our customary ways of looking at our work.

CORDT: the federal government's monitoring system

One of the most dramatic historical developments in relation to the DRG reforms is the introduction of the Central Office and Regional Dispersal Terminal Network (CORDT) as an example of the measures which the Federal government is adopting to enforce this transition. Tucked away in an office in HCFA's Baltimore headquarters is the nucleus of a nationwide network of computers to track hospitals' every move under the prospective payment system. This will enable HCFA, its regional offices, and soon fiscal intermediaries, to keep close tabs on the hospitals covered by the Medicare payment system. This Central Office and Regional Dispersal Terminal Network (CORDT) will enable HCFA to have the necessary data to prove or disprove that proprietary hospitals will make a windfall profit under the Prospective Payment System (PPS). This will be accomplished by monitoring a hospital's case mix history. Indeed, the centerpiece of the CORDT system is the Admission Pattern Monitoring (APM), which is CORDT's most effective means to detect admission abuses. It is more than a policing system. Like the DRG system itself on which it is based, CORDT is also a tool that can streamline management in the hospitals on the system. But let us understand some of the details of the CORDT system.

Approximately 1500 hospitals are currently under the HCFA prospective payment system and they are monitored by CORDT. Further, all individual acute care hospitals will be on the prospective payment system network by fiscal year 1984. The CORDT network monitors every readmission executed within seven days of discharge, with the rationale that this kind of return of patients for further treatment tends to avoid cost ceilings as they are currently imposed. Other cost-increasing activities monitored are transfers from acute-care units to distinct units that are excluded from the Prospective Payment System's ceilings. These are watched closely by CORDT in each hospital on the system.

Further, all transfers from Prospective Payment System hospitals to those still based on cost-based reimbursement will be closely monitored to prevent avoidance of payment ceilings. As a further measure, 5% of all admissions will be sampled randomly by the CORDT system to determine whether services are necessary and appropriate. All day and cost outliers will be watched for their tendency to avoid cost ceilings. Also, all permanent insertions of pacemakers as well as all other surgical procedures will be closely scrutinized for possible misclassification of other less costly operations in these high-level reimbursement slots.

A little more detail here with regard to APM will also help to clarify the degree to which this system will be able to effectively enforce the prospective payment system. Admissions Pattern Monitoring (APM) involves entering data generated from reviews of hospital admissions records either by the fiscal intermediary or the Professional Review Organization (PRO). These data are fed into an IBM 4341 computer located in Baltimore. These data together assemble a profile of each hospital, compared with the hospital's previous history. This is also compared with other hospitals in their various regions, their states, and nationwide. If hospitals are found to have questionable admissions patterns, APM triggers a corrective action program. PSRO/PRO or fiscal intermediaries discuss educational activities designed to correct the questionable admissions patterns. In addition, the PSRO/PRO or intermediary intensifies its review of all of the hospital's future admissions, focusing on specific diagnoses or physician cases. These intensifications may even involve preadmissions reviews as well as payments for inappropriate admissions. The most punitive step is civil monetary penalties, which may be imposed on the hospital with the questionable admissions policies. Some leading authorities see steps taken by HCFA to safeguard quality of care as being no more than a pretext for cost containment without real impact on quality.

But we are meeting here to discuss the impact of the new DRG prospective payment system on "Health Care Management and the Health Professions." So now I will turn to how the new system will affect us as managers.

CONCEPTUALIZING DRG: CATEGORIES AND STRATEGIES

The DRG system has been approached by health care professionals with a sense of mystery that the complexity of its origin has generated. I would like to dispel some of this sense of mystery by outlining the goals of DRG, its principal categories, and the strategies for their implementation.

The hospital product

First, and most important, DRG is an attempt to define and conceptualize a "product" of an industry that had previously neglected to do so. This product is comprised by the specific set of outputs received by patients. The "output" that the hospital provides is defined in terms of hours of nursing care, medications, laboratory tests. The costs, or "inputs" required for the creation or provision of this service-output are labor (including nursing and other staff salaries), material, and equipment used (Fetter and associates, 1980).

Different patients receive different amounts and types of services which heretofore were priced inaccurately under the per diem system of reimbursement. By conceptualizing the hospital output as "products" used by different patients, the authors of the DRG proposal conceptualize the hospital as a multiproduct firm, "with a product line that in theory is as extensive as the number of patients it serves" (Fetter and associates, 1980). The particular product purchased, selected, or provided is defined by the researchers in terms of diagnosis. Some "products" require more hospital resources than others and are therefore considered to be more complex—and expensive. The relative proportions of the various types of cases treated by a particular hospital are called its case mix.

Internal management of efficiency and effectiveness are not served by the per diem criteria of hospital performance, which have been aggregate indicators: cost per patient-day, percent occupancy, and mortality rate. Patient-days of care and number of admissions or discharges have been used to describe hospital output under the per diem system. According to Fetter and associates (1980), diagnosis related groups were developed "to evaluate, compare, and provide relevant feedback regarding hospital performance." To do this they require identification of the specific products provided by the institution. In order to treat the large numbers of consumers demanding hospital products, the "consumers" must be classified by type. The method that Fetter and associates (1980) follow in defining these consumer types is classification by case diagnosis, demographic characteristics, and therapeutic attributes. The researchers note

The means of defining hospital case mix for this purpose is the construction and application of a classification scheme comprised of subgroups of patients possessing similar clinical attributes and output utilization patterns. This involves relating demographic, diagnostic and therapeutic characteristics of patients to the output they are provided so that cases are differentiated by only those variables related to the condition of the patient (e.g., age, primary diagnosis) and treatment process (e.g., operations) that affect his utilization of the hospital's facilities.

Management information implications inherent in DRG

The researchers (Fetter and associates, 1980) then note, in one sentence, the major cost-saving and managerial component of the DRG system. "These groups or patient classes may then be useful for certain applications in patient care *monitoring, budgeting, cost control, reimbursement, and planning*" (emphasis added). These cost control features, oriented to clinically based diagnostic categories, assign cost accounting indexes and managerial strategies to the hospital product. For the first time, the hospital has become an industry with a product the price of which can be managed and monitored by the caregivers themselves as the product is dispensed.

The researchers determined that the classification scheme should have the following attributes:

1. It must be interpretable medically, with subclasses of patients from homogenous diagnostic categories. That is, when the patient classes are described to physicians, they should be able to relate to these patients and be able to identify a particular patient management process for them.
2. Individual classes should be defined on variables that are commonly available on hospital abstracts and are relevant to output utilization, pertaining to either the condition of the patient or the treatment process.
3. There must be a manageable number of classes, preferably in the hundreds instead of thousands, that are mutually exclusive and exhaustive. That is, they must cover the entire range of possible disease conditions in the acute-care setting without overlap.
4. The classes should contain patients with similar expected measures of output utilization.
5. Class definitions must be comparable with similar expected measures of output utilization.

The classification categories were coded using the International Classification of Diseases, Adapted for Use in the United States, Eighth Revision (ICDAS) and the Hospital Adaptation of ICDA, Second Edition (HICDA2).

These coding schemes "provide a classification of conditions of morbidity and mortality for statistical reporting purposes as well as for information retrieval" (Fetter and associates, 1980). Hence the numbers attached to each diagnostic category that have traditionally alienated large numbers of persons intimidated by computer data.

Let us now see how this research has been translated into practice by the new prospective payment system.

DRG AS A MANAGEMENT INFORMATION SYSTEM

It should be noted, first and foremost, that the Yale researchers who designed the DRG system conceptualized it as a management tool. In their statement concerning the major cost saving and managerial component of the DRG system, Fetter and associates (1980) noted, "These groups or patient classes may then be useful for certain applications in patient care *monitoring, budgeting, cost control, reimbursement, and planning.*" Similarly, Bisbee and Bachofer (1980) underline the importance of the very structure of the DRG system itself as a management tool. They note

> Case mix is important for management purposes because, along with the volume of patients admitted during the year, it influences the resources that a hospital will use. Staffing levels, capital equipment and the type and quantity of supplies to be ordered are all influenced by the type of patients that will be admitted to the hospital. An effective case mix system could enable the administrator to analyze the types of patients being admitted, to estimate the amount and type of resources required to treat those patients, and to monitor performance based on the types of patients actually admitted.

And they continue

> There are four potential management applications of case mix information:
> 1. Resource allocation including planning and budgeting
> 2. Pricing including rate setting and financial planning
> 3. Cost and efficiency control including standard setting, measurement of performance and productivity management
> 4. Quality control including utilization review and quality assurance

Thus the architects of the DRG program themselves find, inherent in the system's structure, a management information function.

The prospective payment system has been applauded by proregulation forces as an effective cost-containment mechanism and a fair way to balance the books. But we now have seen that it is a management tool and that this is primarily true because it encourages the integration of clinical and financial records into one document: the patient discharge record now located in the medical records department. The issue which we must now entertain is: how will all of this alter the nature of the modern hospital environment? How will the places where we work day-to-day be altered by the introduction of the prospective payment system? To best answer this question we should briefly

examine the results of the system's piloting in hospitals in the state of New Jersey. These results were most prominently achieved in the areas of
- Decentralization of authority
- Organizational flattening or restructuring
- Increased involvement of physicians in management
- Increased computerization
- The development of the team approach to management

From the results that were observed after two years of operating under a HCFA pilot system, we can draw some conclusions and make some predictions concerning the effect of the national DRG management information system.

New Jersey model

In New Jersey we saw changes in hospitals involving decentralization or flattening out of the organizational structure that comprises the hospital environment. This involves increased participation in the management process as the result of increased accessibility to the clinical and financial records' combination in the medical records office. Information is now available to all by the nature of the computer systems which use prospective payment categories to manage the hospital product.

Many organizational changes are gradually falling into place as a result of the new system. The most prominent of these is participative management and decentralization. There is particularly noticeable a movement downward in allocation of management authority. The head nurse and first-line managers, for example, become much more important because they control allocation of resources. If these individuals have the information based on the case and cost per case and cost and utilization of resources per case they can become more cost conscious and therefore productive in the allocation of nursing resources. The head nurse is, then, in a pivotal position to control cost.

Because of this decentralization of authority, all other departments must enhance their collaboration with medical records; the medical record is newly appointed financial record of today. Nursing—and all of the other departments for that matter—must work out a good relationship with the medical records department to assign staff correctly. Either medical records personnel or nursing personnel may be responsible for accurate record keeping, but *who does what* must be firmly established and the personnel responsible must be checked to determine whether the information recorded is accurate.

A good example concerning the far-reaching effect of the new system in all departments is seen in the case of a hospital whose laboratory work had been performed *after* patient admission under the old, retrospective payment system. Under the new system, however, much more of the testing is currently conducted *before* admission in new laboratory facilities designed for faster turnaround. While there was an initially larger cost outlay for new lab equipment, the patient length of stay was significantly reduced for a long-run overall saving. The point of this is that, under the old system, these kinds of issues never surfaced from beneath the logjam of day-to-day operations to permit strategic planning for cost reduction rather than moment-to-moment reacting to one short-run crisis situation after another. Under the new system we can conceptualize the management of information in this way for cost-saving decision making by one department after another. In this way we can begin to understand DRG will multiply savings geometrically, not only in New Jersey, but nationwide, after a relatively short time.

Other developments that are resulting from case mix include the extension of hospital services out into the community to reduce length of stay by keeping certain types of treatment out of the hospital altogether. Instances of the replacement of costly hotel-type room and board hospitalization by free-standing ambulatory surgery centers, occupational health centers, and rural health care clinics are multiplying because alternatives to long-term length of stay are increasingly sought.

Let us take a look now at the way in which this changing environment is altering the roles of the actors within it. We will examine the effect of the new prospective payment system on the Board, the chief executive officer, the doctors, the nurses, and a new actor, the DRG Coordinator.

BOARDS OF TRUSTEES

Before the prospective payment system's inception, hospital boards remained aloof from the day-to-day operation of the facility. Under the new system the boards will become more actively involved in running the organization day to day and will hold the chief executive officer more accountable than previously. The previous image of the typical board member will alter from that of the philanthropic community-minded person to that of the businessperson or executive. The board will actively recruit businesspeople in order to increase cost consciousness, but it is hoped that this will not be accomplished at the expense of attention to quality of care. As we will see later, nursing can play an active role in this area. Indeed the board's relationship with the medical and nursing staff will remain paramount. Increased controls that will be placed on medical staff to reduce costs will inevitably cause conflicts. It should be noted particularly that the granting of hospital privileges to physicians will be scrutinized more carefully and the individual physician's case mix efficiency record will be evaluated. The physicians who consume a higher percentage of hospital resources by treating cost-ineffective patients will be less likely to be granted hospital privileges.

The major issue will be: who really controls the hospital—the physicians or the board? We know that the court has ruled in the *Darling* case that the board of trustees has full responsibility and accountability for governing the hospital.

IMPACT ON CEOs

A recent statistic shows that, since the inception of the prospective payment system, there has been a 40% turnover among hospital administrators nationwide. Can anyone point to a *more* significant statistic concerning the impact of the new system? To more fully understand the changing role of the CEO, it is important to obtain an understanding of the changing position that hospitals occupy both in the economic community and in the community-at-large. In this connection, Johnson (1982) indicates that the general freestanding community hospital will no longer be the cornerstone of the health care field. It will have been replaced either by a vertically or horizontally integrated health care delivery system. The vertical system will most likely result from the evolution of community hospitals. The horizontal systems will be the result of regional or national hospital chains that will be investor-owned or religious. More independent hospitals will take shelter in multihospital systems and networks. In essence, the hospital environment is changing to become more like the huge, multinational corporate environment.

Therefore, the role of the hospital chief executive officer will be more structured and less autonomous. The new prospective payment system elevates the responsibility of chief executive officers insofar as their role will now extend to encouraging admission of more profitable patients and discouraging admission of less profitable patients. In essence, the CEO will become more similar to his counterpart in the rest of the business world. In this regard, he will be held more accountable for his administrative decisions, and to the extent necessary to meet this accountability, he will hold the physician responsible for contributing his share to the institution's profits. This will inevitably lead to conflict between the CEO's new role and that of the physician. This diminishes the role of some doctors and other health care providers in making these decisions.

While the CEOs may be members of the hospital board, they must primarily be visible and accessible to the hospital community. This is crucial to assess the efficiency with which it is meeting the health care needs of the community at large. This visibility represents a shift away from the primarily financial role that the CEO used to assume; the large corporate staffs available for provision of financial expertise will provide all of the computational and economic expertise that any top manager could desire. What the corporate structure will require, however, will be someone who can talk to medical personnel with clinical expertise. According to Johnson (1983): "Successful CEOs will need developed political skills. One highly valued skill will be the ability to negotiate and compromise among diverse viewpoints and still maintain progress. Such consensus-building skills require knowledge of who to involve at what moment, and how much to expect of each party."

CEOs will also want a management team that can scrutinize operations as well as resolve battles, and initiate corrective actions to keep costs down without reducing quality. First, from a top management perspective, the hospital has traditionally been divided into distinct departments conceptualized as medical staff, administration, finance, nursing, and laboratory. Under the new system, however, a new department, actually in existence before but previously understood as part of the financial department, emerges in its own right. This is the medical records department.

This organizational change is important for a variety of reasons. The most important of these, however, is that the new system operates on a practical, day-to-day basis to merge clinical and financial data in the same computerized system and in the same management information reports. This never happened under the old system which organized the financial data separately from the clinical data. Under the old system, the medical and the financial information systems operated separately as two autonomous organizational spheres of influence connected only by limited communication at the time of discharge and billing.

We now turn to examine how the clinical side of this new equation is becoming more closely integrated with and affected by cost consciousness.

IMPACT ON MDs

Physicians will hardly emerge unscathed by the new DRG system (Maraldo, 1983). Medical practice will be restructured to some extent as hospital administrators are forced to intervene in the clinical management of patients. Economist Paul Feldstein predicts increasing competition among physicians for positions in hospitals, as well as with other health providers in the future. And he predicts the further erosion of real physician income. A freeze on physicians' fees is becoming reality. For example, in California, physicians recently volunteered to freeze their salaries, and, on the national level, the new Reagan budget also encourages caps on physicians' fees. Further, the new prospective payment law mandates a study on physicians' fees to be completed by 1986. Certainly, the political repercussions among the medical community in reaction to this government intervention in the determination of their income are predictable.

Because the physician prescribes for the consumption of most hospital resources, the medical staff must be educated concerning the implications of the new payment system. CEOs are cognizant of this resource consumption pattern. Therefore, on a national level, they are replicating New Jersey's policy of employing medical directors who will be responsible for monitoring physicians' practice for cost effectiveness. Using DRG data the medical directors, working with the department chiefs will police physicians' practice and will require corrective action for those physicians who are "cost" or "length of stay" outliers, themselves. Major hospital chains, such as NME, have already begun developing physician practice protocols using DRGS. Physicians will recognize that their practices are being monitored and will need ongoing feedback concerning what inpatient cases cost.

The AMA, recognizing that the new payment system will place controls on medical practice, will probably encourage physicians to look to the system to identify areas in which they can gain positions of control. For this reason there is already an increasing trend for physicians to become hospital chief executive officers. From this position chief executive officers can exercise power, influence, and control. For this reason the AMA is encouraging physicians to take courses in hospital economics and organizational management. And with physicians in the CEO position the hospital management picture will resemble hospital management in the past and even now in both military and public hospitals. The physicians of the future who will enter these CEO positions will be better prepared in hospital management and organizational dynamics than their predecessors.

While some physicians will aggressively resist the prospective payment system, others will recognize it for what it is and will work with it. Physicians must be actively involved in utilization review and the hospitals' quality assurance program. They will recognize that the payment system is not designed to encourage a reduction in quality. Indeed, some physicians are "movers" and "shakers" under the new system. I would like to point to one such individual, Dr. Nester, Vice President, Quality Assurance, Overlook Hospital, Summit, New Jersey. Dr. Nester has become a spokesman for the medical community concerning how quality can be maintained and enhanced under the prospective payment system. I am sure that there are many other physicians like Dr. Nester and that this group will continue to increase in numbers.

The "unbundling" process involves the offering of a service in private physician office settings that was previously available primarily in the hospital. This unbundling process takes business away from the hospital and will ultimately cause conflict between the Board of Trustees, the CEOs, and the physicians. This conflict will increase with a continued loss of income to the hospital. The federal government is currently applying limits to the unbundling process through regulation.

During the past several years there has been much delegation of services once performed by physicians themselves, to nurse practitioners and physician assistants. There is now an extensive literature comparing the primary care services provided by nurse practitioners and physician assistants with those provided entirely by family practitioners and general internists. The research contains two major findings: (1) nurse practitioners and physician assistants provide care that is comparable to that provided by family practitioners and general internists, and (2) nurse clinicians and nurse practitioners provide a more personal kind of care that measurably inproves compliance, reduces symptomatic complaints, eliminates return visits, and shortens hospitalization. The productivity and cost benefit figures are favorable when nurse clinicians or nurse practitioners render these services. As the competition between physicians and both nurse clinicians and nurse practitioners increases, these findings will be useful in antitrust proceedings before the Federal Trade Commission in support of the validity of treatment and services rendered by nurse clinicians and nurse practitioners.

IMPACT ON NURSING

The impact of the prospective payment system on nursing must be related to what has happened in New Jersey. There, (1) organizational flattening, (2) decentralization of authority, and the (3) introduction of the team approach have characterized the transition to the prospective payment system. These three areas are not new to nursing. As a matter of fact, they have been identified as major concerns in the nursing community by three national studies: (1) the recently conducted National Commission on Nursing study, (2) the Institute of Medicine Study, and (3) the Magnet study. The findings of all three studies support nursing's quest for involvement in the decision making process in both the clinical and administrative realms.

Nursing, because of its percentage of the hospital budget and its labor-intensiveness, is usually the first area in which a hospital administrator will cut costs. Many key hospital officials have made public statements regarding the potential cost savings that would accrue from using cheaper labor in lieu of registered nurses. To cite an example, when the Medicare cutbacks began, National Medical Enterprises dispatched a team of corporate consultants to their 90 hospitals. The team discovered that a number of hospitals could improve the "effective level of operation by altering the mix of staffing" in the nursing department, largely through increased use of LPNs and aides instead of registered nurses. Superior Care, Inc., stated in an interview with *AMA News* that, to keep expenses down, Superior Care would use an increasing number of unskilled aides rather than LPNs and RNs. Eventually, they believed, insurance contracts would probably even stipulate the use of skilled aides instead of costly nurses.

In some areas only a long-run understanding, coupled with some hard lessons, will create a bond between nursing and management. But it must be remembered that the bond will come because management needs nursing's clinical expertise. For example, the nurse executive's relationship with the CEO will be strengthened once the nursing executive demonstrates that cutting nursing staff can only bring short-run financial gains. While it may take time, the CEO must be shown in dollars and cents in computerized management reports, that short-run savings from cutting nursing staff generally evaporate as the patient's length of stay increases and quality of care is diminished. The future health care system with a cost-conscious chief executive officer at the helm will have found that quality of care is the competitive edge. The wise chief executive officer will also rapidly find that the best insurer of quality care is the nurse executive.

Similarly, interaction between nursing and medicine under the new prospective payment system will produce positive and negative outcomes depending upon the choices made by members of both groups. On the positive side, nurses and physicians can begin to collaborate and to appreciate mutual goals in practice. Nurses and physicians can cooperate to improve the hospital's efficiency by collaborating more in discharge planning and patient education. They will need to communicate better to help to improve their respective treatment protocols. The kind of integrated medical record system that will be found increasingly in computerized departments will be mutually advantageous to doctors and nurses in problem solving in both patient care planning and treatment.

The most singularly identifiable negative components that will affect the physician/nursing relationship during the coming years will be the oversupply of physicians and the search for cost-effective providers of health care. As a result of the work performed by Fagin, nursing is being identified by third-party payers as an alternative to more expensive health care provision. Major insurance company executives share this awareness. They see that, in this new situation, physicians will attempt to reclaim activities previously classified under the domain of nursing that will now be considered to be under the domain of medical practice. We can anticipate that the AMA will lobby for increased gatekeeping to screen out nurses and other cost-effective alternative health care providers. Nursing and medicine will become competitors in the health care marketplace. The time is ripe to establish joint practice committees to redefine professional territorial imperatives.

Nursing's professionalization can occur under the new prospective payment for several reasons. I will, however, draw your attention to only two major reasons:

1. Patient stays in the hospital will be shortened, forcing sicker patients into the community.
2. Emphasis will be placed on wellness and prevention.

These two factors will affect the two goals of nursing that distinguish it from medicine: (1) promotion of wellness and (2) orientation to the community. That is not to say that we will abdicate our role in the hospital. On the contrary, nursing's function in the inpatient setting will become, as mentioned earlier, pivotal. Nursing will be recognized as the coordinator of inpatient services on the health/wellness continuum on a 24-hour basis. For those nurses who continue to practice in the hospital, the professional skill mix will change. While there will probably be fewer registered nurses, expert nursing clinicians will nonetheless be needed to care for the complex short-stay patients. What this means to nursing and the health care manager is that nursing will be recognized as the hospital's competitive edge. Those executives who invest in nursing will certainly obtain a substantial return.

Nursing, however, must gear up for this change. We must define for everyone what nursing is and place a price tag on the product. Nursing must begin to market itself, approaching all clients with the attitude that nursing provides the valuable services that they need on a 24-hour basis. It is nursing's quick assessment and proper intervention that prevent death in life-threatening situations because nursing is on the front lines in all such situations. Nursing must educate consumers concerning its valuable role so that they will become nurse advocates in the same way that nursing is the patients' advocate.

One thing is certain, however, and that is that the nurse will continue to be in a pivotal position to make the new system work. The nurse is the link between quality and cost. But first she must be able to identify nursing as a revenue-producing cost center rather than as part of overhead and to identify areas of cross-subsidization and downward skill substitution. In this regard, Shaffer (1984) has suggested a protocol for nurse executives entering the prospective payment system. Some of the protocol includes

- Identification of the nursing case mix profile
- Identification of the staff mix needed to care for the case mix identified
- Identification of nonhuman resources needed to care for those patients
- Development of standards of nursing practice for case mix
- Identification of nonnursing activities performed—cross-subsidization and downward skill substitution—by staff nurses themselves
- Determination of which support services should be available on a 24-hour basis
- Utilization of case mix to collaborate with admitting in the assignment of rooms
- Assessment of work flow into nursing and what nursing care flows out of the nursing department
- Determination by case mix where decentralization can be employed
- Utilization of management information reports to invoke cost consciousness on the part of nursing staff
- Utilization of quality assurance audits to correlate length of stay with nursing cost
- Correlation of nursing productivity and case mix to examine correlate productivity with DRGs for hospitals nationwide

This protocol presents the major areas requiring in-depth analysis within the nursing division. It will provide some insight into the areas of nursing that need both internal and external assessment.

DRG COORDINATOR'S ROLE

With this kind of change to cope with, some hospitals have found it expeditious to supplement the efforts of the administration with the appointment of a

DRG Coordinator. Beginning with the prospective payment system's start-up in New Jersey in 1980, these new figures have helped to smooth the transition by discouraging inefficiency in the hospital's various departments and showing by example how computerized reports can raise cost consciousness and increase quality of care. By monitoring case mix and utilization patterns, the DRG Coordinator can interface with physicians to improve the hospital's financial position. While the DRG Coordinators can be described as technicians and watchdogs they really are medical records technicians who are responsible for analyzing the DRG reports and identifying physicians or ancillary departments that are causing their facilities to lose money. While some background in financial areas is important for this position it is also commonly occupied by clinical personnel, including nurses and even retired physicians.

Different kinds of reports are required for management personnel in different positions—data alone are meaningless unless they are organized and presented as meaningful information. The key to accomplishing this indispensable function afforded and required by the prospective payment system is a sophisticated information system, and the DRG Coordinator can play a pivotal transitional role in interpreting and implementing such a system under much more of a team approach. Indeed, only the reduction of the time lapse between the collection of data and their availability for management's use afforded by *computers* has made the DRG system possible in the first place.

COMPUTERS

So in a sense, the computer revolution is the historical spawning ground that has brought the prospective payment system into existence, and in many ways the learning process involved in becoming *computer literate* parallels the learning process involved in becoming familiar with and expert at using the new prospective payment system. Computer reports—the fruit of an information management system—intimidate many people in organizations undergoing management transitions in the same way that computers have traditionally been used to intimidate everyone from the top to the bottom of the society at large.

Management personnel have traditionally understood that getting information and getting hands-on contact with reports, files, records, data, facts, and statistics is power. Now, these sources of power are changing, and this is causing an enormous increase in anxiety. Well that it should, because power relationships are entirely reconfigured by the implementation of new technology.

Errors in coding patients' diagnoses according to the DRG system constitute the most difficult problem in the system's implementation. To rectify this pitfall, as in other problem areas of the system, not only the medical records department but also the financial and medical staff must be involved. The accurate completion and coding of the medical record and the patient's bill is paramount for the success of the DRG system and for the continued solvency of the hospital under the new federal monitoring constraints. The DRG Coordinator also plays a key role in coding these records.

THE CONSUMER

While I was specifically asked to address the impact that prospective payment will have on management and health care professionals, I would be remiss if I neglected to address the most important component in the delivery system: the consumer. It must be noted that the education of the consumer is imperative under the prospective payment system. Under the retrospective payment system the consumer was insulated from the true cost of health care. This will not be the case under the prospective payment system. In fact, the consumer will be expected to make choices between more and less expensive health care alternatives. In this connection it may safely be hypothesized that cost conscious consumers will choose less expensive options previously ignored. This choice may well be forced upon them as the trend among employers and insurance companies moves toward "wellness packages," such as weight control and exercise programs, as opposed to "illness options," such as hospitalization.

Competition in medical care, then, is likely to grow, not only because of the increase in the supply of physicians but also because groups of powerful consumers who have the means to shop for cost-effective care are applying their initiatives in the health care market for the first time. These consumers include corporations, unions, and state and federal governments. There are also increasing numbers of consumers, including business coalitions who are not only asking such key questions as "Why are your prices higher in this hospital than in other hospitals?" but who are also publishing the answers to these questions for all to see.

Recognizing the importance of the consumer's role in this system, the Health Care Financing Administration (HCFA) in a *Federal Register* request for proposals, called for demonstration projects and studies directed toward educating the consumer. HCFA also encouraged studies that would extend the prospective payment system to alternatives to hospitalization such as: (1) hospices, (2) continuity care centers, (3) skilled nursing facilities, and (4) long-term care. HCFA has recently awarded a grant to Rensselaer Polytechnic Institute for the use of DRGs in the long-term care setting. This model is based on Resource Utilization Groups (RUGs), an alternative diagnosis related group system based on the resources consumed in the performance of the activities of daily living.

ETHICS

We already know that the prospective payment system is going to produce (1) cases that are profitable and that are therefore winners and (2) cases that are not profitable and that are therefore losers. According to Dowling (1979), the provider is now at risk: the system sanctions rewards for efficient management and sanctions losses for inefficient management. Therefore, in order for the hospital to remain solvent it must maximize profitable admissions. The multihospital system looks upon the prospective payment system as an encourager of competition and an enhancer of profits based on economies of scale. This creates the dilemma, "Who cares for the cases labeled as 'not profitable'?" This question cannot be answered within the scope of this presentation. I will, however, raise several issues that need be addressed in an examination of the ethics involved in an environment of scarce or limited resources. These include (1) the technological imperative, (2) criteria for allocation of scarce resources, and (3) limitations upon utilization of these resources once allocation decisions are made.

The technological imperative

We already understand the paradox that the very technological advances that have advanced health care have also caused its costs to skyrocket. The question arises, "Are we obligated to use the technology that we create?" Should every hospital have an NMR or a CAT scannner?

Criteria for the allocation of scarce resources

We know that the prospective payment system does not currently address kidney acquisition. We also know that the system closely monitors the insertion of pacemakers and the readmission of patients within seven days after discharge. These instances of allocation of scarce resources represent decision-making implicit within the system that must become more explicit as time goes on. With the advent of intensive care units we must examine the criteria for admitting patients to these units when the beds are filled. Some patients are being refused open heart surgery because they are smokers.

Limitations upon utilization of these resources once allocation decisions are made

On a daily basis, in almost every hospital in the United States, the questions arise, (1) "to resuscitate or not to resuscitate," and (2) "when shall we pull the plug?" The well-known Quinlan example cannot be ignored any more than "Baby Doe." Hospitals have a duty to assist their staff in making these kinds of decisions by providing protocols such as "Do Not Resuscitate Criteria" as well as consultants and inhouse Ethics Committees consisting of clergy, psychologists, and other counselors.

Summary

Physicians, government regulators, and third-party payers all agree that health care must be rationed, but they don't want to be the ones to do it. If we say that hospitals are the ones that ought to be responsible for rationing health care, then we must learn to be very specific in identifying who we mean by "hospitals." Do we mean the Boards of Trustees, do we mean the doctors, or do we mean the nurses? People who have spent their entire careers trying to save lives unconditionally are now, in a time of scarce resources, being asked to decide who should or should not be saved. These health care professionals are thus being confronted with new kinds of dilemmas for which they have received little or no training or preparation. Our duty, then, must be to seek out and provide these professionals with this training and preparation, to meet the new kinds of decision-making that the system's increasingly limited resources will demand. This is as much the responsibility of the health care education process as is educational preparation for practice.

One thing is certain: hospitals must lobby for policy and legislative enactment reflecting societal consensus on the standards used to ration health care. This should create a more realistic climate in which people will understand the limitation inherent in our health care delivery system: everyone is not going to receive maximum optimal care provided in an equitable way across society. In all fairness, however, the consumers themselves must be involved in the hard decisions that determine the choices in the midst of scarce resources. This has already been initiated in family involvement in such decision-making as, "When should we pull the plug?"

CONCLUSION

As I noted at the beginning of this presentation, the Prospective Payment Assessment Commission (PROPAC) Commission is scheduled to recalibrate the DRGs in 1986 and the changes that we are experiencing will continue until cost effectiveness in health care is achieved. In the interim years, coping strategies are required to contain and alleviate the anxiety that we all face during what will prove to be a transitional era. To turn this anxiety to productive ends we must adopt a patient insistence and a firm hand to demand that *all* personnel learn to read the appropriate computerized reports. This is not possible without two prerequisites: (1) an effective information management system, and (2) a confused, anxious, but courageous group of employees highly motivated to be educated. These prerequisites explain my beginning this discussion of the prospective payment system with a review of developments at top management. This is the level at which the dollars currently exist in sufficient quantity to purchase the sophisticated computer technology required to properly manage a large organization in the closing decades of the twentieth century.

The new system has presented a nearly unprecedented opportunity for nursing and other hospital management personnel to establish closer ties. This includes both medical staff and financial staff. Physicians, heretofore excluded from the financial management of the hospitals, are becoming medical directors. Nursing managers will be working more closely with the physicians and financial administrative team as well as the medical records department.

In closing, as we have seen, the *raison d'être,* or in the terminology of the prospective payment system, the *product* of the hospital is patient care. This is what the institution sells and this is the commodity for which it is reimbursed. Nurse executives are the linking pins between quality and cost because they alone are in contact with the patients seven days a week, 24 hours a day. The nursing department is the leading edge for the hospital's public relations on a 24-hour basis. Nurse executives must learn that their staffs can no longer afford to be all things to all people at all times. They must develop a marketing plan for the products that they offer to the community. As competition increases, the patients will be drawn by the quality of patient care. The nurses have to understand how valuable the client contact is in this marketing approach that hospitals must increasingly adopt to remain competitive for scarce resources. There is one thing for us to keep in mind as we go out into the community: cost effectiveness and improvement in quality can go hand in hand under the prospective payment system. And if we in nursing play the game by the new rules, we can be the ones to prove it.

REFERENCES

Bisbee, G.: DRG concept generates mixed reaction in hospital industry as research continues, Fed. Am. Hosp. Rev. **13**(3):15-19, 1982.

Bisbee, G., and Bachofer, H.: Usefulness of case mix systems as a tool in hospital management must be determined, Hosp. Serv. Res. **2**(2):28-31, 1980.

Dowling, W.: Prospective rate setting: concept and practice, Top. Health Care Financ. **3**(2):7-38, 1979.

Fetter, R., Shin, Y., Freeman, J., Averill, R., and Thompson, J.: Case mix definition by diagnosis-related groups, Med. Care **18**(2):1-53, 1980.

Johnson, R.L.: New systems taking over as field's keystone, Mod. Healthcare **12**(1):47-50, 1982.

Johnson, R.L.: Era of responsibility: competition challenges CEOs to be tough-minded and to take risks, Hospitals, June 16, 1983.

Maraldo, P.: The world according to DRGs, National League for Nursing Public Policy Bulletin, vol. 2, no. 2, 1983.

Pointer, D., and Ross, M.: DRG cost-per-case management, Mod. Healthcare **14**:109-112, 1984.

Shaffer, F.: Nursing gears up for DRGs: management strategies. In Shaffer, F., editor: DRGs: changes and challenges, New York, 1984, National League for Nursing.

DRGs and nursing diagnosis

LUCILLE A. JOEL, Ed.D., R.N., F.A.A.N.

Prospective rate setting based on case mix calculations, infamously known as Diagnosis Related Groups (DRGs), promises to change the face of the health care delivery system. The reimbursement model put in place by Medicare in October of 1983 builds on these elements and additionally incorporates an incentive system for efficient management, and sequential steps in rate blending which eventually result in national standardization of cost. The nation has been propelled into this model with unprecedented speed. As we all strain to gear up for DRGs, one can look to the effect similar reimbursement mechanisms have had on nursing and health care in New Jersey. Various aspects of the case mix classification system (DRGs) and the reimbursement methodology were put into place in New Jersey before national adoption. As of January, 1984, some New Jersey hospitals have operated on DRGs for over three years. Though the reimbursement models are not mirror images of one another, there is enough similarity to extrapolate. The New Jersey system establishes identical rates for all third-party payers. The Medicare system addresses only 40% of the inpatient population in most states. The New Jersey Department of Health provides hospital-specific management reports and a formal process for grievance and appeal. Despite these minor variations in a theme, our experience will be similar.

Hospitals which survive, and even flourish, under DRGs become characterized by short length of stay, high volume, and complex case mix. These characteristics place a serious drain on the resources of the nursing department. Let us consider each characteristic separately. In these days of sophisticated technology, medical diagnosis, prescription, and stabilization of the treatment regimen can be accomplished quite expeditiously. Those patients who have an extended length of stay are more usually confined for care which has traditionally fallen within the province of nursing. At some point during a hospital confinement there is a shifting of balance from medicine to nursing as a priority. Patients are admitted for pathophysiological needs but remain because of deficits in self-care, the need for teaching and counselling, the development of community and family support systems, and so on. Complexity and cost within the DRG system is largely equated with length of stay. Those patients who are most costly and most complex are actually nursing intensive. The pressure from more nursing intensive patients is heightened by a pervasive pressure on every caretaker within the system to decrease length of stay. This fact is relative to both costly long-length-of-stay patients and shorter-length-of-stay patients whose time in the hospital must be further decreased. The high-volume characteristic presents additional problems. High volume refers to the number of individuals serviced within a reporting period, regardless of their length of stay. Shortened length of stay, together with the pressure to fill beds or operate at maximum capacity, creates more new admissions. Those of us who have nursed know that there is a certain amount of resource investment in new admissions which is unavoidable, regardless of the priority which nursing personally assumes for them. To confound this whole picture, sophisticated directors of nursing in our state report that sicker patients are being admitted. This remains opinion, but it would make sense. Physicians who serve as the hospital gatekeepers are trying to avoid admission where possible. Additionally, professional review organizations (PROs) focus on admission as well as discharge as crucial points in assessing utilization. It is likely that the result could be sicker admissions. The capacity issue speaks for itself. Where several years ago hospitals operating below 75% capacity were considered in jeopardy, leaders in nursing service administration in our state currently fear for any hospital that displays less than 85% occupancy. Indeed the most cost-efficient facilities are operating at over 110% occupancy. Day-of-admission programs have flourished.

It has been my objective to set the stage for the observation that nursing can no longer remain anonymous within a health care delivery system that predicts such an increased need for its services. Though common sense tells us the dramatic demand for nursing that the future holds, we have been negligent in developing any mechanism to quantify nursing resource use on a patient specific basis. This now holds serious implications for the profession. Moreover, until nursing can be detailed according to case mix, the reimbursement methodology will be unable to achieve maximum budget control. The DRG system predicts reasonable and usual hospital resource consumption on a patient specific basis. It becomes possible, drawing on the case mix information in the base year, to predict the extent to which laboratory, radiation, physiotherapy, oxygen therapy, and so on will be used in a budget period. The number of inpatient days can be likewise predicted. It becomes impossible to predict the extent of nursing resource use until that variable can be made case specific. In other words, 35% to 50% of the direct care budget in a hospital, which usually characterizes nursing, remains uncontrollable. This becomes a significant problem to rate setting.

What is needed is a case-specific measure of nursing resource consumption and, more specifically, a DRG-specific measure—since DRGs have become the unit of analysis. The New Jersey Department of Health has sought to begin to address this problem through its Relative Intensity Measures of nursing methodology (RIMs). Due to financial constraints which developed in their developmental period, RIMs reflect only the minutes of nursing resource invested in the care of patients. The independent variables used in calculations

---

BOX 1   **Case mix nursing performance study***

Need assessment categories and nursing diagnoses
A. Individual physiological integrity
    1. Cardiovascular function/activity
    2. Fluid-electrolyte levels
    3. G.I. function/activity
    4. G.U. function/activity
    5. Inflammatory response and immunity
    6. Mobility
    7. Nutritional pattern
    8. Respiratory function
    9. Skin integrity
    10. Sleep/rest activity
B. Interaction with immediate environment
    11. Physical comfort
    12. Communication pattern
    13. Consciousness
    14. Orientation
    15. Sensory functioning
C. Psychosocial
    16. Anxiety/fear level
    17. Aggressive behavior
    18. Body image
    19. Coping behavior, patient
    20. Coping behavior, family/significant other
    21. Self-acceptance
    22. Sexual functioning/sexuality
    23. Grieving
    24. Parenting behavior (toward pediatric clients)
D. Health education
    25. Ability to set health care goals
    26. Knowledge of health care regimen
    27. Self-care activity

---

*State of New Jersey, Department of Health.

are primary diagnosis, comorbidity or complications, surgical procedure, age, and admission status. Though much nursing relevant data was collected during the study period, none of it was used in the development of the RIMs allocation statistics. It is not that organized nursing in the state of New Jersey and consultants to the Project agreed that these variables were the most relevant but rather that there was no money to go further or to do differently. The New Jersey project, conducted in the late 70s, gathered data on 3500 patients and 64,000 shifts in eight hospitals. Nurses diagnosed the human responses they observed in their patients, and designated the acuity of the diagnosis. Diagnostic labels were selected from the list presented in Box 1. The acuity scale

BOX 2   **Nursing diagnosis (acuity) rating scale***

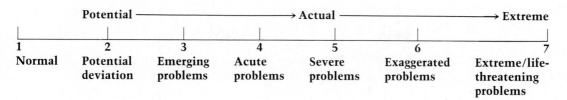

Potential ——————————————→ Actual ——————————————→ Extreme

1	2	3	4	5	6	7
Normal	Potential deviation	Emerging problems	Acute problems	Severe problems	Exaggerated problems	Extreme/life-threatening problems

    1 = Normal or no change (client able to move about freely with full range of motion of all extremities, good muscle tone, and no constraints or confinement related to pathology and/or treatment)

    2 = Potential deviation from normal

    3-4 = Actual deviation from normal (may be partial interruption, interference, or distortion of balance, locomotion, and/or muscular activity)

    5-6-7 = Severe deviation from normal (complete interruption, interference, or distortion of balance, locomotion, and/or muscular activity)

*State of New Jersey, Department of Health.

and its application to the category of mobility can be found in Box 2. The design was visionary for its time. Planning for primary analysis of this data are currently in process.

Case mix analysis to predict nursing resource use should begin with acute care, but not be limited to that setting. Long-term and home care will eventually face the case mix guillotine. In these settings nursing is more clearly a priority from the first patient contact. Investigation has already shown us that medical diagnosis bears little relationship to resource use in long-term care (Katz and associates, 1979). The predictive or independent variables should be simple, easily retrievable from summary abstracts, patient oriented, limited in number, and universal. It is likely that one variable could serve as a proxy for several others. It becomes questionable whether any nursing case mix system will find itself in favor if we are dealing with terms that are unintelligible to most practicing nurses. Should these variables be nursing diagnoses? They will be those factors in patients which are most predictive of nursing resource consumption. If nursing diagnoses hold that predictive ability, it would be logical to use them. In fact, the construction of resource allocation statistics using nursing diagnoses as the major variables could provide a test of their utility, and the degree to which they reflect the realities of practice. I do feel that there will be other elements which enter into the equation. In the acute care setting the medical diagnosis will always be a factor in calculating the nursing intensity, since one dimension of nursing activity is the dependent execution of the medical regimen. Additional factors are the functional status and self-care ability of the patient. The egalitarian relationship and self-care approach of nursing establish a situation where the patient and the nurse function as a singular unit. The nursing resources a patient uses to supplement, complement, maintain, or develop self-care ability are central to the relationship and resource consumption.

I am sure I have created more questions than I have answered. I would like to emphasize the need for immediate data collection to tease out those factors which are most predictive of nursing intensity. I urge us to let go of the defensiveness of our development years; display a new ego strength; and accept where medical diagnosis may continue to be a major element in calculation. I urge us to seek common language and maximum understanding at the bedside. I urge us not to "hold out" until we are able to predict all of the nursing resource use. Be content if our predictive control addresses 30 or 40 or 50%, or anything significant. The work of Dr. Brant Fries from Yale and Rensselaer is particularly impressive as he has developed the Resource Utilization Groups (RUGs) system to case mix long-term care (Fries and Cooney, 1984). The variables he defines in his work build on the proxy concept. He identifies four variables which predict about 40% of the resource use in long term care. His methodology is based on the logic that functional ability in one area may closely reflect human capabilities or limitations in others. Let us begin to search for answers; value the efforts of those who have been pioneers and risk takers; aim for simplicity because nothing else is useful; and postpone perfection. Remember that DRGs were painfully simplistic in their first application and refined through use. Any case mix methodology which nursing produces deserves equal courtesy and time to develop.

REFERENCES

Fries, B.E., and Cooney, L.M., Jr.: Unpublished report of research, Troy, N.Y., 1984. Rensselaer Polytechnic Institute.

Katz, S., Hedrich, S.C., and Henderson, N.S.: The measurement of long-term care needs and impact, Health Med. Care Syst. Rev. **2:**1-21, 1979.

Nursing diagnoses: key to quality assurance

ANN McCOURT, M.S., R.N.

At our National Conference in 1980, I stated that one of the newer and more challenging aspects of nursing diagnosis was its use in nursing quality assurance programs (McCourt, 1980). In the interim, both nursing diagnosis and nursing quality assurance have enjoyed increased professional acceptance. Both are still in various phases of implementation.

Quality assurance (QA) has taken on new dimensions and has been viewed from many perspectives. For some, it is a management information system; for others it is a tool for determining utilization of resources or a risk management system to decrease hospital liability. Nursing quality assurance (NQA) is a process used to evaluate and improve nursing care: evaluate by monitoring standards, improve by identifying and correcting problems. How better to assess the effectiveness of nursing care than to evaluate outcomes of the health problems which nurses diagnose and treat? I will focus on the relationship between nursing diagnosis and nursing quality assurance and address four distinct areas: the development of standards for nursing diagnosis; the application of standards to quality assurance; the influence of external controls; and future directions of nursing diagnosis and quality assurance.

Before nursing diagnosis can be effectively used in quality assurance, a firm foundation in nursing process must be laid and an NQA program must be fully implemented. In the nursing process, each patient should be assessed, his nursing diagnoses identified, and specific interventions documented. The effectiveness of the documented interventions should be routinely and systematically evaluated. Nursing quality assurance must be integrated with, but distinct from, the hospital-wide quality assurance program. Nursing must have its own quality assurance committee which sets priorities, determines topics for study, and facilitates changes in nursing practice. The complete commitment and support of nursing administration is essential.

Once nursing process and nursing quality assurance are operational, standards must be written for each nursing diagnosis. Standards should include both process and outcome criteria. The volume of nursing literature relating to process and outcome criteria for nursing diagnosis is increasing steadily. Most of the literature is helpful because it reflects critical thinking for guiding nursing care and teaching. Quality assurance nurses should be reluctant to adopt or adapt published criteria for *evaluation* purposes, unless there is clear

---

Examples of nursing diagnoses in this section are based on those used at New England Sinai Hospital, Stoughton, Mass.

evidence that the criteria have been clinically tested and are valid and reliable indicators of quality care. The consequences of accepting poorly written criteria could be disastrous and produce unreliable data on the quality of care delivered. There is no short cut. Writing process and outcome criteria for nursing diagnoses is one phase of development. Clinically testing the criteria is another. Evaluation of the criteria over a long period of time and in different settings is yet another. This is the direction we must pursue to produce standards/criteria which truly reflect the appropriateness and effectiveness of nursing care.

Using nursing diagnoses in nursing quality assurance is at once interesting, challenging, complex, and frustrating! A key to success is to have the quality assurance committee as well as the staff convinced that it is in their best interests to have criteria for guiding care. The staff must also realize that the same criteria will be used to evaluate their effectiveness as providers. Standards for nursing diagnoses can be used for both nursing process and for NQA.

Our experiences at New England Sinai Hospital may help demonstrate some aspects of the growth process in using nursing diagnoses in nursing quality assurance. New England Sinai Hospital is a 200-bed, JCAH accredited, chronic disease/rehabilitation hospital. Currently, standards are written for seven nursing diagnoses—all of which have been ratified by the staff and are in various stages of implementation. We have declared a moratorium on using additional standards for quality assurance purposes until the standards already implemented have been thoroughly tested. The completed nursing diagnosis standards include

Alteration in skin integrity: potential for decubitus ulcer
High risk for physical injury: potential for slips and falls
Self-care deficit: feeding, bathing, dressing, and toileting
Alteration in skin integrity: actual decubitus ulcer
Ineffective airway clearance
Ineffective breathing pattern
Alteration in comfort: chronic pain

The order is significant because it represents the priority-setting of the nursing quality assurance committee. The first two represent areas of risk management, areas which enjoy support from both nursing and hospital administration. Evidence of positive outcomes from implementation of these standards gained the nursing quality assurance committee's continued support for using nursing diagnosis. The third diagnosis, self-care deficit, represents the most common nursing diagnosis at New England Sinai. Over 90% of our patients have documented problems in this area. The remaining standards reflect special interest areas of the rehabilitation, pulmonary, and oncology nursing staffs. In some standards, the diagnostic category is listed first, followed by a specific diagnosis. This occurs when we find the category too broad for guiding interventions or measuring outcomes.

BOX	**Model for writing standards/criteria for nursing diagnoses**[*]

1. Diagnostic category (taken from NANDA approved list)
2. Specific nursing diagnosis (related to category)
3. Assessment criteria (defining characteristics of nursing diagnosis)
4. Etiologies or risk factors (major cause of health problems)
5. Process criteria (interventions) (statements to guide nursing care of groups of patients)
6. Outcome criteria (projected goals) (changes in health status resulting from nursing interventions)
7. Review of literature (significant references)
8. Standards Committee, New England Sinai Hospital (date)

New England Sinai Hospital, Stoughton, Mass.

Before writing standards/criteria, it is helpful to have a model to lend consistency to the project. Let me share the one which we developed and modified several times. This model (see box) represents only one possible example. There are others which are being effectively used elsewhere.

Including etiologies as an element of the standard helps to focus the interventions and provides a quick reference for guiding care. In describing *potential* health problems, risk factors are used instead of etiologies. Using the nursing diagnosis of self-care deficit as an example, observe that interventions for the etiology of activity intolerance are different from those relating to cognitive impairments.

Etiological factor	**Process criteria**
Intolerance to activity	Assistance and teaching as indicated
	Energy conservation techniques
	Positioning to minimize energy expenditure
	Scheduling sufficient time to complete activity
	Encouragement and emotional support
Cognitive deficit	Assistance and teaching as indicated
	Supervision for thoroughness
	Perform task analysis if indicated
	Establish set routine
	Positive reinforcement for small gains
	Structured and controlled environment

In all areas of clinical practice, self-care deficit is a widely used nursing diagnosis. Writing process and outcome criteria for self-care deficit presents difficulties. Although the standard has been implemented for a long time, we continue to refine it. We have added to the etiologies found in Gordon's (1982) *Manual for Nursing Diagnosis* and have written accompanying process criteria. We found it to be particularly difficult to project reasonable outcomes for large groups of patients with self-care deficits. Just as people who are ill do not all recover, people who are disabled do not all regain functional independence. A significant outcome indicator for patients with a self-care deficit appears to lie in the etiology of the nursing diagnosis. In our population, patients whose self-care deficit relates to activity intolerance tend to achieve a higher level of independence than those whose self-care deficit relates to impaired cognition.

Etiological factor	Outcome criteria
Intolerance to activity	Independent in self-care with or without equipment
Cognitive deficit	Performs self-care with supervision or minimal assistance

Etiology is not the only factor impacting outcome. There are many variables; but, regardless of our ability to control them, we must still try to predict outcomes which are reasonable, achievable, and measurable.

All QA programs are influenced by external controls, including those required for hospital accreditation. A new quality and appropriateness standard has been introduced in the 1984 Joint Commission on Accreditation of Hospitals (JCAH) Accreditation Manual (JCAH, 1984). The new standard emphasizes monitoring and evaluation of patient care as an ongoing and systematic process, using defined, objective criteria. The manual defines objectives but does not describe the mechanisms to meet the objectives; these are left to each hospital's discretion. The JCAH's QA Director, in discussing the new standards stated: "The key issue for hospitals now is to develop a system to monitor providers' judgment, performance and decisions about patient care" (Walczak, 1983). The JCAH Vice-President further emphasizes: "Aspects of care, which are monitored, should be carefully chosen to reveal the level of skills, performance and judgment of each health care practitioner" (Roberts, 1984). Although no mention is made of nursing diagnosis, monitoring outcome criteria related to nursing diagnosis would certainly facilitate evaluation of the nurses' judgment, performance, and decision-making ability.

Criteria based on nursing diagnosis should not be used for evaluation purposes until there has been sufficient time for implementation. Initially, outcomes should be evaluated through NQA studies. When the results are satisfactory and indicate that no critical problem exists, nursing diagnoses can be put on a monitoring schedule. Monitoring implies collection of information at regular intervals. Some nursing diagnoses will need continuous monitoring, perhaps on a monthly basis. Others may be monitored less frequently. Remember, the new JCAH Standard calls for continuous monitoring and not periodic auditing as in the past.

Monitoring outcomes of care to identify problem areas helps assure that the care provided is appropriate and effective. From writing criteria for nursing diagnoses, to preliminary evaluation studies, to ongoing monitoring of outcomes, is a series of giant steps. Accomplishment is a lengthy process.

Nursing diagnosis standards are applicable to many aspects of QA, including multidisciplinary auditing. Multidisciplinary auditing, or program evaluation, implies the use of criteria from all involved disciplines. This is not to be confused with the practice of nurses developing process/outcome criteria for nursing diagnoses associated with a specific medical diagnosis. This practice is not helpful in NQA because the study topic then becomes the medical diagnosis.

Joint quality assurance efforts are meaningful *if* they represent a coordinated approach to patient care. Individual disciplines submit their criteria in accordance with the overall objectives of the program being evaluated. For example, in evaluating the effectiveness of a stroke program, many disciplines might be involved. Nursing might submit criteria related to self-care deficits, ambulation deficits, and alteration in elimination: urinary incontinence.

Program objectives	Outcome measurements (discharge)
Maximize independence in self-care: feeding, bathing, dressing	Patient requires no more than minimal assistance with feeding, bathing, and dressing
Maximize independence in transfer and ambulation	Patient requires no more than minimal assistance with transfer and ambulation
Maximize independence in urinary continence	Patient has catheter-free controlled pattern of urination

The program objectives would include maximizing independence in self-care and ambulation so that, upon discharge, no more than minimal assistance is required. Minimal assistance is defined as the patient doing at least 75% of the work (NESH, 1983).

Other disciplines might also be concerned with these same health problems, particularly the first two. Projected outcomes should be the same. *Process* criteria would be different, reflecting the contribution of each discipline. When program evaluation indicates that projected outcomes are not being met, the process criteria or interventions of the involved disciplines are reviewed.

Outcomes of care have assumed new significance. No longer are they merely changes in the health care status of patients, reflecting appropriateness and effectiveness of care. Consideration is now being given to the feasibility of using outcomes as indicators for reimbursement, for determining level of nursing home placement, and even for licensure of long-term care facilities. This thinking reflects the rapidly changing climate of professional accountability. Who is going to determine the outcome criteria for nursing? The effort should be systematic, concerted, and coordinated by nurses and their professional organizations. The American Nurses Association has assisted the effort by publishing *Standards of Practice* (ANA, 1973) and a *Management/Learning System for NQA* (ANA, 1982). The North American Nursing Diagnosis Association is contributing by sponsoring conferences such as this to fulfill its purpose to develop, refine, and promote a taxonomy of nursing diagnostic terminology (NANDA, 1982). Specialty nursing organizations need to further delineate the major health problems of concern to their own memberships. Above all, nursing must control the outcomes relating to nursing diagnoses.

I have attempted to point out the relationship between NQA and nursing diagnosis. In closing, I ask you to ponder the question: From the practice perspective, is nursing diagnosis the key to quality assurance or is quality assurance the key to nursing diagnosis?

REFERENCES

American Nurses' Association: Standards of nursing practice, Kansas City, Mo., 1973, The Association.

American Nurses' Association and Sutherland Learning Associates: Nursing quality assurance management/learning system, North Bridge, Calif., 1982, Sutherland Associates.

Gordon, M.: Manual of nursing diagnosis, New York, 1982, McGraw-Hill Book Co.

Joint Commission on Accreditation of Hospitals: Accreditation manual for hospitals, Chicago, 1984, The Commission.

McCourt, A.: Models, activities and issues: nursing diagnosis in nursing practice. In Kim, M.J., and Moritz, D.A., editors: Classification of nursing diagnoses—Proceedings of the Third and Fourth National Conferences, New York, 1982, McGraw-Hill Book Co.

New England Sinai Hospital: McCourt Index of functional ability in long-term care, Stoughton, Mass., 1983, The Hospital.

New England Sinai Hospital: Unpublished standards for nursing diagnoses, Stoughton, Mass.

North American Nursing Diagnosis Association: ByLaws. Article I. Section 2, St. Louis, 1982, The Association.

Roberts, J., and Walczak, R.: Toward effective quality assurance: the evaluation and current status of the JCAH Q.A. standard, Qual. Rev. Bull. **10:**11-15, 1984.

Walczak, R.: JCAH's new standard calls for more deliberate QA activities, Hosp. Peer Rev. **8:**155-158, 1983.

Discussion

Toni Welsel: Toni Welsel from New York. This question is directed to Dr. Shaffer. You made a reference to New York as being a waivered state. Could you explain that?

Frank Shaffer: There are four waivered states in the United States. New York is one, meaning it is an exception. However, I do not think it is going to be waivered long. In 1986, I do not think it is going to be waivered again. Thank you.

Pauline Green: Pauline Green, from Doctor's Hospital, Prince George's County, Lanham, Maryland. I have a few comments I would like to make. One is that I am very concerned about the nursing profession and nurses as individuals responding to the DRG issue in a very critical way. I am concerned that it will adversely affect patient care delivery by nurses. I think that nurses should not swallow all statements they see in the printed word as fact. It might be good to have an outlook of suspicion that this administration is making a deliberate effort to decrease the availability of health care. Also, nurses should read the health-related articles that appear in magazines, in a very critical way, and look at DRGs for the consequences that they have for the vulnerable people in society: the elderly and children. In response to Mr. Shaffer's questions, I do not think that many staff nurses are educated in ethical, moral decision making and they will not feel confident making those decisions. I think we should remember that a moral decision is a choice between right and wrong; an ethical decision implies a vision of the future that you would like to see created. You can ask two questions: are we obligated to use technology when available, and will we cease providing health care to patients who have not practiced wellness? I think if anyone answers these questions affirmatively, it is with a callous attitude and would be a tragedy for nursing as a profession.

Frank Shaffer: In response to the two ethical questions, I was trying to give a frame of reference for the very futuristic environment that we are moving into. I totally agree with you. I would have liked to spend more time talking about the educating that we need to do in ethics and morality. We, as educators, nursing service administrators, and hospital administrators, have an obligation to prepare our staff for this role because today around this United States decisions are being made in every hospital when to pull the plug, who gets what service, and when do they get that service. The nurse is on the firing line all the time already.

Pauline Green: The reason I came to the mike is my concern over just that realization; I think we are being worn down, and I think after 3, 5, 10, years of this, perhaps people will get tired to the point where they will say yes to those questions. I think we have to continue to have an outlook of providing for the least capable in our population.

Frank Shaffer: Well, I think probably some of that is true. I do think a lot of it is going to go, however, into the legislative realm of things. Examples are Baby Doe and the Quinlan case.

Bill Windells: Bill Windells from Vermont. This is to Dr. Joel. Is the intent of the Maine legislation to make nursing services a line item cost to the patient, rather than just a cost center?

Lucille Joel: As far as I understand, the Maine legislation is a provision in the enabling regulations that nursing shall be costed out. It was a caveat put in there to allow for the development of allocation statistics. In other words, they are not prepared to move on it, just as we would never suggest RIMs be used anywhere right now. They have to be perfected and looked at in one place. But as I understand, there is not the mechanism in place to do what is called for in the Maine regulations. It is just that they wanted it there to protect nursing for the future. So it would be the same concept, having nursing in some way costed out separate from the patient day as you go on to case mix.

Bill Windells: That appears to be the utility of doing this whole thing: the RIMs, or trying to measure in some way what part . . .

Lucille Joel: You are saying is it useful? It is very possible, and a rate set is dreamed of because it begins to control that large portion of a budget on a patient specific basis. It now becomes the obligation of the profession to move fast enough to have a proposal ready to be considered seriously rather than rate setters coming up with a proposition.

Bill Windells: Okay. In order to convince the controller at my own hospital about the potential and viability for this, I need information as to the costs and utility of doing this as well as the value to nursing. Is it worth investing in? Maybe if you could just say something about this.

Lucille Joel: Yes. With runs on our RIMS, which are not the best, there have been statistically significant shifts in the cost of nursing DRG to DRG. There are patients who definitely consume more nursing, even with our only beginning statistics. It is a totally computer-driven system. In other words, it is not a bookkeeping thing. It is a computer-driven system where rates are calculated the same as DRGs. So, you need the computer capacity to do it. That's the problem in our state right now. Our computers are decent but not superb, and so there is trouble getting these data out of the computer. If you have a good computer system, it is relatively simple. All you need is a programmer and the information from a base. Medical records is central in all this. They are the people who, if the physician does not provide the information, currently keep it out of the chart.

Judy Kieffer: Judy Kieffer, the University of Louisville in Kentucky. I have had senior students this past year studying in a hospital that is under the prospective payment system and in another which is not. I cannot tell any difference between them, but I wonder if you might comment on any changes you expect will occur under the prospective system in relation to nursing students using these clinical facilities.

Lucille Joel: Nursing, indeed, is sharper and more fine-tuned under DRGs, which is good for students to see. I do not see it as a negative, and I refuse to "bad mouth" the system. That will do us no good. As far as the cost of having students, the future success of DRGs for nursing is dependent upon clinical sophistication. That's where our hope lies, that and data. But clinical sophistication is necessary, so if I were a hospital, I'd look for an affiliation with schools of nursing, and I would give courtesy to those students because I need those faculty. Faculty are supposed to have a cutting edge on clinical knowledge. Now we will find out, will we not? Clinical knowledge is what will enable you to decrease length of stay, avoid complications, etc. I would value a school of nursing. Now that is probably not the type of answer you wanted. As far as the cost of nursing education, I feel that cost should be averaged among all patients. It's not simply entry level education but professional development that is necessary to maintain safe care. Right now the cost of education is being passed through, but, as Frank said, that is definitely in jeopardy. How do you get around that? I think faculty are going to have to give to service agencies. They will give by way of their clinical knowledge, which will help service agencies become more cost efficient.

Mary Ann McNeal: Mary Ann McNeal, Memorial Sloan-Kettering, New York City. I would really like to just offer some comments to Dr. Shaffer and to the group at large. I would propose to you all that a for-profit motive has always been in health care. Up till now it has only been with Blue Cross, Blue Shield, and the physicians. Now it has shifted to the hospitals. But the ultimate victim of this is the consumer, and someday that is going to be you or me, perhaps in a hospital bed on a respirator. I would like to ask everyone how they feel about a dual health care system? How do they feel about the poor in this country, the elderly and the young, who are going to receive second-class treatment? And I would suggest to President Reagan and to the administrators that, yes, we need cost containment, but is it at the expense of the consumer? Thank you.

Lucy Brand: Lucy Brand, Traverse City, Michigan. Ann, my greatest experience currently is with the home health care agencies, so I must address this question. I am sure that many of us are aware of the fact that HCFA does reimburse on the basis of skilled nursing. Skilled nursing is defined as direct care, teaching, monitoring, and supervision. Therefore, I'm very much oriented to this kind of thinking. You said you design your interventions based on etiology. Going back to my former experience as a teacher-educator, every time I see an intervention I ask how that intervention achieves that outcome. If it does not, then I wonder how worthwhile the intervention was. In the example you gave in terms of independence—I cannot remember just how it was stated—one of the interventions was to teach and assist in the activities of daily living. Well, we could teach and assist forever, and they would not become independent. In terms of our documentation, unless we identify in home care that people indeed are not able to perform because they lack a knowledge base or understanding of that, we cannot teach. And we have to identify what their level of understanding is. Do you understand my confusion? I have a real need to design my interventions on the basis of projected outcomes. Do you have a problem with that?

Ann McCourt: No. None whatsoever. I give a very small sample here, and you cannot assist and teach forever and have nothing happen. There are other interventions, and I would be happy to talk to you about that later. You're going to see more and more of this. I think one of the most important things that you have mentioned is to concentrate on functional areas because they are the ones we will be reimbursed for. But certain interventions we do know lead to certain outcomes. We have a list right now of eleven etiologies, and we have had a lot of experience with the outcomes. You also have people with bizarre types of behavior, and the outcomes are going to be very different. The interventions are going to be very different, but hopefully we can reach that. I do not have a problem with that, and I'd be happy to discuss it with you later.

Margaret Lunney: Margaret Lunney from New York. Would you comment on a problem which I see as a really common problem, and that is setting outcome criteria by symptoms, such as the patient's blood pressure will be between this and that. Would you comment on that?

Ann McCourt: Yes. We do not set outcome criteria by symptoms, because we are not reimbursed for that. The name of the game is reimbursement. You have to have outcomes which are going to show the person reviewing your records that indeed the patient needed your services. In other words, alleviating symptoms is not going to do anything unless it affects your level of functioning. We cannot have goals that, for example, strength and endurance will increase. We will decrease flaccidity.

We will increase coordination. You have to have a goal that relates to the fact that it will improve their level of functioning. Does that answer your question? It is a reimbursement issue. It is very reality based. We also do not get paid for assisting people to cope unless we can show that by assisting them to cope we indeed are enabling them to function better. I would encourage you to write standards for functional disabilities using other nursing diagnoses as etiologies only because it keeps it simplistic. I am not saying that is the only route to go. It keeps it simplistic, and it does allow for reimbursement.

Eleanor Kirsch: Eleanor Kirsch from Wisconsin. Maybe I missed this, but how did you check for validity for etiologies, and process and assessment criteria in your model?

Ann McCourt: We did not. Now what's your real question? What are you saying?

Eleanor Kirsch: We are doing the same type of thing, at least we are trying to look at that now, and we wonder if we need to have some type of validity and reliability in our model.

Ann McCourt: I think the model is certainly a valid model, and the quality assurance literature would indicate that. I would refer you to ANA's *Management Learning System for Quality Assurance.* We get into the validity of models in that reference.

CHAPTER 5

Implementation

Implementation of nursing diagnosis: acute and long-term care settings

JANE LANCOUR, M.S.N., R.N.

To speak on the topic of implementation of nursing diagnosis in acute and long-term care facilities in 45 minutes is indeed a challenge. However, it is not the challenge that nursing service leaders meet as they attempt the change process in either type of health care settings.

Administrative personnel and staff involved in this practice change are confronted with numerous challenges for two reasons: (1) the state of the art of nursing diagnosis and (2) the state of the art of clinical nursing practice. Because of the evolution of nursing diagnoses, nurses in clinical settings experience disbelief, confusion, and frustration. Many nurses are seeking absolutes, black or white situations, a traditional cookbook approach to practice which is neither real or possible.

The state of the art of clinical nursing is one of flux. Traditional practice flows from systems that support the medical model, with little consideration or recognition of a nursing model. In addition, all levels of nurses are practicing as registered nurses, since all levels become licensed with the same examination.

The incorporation of nursing diagnosis presents difficulties because nurses are forced to rethink their practice; administrators are required to examine methods/systems of operation now in place and the education and experience of nurses they have employed.

In examining long-term care and acute care, differences in the implementation of nursing diagnosis lie in the dissimilarity of the patient populations, the medical services required, framework for practice, length of stay, and nursing care required. These are compared as follows:

	Long-term	**Acute**
Population	Individuals generally experience problems with responses that impair functional ability. Patients share similarities in age and developmental stage.	Individuals experience exacerbation of a chronic situation or a crisis situation in which rapid changes are occurring. Age and developmental stages are diverse.
Medical services	Primarily medical in nature, therefore generic in focus.	A wide variety of medical services and specialties
Framework for practice	A generic framework can be utilized without difficulty for the entire patient population.	A variety of frameworks may be required because of the diversity of patient population.
Nursing	A high percentage of independent function. Major focus is on the individual's response to health state.	A high percentage of interdependent function. First efforts are toward achieving a state of homeostasis; second efforts are toward responses to illness.
Patient stay	Extended over long period of time, often months or years; many long-term care facilities become the final home of a large segment of our population.	Acute care stays are shortening to merely a few days.

In summary, long-term care has a generic patient population featuring chronicity with specific emphasis on response to illness or developmental stage, extended stay, and a high degree of independent nursing. This creates a stable situation that leads to ease in the use of nursing diagnoses. This is a sharp contrast to the instability, diverse patient population, and low degree of independent nursing that is found in acute care where use of nursing diagnosis becomes a greater challenge.

The rest of the discussion in this paper has application to both long-term and acute care settings.

In order to overcome some of the ambiguity, controversy, conflict, and questions without answers in the implementation process, it is important that nursing service directors, managers, educators, and staff nurses identify specific objectives. These objectives can serve as a means of maintaining focus throughout the change process. When problems or questions arise, the objectives serve as a basis for decision making. The objectives could be as follows:

1. To articulate what nursing is to the patient, society, and other health care workers
2. To demonstrate a difference in the state of the patient, attributable to nursing (The difference in the state of the patient may be maintenance, restoration, or facilitation of a change.)
3. To provide a system for use of the nursing process, including analysis and synthesis, which is efficient, effective, and realistic for staff nurses
4. To build a system for identifying costs of nursing care
5. To provide a basis for third-party reimbursement
6. To provide a means for documenting nursing diagnoses that will allow

for retrieval of data for research, so as to contribute to the ongoing development of the science of nursing

Having determined the objectives, it is essential to commit to the hard decision of a definition of a nursing diagnosis for the department of nursing. What is the focus expected of the staff for developing a nursing diagnosis? Is it to include all that nursing does, or is it to include only those human responses for which nursing has a high degree of independent function, and therefore can be held accountable for the outcome of the state of the patient as it relates to these specific human responses? Even though a standard definition of nursing diagnosis has not been decided nationally, a nursing department must grapple with a definition for their department since it serves as a basis for determining expectations and accountabilities that can be drawn on in the evaluation process. With new knowledge, revisions can be made. Making the decision, however, will reduce the ambiguity that staff will experience.

Having identified specific objectives and having made a commitment to what a nursing diagnosis is, an assessment of the practice setting is essential. The assessment provides information for planned change that will need to occur in the nursing department, or in a particular unit, which will culminate in the final use of nursing diagnosis. Realizing that nursing diagnosis is not an entity unto itself and cannot be utilized in a vacuum, but is a means of highlighting the focus of nursing and is useful only within the nursing process, the following assessment areas need to be addressed:

Philosophy
- What is the philosophy of the nursing department or unit?
- Is the philosophy apparent in everyday practice, or is it merely a piece of paper in the nursing administration policy manual?
- Does the philosophy support the use of the nursing process?
- Does the philosophy include a definition of nursing?
- Is the definition of nursing, as it appears in the philosophy, compatible with nursing diagnosis?

Staff
- What categories of staff function within the nursing department?
- What percentage of the staff are registered nurses: 20%, 40%, 60%, 80%, 100%?
- What percentage of the registered nurses are baccalaureate prepared?
- What is the staff's knowledge and expertise in the use of the nursing process?
- What attitudes and beliefs about the autonomy and accountability of nursing permeate the registered nurse staff?
- What is the staff's knowledge or expertise in the use of nursing diagnoses?

Standards of nursing practice
- What are the standards of nursing practice for the nursing department; for each unit?

- Are the standards clearly articulated?
- Is present practice congruent with written standards?
- Have the written standards been operationalized?
- Is there an active quality assurance mechanism in place?
- Is staff involved in the evaluation of nursing practice?

Resources
- Does the present management structure support a major change in nursing practice, or is it a thrust that reflects the interest of a speciality group, such as clinical nurse specialists, or the education department?
- What is the availability of clinical role models for the identification and validation of nursing diagnosis in specific patient situations?
- Is the education department supportive and available to the nursing department, and is the nursing department aware of the goals or interests of the education department?
- Is there a commitment of monies to the completion of a major change in nursing practice?

Job descriptions and performance appraisals
- Does the organization have criterion-based job descriptions?
- Are these job descriptions congruent with the philosophy of the nursing department?
- Does the job description for the professional nurse include the expectation of use of the nursing process in practice?
- Does the performance appraisal support the criterion-based job description?
- Are both the job description and the performance appraisal criteria specific to each step of the nursing process, versus a general criterion that states: "Utilizes the nursing process in practice"?

Delivery of care and documentation system
- What type of documentation system is now in place?
- Will the present documentation system support the projected change without becoming a burden for staff?
- What changes might be anticipated to prevent increasing the workload for staff?
- Is the admission history and assessment constructed so that collection of data can lead to the identification of nursing diagnoses?
- What is the modality for the delivery of care: functional, team, modular, total, primary? (If a department is using a functional approach in the delivery of care, it would be prudent to change this modality first; after that change had occurred, a reassessment as outlined would be in order.)
- Does the format for documentation of the nursing process include an area for nursing diagnoses, expected outcomes, evaluation date, interventions, dates, and signature?

Change process

- What methods of change have been successful in the nursing department in the past?
- How much change is going on *now* in the organization; in the nursing department?
- What might enhance the introduction of nursing diagnosis?
- What factors could lead to resistance or inhibit the implementation process?
- How have changes been evaluated in the past?
- Would the same method for evaluation be appropriate in this change?
- If the same method is not appropriate, what might be?
- What type of reactions could be projected from various groups in the organization, i.e., physicians, other disciplines, nonprofessionals?
- What groundwork or politicking might be carried out which would lead to support by these groups?

This assessment provides data for the detailed planning of the change process. As primary nursing is not just a different way of making assignments, so also nursing diagnoses are not just categories for documenting. Both primary nursing and the nursing diagnosis flow from a philosophy and a commitment to the professional practice of nursing which requires the use of cognitive and creative skills and which establish accountability for the individual nurse. Assessment of appropriate areas and action in keeping with the findings of the assessment provide a department of nursing with direction in carrying out its commitment to professional practice.

As change ensues, it is helpful to be aware of possible pitfalls or barriers that can be encountered in the change process. Following is a brief description of some of these:

1. Lack of articulation of a definition of nursing and lack of commitment to a definition of nursing diagnosis result in dubiousness.

2. Lack of involvement of staff nurses in the planning process can result in a system that has little relevance to clinical practice.

3. Frustration of staff that is not dealt with, can thwart the change process. This frustration can stem from the ambiguity or lack of certainty that occurs in an evolving body of knowledge. Limiting the use of nursing diagnosis to the "list of approved diagnoses from the national conferences" (Kim and Moritz, 1982) impedes the advancement of the body of knowledge of nursing and puts nurses in a situation in which they are compelled to use diagnostic labels that are inappropriate for specific patients. All diagnostic categories that nurses treat are not diagnoses that have been brought to the conference groups and "approved" for clinical testing. The body of knowledge of nursing far exceeds the "list." Nurses need to add to the list by identifying pertinent diagnostic labels with patients, validating the critical defining characteristics, and sub-

mitting this information to the North American Nursing Diagnosis Association for further evaluation and approval.

4. Lack of resolution of documentation issues can cause havoc in the clinical setting. Many systems for documentation do not support the use of nursing diagnoses. There is also a lack of vision in developing efficient, effective means of documenting, consistent with the use of nursing diagnoses. Every effort must be made to create methods that decrease nurses' writing work load, so that nurses have adequate time for the cognitive processes essential to professional practice.

5. Another pitfall results from major deficits in the use of cognitive processes required in diagnosing. Too little attention has been given to planning this portion of the change process.

6. Inadequacies in evaluation methodologies result in unawareness of the "state of the art" of the use of nursing diagnoses and the nursing process on a particular unit or within a department. Without follow-up evaluation, what is believed to be operational within a setting can be different from what is occurring in practice. To say that a unit or department is using nursing diagnosis is one thing; to validate the existence of nursing diagnosis in actual clinical practice is another. Some departments that claim to use nursing diagnosis have only a system whereby nurses use categorical headings for organizing and documenting their clinical data.

7. A final pitfall that occurs is based on the belief that sending nurses to a workshop on nursing diagnosis will be adequate for the implementation of nursing diagnosis in a particular agency. This is a myth. Nursing diagnosis as a concept, and as the basis of the practice of nursing, has ramifications for an entire organization and nursing department. Its use requires highly complex cognitive skills in an environment that supports the professional practice of nursing. A 1-day workshop merely exposes nurses to the concept.

Successful implementation and ongoing use of nursing diagnosis require that change agents avail themselves of all types of strategies that could contribute to successful change in a particular setting. The following have proven to be effective:

1. Designing a system for change based on identified assumptions of how people change and how people have changed in a specific setting requires knowledge of the elements of the change process. Designing a grid for change, with deadline dates for achievement of particular goals and an action plan designating who is to carry out specific activities, is also essential. A commitment to a deliberate collaborative process, with all individuals responsible for the change, is essential.

2. Realizing that the process of diagnosing is different from intuition or problem naming puts an onus on change agents to allocate time and energy for nurturing the development of diagnostic skills that will be required by practitioners.

3. Some diagnostic categories represent areas that are not familiar to certain practicing nurses. Identifying diagnostic categories common to a particular group of patients and strategizing to developing expertise in individuals within those defined areas serves to narrow the gaps that exist.

4. Based on the assessment completed within the department of nursing, it is essential to define, for all concerned, the expectations that are to be met. Recognizing the ambiguity of the evolving science of nursing requires the need for a department to make a determination on its philosophical position as it relates to the particulars of nursing diagnosis. It is helpful to create an atmosphere of defined expectation, of openness, and of creativity for individual nurses.

5. Developing resource tools to ease the use of nursing diagnoses, i.e., standard care plans for particular common nursing diagnoses in a particular patient population, can be helpful in the education process. At the same time awareness of the pitfalls of standard care plans and monitoring in this regard can assure that care plans are individualized.

6. The use of nursing diagnoses in care planning is most effective in those practice settings where the modality of the delivery of care takes into account continuity of assignments and accountability by the nurse for outcomes with specific patients.

7. Last, the change process is not completed when nurses start writing nursing diagnoses on care plans. Change occurs over a long period of time and is completed only when individuals internalize the change to the point that, on a continuum, nursing care is personalized, expected outcomes are met, and care plans are updated and revised, based on new data, new knowledge, and new insights. Evaluation methods must be used to determine the degree of internalization that has occurred not only on a particular unit but also by individual nurses.

In a research study by McLane, Lancour, and Gotch (1984), titled *Nursing Diagnoses in Clinical Practice*, 228 respondents identified the following areas as problematic in the use of nursing diagnoses (respondents could identify more than one area):

a. Inadequate knowledge—72%
b. Absence of a classification system for diagnostic labels—41%
c. Time constraints—40%
d. Absence of a practical system for documenting nursing diagnoses—39%
e. Absence of standardization of diagnostic labels—39%
f. Insufficient organization support—36%

Of the 228 respondents, primarily from acute care settings, 146 indicated that nursing diagnoses had been integrated into their practice setting, 54 were in a situation in which planning for implementation was occurring, and only 28 indicated no integration and no planning.

These findings are exciting at a point in time where we stop to take a Janus view. Nursing has come a long way, struggling; as the evolution continues, information is emerging that can offset the challenges and pitfalls of implementation.

Nursing administrators, educators, managers, and staff in service settings must be supported in their continuing efforts to recognize nursing diagnosis as the core of the professional practice of nursing and a viable means for nurses to demonstrate their contribution and accountability. Furthermore, at a point in time when health care costs are of great concern to our entire nation, nursing diagnoses can serve as a means for costing out what we as nurses are worth in the health care delivery system.

Service settings provide the "real world" of nursing, and it is in these settings that the furthering of the body of knowledge of nursing must take place through clinical nursing research. Unless service settings can provide a basis for research, the development of the science of nursing will be stymied.

Change in nursing will continue as the administrative leaders make the decision to uphold the professional practice of nursing. In addition, the commitment to professional nursing must be made at the staff nurse level. The use of nursing diagnoses in clinical practice is the means to show to the patient, family, and society nursing's accountability within the health care system.

REFERENCES

Kim, M.J., and Moritz, D., editors: Classification of nursing diagnoses—Proceedings of the Third and Fourth National Conferences, New York, 1982, McGraw-Hill Book Co.

McLane, A., Lancour, J., and Gotch, P.: Nursing diagnosis in clinical practice. Unpublished research study, 1984.

Implementation of nursing diagnosis in a community health setting

DELANNE A. SIMMONS, M.Ph., R.N.

I am pleased to be with you today. I always enjoy sharing our agency's experiences with the concept of nursing diagnosis, because I am so strongly committed to its value. During my presentation, I will describe the stage (our agency), the actors and actresses (our staff from 1970 to present and others involved with us), and the plot (the development and use of the problem classification scheme).

The Visiting Nurse Association of Omaha was founded as a voluntary nonprofit organization in 1896. In 1946, agency staff was instrumental in establishing the Omaha–Douglas County Health Department. Since that time, our agency has served as the Health Department's Division of Public Health Nursing. This combination has enabled the agency to provide all community health nursing services commonly associated with both official and voluntary organizations.

Our 150 employees serve individuals, families, and groups of all ages in the urban areas of Omaha and the rural areas of Douglas and Sarpy Counties. Programs available to the 500,000 population base include intermittent and extended home health care, maternal care, infant and preschool health, handicapped child services, school health, communicable disease control, mental health, mobile meals, child health clinics, and health maintenance centers. Agency staff is decentralized in five locations throughout the service area with a generalized home visit caseload.

The increase in both size and complexity just described has necessitated changes in documentation by the staff. While the agency's administrators, supervisors, and staff acknowledged the value of complete, timely, and accurate recording, they also experienced the difficulties with such recording. The frustration level of one nursing supervisor and her staff became sufficient in 1970 to begin the search for a solution. Thus, in 1972, a problem-oriented method of recording, originally developed by Weed, was introduced (Weed, 1968). I encouraged a staff committee to initiate the first in a series of revisions that eventually became a family problem-oriented record of community health nursing. However, the lack of a standard classification of health or health-related problems soon became apparent. The lack of such a classification system hindered not only the documentation of nursing services but also the development of specific nursing interventions, communication among health disciplines, and nursing research efforts. Therefore, agency personnel committed themselves to the goal of developing such a classification.

A contract to develop a classification of client problems addressed by nurses in a community health setting was negotiated between the Visiting Nurse Association of Omaha and the Division of Nursing, DHEW, Washington, D.C., in 1975. An advisory committee was formed which included representatives of ANA, NLN, nursing education, and nursing research. At this period of time, many staff nurses were anything but happy to be involved in a *research* project. That attitude has changed dramatically over time to the point where involvement is now an *honor!*

Data used to develop the Problem Classification Scheme were derived empirically from a 100% sample of families admitted to service during a 3-month period. A total of 1341 nursing problems, or 3.97 per family, were identified. These data were consolidated to develop a classification which contained 49 problem names with mutually exclusive descriptors, classified according to selected categories of the data base.

The scheme was then tested by 16 PHNs who did record reviews of selected open records, identifying problems and their descriptors using the problem classification. The nurses identified an average of nine problems per family. This increase was felt to be due, at least in part, to greater specificity provided through the use of the classification. The ability to identify problems amenable to nursing intervention is the first step in providing that intervention, thus improving quality of care. The classification was refined again as a result of the testing.

The initial contract was completed in May of 1977. A second contract, completed in 1980, allowed us to begin work on the development of expected outcome–outcome criterion schemes; to test the problem classification scheme in three other community health agencies; and to further refine the scheme. The three agencies were chosen to represent the diversity of geographical and structural organizations in which community health nurses practice. The DesMoines Public Health Nurses Association represented the combined agency; the Dallas Visiting Nurse Association, the voluntary agency; and the Delaware Department of Health and Social Services, the official agency. Results of this testing and two years of experience with use of the scheme at the VNA were used to revise the scheme. Additionally, the contract financed development of a manual designed to act as a guide for agencies wishing to implement the scheme. The manual was published by the Division of Nursing as *Volume 14, Nurse Planning Information Series.* The positive response to the manual nationally necessitated second and third printings. The manual is no longer in print from the Division of Nursing but is available through the National Technical Information Service (NTIS) (Simmons, 1980).

Notice that I began my presentation referring to nursing diagnosis and switched to nursing problems. We used the terminology, nursing problems, for two reasons. First, the term problem was congruent with problem-oriented record terminology. Second, nursing diagnosis was not yet a well-accepted term, and the federal government indicated willingness to investigate nursing problems rather than nursing diagnoses.

The problem-classification scheme as it exists today is comprised of 38 problem labels, each with signs and symptoms. It is divided into four categories or domains representative of community health nursing practice. First, the environmental domain refers to the material resources and physical surroundings of the home, neighborhood, and broader community. Second, the psychosocial domain refers to patterns of behavior, communications, relationships, and development. Third, the physiological domain refers to the functional status of processes that maintain life. Finally, the health behaviors domain refers to activities which maintain or promote wellness or recovery or maximize rehabilitation.

Problems may be designated as family or individual and as actual or potential. The signs and symptoms denote the actual state of the problem. There is an assumption that the nurse has a knowledge base of risk factors and will identify a problem within a continuum of time. Similarly, the scheme does not include etiology. Again, it is assumed that the nurse has the ability to identify etiology.

To this point, I have described the stage and the actors and actresses. I have described the plot as it relates to the development of our problem classification scheme. Now, I have reached the heart of the plot, the use of nursing problems or nursing diagnosis within our agency. In our minds, use of nursing diagnosis is always planned and structured to benefit our clients and to improve their health status.

When a new community health nurse begins employment, the orientation schedule includes various opportunities to observe others making home visits and recording. A recording session is scheduled for one morning of the second week. A description of the problem classification scheme and actual practice with a clinical record are significant portions of that morning. Then, as the new nurse begins to independently make home visits and to record, the problem classification scheme is an essential tool. The problem classification scheme has improved orientation and assimilation of our new nursing staff. It speeds the process of introducing and describing the world of community health nursing to that staff.

The agency's clinical record offers a valuable supervisory tool which enables visualization of the family nursing process from collection of data through evaluation of outcomes of care. Thus the supervisor can assist the staff nurse who is experiencing difficulty with the process. The clinical record provides supervisory access to data about the family and individuals gathered by the practitioner and used to identify nursing diagnoses. All diagnoses, both medical and nursing, actual and potential, are listed on the problem list, which serves as an index of family health status. The supervisor is able to independently assess the data and compare his or her findings or diagnoses with those identified by the nurse.

In addition, the supervisor reviews the staff nurse's projected outcomes of nursing intervention and plans. These are recorded only for those nursing diagnoses for which intervention will occur. By comparing the master problem list with the expected outcome and plans, the supervisor is able to identify the priorities established by the nurse. Our supervisors unanimously see review of clinical records and follow-up conferences with staff as an important and critical means of monitoring, improving, and ensuring high-quality nursing care for our clients.

The VNA has been involved with modest mechanical systems of data gathering since the late 1950s. It was not until 1974, however, that we made an emotional and financial commitment to the development of a total management information system. At that time *Management Information Systems for Public Health–Community Health Agencies* was published (NLN, 1974). This book was a compilation of papers presented at an invitational conference sponsored by the National League for Nursing and The Division of Nursing, Bureau of Health Manpower. In viewing those presentations I was struck by two specific quotations. The first, by Alice Mary Hilton, a modern-day philosopher, stated, "We have what humanity never knew before, slaves that are not human, and we need not be ashamed to employ what they produce. For the first time in human history, man can be free. Human beings who learn to use the machine wisely will be freed by the machine to achieve excellence." The other quote was attributed to Coach George Allen, who said, "The future is now." The Board of Trustees and the management staff of the Visiting Nurse Association realized that the future was yesterday, not today. We realized we had to invest in tomorrow if we were to survive in today's complex milieu of community health agencies. Based on several studies, the agency made the decision to develop its own system rather than utilize a service bureau. We knew that we wanted to use our family problem-oriented record and classification of client problems as the pivotal input document of our entire system.

After much deliberation, we decided to use the services and hardware of IBM. We began with an IBM System 32, until the IBM System 34 became available. Other community health agencies expressed interest in purchasing software developed in our agency. Thus, Omaha Health Resources, a wholly owned subsidiary, was formed to market software and on-line computer services. In June of 1983, we began the conversion to an IBM System 38. That system has a main core of 1.75 mega-bytes and a disk capacity of 500 mega-bytes.

Our system is now complete and appears deceptively simple. Requests for service are received in central intake; the client record is initiated and is transmitted via telephone line and printed in the branch office. Simultaneously the family identification data are transmitted to central processing, and stored for future use. After making the visit, the nurse dictates via any telephone (a touch tone allows maximum utilization of word processing dictation) and completes any additional identifying information, as well as the family data base, the problem list, the expected outcomes/plans, and the progress notes. All of the data are recorded and transcribed by central processing staff into the CRTs. Pertinent identification, financial, and statistical data are extracted and stored in the central processing unit (CPU). During the night all narrative data are printed in the branch offices and are available to the service delivery staff the following morning.

Information from the record and from a data input document completed by each staff member each day is used to generate statistical data. These data are combined in various formats to provide information on the numbers, distribution, demographic characteristics, medical and nursing diagnoses, service problems, costs of services, etc., for the agency's caseload. Thus nursing diagnosis is an essential component in our agency's program planning and evaluation process.

Nursing diagnosis facilitates emphasis on nursing within our agency's quality assurance program. Throughout our clinical record and management information system I have just described, the focus is *nursing*. Our quality assurance system includes two major components. First, a utilization review committee meets quarterly to review care delivered within the home visit caseload. Length and frequency of service, level of staff assigned, and use of other community resources are examined. Second, supervisory review occurs both in a group setting and individually. Quality of care delivered and accuracy of recording are examined.

The concept of nursing diagnosis has become a reality at the Visting Nurse Association of Omaha. I have described how it relates to our clinical record, our orientation plan, our computerized management information system, and our quality assurance program. In addition to the impact on our agency, the problem classification scheme has been well accepted by community health nursing in general. The scheme is currently used by approximately 65 individuals, agencies, or institutions in 24 states. This widespread use indicates the value of the scheme and its applicability for community health nursing.

REFERENCES

Martin, K.: A client classification system adaptable for computerization, Nurs. Outlook **30:**9, 515-517, 1982.

National League for Nursing: Management information system for public health–community health agencies, New York, 1974, The League.

Simmons, D.: A classification scheme for client problems in community health nursing, Washington, D.C., 1980, U.S. Department of Health and Human Services, Bureau of Health Professions, Division of Nursing, Publication No. HRA80-16.

Weed, L.: Medical records that guide and teach, N. Engl J. Med. **278:**593-600, 652-657 (March) 1968.

Discussion

Laura Rossi: I am Laura Rossi from Boston. I have a question for the first speaker. You commented or referred to systems of documentation that somehow facilitated implementation. I wonder if you could be a little bit more specific.

Jane Lancour: Okay. Systems that could facilitate implementation. By that I mean taking a look at what kinds of things you are doing that could lend themselves to flow sheets. Keep cleaner, if you will, that which demonstrates the aspect that diagnosis is all about. It's much easier to view those interdependent functions, such as data collection, on an ongoing basis, as a means of obtaining information to put on flow sheets and make decisions about rather than trying to take all of them and put them under some diagnostic category. That has been an unbelievable help in many organizations allowing for documenting nursing diagnosis in some type of a problem oriented approach. The "A" of the SOAP is utilized to focus on where the particular patient or resident is in relationship to the expected outcome. Furthermore, to consider not being too dogmatic in terms of the expectation regarding documentation but rather believe in the nurse, to make a judgment regarding when or when not to document something. There are a lot of policies floating around in regards to charting. For instance, there must be a SOAP note on one problem every shift. Could we loosen up a little bit in that regard? Trust the nurse to decide when documentation fits for this particular patient in terms of what we are trying to demonstrate. We might get away from an exercise in writing and move toward demonstrating what we are doing.

Laura Rossi: I asked because I think it particularly becomes an issue with regard to time constraints and developing writing skills.

Jane Lancour: There are various types of flow sheets that can be developed for gathering assessment data that would be invaluable in terms of arriving at a diagnosis when certain things come together and show a pattern. The data may not, at an earlier point in time, necessarily fit under a diagnostic category. I am finding that people are feeling this terrible need to put everything they are doing under a diagnostic category. In the end all they have is a heading to categorize what they are doing rather than gathering data in some fashion that is easier, smoother, and preprinted in some regard. There are a lot of different assessment formats that you can develop that will allow you to make correlations much easier, and realize when you are arriving at something. I think we need to take a fresh look at what all the options are rather than getting entrenched. Another possibility would be to use a problem-oriented record. I think we need to allow for some flexibility: a problem-oriented record along with narrative possibilities for the unforeseen, for the dramatic happening that might have occurred, or for some data that right now we are just not sure about but we are looking at.

Eleanor Kirsch: Eleanor Kirsch, St. Michael Hospital, Milwaukee, Wisconsin. In regard to acute care settings and the impact of DRGs on length of stay, do you think that every patient should have a nursing diagnosis? If they don't, does that then mean that you do not need a professional nurse carring for them?

Jane Lancour: I am totally against a policy statement that says every patient that comes in must have a nursing diagnosis, because I think it is ludicrous. The nursing diagnosis depends upon the client's health history. Also, situations change minute to minute. Among the variables that contribute to making a nursing diagnosis is the perspective of different nurses who have a different body of knowledge and/or a different relationship with the patient.

Eleanor Kirsch: Second question. If people are looking at staffing according to patient needs and nurses are not documenting nursing diagnoses on these people, then do they need professional nurses to care for them?

Jane Lancour: Well, I guess my question is: Do you need a professional nurse in order to do assessment? We need to do more assessment in order to perhaps arrive at a nursing diagnosis if indeed there is one.

Eleanor Kirsch: So a professional nurse is needed in every instance to determine the patient needs to begin with.

Jane Lancour: Yes.

Vivian Barry: Vivian Barry. I am with the Board of Education in Chicago. My question is addressed to DeLanne Simmons. You do a generalized public health program, if I understand correctly, in Omaha, so that you cover the schools also. In evaluating your program, do you do it by families or do you do some breakdown in terms of the school-age child?

DeLanne Simmons: We do a breakdown in terms of the school-age child, and we break down different categories and different kinds of activities within our school nursing program. Let me also tell you our school nursing program is not generalized.

Vivian Barry: I see. Do you break down in accordance with Public Law 142 regarding special education, the health component, in terms of the utilization of nurses' time?

DeLanne Simmons: No, we have not.

Vivian Barry: Thank you.

Lucianne Nolan: Lucianne Nolan from Augusta, Georgia. I have a question for Ms. Lancour. What is the role of nurses who are not baccalaureate prepared? Also, do you have any recommendations for overcoming some of the barriers when people say "Gee, it takes too much time. We do not have time to do that. I am busy doing other things."

Jane Lancour: In some geographic areas there is a certain percentage of nurses not baccalaureate prepared. Is there a possibility that in the future non-baccalaureate prepared nurses will be focusing on some predetermined nursing diagnoses that fit within certain categories, such as potential for skin integrity breakdown or skin impairment or impaired skin integrity? There might be certain things that they can focus on that are in keeping with the level that fits their preparation, if you will. They might not make the diagnosis itself but they can work it through, say, for example, impaired parenting. Regarding barriers to nursing diagnosis in terms of time, I would suggest first of all you admit that admission does take time and explain why it does take time. The new cognitive skills that you are asking these individuals to carry out takes time. So admit that. Facilitate that operation as best you can via situations where people work in groups with data to attempt to arrive at diagnoses. Perhaps initially expect that they identify the most important high priority nursing diagnoses on each client in a situation where indeed a nursing diagnosis exists. That helps take some of the burden off of them initially. I have found that to be helpful. After they feel comfortable with doing at least one for each client, they begin to become more experienced with the process and it takes less time to develop diagnoses.

Don Hudson: I am Don Hudson from San Francisco. I have one more question for Ms. Lancour. In my facility, frequently the taxonomy is ridiculed by a host of people from physicians to nurse managers, and I believe this encourages staff nurses learning to use it to reject it. Can you give me some advice for dealing with that?

Jane Lancour: Well, I guess first of all we need to find out the basis of the ridicule. Is it lack of knowledge? That would be one place to start. I think the other place to start is to attempt to determine what the level of understanding is of the nurses from a nursing perspective versus a medical perspective. I think lack of knowledge on both sides is really a big problem. It is easy to ridicule something you do not know anything about. Now if they have something very specific that they are ridiculing, then it is going to be easier to deal with the specifics, but it's very difficult to deal with generalities. It is very difficult to deal with the list. The other point, I guess, would be, are they aware of what that list represents? Do they really believe that it contains the body of knowledge that is nursing? A lot of people believe that is all of it. A lot of people do not understand the history of the list. A lot of people do not have an awareness of why the list exists. Maybe providing some of that information would help.

Don Hudson: So basically you see it as an educational problem.

Jane Lancour: Oh, I think a lot of politicking too. Education by itself is not necessarily going to do it. I think you need to capitalize on people who have an interest. Get a group of people to network among themselves; even utilize segments of it. Develop cores of people. Small groups make up larger groups after a period of time. That gives you strength.

CHAPTER 6

Research and computerization

Nursing diagnoses research methodologies

JACQUELINE CLINTON, Ph.D., R.N., F.A.A.N.

The tasks of identifying and articulating nursing diagnoses research methodologies are not as awesome as they first sounded when I was invited to prepare this paper to present before you today. This is because the rules of evidence that govern science are applicable to all disciplines, including the most complex applied sciences where phenomena of interest are multivariate and holistic, such as explaining human responses to actual and potential health problems.

Before I outline the specific research tasks appropriate for the testing and refinement of nursing diagnoses, I want to share some of my own opinions about the heuristics of developing standard diagnostic nomenclature within nursing. I take issue with Gebbie (1982), who indicated that the goal of developing a nursing diagnoses classification system is to establish nursing as a full profession. I argue that the goal is twofold: (1) to unequivocally inform the public about what we are able and willing to be accountable for, and (2) to systematically demonstrate that nursing's influence within these domains has a positive impact on the public's welfare. These two goals are prerequisite conditions for professional status and privilege.

I concur with Kritek (1982), who voiced concern that "prescriptive theory has been generated without adequate care being given to the prior stages of theory construction." Hence, my recommendations for research exploration in this paper concentrate on pre-prescriptive theory testing. There is an intentional omission of experimental and quasi-experimental strategies for testing the effectiveness of nursing interventions that may be associated with nursing diagnoses nomenclature. Premature experimentation is like infanticide: it brings an early death to promising theory.

A substantial amount of descriptive research on nursing diagnoses is currently underway. I consider these epidemiological studies in that frequencies or incidences of certain diagnoses and their critical indicators are being tallied for different aggregate populations. Therefore my paper will not outline the need and rationale for such work.

Within the parameters of pre-prescriptive theory generation and testing, I believe it is advisable to pursue both inductive and deductive methodologies concurrently. An exhaustive nomenclature does not have to be in place before deductive approaches can be pursued. I argue that, in any science, classification and nomenclature are *never* complete, for that is the open and evolving nature of science itself. If this were not the case, science would become a religious or political institution predicated on shared beliefs rather than theoretical explanations that are submitted to repeated testing and revision.

Now for the task at hand. I see four major categories of research that need to be pursued in nursing diagnosis at this time: (1) practical feasibility, (2) reliability, (3) validity, and (4) sensitivity. I will speak to each of these in turn. Since I perceive "sensitivity" as a special case of validity, it will be presented in that discussion.

PRACTICAL FEASIBILITY

It is indeed apparent that the use of nursing diagnostic nomenclature in the clinical setting is highly feasible, especially in the acute care setting, where the system has been incorporated as a standard of practice in many hospitals across the country. Computer technology has had a significant impact on the practical feasibility of using such a system. It is less apparent that the standard nomenclature is equally feasible in other settings and the issues in doing so should be addressed.

I believe it would be useful to survey institutions that have integrated the nursing diagnoses structure to find out what factors facilitate its use and what factors deter its implementation. Such data could prove useful to administrators and clinicians in agencies that are moving toward the adoption of such a system for classifying recipients in order to determine nursing resource allocations.

The fact that we know it can and has been implemented in agencies across the country also leads to the question of what is being done with all these data. At this point, multiple institutions generate comparable data (thanks to NANDA). The next step is to create a mechanism for establishing a nationally generated, nationally accessed database of nursing diagnoses. Much of the research work I describe herein could be done by different researchers taking various pieces of a large national database.

I have personally observed that, in many agencies, nursing diagnoses and their indicators, expected outcomes, and achievement of expected outcomes are computerized. This is a scientist's dream come true if only one has access. Many agencies are storing these data on tapes, with few clues as to what to do with them. I recommend that a mechanism and funding for accessing such data be pursued and negotiated between scientists, administrators, and clinicians, with details of benefits and sharing of publication rights worked out from the beginning.

I do have some thoughts about outcomes and how they can be standardized. Survey research could be useful for discovering the outcomes relevant to each nursing diagnosis, how they should be scaled, and at what time and at what level outcomes can be reasonably expected to be achieved.

RELIABILITY

In terms of reliability, I will address three forms: internal consistency, interrater reliability, and intrarater reliability. This deliberate ordering of procedures, that is, testing for reliability first and validity second, is important because reliability is a necessary but not a sufficient condition for validity to exist.

When one thinks of internal consistency for nursing diagnoses, attention focuses on the extent to which a set of indicators for a given nursing diagnosis is dependable over different populations and settings. This is the most basic of reliability measures and is easily accomplished. It is expected that relationships also exist between and among the various nursing diagnoses and that there is some internal consistency to these relationships. One can do predictive validity testing as well as reliability testing on nursing diagnoses data alone. That I have progressed to speaking of validity here shows how reliability and validity are inextricably linked.

Previous research by Halloran (1981) has already demonstrated the high degree of agreement between different nurses fourmulating nursing diagnoses for the same individual. Such findings should be replicated in other populations and settings.

Intrarater reliability testing is a bit more tricky. The task is to find out if the same nurse derives the same diagnoses given the same stimulus at different points in time. Since client status and associated nursing diagnoses change over time in the same individual, intrarater reliability requires some sort of documentary evidence such as case description or simulation type testing.

VALIDITY TESTING

Three different approaches to validity testing should be applied to nursing diagnoses: (1) exploration of underlying data structure or construct validity testing, (2) analysis of the capacity to predict external events or external criterion validity testing, and (3) analysis of the capacity to detect differences in populations whose characteristics are hypothesized or known to vary with nursing diagnoses or discriminant validity testing.

Exploration of the underlying data structure involves the interrelationships among nursing diagnoses and/or their indicators and finding ways to represent these relationships in a logical, efficient, clinically relevant manner. Factor analysis is a useful tool that would allow investigators to explore underlying data structure, as well as confirm theory-generated hypotheses held by nurses working in this area.

The application of factor analysis to either explore or confirm the data structure of nursing diagnoses means that the investigator is seeking to accomplish three things: (1) statistical parsimony, (2) some lawful way to combine variables that represent a theoretical construct in a few mathematical expressions that take into account the relationships among variables and also account for a significant degree of variance, and (3) a group or groups of variables which one can generalize and which can be given the same name (Muliak, 1972; Nunally, 1978).

I would also voice a word of caution in the misuse of factor analysis, lest I put forth the impression of a rampant, crazed empiricist. One should also have a priori decision rules about when *not* to use the products of factor analysis. I have three rules. First, factor analysis should not be used when the results of the procedure do not clearly define a conceptually meaningful or interpretable data structure. Second, it should not be used when the procedure failed to condense the data. Third, it should not be used when assumptions required of the procedure itself were violated, such as the appearance of commonalities less than their corresponding R-square values. Amply warned by Armstrong (1967), in his essay entitled "Tom Swift and His Electric Factor Analysis Machine," about the misguided researcher who practiced shotgun empiricism in the name of scientific theory, these decision rules should be strictly adhered to by those involved in the validation testing of nursing diagnoses.

Before discussing a second alternative to construct validity testing for nursing diagnoses, I believe it is paramount to delineate a critical argument for treating nursing diagnoses data as legitimate interval-level data. This is implied in my suggestion of using factor analysis procedures. Stevens (1951, 1968) has taken the position that the findings of parametric analyses are meaningless unless applied to measurement having at least interval scale properties. Yet Labowitz (1967) and Harris (1975) both speak to the robustness of parametric procedures in large samples. They have also demonstrated that there is little mathematical evidence of error, even when an interval level measurement scale assumption is violated. Hence, the only criterion I use for employing non-parametric statistics is when there is evidence that an assumption of parametric procedures has been violated, such as that of homogeneity of variance.

The second alternative I suggest for testing construct validity of nursing diagnoses should ease the minds of skeptics who hold a conservative opinion about manipulating measurement levels of existing data. This second alternative, called "IDEA," has no assumptions about scaling. In other words, it allows researchers to undertake construct validity testing with nominally scaled data.

IDEA is an interactive computer program for *I*nductive *D*ata *E*xploration and *A*nalysis. It was originally created and tested by Press (1967) at the

University of California at Los Angeles and further developed by Rogers and Shure (1971). It was designed to detect and summarize the structure or patterns existing in a multivariate database. It produces a decision tree which represents partitioning of the multivariate space into exhaustive, mutually exclusive regions. The need for and potential usefulness of this program can best be understood if one considers the limitations of classical statistical approaches to exploring data structure and the heuristics of the IDEA program itself.

Rogers and Shure (1971) explain that IDEA was developed as an alternative to classical inductive algorithms such as factor analysis, multiple regression, and cluster analysis. Press (1967) points out that the limitations of these models lie in their assumptions that: (1) All variables are scaled at least at an interval level of measurement. (2) The contribution which any component makes to a given value of the dependent variable is a linear function. (3) A single model fits all the data. (4) Every component is employed in predicting the dependent variable in a uniform way for all the data points.

IDEA is different from these classical techniques in several important ways. *First*, it is free from assumptions concerning level of measurement and distribution shape. When confronted with nominal data (as is the case in nursing diagnoses), the researcher using any of the classical procedures may elect to employ dummy coding. Press (1967) warns, however, that this leads to maximally complex results which are extremely difficult to understand and interpret even for experts. In IDEA, any characteristic of a variable which can be made explicit can be accounted for in a unique inductive routine.

The *second* contrast is that, unlike the classical models which predict a dependent variable by summing weighted contributions of several independent variables, IDEA is not an additive model (Press, 1967). If a given variable does not significantly contribute to the dependent variable in certain subjects, it is not calculated into the model for those subjects. In other words, the provision is made to drop variables once they no longer significantly account for the dependent variable. This unique feature of IDEA means that there is nothing in the procedure itself that requires the model for one region of the data structure to resemble that of another. In essence, it searches for models that best fit various regions of the data space. This feature provides a means of discovering which indicators are significant in contributing to nursing diagnoses in different subjects.

The *third* contrast is the amount of human control that is allowed in a procedure. In cluster analysis, multiple regression, and factor analysis the investigator has input only at the beginning of the procedure. IDEA requires human input at every decision point of the analysis. Press (1967) stresses the importance of human-directed analysis in terms of its contribution to theory development and expansion:

Data analysis should not consist of blind computation on an unfamiliar array of numbers. With IDEA the investigator may interpret his results and plan subsequent analysis in the light of the broad theoretical framework of his discipline, of his knowledge of the artifacts of the data analysis techniques being used, of his knowledge of the precision of the measurements which yielded his data, of the purpose of the current analysis, and finally, of the results of previous steps in the analysis.

IDEA is particularly useful in situations where a study population is complex and not readily summarized or easily explained with a single, simple model or where prediction is desirable and the researcher has little or no control over independent variables. Both of these situations exist in the study of nursing diagnoses.

The following key features of IDEA are offered to give you a basic knowledge of how it works. IDEA searches out patterns in the data structure in a way that favors strong main effects. This is accomplished by a series of significance tests. In the case of nominal level data, the partitioning of independent variables is ranked by the significance level of their corresponding chi-square values. For interval level data the order of partitioning corresponds to which independent variable produces the largest reduction in unexplained variance. These partitions are represented graphically in a decision tree. An IDEA tree has nodes (circles), which represent a given independent variable; paths or branches (lines), which represent certain values of the independent variable; and leaves (boxes), which represent the point at which partitioning was terminated. Inside each box (leaf) is the distribution on the dependent variable for those subjects partitioned to that leaf.

To summarize, IDEA is an inductive computer routine that involves interplay between the investigator and the data. Its purpose is to search for homogeneous criterion subjects in a multivariate dataset allowing the researcher to discover empirical models that predict a designated dependent measure in a way that best fits different subjects within a given sample. IDEA has been found to be most useful in those situations where data are scaled at a nominal level of measurement, and when the population under study is not easily summarized in a single, simple mathematical expression.

The first step in testing the construct validity of a nursing diagnostic classification system with IDEA technology would be to create a large database of nursing diagnoses, indicators, and selected client characteristics considered to be linked to nursing diagnoses. Next, the IDEA program can be brought on line and informed that the variable "nursing diagnosis x" is the dependent variable and that x number of "indicators" are to be considered independent variables. Then IDEA should be instructed to start its search for patterns in the dataset. At each node, IDEA will rank-order all indicators in terms of their chi-square significance values and suggest to the researcher the next indicator to use in building the tree or model. At these decision points, the investigator can direct IDEA to continue to build the tree as long as the independent variable it suggested for partitioning the data continues to significantly contribute or account for the dependent variable (nursing diagnoses). In other words, the investigator can allow the search to continue contingent upon a predetermined p value. When a point is reached where no other indicators significantly account for a given nursing diagnosis, IDEA is then instructed to make the partition a terminal leaf. This process continues until all significant contributions to a nursing diagnosis are exhausted. Subjects who emerge on the different leaves of the model can then be examined for commonalities and differences in other characteristics such as gender, developmental level, ethnic group, and so forth. Hence I suggest that the application of IDEA would serve to refine nursing diagnoses in a scientifically lawful and clinically relevant fashion.

Establishing external criterion validity is somewhat simpler. The question here is what direction, strength, and significance of association exist between specific nursing diagnoses and other theoretically related phenomena. For example, some I have thought about are as follows:

- What is the association between nursing diagnoses and consumption of nursing resources?
- What is the association between nursing diagnoses and cost of nursing care?
- What is the association between nursing diagnoses and standard measures of social and physical functioning?
- How well do nursing diagnoses at discharge predict health care utilization post-discharge?
- What is the congruency of nursing diagnoses with client perceptions of need for nursing care?

These questions clearly reflect my own underlying expectations and assumptions about the nature of nursing itself as well as the value inherent in a classification taxonomy for the discipline. That is, I expect that nursing diagnoses and related outcomes are highly amenable to nurse influence by autonomous action. It is also reasonable to expect that the degree of nursing effort expended should be related to nursing diagnoses.

My last example is perhaps the most important. Given our proximity to recipients of care and nursing's traditional value placed on incorporating the client's world view into the caring process, it is imperative that nursing diagnoses have a strong, positive correlation with emic perceptions of our clients. The question I raise here is: to what extent do professionally defined needs correspond with needs as perceived by clients themselves? This view also reflects the notion that scientific advances are inseparable from the social and political milieu in which they are developed. Thus my suggestion speaks to the development of nursing science within a broad social context.

SENSITIVITY

Now I turn your attention back to validity testing, which involves analysis of the capacity of nursing diagnoses to detect differences among various aggregate populations. This is discriminant validity and the task is to assess the capacity of a given construct to detect differences between or among subjects when stratified on various dimensions thought to affect the dependent measure—nursing diagnosis. This form of validity testing really addresses the sensitivity of nursing diagnosis measures.

Selection of stratifying variables for the conduct of discriminant validity testing can be guided by three knowledge-based sources: previous empirical research, intuitive clinical knowledge, and common sense. Following is a list of stratifiers I believe are particularly germane to discriminant validity testing for nursing diagnoses:

Developmental stages
Gender
Setting
Social class
Ethnicity

I select these particular stratifiers because there is reason to expect that certain groups stratified on them are more "at risk" for certain nursing diagnoses than others.

For those familiar with my own research background in ethnicity and health in urban America, it is not surprising that I wish to say a few more words about cross-cultural validation issues. My message is a word of caution not to confuse the concept of social class with ethnic group. This is a serious issue in the majority of previous health studies on ethnic populations in the United States. Both scientists and professional health personnel too often inaccurately equate the concept of culture with socioeconomic status. Originally formulated by Oscar Lewis (1966), the idea of a "culture of poverty" has resulted in research which fails to differentiate between patterns of health behavior that occur as a result of inadequate resources versus those that exist as a function of a cultural heritage. Response patterns resulting from economic deprivation is not something any group desires to perpetuate. In contrast, traditions or patterns of responses and beliefs handed down by grandparents are often voluntarily maintained over time even as younger generations achieve economic mobility. The failure of health professionals to recognize the differences between ethnicity and social class has led to ill conceived or nonexistent groups often referred to as the "culturally deprived" or the "culturally disadvantaged."

Fortunately, the nursing profession has a well-qualified cadre of nurse anthropologists whose talents should be brought to bear on the development of nursing diagnoses, particularly if the eventual goal is to create and validate a usable taxonomy for the discipline. It is particularly salient, given that the American public is the most culturally diverse population in the world.

There is yet another stratifier that would prove useful to validity testing for nursing diagnoses. That is the Diagnostic Related Group taxonomy, for it is reasonable to expect that nursing diagnoses are related to the health or disease status of individuals as well as physician-initiated procedures. This is especially true in the acute care setting when individuals are in an acute phase of illness. The care-cure dichotomy is not as clear-cut as some nurses want it to be. I personally have witnessed many physicians "caring" and many nurses "curing," and I am quite comfortable with the overlap in roles. And as a scientist, I am alert to discriminating scientific issues from professional or political issues.

SUMMARY

I have outlined the major research strategies that I see as useful for the development and testing of nursing diagnoses appropriate for the current level of theory testing in the area. The intent is to access the profession to already existing standards of scientific inquiry as well as new technologies that fit the complexities of phenomena of interest to nursing. I hope my ideas and visions prove useful in advancing this important work you are doing.

REFERENCES

Armstrong, J.S.: Derivation of theory by means of factor analysis, or Tom Swift and his electric factor analysis machine, Am. Statician, pp. 17-21, December, 1967.

Gebbie, K.M.: Toward the theory development for nursing diagnosis. In Kim, M.J., and Moritz, D.A., editors: Classification of nursing diagnoses—Proceedings of the Third and Fourth National Conferences, New York, 1982, McGraw-Hill Book Co.

Halloran, E.: Analysis of variations in nursing-workload by patient medical and nursing condition, Univeristy of Illinois at the Medical Center, 1980, Doctoral Dissertation.

Harris, R.J.: A primer of multivariate statistics, New York, 1975, Academic Press, Inc.

Kritek, P.B.: The generation and classification of nursing diagnosis: toward a theory of nursing. In Kim, M.J., and Moritz, D.A., editors: Classification of nursing diagnoses—Proceedings of the Third and Fourth National Conferences, New York, 1982, McGraw-Hill Book Co.

Lewis, O.: The culture of poverty, Sci. Am. **215:**19-25, 1966.

Lobowitz, S.: Some observations on measurement and statistics, Social Forces **46:**151-160, 1967.

Muliak, S.A.: The foundations of factor analysis, New York, 1972, McGraw-Hill Book Co.

Nunally, J.: Psychometric theory, New York, 1978, McGraw-Hill Book Co.

Press, L.I.: IDEA: a technique for inductive data exploration and analysis, Unpublished doctoral dissertation UCLA, 1967.

Rogers, M.S., and Shure, G.H.: A user's guide to IDEA in the CCBS system. Los Angeles, 1971, UCLA Center for Computer-Based Behavioral Studies.

Stevens, S.S.: Handbook of experimental psychology, New York, 1951, John Wiley & Sons, Inc.

Health information systems: toward computerization of nursing diagnosis

MARGARET R. GRIER, Ph.D., R.N.

In this paper a historical perspective on nursing diagnoses and computers will be presented, followed by a series of considerations in moving toward the computerization of nursing diagnoses. But, first, I would like to commend the North American Nursing Diagnosis Association for its diligent and noteworthy work over the past 10 years. Although the need to identify and describe phenomena basic to nursing has long been recognized, nursing has not made a concerted effort to address the problem. A favorite response to the idea of nursing diagnoses has been, "the world is not ready for that." Well, 100 years is a long preparation time, and the world now waits for descriptors of the nature of nursing, a task the Nursing Diagnosis Association undertook 10 years ago.

HISTORICAL PERSPECTIVE
Nursing diagnoses

Florence Nightingale, our eminent scientist, said that observation and reflection were essential to nursing, and implied that nursing diagnosis, action, and evaluation resulted from these processes. I quote from her 1894 publication, *The Training of Nursing:*

> Observation tells us the fact, reflection the meaning of the fact . . . Observation tells how the patient is, reflection tells what is to be done . . . Telling the nurse what to do is not enough and cannot be enough to perfect her, whatever her surroundings. The trained power of attending to one's own senses, so that these should tell the nurse how the patient is, is the *sine qua non* of being a nurse at all.

While Nightingale did not use the term diagnosis per se, she did say that the nurse must judge the condition of the patient and that this diagnostic process was an essential and indispensable prerequisite to the practice of nursing.

In a 1925 publication the Committee on Records of the National Organization for Public Health Nursing was more specific than Nightingale as to the nature of nursing judgments, and presented what I believe to be the first set of nursing diagnoses. This Committee said that the nurse must determine if the patient's condition is (1) satisfactory, (2) unsatisfactory and needs watching, or (3) serious and needs medical attention. The Committee spoke to the difficult cognitive processes in choosing among these alternatives, and to the necessity for complete and precise documentation of the basis for the judgment.

Investigations of nursing diagnoses were among the first formal investigations in nursing. One of the first studies approved under the first federal grant program for nursing research was a study of nurse record keeping (Arnstein, 1956). Unfortunately, no report of this work could be found. In 1957, Abdellah reported on her study of methods for identifying patient problems so as to make nursing diagnoses. And then in the 1960s there was the work of Kelly (1964, 1966) and her colleagues on the diagnosis of pain. Among other things, they described the complexity of one nursing inference and suggested methods for studying nursing diagnoses and intervention choices. Since the 1960s there has been a growing interest in describing nursing diagnoses by groups and individuals such as yourselves, and I think now there is awareness among some nurse leaders that this work is a necessary task for the future development of the discipline.

Computers

During this time that the world was preparing for nursing diagnoses, a drastic change was occurring in how information was processed. The first revolution in processing information gave us written language, while the second revolution gave us the printing press (paper, books, typewriter, mail; compilation and reproduction of ideas). The third revolution, in which we are now engaged, began in the 1800s and has had three phases. The first phase concerned the transmission of auditory information, and produced the telegraph, telephone, phonograph, and radio (rapid and wide communication of ideas). The second phase involved visual information, and resulted in photography, moving pictures, and television (more efficient and effective communication of ideas). The third and current phase of the third revolution is more dramatic than the auditory and visual phases, in that mental processes are involved. Computers are the first innovation that extends the human intellect, allowing humans to develop and analyze ideas which are difficult or impossible to observe in the real world. The potential results of the computer's ability to automatically carry out functions previously done only by the human brain are just being glimpsed (Simon, 1977).

To date, nursing has not exploited the processing methods that resulted from this third revolution. Except for a few isolated and limited instances, even the earlier auditory and visual devices have not been used for processing patient care data, even though these tools provide more rapid, wider, and effective dessimination of information. Nightingale understood the importance of conveying information visually, as shown by her innovative use of graphs (Cohen, 1984; Grier and Grier, 1978). The Committee on Records (1925) appreciated the cognitive activities in nursing, and the important role of nurses in acquiring and recording public health data was recognized in the early part of this century (Montanye, 1918). While there were attempts to identify and describe nursing data and its processing in the 1950s and 1960s, nursing was unable and/or unwilling to build on this work. The reasons for nursing not benefitting from the revolution going on around us are many, but relate to: failure to recognize and support the important nursing function of processing information about health care, lack of appreciation of the cognitive activities that underlie nursing practice, and a woeful lack of resources for attacking what is a resource-intensive problem.

Meanwhile, health data have increased exponentially, as has the paper on which they are recorded. And nursing's continuing reliance on print for information processing is detrimental to patient care, as so sadly demonstrated by the recent emergency situation in Dallas when the nurse delayed sending emergency care for 15 to 20 minutes and the patient died. The emergency triage nurse in Dallas used a standard protocol, and while protocols for individual situations were available on a card file, such paper protocols are too inefficient for the complexity of present-day health care. If a computerized system of protocols such as that developed by Moreland and Grier (in press) at St. Paul–Ramsey Medical Center had been in use, the Dallas nurse automatically could have moved to a protocol for evaluating her hypothesized judgment of hyperventilation, been aided in assessing the problem, made a judgment, and dispatched emergency care within 90 seconds.

In the past, computers have been used chiefly to perform mathematical calculations, and until recently 95% of computing power was spent in calculating and record keeping. The capability of the computer to aid in or actually to solve problems and make decisions is their real novelty, however. Computing is no longer confined to calculations with numbers, but also can be used to manipulate and process information, as well as to control other machines in real time (Simon, 1977). Thus the third revolution in the processing of information makes available a device that nursing can use to describe and document the basis for nursing practice, in that: large amounts of complex data can be rapidly and automatically evaluated and analyzed; information can be transmitted to and from various sensory modalities; and complete, precise, and clear documentation can be generated automatically. Now that the world is ready for nursing diagnoses, the question is: How can this revolutionary device be exploited to best aid the nurse in making such decisions?

Computerization steps

1. The first step in computerization is to recognize that the purpose of an information system is to provide the data necessary for making decisions. Nurses must choose actions for health problems. Thus the basic set of data that nurses need is information about the health problem for which they must act; specifically, diagnostic labels for and descriptors of the actual or potential health problems of patients (Grier, 1981). The establishment of this fundamental set of data, along with the desired outcomes and alternative nursing acts, is the major task facing the profession today. It is these three datasets

that provide the data for subsequent decisions on staffing, resource allocation, quality assurance, and costs. Therefore the first step in developing a computerized information system is to describe what decisions must be made and what data are necessary for making those decisions. The computerized information system should then be designed to provide appropriate persons the data they need to make the decisions for which they are responsible.

The first and most fundamental of these decisions is a nursing diagnosis. The work of describing nursing diagnoses builds theory at the nominal or most basic level and is the inductive approach to theory development. The work is slow and resource-intensive; dramatic results will not occur rapidly. While grand or meta theories may guide the describing of nursing diagnoses, I believe that the true nature of nursing is more likely to be captured from the gradual discovery of fundamental facts over time.

At the University of Illinois we are using the four concepts of healing, regulation, cognition, and perception to organize the analysis of nursing decisions. While nursing diagnoses fit within these classes, the concepts have little utility for reflection on nursing problems. Eight out of ten graduate students in a recent seminar identified nursing diagnostic labels from medical diagnoses, and the other two from a psychosocial or care delivery perspective. These students said that in clinical practice they think in terms of medical diagnoses. Until nursing has a clinically meaningful approach to the cognition of health care, we have little choice but the perception of health in terms of disease entities or problems in care delivery. Even so, nursing knowledge differs from that of medicine as described from the system developed at Creighton University in Nebraska (Evans, 1982). Only nurses know the information they need; and it is the nurses themselves who must undertake the task of describing their knowledge base.

2. The scope of data included in an information system must be limited to those data items that best discriminate between diagnoses. In conceptualization of initial implementation of a system, all possible data might be included, but the ultimate goal should be to delete data items that are not used and that are irrelevant. Cognitively the system should be limited to five to nine patient characteristics that are highly related to each diagnostic label (Miller, 1956).

3. For each diagnostic label selected for computerization, an algorithm or model describing the logic for arriving at that particular diagnosis, as well as the desired outcome of care, nursing actions for achieving the outcome, and subsequent administrative decisions, should be developed and coded. I found that specifying the desired outcome for a diagnosis frequently leads to clarification and greater precision of the etiology and/or diagnostic label. Perhaps because of the lack of a scientific base, there is little opportunity or attempt in nursing to explore the rationale for nursing judgments and actions. Night-

ingale (1894, 1907) spoke to the necessity of reflection in nursing care, the Committee on Records (1925) spoke to the complexity of the cognitive processes underlying the documentation of care, and Abdellah (1957) spoke to the need to identify the relationships between steps in the nursing process. Yet we still provide little time in clinical settings to reflect on practice, and give little attention in education settings to the logic of nursing decisions.

But computerization of nursing data requires logic and precision. Certainly nurses have been omitted from crucial decision-making about computer systems. But even when included, if nurses could not provide algorithms or flow charts describing the logic of data processing, computer scientists naturally concentrated on more defined data sets and excluded those of particular interest to nurses.

Coding is a particular problem in most computerized health care information systems. At best, flexible retrieval of health care data from computer storage is inefficient and costly. Aggregating and retrieving data from one computer system is difficult; aggregating and retrieving data across institutions, almost impossible. Medicine uses the International Classification of Diseases for coding medical diagnoses, but nursing has not identified a coding scheme. If this problem is not addressed soon, and on a national scale, we will be severely retarded in developing nursing knowledge and in charging for nursing services. Rather than having a coding system mandated by interests outside of nursing (such as computer vendors), the nursing community should determine a system that is appropriate to our needs.

4. Once the possible diagnostic data are computerized, the automatic processing, storage, and retrieval capabilities of the system can be used to evaluate the diagnostic concept. Easily determined by computer, both across patients and across nurses, are the selection of diagnostic labels, the frequency with which each descriptor is used with a diagnostic label, the type and number of times a descriptor not included is written into the system, and the importance rating of a given descriptor in making a diagnosis. After a trial period the computerized listing can be altered to include those descriptors written into the system and to exclude those not used or not rated as important in making a diagnosis. A process of clinical use followed by conceptual refinement can continue until all the important descriptors used by nurses in making diagnoses are listed and all those unimportant and not used are excluded—in other words, until a list of the most essential diagnostic data are identified.

After a suitable period of using a refined listing, the computer can be used to evaluate the collected data, such as the reliability of a diagnostic label across patients and across nurses, the sensitivity of a descriptor to a diagnostic label, and the inclusiveness of a set of descriptors.

In addition to this basic evaluation, other approaches also should be explored.

Simulation of a particular diagnosis could be useful, particularly for one that is difficult to describe. One of the greatest benefits to nursing from computerization is the forced description, precision, and logic of variables. The refinement of diagnostic concepts to the extent possible prior to clinical testing is necessary for efficient evaluation. The problem with simulation is generalizability to the real world, but this problem is aided by simulating a random selection of actual cases.

The techniques of *artificial intelligence* should be considered. These computer systems, which mirror the cognitive processes of experts, can be used to describe and make diagnostic judgments and care decisions. To my knowledge such a project has not been undertaken in nursing, although there have been efforts to describe the cognitive processing nurses use to make diagnostic judgments and choose appropriate actions (Corcoran, 1983). Such techniques have promise for identifying and describing nursing diagnoses.

Another approach that should be explored is *signal detection theory*. From methods used to detect and analyze radar signals, a methodology for evaluating diagnostic performance has been developed (Swets and Pickett, 1982). In contrast to the descriptive approaches mentioned above, the signal detection approach is prescriptive. In other words, rather than to describe diagnosing, this method is used to evaluate and guide diagnostic performance.

5. As I have said several times, computerizing nursing data is resource-intensive. The first thing required is a good manual system of information. A computerized system will be little better than the manual system that is automated. Regardless of plans for computerization, every clinical setting should refine the manual information system to include advances in nursing knowledge and to improve precision and efficiency.

A lot of nursing time is required either to refine or to develop an information system; both conceptualizers and operationalizers are necessary for the task. Nurses with expertise in the diagnostic concept, and with understanding of that process, should identify and refine diagnoses with input from the practice setting. This is *not* a task for students, who lack both the knowledge and the experience necessary for expertise in making nursing judgments. Ideally, clinical specialists will be used, but this may not be feasible. One approach might be initial development using a Delphi technique, with about five clinical specialists, interspersed with evaluation and refinement of the results in a clinical setting.

The development and testing of nursing diagnoses are ideal for a research program, in that a set of diagnoses for a given type of patient can be developed and tested individually and then combined into a computerized system for that type of patient. Groups of clinical nurses have been enthusiastic about such a project and, with the appropriate leadership and resources, are ideal for the task.

In addition to nurse scientists and practitioners, both a computer scientist and a computer programmer are needed. Or computer science expertise might be acquired through the vendor of a predeveloped system. Whether the system is self-developed or purchased, however, computer expertise should be sought with algorithms for the diagnoses and other decisions in hand. If nurse practitioners, administrators, and researchers do not know what data to computerize, others will not know either. Other personnel who can be useful are information scientists and evaluation experts, as well as experts from other clinical fields and settings such as medicine, pharmacy, clinics, public health departments, etc., the various areas with which nursing must interface.

Hardware, along with site provisions and alterations, will be needed. Currently, most health care information systems use large mainframe computers, but this type of technology is becoming outdated. In all settings, nurses need to look toward networking tabletop, portable, and/or wearable computers located where the data are acquired. Individual patient data collected in portable computers can be transmitted by modem and cable to a tabletop or minicomputer for aggregating on a group of patients. In turn, these aggregated data can be transmitted to other computers for administrative analysis and decision-making on larger patient groups.

In addition, support in terms of money, time, and leadership are necessary, as so well described in the paper by Simmons. The development, design, and implementation of computerized systems of information takes long-term commitment. Individual nurses must, and will, provide some of their own support. Organizations and institutions also must make a considerable investment in the development of a system. However, there are indications that benefits acrue in the social milieu of nursing practice, the cost of nurse staffing, the quality of care, and the status of the implementation site.

Some of the problems we must address in computerizing nursing diagnoses are

1. Ascertaining the reliability of nursing diagnoses across patients and across nurses (requiring large samples of a lot of data)
2. Sampling diagnostic data when the sensitivity of patient characteristics for diagnostic labels is unknown and large numbers of descriptors are specified
3. Determining the validity of a nursing diagnosis
4. Analyzing nursing data when there is both co-morbidity and co-activity; in other words, more than one nursing diagnosis within a patient and the nurse simultaneously taking more than one action for one or more diagnoses
5. Determining the benefits of a computerized system of information when so little is known about the manual system, and the manual system is poorly controlled

6. Developing within nursing, and attracting from other disciplines, the expertise necessary for developing and testing computerized information systems
7. Critiquing and communicating in a timely fashion the advances made in describing and computerizing nursing data

SUMMARY

The considerations necessary when computerizing nursing data are
1. Specify the decisions that are necessary in the practice, administration, and/or investigation of nursing care.
2. Work toward identifying a limited set of the most essential data (three to five items) for making those decisions.
3. Develop an algorithm or model (with codes) describing the logic for each decision.
4. Identify and acquire the necessary resources.
5. Plan and implement an evaluation program appropriate to the purposes for which the system was developed and designed.

We can document efforts throughout the history of modern nursing to cope with the processing of health care data. The work of this group over the past 10 years is salient in that history. As demonstrated over time, nurses have the commitment to conceptualize nursing diagnoses and health care. What we need are the resources and expertise necessary to test, analyze, and use those conceptualizations to improve health care. We were unable to capitalize on the developments in processing auditory and visual information, but we must not let advances in mental processing elude us. Dr. Werley once told me to think big, so I would like to leave you with some big ideas:
1. Introducing a resolution before the ANA House of Delegates to establish a national program for identifying and standardizing diagnostic labels and descriptors of actual and potential health problems
2. Requesting the Division of Nursing, National Library of Medicine, and/or the National Center for Health Services Research to set aside funds, and issue proposal requests, for research and development of computerized nursing information systems
3. Asking the United States Congress to appropriate funds for the establishment of a national patient-care data base for nursing

If achieved, such acts would provide resources; and if resources are available, expertise will follow.

REFERENCES

Abdellah, F.G.: Methods of identifying covert aspects of nursing problems, Nurs. Res. **6**:4-23, 1957.
Arnstein, M.G., editor: PHS Research grants program in nursing: progress and direction, Nurs. Res. **5**:46, 1956.
Cohen, I.B.: (1984). Florence Nightingale, Sci. Am. **250**:128-137, 1984.

Corcoran, S.A.: Nursing care planning by hospice nurses (doctoral dissertation), University of Minnesota, Dissert. Abstr. Int. (In press.)

Evans, S.: Differentiation of the information needs of health professionals using expert systems, Proceedings of the First IEEE Computer Society International Conference on Medical Computer Science/Computational Medicine, Philadelphia, 1982, IEEE.

Grier, J.B., and Grier, M.R.: Contributions of a passionate statistician, Res. Nurs. Health **1:**103-109, 1978.

Grier, M.R.: A model of processing information for making patient care decisions. In Werley, H.H., and Grier, M.R., editors: Information systems for nursing practice, New York, 1981, Springer Publishing Co., Inc.

Kelly, K.: An approach to the study of clinical inference in nursing, Nurs. Res. **13:**314-315, 1964.

Kelly, K.: Clinical inference in nursing, Nurs. Res. **15:**23-26, 1966.

Lewis, E.P.: An opening door, Nurs. Res. **4:**3, 1955.

Miller, G.A.: The magical number seven plus or minus two: some limits on our capacity for processing information, Psychol. Rev. **63:**81-97, 1956.

Montanye, B.: Records and statistics, Public Health Nurse **10:**165-169, 1918.

Moreland, H.J., and Grier, M.R.: Telephone consultation of the older adult, Geriat. Nurs. (In press.)

Nightingale, F.: Training of nurses. In Nutting, M.A., and Dock, L.A., editors: History of Nursing. Vol. II, New York, 1907, G.P. Putnam's Sons.

Simon, H.A.: What computers mean for man and society, Science **195:**1186-1191, 1977.

Swets, J.A., and Pickett, R.M.: Evaluation of diagnostic systems: methods from signal detection theory, New York, 1982, Academic Press, Inc.

Discussion

Marie Gould: Marie Gould from Chicago. Would you clarify a point for me, Doctor Clinton. Is the belief that indicators are population specific inconsistent with the idea that there are critical indicators for each diagnosis?

Jackie Clinton: Well, you see, they are sort of inseparable. There might be some. The question I'm raising is that all indicators might not be indicators for given diagnoses for all people, all times, all places, and all settings. Are you with me? It is naive to think that all indicators will somehow significantly contribute to the variance in a nursing diagnosis. We have some technologies available that would let us test that out. Maybe there are some indicators, for example, if you are a certain age, that you do not have to think about. It would be nice to know that as a clinician. That is what I am addressing.

Marie Gould: So, then, the critical indicators are within the population, as opposed to critical indicators within the diagnosis?

Jackie Clinton: I'm saying that you can test critical indicators as identified by clinicians related to a diagnosis. Then you can see if in relationship to that particular diagnosis all those indicators are applicable across all populations. In some cases they may not be. In some they would be. But clinically it makes sense to me. Does it make sense to you?

Marie Gould: Yes. Thank you.

Jackie Clinton: In addition, it might be cost effective over time if from data collection you knew you did not have to do all critical indicators in terms of populations.

Richard Fehring: Richard Fehring of Wisconsin. I just wanted to clarify something. In the beginning, you mentioned that you thought it was premature for experimental research. I can understand that from a theoretical and a research perspective as well as developing our body of knowledge. However, in a practical sense, we have nurses who are diagnosing and treating using interventions, and we need to do that every day. So, from the standpoint of intervention, is experimental research premature?

Jackie Clinton: Well, all I'm saying is that it is very important to name things. It is very important to find an indicator. What happens if a lot of experiments are rolled out, and for some reason because of the way that indicator or the way that nursing diagnosis was conceptualized or measured the investigator finds that they had no impact on the welfare of that subject relative to that diagnosis? Must there be something wrong with the diagnosis? Must there be something wrong with the intervention? Maybe not. Premature, really creative, interventions can get ditched quickly. Are you with me? And so do the diagnoses. My fear is because we have for so long, in our adolescence as a scientific discipline, reached for what was valued in the physical sciences, we will cut ourselves short. Of course that is going to go on. But I think the major bulk of the work, and I am talking about prediction which gets us really close to experiments—you know, that kind of predictive level theory— I am saying we can do a lot in predicting things without really going to the expense of doing experiments. This is not saying no experiments for the rest of our lives. Right now, I think we would be better to play it safe and not kill some of our bright ideas.

Joanne McCloskey: Joanne McCloskey, the University of Iowa. I have a comment on this same topic. I heard you and also Phyllis Kritek yesterday say that it is premature to work on the testing of nursing interventions. At the same time, most of your presentation, in my opinion, was talking about nursing interventions. For example, the need for practical outcomes; the interrelationship between an inductive and a deductive approach; the consumption of nursing resources; the use of post-discharge health care resources. The reason why anybody makes a nursing diagnosis is to go on and do interventions. The research on nursing interventions and on particular interventions is much older than much of the research on nursing diagnosis. I appreciate the hesitancy to have any premature predictive theory, but I think we need to promote research on interventions and the relationship between interventions and diagnoses.

Jackie Clinton: I am saying that you can get to predictive level theory without ever doing an experiment. Today I have only talked about purely descriptive associational hypothesis testing. There has not been one mention of any other kind of approach methodology. Being deductive does not mean experimental. By being deductive, I mean that we have instruments, we are measuring, we have predetermined hypotheses, and we are going in there. For some things we have names. I am purely at a descriptive survey associational level in all of the things that I have mentioned. One can monitor or watch for the outcomes passively without manipulating anything. And I am saying we can get to a very high level of theory development without going to the expense of quasi-experimental studies.

Joanne McCloskey: I don't think we disagree. It is just simply that statements that you made earlier sound like one should not be working on interventions, and I don't think you mean that.

Jackie Clinton: Yes I do. Right now intensively. Absolutely.

Joanne McCloskey: Oh, you do. Well then, I do disagree with you.

Jackie Clinton: If there is to be money and funding in terms of the developmental levels in science, we would do well to move toward predictive associational hypotheses lest we throw out some very creative nursing diagnoses prematurely. Clearly, there are going to be people running around experimenting. They will take care of themselves. I am saying the major thrust should be at this level, and it makes sense and is in concert with how scientific inquiry is developed.

Joanne McCloskey: I think I need to talk with you more later.

Mary Lou Kiley: Mary Lou Kiley from the University Hospital of Cleveland. I would just like to say I enjoyed your paper very much. It had great breadth and was very thought-provoking. I would like to ask in relation to the IDEA approach to this, are you familiar with the autogroup process that was used with the DRGs?

Jackie Clinton: Yes I am. It is very similar to this technology: The clinical input, the clinical judgment input, and also the technology of computers.

Mary Lou Kiley: Do you think IDEA is more appropriate for nursing, or did you just happen to be more familiar with it?

Jackie Clinton: The thing that intrigues me about IDEA is that it will handle data that are not scaled. It also entertains the idea that you do not have to have matching levels of data. If you have a hemoglobin over here and how I feel today over here, it will entertain all of the multiple levels that interest me as a clinician.

Mary Lou Kiley: Thank you.

Jackie Clinton: Well, you are doing some nice stuff in Cleveland with nursing diagnosis and DRGs too.

Margaret Grier: Jackie, first I would like to say that I wholeheartedly support your idea that what we need to be about is the description of nursing diagnosis before we move into experimentation in relation to nursing actions. And that is coming from one whose work has been in the area of choosing nursing actions. But believe me, nursing *must, must* get about the task of describing nursing and get about the task of describing nursing diagnosis or the basic phenomena in practice, which all of our activities surround. My question in regard to your paper, which I thoroughly enjoyed, is: could you please speak to sample size in relation to the analyses that you presented?

Jackie Clinton: Well, I come from a place where, if you don't have a cast of a billion, you are no good. The reason why I suggested a national data base is to take care of the issue of sample size. Margaret, IDEA will deal with a sample size as little as fifty or as large as a billion. It will deal with as many as a hundred independent variables and a hundred indicators for one dependent variable, e.g., one diagnosis. So the technology is there. The other thing I am thinking about is how to get a large n for nursing diagnoses' descriptive data. Let us look at hospital subjects, and diagnoses by day of hospitalization. The average length of stay is about eight days for people with chronic illness. Your n gets high very quickly if the unit of analysis is day of hospitalization. That is what we are doing in the ANA study. We are thinking of ways to deal with that, looking at how many days of hospitalization did this person have a given nursing diagnoses, what the indicators were, and what was the pattern of those diagnoses over time. Certainly, they would change, and one could predict them in certain patient populations. So I am talking large ns, very large. One needs to have a mechanism for upping the n very quickly.

Lark Kirk: Lark Kirk, Case Western Reserve University student. I, too, found your discussion of IDEA provocative, and I have a question that is rather size related, also. Am I correct in understanding that IDEA is a program for large system implementation, main frame computers? And, if so or if not, do you see a place for microcomputer usage? Can that expand the work in data base management?

Jackie Clinton: I think IDEA is eclectic in that it has been used by scientists. Agencies want to tally things, keep them on record, and retrieve them as opposed to doing some sort of analysis. So it is predominantly used by scientists, social scientists, to predict certain things.

Lark Kirk: Is it primarily available in a university setting at this time?

Jackie Clinton: It can be bought. UCLA marketed it to me. The computer laboratory at UCLA has developed it over time, and kept track of who has used it and why. I was first drawn to it because of how much sense it made to me dealing with clinical nursing data, and I was so tired of factor analysis doing strange things that did not make sense to me as a clinician. I could not label it. It was useless to conduct those analyses when I could not name the phenomena, and with IDEA it seemed better to me.

Lark Kirk: Thank you.

Ann Marie Voith: Ann Marie Voith from Wisconsin. Going back to what you said about reliability, I was wondering if you have recommendations on what level of nurse you would like to see used as the sample for these studies?

Jackie Clinton: I see that as an empirical question. I would check it out and see if there is an associational relationship between level of preparation and the nursing diagnoses and the indicators that nurses identify. I have no evidence in my world that anybody has studied that.

Mary Lou Kiley: Mary Lou Kiley. When I was up here before, I forgot to say that I certainly support your recommendation for a national database. In our work thus far, we have about 1294 cases. We think in order to make our position clear, we need at least 60,000. In our hospital we would collect about 25,000 in 1 year, which certainly makes multi-institutional data collections desirable, as does making the databases available to everyone.

Jackie Clinton: Right.

Harriet Werley: I enjoyed your paper, but I am a little confused by comments, questions, and responses so I seek clarification. I understand you to say that though you see the major thrusts being in one direction, you are not opposed to people pursuing a well-constructed piece of research on interventions, etc.

Jackie Clinton: That is exactly what I'm trying to say, Harriet. There is a lot of descriptive work to be done, and it should not be overlooked because we are into experimentation. There is a lot to be done that would even improve our experimentation. One of my concerns is the premature termination and killing of great theory because you have not taken time enough to learn how to measure or describe it yet. That is a danger. It has been a danger in our discipline. It is not particular to nursing diagnoses, by any means.

Mi Ja Kim: I was very pleased to hear that in your ANA study you looked at nursing diagnoses as a part of and in relation to the DRGs. However, on the one hand, though you emphasize the need for descriptive study with reliability, validity, etc., the problem, at least from my vantage point, is that the diagnoses do not have reliable, valid defining characteristics. How did you handle that in your study?

Jackie Clinton: In the DRG study?

Mi Ja Kim: Yes. How do you know that the nursing diagnoses that have been generated by these nurses are indeed valid and reliable and clinically useful?

Jackie Clinton: Well, first of all, when did I say we were doing all of that? Number two, we are looking at some external criteria, such as other measures that indicate the use of nursing resource consumption. The underlying premise is that nursing diagnoses are related to nursing resource consumption. We are looking at external measures that are not generated from the same individual in most cases.

Mi Ja Kim: I guess what I am concerned about is that, with the current status of the nursing diagnoses, this is the only way to operate. But I just do not want to get short-changed in the outcome of the study. It may not really reflect what nursing diagnoses are, and that is my concern.

Jackie Clinton: Yes, and I share that concern.

Mi Ja Kim: Thank you.

Cindy Koviac: Cindy Koviac from Grand Rapids, Michigan. I am interested in the portable mini-main frame computer model that Dr. Grier described. Are there systems such as this in use somewhere in the United States or in other countries at this time?

Margaret Grier: There is a project that is probably reaching completion at the University of California, San Francisco, networking computers within acute care settings, specifically a university hospital there. The technology for doing that is available. The reports coming from that particular project suggest that the networking hardware, etc., is simplistic. What is going to be difficult is pulling together and standardizing the information that is networked across various disciplines, such as nursing, medicine, and pharmacy. In fact, in the last description I heard of that project, the investigators were almost saying that it looked like it could be practically an impossible task. But nursing, and in fact nursing in terms of network, may sit in an interesting and rather unique position. I think the possibility of networking within one discipline is readily available already. And the interesting thing about nursing is that nursing already interfaces with practically all of the other disciplines. So it is an interesting idea, I think.

Betty Chang: I am Betty Chang from the University of California, Los Angeles. I was interested in your presentation. I am especially interested in the fact that you point to our need for a list of defining characteristics which would eliminate the need for excess information. To this end, I wonder if you could share with us how hospitals could reconcile their use of different nursing models. If you use one nursing model, the assessment tool is different from that of another.

Margaret Grier: I think one of the major strengths in nursing is our diversity. I happen to believe that one of the most feasible ways for developing computer systems is by unit, even though models or philosophies of care may differ from unit to unit. The characteristics and the type of care required by a given group of patients can greatly differ from that of patients on another unit. I think developing a nursing information system for a limited number of patients using a given model can be very useful. And in fact nursing needs that.

Betty Chang: But what if there's a system that could be developed that we would like for more than one hospital to use, because it takes quite a bit of work to develop the system?

Margaret Grier: I would agree. I think one of the projects that the entire nursing profession needs to be concentrating on has to do with the establishment of a national data base. The task of aggregating data across institutions is going to be a huge problem that is going to take a lot of effort, a lot of time. Florence Nightingale even undertook that and, as far as I can determine, it is about the one thing she failed in among all of her efforts. I do not think we have advanced in aggregating data across institutions over what Nightingale did. But nursing, in tackling that problem, could make some advances. One of the concerns about existing medical databases has to do with the generalizability of that data to other settings. When those databases were initially developed, the idea was that they would provide information that could be used to look at patient characteristics, medical diagnosis treatment, etc., and of course the federal government provided huge sums of money for their developments. Currently there is a lot of concern that that is not going to happen. The feeling is the databases are in fact unique to the setting in which they were developed.

Harriet Werley: I just want to alert you to the fact that there is a group within nursing that is working to establish a national nursing information network. Some of the representatives are from the Association of American Colleges of Nursing, the ANA, and the NLN. Perhaps your president might want to pursue this information. I would suggest it.

Margaret Grier: Yes, I think so. It sounds like that group should be considering, and will be considering, some of the fundamental kinds of problems that I think have to be addressed in preparation for establishing a national database.

Mary Lou Kiley: Mary Lou Kiley. I am interested in your concerns about inter-institutional data. I agree with you that it is a difficult task, but if one had a list of data that was to be obtained and a method for entering it into a database, I do not see that it is as difficult as you suggest.

Margaret Grier: I think my concern is that if five years down the road nursing decides that we are going to standardize a particular coding scheme and then use that coding scheme to aggregate data into a national database, the institutions who have put millions of dollars into establishing a computer system are not going to be willing to go back in and change their coding scheme. That's why I think nursing needs to address some of the standardization issues soon.

Mary Lou Kiley: I think that nursing needs to look at its own data before we can determine our interface with medicine, pharmacy, and the other disciplines.

Margaret Grier: That's a good point.

Harriet Werley: I wanted to ask Margaret if she has some documentation for the study that indicated there would be this limited number of characteristics. You cited it as though it were something that had been the result of research.

Margaret Grier: I cannot give it to you. It has been long known, perhaps for a hundred years. In the area of human behavior, it is well accepted apparently by the psychologists. One can raise some questions about it, but it is still considered a good guideline in terms of cognitive limitations.

CHAPTER 7

Validation

Validating diagnostic labels: standardized methodology*

RICHARD J. FEHRING, D.N.Sc., R.N.

A diagnostic validity gap exists between diagnoses on the alphabetized list sanctioned by the North American Nursing Diagnosis Association (NANDA) and the diagnoses actually used in clinical practice. The so-called accepted diagnoses >50 are not valid in the usual sense of the word. Acceptance by NANDA means that the diagnoses should be studied and tested. Many nurses use the diagnostic labels "as if" they were generated from rigorous research. Other nurses find that the diagnostic labels are not relevant to their clinical practice.

One of the reasons that a validity gap exists is because of the way in which the current list was generated at regional and national classification conferences. Participants at the conferences signed up to work in small groups on diagnostic labels of interest. The group members retrospectively identified definitions, labels, etiologies, and characteristics of a given diagnosis. Although group members were asked to bring clinical data and research to support work on a particular diagnosis, many participants contributed to developing diagnoses without sufficient evidence of expertise. At the Fifth National Classification Conference the problem was addressed in three ways: (1) no changes were made on existing labels, etiologies, and defining characteristics without supporting data; (2) new diagnoses were accepted on the basis of supporting data; and (3) members of small groups developed research questions to help validate existing diagnoses.

Another cause for the diagnostic validity gap is the paucity of studies which could contribute to diagnostic validity. What this means is that virtually every

---

*I wish to acknowledge Audrey McLane, Ph.D., for her encouragement and assistance in writing this article, and Judith F. Miller, for her editorial assistance.

diagnostic label on the accepted list needs to be validated through clinical research.

One reason for the few diagnostic validation studies is the absence of practical validation models. Gordon and Sweeney (1979) presented three models that could be utilized to identify and validate diagnoses, and Avant (1979) listed a seven-step approach for diagnostic identification and validation. Although these models are useful, they might be confusing to a nurse unprepared in research methodologies. The models are also somewhat impractical for the beginning researcher, since geographical representation and large sample sizes are required. Geographic representation is recommended in order to establish generalizability for a given diagnosis. However, smaller studies that can be replicated for generalizability might be more practical and might provide the motivation for more nurses to contribute to validation efforts.

Nursing diagnosis interest groups, now forming throughout the country, are a tremendous resource which can be mobilized to assist with validating existing diagnoses. Many times the goals of the regional, state, and local groups are to validate diagnostic labels. Practical validation models are needed to provide direction for such heterogeneous groups. The purpose of this paper is to present practical methodologies that could be used to validate and to gather quantifiable evidence for diagnostic labels. These proposed methods are based upon Gordon and Sweeney's models but employ the scientific reasoning used to obtain validity and reliability for scientific measures. A second purpose of this paper is to provide a possible scheme for standardizing validation.

DEFINITIONS OF VALIDATION

According to the dictionary (Webster's ninth edition), something is valid when it is based on evidence and sound reasoning and is able to withstand criticism or objection. Using this definition, validating a nursing diagnosis entails providing evidence and sound reasoning that a diagnosis exists. The evidence would be provided to convince professional nurses and/or the members of the Diagnosis Review Committee of NANDA that a given diagnosis should be placed on the accepted list. According to Gordon and Sweeney (1979), validation of a nursing diagnosis consists of providing evidence that the cluster of defining characteristics to which the label refers actually occurs as an entity in clinical situations. Their statement about validation flows from their definition of a nursing diagnosis. Gordon stated that there are three components to a diagnosis: the structural, the conceptual, and the competency components. The structural component refers to the observable characteristics of a diagnosis, the conceptual refers to the type or focus of the health problem, and the competency refers to the ability and expertise of the nurse who makes the diagnosis. All three of these components are important and must be taken into account when validating a diagnosis. Validating a diagnosis means more than providing evidence that a label refers to a clinical entity; validating also means that the defining characteristics of a diagnosis occur as a cluster and that nurses who determine the defining characteristics of a given health problem have the expertise and experience to do so.

Validation is a common topic in scientific research. It is of concern throughout the research process but especially during the design phase and when selecting measurement tools to gather data. In reference to research design, there are two types of validity; internal and external. Internal validity refers to whether an effect can be attributed to the independent variable in an experiment, and external validity refers to whether the results of an experiment can be generalized to the entire population of concern. Both internal and external validity can be applied to nursing diagnoses research. Internal validity has relevance when a researcher designs an experiment to determine the effectiveness of an intervention to treat a diagnosis, and external validity has relevance both to the generalizability of such research and to whether a given diagnosis has geographical representation.

Validity of a measurement tool usually means the degree to which that tool measures what it is supposed to measure. There are three general types of measurement validity: content, criterion-related, and construct. Content validity refers to whether the items of a tool are representative of the universe of items that could be used to describe a given concept. Evidence that a measurement tool has content validity is commonly obtained through the literature or by a panel of experts. The experts are asked to judge whether the items of the tool represent the concept that the tool is purported to measure. Content validity has relevance for nursing diagnoses in that diagnoses are essentially phenomena (concepts) that represent some type of health problem. Just as content validity refers to whether items of a tool are representative of a concept, with nursing diagnoses it refers to whether the characteristics (that is, the signs and symptoms) of a diagnosis are representative of the diagnosis and that they actually occur as an entity in clinical situations.

Criterion-related validity also has relevance to validation of nursing diagnoses. Criterion-related validity refers to establishing a relationship between the measurement tool and some other criteria. In relation to nursing diagnoses, this could mean providing evidence that a relationship exists between a given diagnosis and the reported etiologies. For example, the diagnosis of spiritual distress is related to the etiology of separation from religious/cultural ties. If this is so, then there should be some type of (positive) correlation between people who are separated from religious ties and the incidence of spiritual distress as evidenced by the defining characteristics.

The final type of measurement validity, construct validity, requires the provision of evidence for the theoretical basis of a given concept or construct. One of the methods for providing this evidence is called the "known groups" technique. This technique entails measuring an attribute in a group that is suspected or known to have the attribute and in a group that probably does not have the attribute. The results are then compared. This technique could be easily applied to validating a nursing diagnosis. For example, you would suspect that people with severe back pain or who are bedridden due to congestive heart failure would exhibit characteristics of the diagnosis "impaired mobility." A healthy group of college students, however, would probably not display these characteristics. Assessing the defining characteristics of impaired mobility in both groups and then comparing the results would help to establish construct validity of that diagnosis.

MODELS OF VALIDATION

The three models of identification and validation that Gordon and Sweeney (1979) have proposed are the retrospective identification and validation model, the clinical model, and the nurse-validation model. The first part of the retrospective model and the clinical model is essentially processes to identify new diagnoses. The second part of the retrospective model and the nurse-validation model is designed to address validation of already identified diagnoses. The validation steps of the retrospective model essentially entail providing a representative sample of expert nurses with a list of characteristics and etiologies without an identified label. They are asked to provide a label. The degree to which they apply the same or similar labels constitutes validation.

The nurse-validation model is the other validation model that Gordon and Sweeney (1979) presented. The model consists of familiarizing a group of trained nurse observers with a given diagnostic label and having them tabulate the defining characteristics observed in an adequate number of patients with a given diagnosis. Coexistence of the observed characteristics of the diagnosis with those characteristics either clinically or retrospectively identified will establish validity. The strength and weakness of the model is the reliability of the nurse observers. Gordon and Sweeney provided examples of how to increase interrater reliability in their article.

I would like to propose two practical models that could be used to validate nursing diagnoses and to suggest a possible third approach. These models are derived from Gordon and Sweeney's (1979) models and from the approaches used to validate research measurement tools. The development of a research measurement tool consists of providing evidence of the tool's reliability and validity. When presenting the tools to the research community it is common to provide evidence of the tools' reliability and validity by citing the established reliability and validity levels. For example, a given tool might have a split-half reliability of 0.78, and a K-R reliability of 0.86. The reliability is often quantified and the researcher can decide from this evidence how much faith can be placed in the tool and the research results. I propose that similar standardized quantifiable evidence be provided on each diagnosis so that nurses can decide how much faith they can have in a given diagnosis. The following models propose ways of standardizing evidence of diagnostic validity similar to the evidence researchers commonly provide for measurement tools.

The three types of standardized validity that I would like to see provided on every diagnosis are (1) diagnostic content validity (DCV), (2) clinical diagnostic validity (CDV), and (3) etiological correlation ratings (ECR). The DCV is retrospective evidence from the perspective of experts on the characteristics of a given diagnostic label, and the CDV is prospective evidence on the characteristics from a clinical perspective. The ECR is statistical evidence of the levels of relationship of a proposed etiology to the diagnosis. For each diagnosis on the classification list, a DCV, CDV, and ECR needs to be established and presented. For example, the diagnosis of spiritual distress might have a DCV of 0.89, a CDV of 0.78, with ECRs of 0.83 and 0.72 for its two proposed etiologies. This example indicates that the diagnosis has high validity and correlation and gives the clinician easily interpretable evidence as to how much confidence to put in the diagnosis.

The establishment of a *DCV model* would be similar to methods employed to establish evidence for content validity of a measurement tool by use of an index of content validity (CVI). With this method experts are asked to rate items of a tool according to how relevant the items are to the concept that is being measured (Waltz and Bausell, 1981). The items are rated on a scale of 1 to 4, with 4 indicating very relevant and 1 indicating not relevant. The CVI equals the proportion of items given a rating of 3 or 4 by both raters. CVI ratings of 0.50 or less are unacceptable ratings. Using this principle of obtaining a CVI for measurement tools, the steps of obtaining a DCV would be as follows:

1. Have an adequate number of "experts" (25 or 50) rate the characteristics of an already identified diagnosis on a scale of 1 to 5. The ratings would indicate how representative each characteristic is of a given diagnosis. The 1 to 5 rating would be interpreted as follows: 1, not at all characteristic; 2, very little characteristic; 3, somewhat characteristic; 4, quite characteristic; and 5, very characteristic.

2. Use the Delphi technique to enhance consensus among the experts. This step would be ideal but would not be necessary, especially if the nurse conducting the study does not have financial resources for multiple mailings.

3. Calculate the weighted ratios for each characteristic. The weighted ratio is obtained by summing the weights assigned to each response and then dividing by the total number of responses. The assigned weights are as

follows: $5 = 1; 4 = 0.75; 3 = 0.50; 2 = 0.25; 1 = 0$. If all of the experts would indicate that the characteristic is very characteristic of a given diagnosis, then the rated ratio for that characteristic would equal 1.

4. Discard the characteristics with a ratio less than or equal to 0.50.
5. Characteristics or items with ratios greater than 0.75 will be labeled critical.
6. Obtain the total DCV score by summing the individual characteristic ratings and averaging the results.

The difficult step in the DCV model is obtaining an adequate number of experts on a given diagnosis in order to have them rate the diagnosis. It is suggested that an adequate number of experts be determined much the same way a researcher obtains an adequate sample for a research study. An ideal number would be 50 to 100. An adequate number, however, would be based on the number of experts available and whether they can be randomly selected. It is suggested that experts be obtained through the literature, through professional societies that have "expert" lists on nursing phenomena (such as the Midwest Nursing Research Society), by soliciting experts on nursing phenomenon from faculty of schools of nursing, or from lists of clinical specialists. Experts might be obtained from members of NANDA or local and state nursing diagnosis interest groups. Although it would be ideal to obtain experts that have a national geographical representation, repeated studies in different parts of the country would be another way of establishing generalizability.

Clinical validity of a nursing diagnosis could be obtained through the use of the *CDV model*. Although this model is similar to Gordon and Sweeney's (1979) nurse-validation model, the intent is to provide quantifiable clinical evidence that a diagnosis exists. The steps of the model are as follows:

1. Two "expert" clinicians observe and assess an adequate number of patients with a previously identified nursing diagnosis.
2. The clinicians check the frequency of the previously identified characteristics of the diagnosis with those characteristics manifested by each patient observed.
3. Calculate the weighted interrater reliability ratios for each identified characteristic by the following formula:

$$R = \frac{A}{A + D} \times \frac{\frac{F_1}{N} + \frac{F_2}{N}}{2}$$

Where A = Number of agreements
D = Number of disagreements
F_1 = Frequency of characteristics observed by first rater
F_2 = Frequency of characteristics observed by second rater
N = Number of subjects observed
R = Weighted interrater reliability ratio

4. Discard the characteristics with ratios less or equal to 0.50.
5. Items with ratios greater than 0.75 would be critical.
6. Obtain the total CDV score by summing and averaging the ratios for each characteristic.

An underlying assumption of the CDV model is that the nursing diagnosis was appropriately identified. The difficult parts of the process, as in Gordon and Sweeney's model, are finding an adequate number of patients with a given diagnosis and demonstrating interrater reliability. The steps of the model, however, should be fairly easy to carry out in a clinical setting. Clinical specialists could have nurses on various units of a hospital notify them when a given diagnosis is made on a patient. Two clinical specialists would then observe the same patients and check off the characteristics manifested by the patients. Interrater reliability is obtained, in this model, by dividing the number of agreements between the two raters by the sum of the number of agreements and the number of disagreements. As in the DCV model, the characteristics with rating ≤0.50 are dropped and characteristics with ratings ≥0.75 become the critical cluster for that diagnosis. It is suggested that nursing diagnoses that have DCV and CDV total scores below 0.60 be further refined and/or rejected and removed from NANDA's accepted list.

The third type of validity is the *ECR*. The basis for this type of validation is the absence of a direct cause and effect relationship of the etiologies with most nursing diagnoses. To reflect the strength of the etiology's ability to predict the existence of a diagnosis, correlation coefficients could be calculated. This would probably be the most difficult type of evidence to obtain because it would entail being able to measure or quantify not only a diagnosis but its etiologies as well. Development of tools to measure nursing diagnoses in practice and research must be given a high priority by the profession. Once tools are developed, it will be easy to obtain correlation ratios between the diagnosis and the etiologies. Measurement tools for diagnosis are also needed in order to evaluate the effectiveness of nursing interventions in treating diagnoses.

Besides the models of validation discussed, there are other approaches to gathering evidence that a diagnosis exists. Potential approaches include qualitative methodologies to establish the existence of new phenomena with the defining characteristics and etiologies, the known-group validation technique for a construct type validity, and single-case experimental designs to validate treatment effectiveness. The approach taken to validate a diagnosis will be dictated by the interests and abilities of the clinician-researcher.

The important point to remember is that validation studies are needed if practicing nurses are to have confidence in diagnoses presented on official lists, and to prevent a validity gap between diagnoses used in practice and those on accepted lists. The purposes of this paper were to provide some practical approaches to validating diagnoses by clinician researchers and to propose a method for standardizing diagnostic validation.

REFERENCES

Avant, K.: Nursing diagnosis: maternal attachment, Adv. Nurs. Sci. **2**(1):45-55, 1979.

Gordon, M., and Sweeney, M.A.: Methodological problems and issues in identifying and standardizing nursing diagnoses, Adv. Nurs. Sci. **2**(1):1-15, 1979.

Waltz, C., and Bausell, R.B.: Nursing research, design, statistics, and computer analysis, Philadelphia, 1981, F.A. Davis Co.

Use of the Q methodology in validating defining characteristics of specified nursing diagnoses

NANCY R. LACKEY, Ph.D., R.N.

Defining characteristics of nursing diagnoses have been defined by Gordon (1982) as the "observable signs and symptoms that are present when the health problem is present or when the diagnostic category is used clinically." Two of the largest tasks facing the proponents of nursing diagnosis are identifying and validating the defining characteristics. Practitioners of nursing care currently find most of the diagnostic categories very difficult to use in daily practice because they lack the concrete signs and symptoms necessary to make a diagnosis, or the critical defining characteristics necessary to differentiate between diagnoses. Nursing researchers need the diagnostic categories operationalized so that they can study the effectiveness of the diagnostic process as well as the validity and reliability of the taxonomy itself.

The purpose of this paper is to present a methodology, the Q technique, that can be used to identify and help validate specified defining characteristics of nursing diagnosis. This paper will be presented in five sections: (1) brief historical overview of the development of the Q methodology, (2) description of the Q methodology, (3) utilization of the Q-sort to validate defining characteristics of nursing diagnosis, (4) statistical analysis of Q-sort data, and (5) advantages and disadvantages of the Q methodology.

BRIEF HISTORICAL OVERVIEW

The Q technique was developed independently and almost simultaneously by Sir G.H. Thomson and William Stephenson. In 1935 both published articles describing the technique. The methodology had been used previously to this time, but was not well developed or accepted. It was written that Thomson himself was skeptical about the future use of the technique. Stephenson was very optimistic about the methodology and could foresee its use in all areas of psychology for testing hypotheses dealing with introspections, moods, sentiments, etc., which up to this time were considered untestable. Stephenson proposed that the Q methodology be used to study the "single case," meaning a case study or a single group of interacting persons (Stephenson, 1953).

The Q methodology did not become popular until the early 1950s. The methodology never achieved the popularity that Stephenson proposed for studying the single case, but instead was used in the study of psychotherapy, personality disorders, and related social problems (Wittenborn, 1961). A review of the current literature reveals that the Q technique is used widely and frequently in all disciplines, particularly education, psychology, sociology, and social psychology.

The first reported nursing study using the Q methodology was done by Whiting in 1959. He studied the importance of various nursing tasks as perceived by nurses, physicians, and patients. Other published nursing studies have used the Q sort to develop an instrument to measure nursing care (Cornell, 1974), to study the impact of baccalaureate degree programs (Stone and Green, 1975), and nursing behaviors related to grief and grieving (Freihofer and Felton, 1976). The Q methodology is also being described and recommended for use in several nursing research design texts (Fox, 1982; Polit and Hungler, 1983; Waltz and Bausell, 1981).

DESCRIPTION OF Q METHODOLOGY

The Q methodology is the term developed by Stephenson to describe "a set of philosophical, psychological, statistical, and psychometric ideas oriented to research on the individual" (Kerlinger, 1973). It is a methodology that makes comparisons among different responses within persons rather than between persons. The Q methodology is implemented by a set of procedures known as the Q technique. The Q sort is part of the set of procedures and involves sorting cards according to specific criteria (Kerlinger, 1973).

In this rank-order procedure cards are printed with statements, concepts, stimuli, or pictures. They are shuffled and then given to an individual or a number of individuals, who are asked to sort the cards into piles according to specified criteria. The criteria for sorting will vary according to the purposes of the research. There is some variation in the literature as to the exact number of cards that should be included in the sort. For statistical stability, most sources agree that between 60 and 140 cards are needed (Kerlinger, 1973; Nunnally, 1978; Polit and Hungler, 1983).

The most common type of Q sort used in research is known as the unstructured Q sort. In an unstructured Q sort a large number of statements are taken from various sources and put together without concern as to the variables underlying the items selected for the cards. In a structured Q sort, however, statements selected for the cards are specifically chosen to represent a specific theory. The cards in the structured Q sort are preclassified before the sort and individuals are then chosen to sort based on their knowledge of that specific theory (Kerlinger, 1973).

UTILIZING THE Q SORT TO VALIDATE DEFINING CHARACTERISTICS

Barr (1982) used the Q sort to develop an instrument whose purpose was to measure the magnitude of environmental stressors perceived by families of intensive care unit (ICU) patients. To obtain the items for her initial Q sort, Barr used content analysis of the literature and informal interviews of families of patients in ICU to comprise her list of 75 stressors. The identified stressors were then each printed individually on cards and given to five professionals who were familiar with the literature dealing with stress and who had worked with families of ICU patients. They were instructed to rank-order the cards from number 1 (the most stressful) to number 75 (the least stressful). The professionals were also instructed to add items that they felt were stressful to these families that were not included in the cards. Six items were added. Those that yielded a mean rank of less than 60 plus the 6 added items were returned to the professionals to be sorted a second time. Again, each was instructed to sort the items from most stressful to least stressful. The items from the second sort that yielded a mean rank of less than 50 were returned to the judges for a third and final sort. All items selected by the professionals that yielded a mean rank of less than 35 were kept for the final instrument.

To further establish content validity, Barr (1982) selected five family members for each of five different patients who were currently in medical, surgical, or cardiothoracic ICUs. They were given an identical set of 75 cards listing the stressors that were previously given to the professionals. The family members were asked to rank-order the cards from number 1 (the most stressful) to number 75 (the least stressful). They were also given the opportunity to add items they felt were stressful that were not on the list. Three items were added. Mean ranks were calculated and the cards were returned to family members for a second and third sort. Again, all items that yielded a mean rank of less than 35 were kept for the final instrument. In all, 51 items were kept for the final instrument by both the professionals and the family members.

Barr next established reliability of the items by asking 20 persons known to her who had had family members in ICU in some previous time frame to sort the cards twice at three-day intervals. The 51 stressor statements that achieved a mean rank of 35 by both the professionals and the family members of patients currently in ICU were printed on cards. Each of the 20 individuals was given the cards and asked to rank-order the cards from number 1 (the most stressful) to number 51 (the least stressful). Three days later, this group was again given the 51 cards and asked to rank-order the cards as they had done before. The data from this sort were analyzed using the Pearson Product Moment Correlation technique. The critical value of r at the 0.05 level of significance was 0.25. Of the 20 judges, 19 showed significant coefficients of correlation. On this basis, the items were considered reliable. Barr then placed the 51 items on a 4-point Likert-type scale and did further testing to establish the reliability of the test as a whole.

Lawson (1983) did a study designed to identify the defining characteristics for the nursing diagnosis of altered levels of awareness of significant others who have experienced psychological impact due to an injury or illness of a loved one and to develop an instrument which would measure these levels. From a review of the literature, the writings of four experts in the area of altered levels of consciousness, and her own personal experiences, she derived a list of 102 behaviors and feelings that she felt were indicative of altered levels of awareness due to psychological impact. These 102 behaviors or feelings were each printed on a card and the cards were then mailed to five experts (professionals who had done research in the area of near-death situations or out-of-body experiences, which are both considered as altered levels of awareness). The experts were instructed to rank-order the behaviors and feelings which they perceived to be significant in determining altered levels of awareness due to psychological impact from the most to the least important. Each expert was to add other behaviors or feelings they felt were important but not included in the list. Those behaviors and feelings receiving a mean rank above 60 were deleted from the second Q sort.

Lawson (1983) then changed the 70 remaining behaviors and feelings from items to statements. These 70 statements, plus 4 identified by the experts, were printed on cards and returned to the experts with the instructions to rank-order these statements as to how well they measured the behaviors and feelings indicative of altered levels of awareness from the most to least important. Those items from the list that yielded a mean rank of less than 40 were utilized to develop the instrument. The 38 remaining items were randomly placed upon a 4-point Likert-type scale with a separate column to indicate if the item could not be recalled. Lawson next established reliability of the test.

The initial defining characteristics for a nursing diagnosis do not always have to be obtained from a review of literature. Jauernig (1983), in a study just completed, obtained her initial defining characteristics for an operational definition of forced fluids from nurse educators. She randomly selected two nursing schools from each state that were accredited by the National League of Nursing. To the coordinators of undergraduate medical-surgical courses of these schools, she sent a cover letter explaining the study and the object content test (OCT), asking for their cooperation. The statement on the OCT was simply, "When I see the term 'force fluids,' it means?" The statement was preceded by instructions for filling out the instrument and was followed by 20 blank numbered lines. Jauernig received a 97% return from this mailing. She next did a content analysis on the answers and categorized the information into an operational definition of force fluids that contained antecendent conditions, defining characteristics, and outcomes. This definition was then returned to the initial respondents for their comments.

After receiving the proposed operational definitions from the initial respondents, Jauernig next printed characteristics for each category on cards and asked three nursing educators to Q sort the characteristics according to specified categories. Correlational coefficients were calculated. Jauernig is currently in the process of writing her results, which will include not only an operational definition of force fluids but a conceptual framework as well.

I believe, based on my knowledge of the Q methodology and my experience with the three above mentioned studies using this technique, that the Q sort is a very reliable and powerful methodology for not only obtaining but also validating defining characteristics of nursing diagnoses. Despite the large number of cards to be sorted, most subjects have reported it to be an enjoyable and challenging experience. To date, we have had no one refuse to take part in a study that has involved the Q technique, and all subjects have completed the total Q sorting process. It is also interesting to note that a high number of subjects who participated in the studies have requested the results.

STATISTICAL ANALYSIS OF Q SORT DATA

Nunnally (1978) stated that the most popular data analysis for Q sorts was simple correlational methods. As the Q methodology has developed, so have the methods of analysis. Currently, Q sort data are being analyzed by more complex methods of correlational analysis such as multiple correlations and various methods of factor analysis. Analysis of variance has been applicable to the data obtained from structured Q sorts.

Throughout the history of the Q methodology, there has been controversy about how the data could be analyzed. Independence is assumed in most statistical tests. This means that the response to one test item should not affect the response to the other test items. Since the Q sort is a rank-ordered, forced-choice procedure, meaning that the placement of one card affects the placement of all the other cards, independence in the statistical test is violated. Kerlinger (1973) raised the question of how serious is such a violation. "Is it serious enough to invalidate the use of correlational and analysis of variance procedures?" He argued that if one feels too much is at risk in Q statistical situations then the Q sort should be accepted at the 0.01 level of significance instead of the 0.05 level.

ADVANTAGES AND DISADVANTAGES OF Q METHODOLOGY

The advantages of the Q methodology are many. It has developed into a very versatile tool that can be used in a wide variety of research designs. It can be used for an intensive study of an individual or to ascertain the political views of groups of people. The task of card sorting, for the most part, is more pleasurable than completing a paper-and-pencil test or undergoing hours of interview. Also, it is a relatively inexpensive method to utilize. Once the data are obtained, they are complete and relatively easy to analyze. The Q methodology is an excellent tool for use in exploratory research. The results of the data frequently generate researchable questions and/or hypotheses. Finally, the Q sort data lend themselves to a variety of statistical tests (Kerlinger, 1973; Polit and Hungler, 1983; Waltz and Bausell, 1981).

There are disadvantages with the Q sort also. One of the difficulties I have experienced is the preparation and handling of a large number of cards. The Q sort can be time consuming to administer and to rank-order. Another disadvantage is that the subjects are placed in a forced-choice situation. The Q technique is not a good method for cross-sectional or cross-cultural studies. It is not a good method for studies that demand large sample sizes. Finally, as discussed earlier in this paper, are the questions regarding the violation of the statistical assumption of independence (Kerlinger, 1973; Polit and Hungler, 1983; Waltz and Bausell, 1981).

REFERENCES

Barr, K.A.: The development of an instrument to measure the magnitude of environmental stressors experienced by families of intensive care unit patients. Unpublished master's thesis, University of Kansas, 1982.

Cornell, S.A.: Development of an instrument for measuring the quality of nursing care, Nurs. Res. **23:**108-117, 1974.

Fox, D.: Fundamentals of research in nursing, Norwalk, Conn., 1982, Appleton-Century-Crofts.

Freihofer, P., and Felton, G.: Nursing behaviors in bereavement, Nurs. Res. **25:**332-337, 1976.

Gordon, M.: Guidelines for reviewing and preparing diagnostic categories. In Kim, M.J., and Moritz, D.A., editors: Classification of nursing diagnoses—Proceedings of the Third and Fourth National Conferences, New York, 1982, McGraw-Hill Book Co.

Jauernig, Sr., P.R.: An operational definition of the concept "force fluids," Unpublished master's thesis, University of Kansas, 1984.

Kerlinger, F.N.: Foundations of behavioral research, ed. 25, New York, 1973, Holt, Rinehart & Winston, Inc.

Lawson, K.: The development of an instrument to measure altered levels of awareness in significant others who have experienced psychological impact, Unpublished master's thesis, University of Kansas, 1983.

Nunnally, J.C.: Psychometric theory, ed. 2, New York, 1978, McGraw-Hill Book Co.

Polit, D., and Hungler, B.: Nursing research, ed. 2, Philadelphia, 1983, J.B. Lippincott Co.

Stephenson, W.: The study of behavior, Chicago, 1953, The University of Chicago Press.

Stone, J.C., and Green, J.L.: The impact of a professional baccalaureate degree program, Nurs. Res. **24:**287-292, 1975.

Waltz, C.F., and Bausell, R.B.: Nursing research, Philadelphia, 1981, F.A. Davis Co.

Whiting, J.F.: Needs, values, perceptions, and the nurse-patient relationship, J. Clin. Psychol. **15:**146-150, 1959.

Wittenborn, J.R.: Contributions and current status of Q methodology, Psychol. Bull. **58:**132-142, 1961.

Construct validity of sleep pattern disturbance: a methodological approach

CHI-HUI KAO LO, M.S., R.N.
MI JA KIM, Ph.D., R.N., F.A.A.N.

Sleep pattern disturbance is one of the common nursing diagnoses identified in patients with cardiovascular disorder and in patients with medical-surgical problems during the acute phase of their illness.

Several studies have suggested that sleep pattern disturbance (SPD) in postoperative patients or ICU patients is due to the interruption of sleep. One study found that the number of potential interruptions of sleep varied from 56 on the first postoperative night to 5.5 on the eighth postoperative night (Woods, 1972). Similarly, an earlier study documented a greater frequency of nurse-patient interactions the first postoperative day, up to 56 in an 8-hour interval, while the greatest number of sleep interruptions was 14 in any 1-hour period (Walker, 1972). McFadden and Giblin (1971) found that patients were deprived of sleep during the first 6 postoperative nights and that the most frequently obtained period of rest was 20 to 30 minutes in duration. Helton and associates (1980) observed sleep deprivation in 56% of their patients during the first day, but the frequency decreased with each subsequent day in the ICU.

Aside from the studies which explored the etiological factors for SPD, no studies have been reported demonstrating the construct validity of the diagnosis itself. If nurses assume major responsibility for dealing with the problem of SPD, nurses need to identify essential defining characteristics that constitute the diagnosis, SPD. This paper describes a methodology which is appropriate for supporting the construct validity of sleep pattern disturbance and which may be applied to other nursing diagnoses. The major purposes of this study were to: (1) describe a method for establishing the construct validity of SPD and (2) report the preliminary results of utilizing the proposed method.

METHOD

Three phases were involved in this method.

During the *first* phase a comprehensive literature review (Fabijan and Grosselin, 1982; Hayter, 1980; Helton and associates, 1980; Hemenway, 1980; McFadden and Giblin, 1971) was carried out which included papers from primary sources, nursing textbooks, and the proceedings of the third and fourth National Conferences on Classification of Nursing Diagnoses. The literature review resulted in 33 defining characteristics for SPD, which were used to construct a tool. Each defining characteristic had a five-point numerical rating scale for the frequency of occurrence, 5 meaning always present and 1 meaning not present (see Box 1).

Box 1   Defining characteristics of sleep pattern disturbance

	Always present 5	Mostly present 4	Often present 3	Less present 2	Not present 1
1. Difficulty falling asleep					
2. Awaking earlier or later than desired					
3. Interrupted sleep					
4. Not feeling well rested					
5. Malaise					
6. Tiredness					
7. Lethargy					
8. Mild fleeting nystagmus					
9. Slight hand tremor					
10. Ptosis of eyelid					
11. Dark circle under eyes					
12. Frequent yawning					
13. Changes in posture					
14. Slurred speech					
15. Rambling speech					
16. Mumbled speech					
17. Restlessness					
18. Irritability					
19. Sensitivity to pain and discomfort					
20. Listlessness					
21. Apathy					
22. Disorientation to time and place					
23. Slow reaction					
24. Poor judgment					
25. Pulling at everything within reach					
26. Attempting to climb out of bed					
27. Hitting anyone within reach					
28. Agitation					
29. Feeling of floating					
30. Disturbed bodily sensation					
31. Illusion					
32. Delusion					
33. Feeling of persecution					

The *second* phase involved 31 nurses drawn from a pool of master's and doctoral students, and medical-surgical nursing faculty who rated each defining characteristic of SPD according to the tool developed in phase one. All nurse raters had medical-surgical background and indicated that they had cared for a total of at least 50 patients with SPD during the past 2 to 10 years. Based on their knowledge and clinical experience, they rated each defining characteristic as to its probable occurrence when patients had SPD.

The *third* phase involved direct clinical assessment by the investigator of 25 patients in medical-surgical units of a 500-bed general hospital for a 2-month period. Patients who had either myocardial infarction or coronary artery bypass surgery and who were transferred out of MICU or SICU were assessed within 24 hours following the transfer. Patients having any complications, such as cerebral vascular accident, acidosis or alkalosis, and unconsciousness were excluded. Clinical assessment was carried out by observation, physical examination, and structured interviews. The 33 defining characteristics identified in phases I and II were used as a guide during the assessment period.

Data generated from all three phases were subjected to three methods of analysis: Cronbach's alpha, interitem correlations, and item-total correlations.

A Cronbach's alpha greater than 0.80 was used as the indicator for homogeneity of items (Nunnally, 1978). In the analysis of item-total correlations, any item that correlated 0.30 with the total score was considered a good item (Nunnally, 1978). For this study we used corrected item-total correlation because the number of items was less than 80 and the number of subjects was relatively small (Nunnally, 1978).

RESULTS

Nurse raters in phase II had a minimum 2 years of clinical experience (range 2 to 10 years) and they indicated that they had experiences in dealing with more than 50 patients with SPD.

In phase II, Cronbach's alpha for the total score was 0.930, and the grand mean and standard deviation of the total score were 2.463 and 0.754 respectively. When defining characteristics were grouped according to similar nature and type, four subconcepts emerged. Items 1 to 4 were grouped and labeled as verbal complaints; 5 to 13 as physical signs; 14 to 30 as changes in behavior and performance; and 31 to 33 as psychotic manifestations. (See Box 1 for items.) All coefficient alphas of the four subconcepts were higher than 0.80 except for the subconcept of verbal complaint. Average interitem correlations for all items were 0.289; and for four subconcepts 0.2285 (verbal complaint), 0.359 (physical signs), 0.374 (change in behavior and performance), and 0.749 (psychotic manifestations). All were statistically significant ($p < 0.05$). All corrected item-total correlations were 0.30 or above except for items 2 and 3 (Box 2). Item 2, with coefficient 0.179, was too low while the negative correlation associated with Item 3 may have been a domain sampling error and suggested the need for deletion of that item. However, it was found that deleting Item 3 did not really increase the alpha coefficient of the total scale (0.933 compared to 0.930) or of the subconcept verbal complaint (0.629 compared to 0.617). Therefore, adding additional items to this subconcept may be the option that can result in a more credible alpha.

BOX 2   Construct validity of the defining characteristics by 31 nurse raters

Grand mean	Standard deviation	Coefficient alpha	Average interitem correlation
2.463	0.754		
		Total 0.930	0.289
		Verbal 0.617	0.285
		Physical 0.830	0.359
		Behavior 0.908	0.374
		Pyschotic 0.895	0.749

Item	Corrected item-total correlation	Alpha if item deleted
1	0.546	0.928
2	0.179	0.932
3	0.011	0.933
4	0.412	0.930
5	0.650	0.927
6	0.620	0.927
7	0.554	0.928
8	0.327	0.930
9	0.480	0.929
10	0.444	0.929
11	0.561	0.928
12	0.539	0.928
13	0.489	0.929
14	0.633	0.927
15	0.674	0.927
16	0.629	0.927
17	0.631	0.927
18	0.614	0.927
19	0.377	0.930
20	0.709	0.926
21	0.554	0.928
22	0.597	0.927
23	0.794	0.924
24	0.667	0.926
25	0.291	0.931
26	0.462	0.929
27	0.598	0.927
28	0.552	0.928
29	0.581	0.928
30	0.491	0.928
31	0.559	0.928
32	0.457	0.929
33	0.473	0.929

BOX 3   **Construct validity of the defining characteristics in 25 patients**

Grand mean	Standard deviation	Coefficient alpha	Average interitem correlation
2.957	1.297	0.821	0.171

Item	Corrected item-total correlation	Alpha if item deleted
1	0.127	0.833
2	0.418	0.813
3	0.493	0.808
4	0.646	0.802
5	0.623	0.812
7	0.217	0.821
8	0.022	0.824
9	0.300	0.818
10	0.277	0.819
12	0.213	0.821
13	0.490	0.809
14	0.558	0.808
15	0.510	0.809
16	0.354	0.817
17	0.482	0.809
18	0.336	0.817
19	0.343	0.816
20	0.664	0.808
21	0.476	0.810
23	0.535	0.807
24	0.472	0.813
25	0.117	0.822
28	0.078	0.827
29	0.233	0.821
30	0.374	0.815
6		
11		
22		
26		
27		
31		
32		
33		

Patients who were assessed during phase III of the study had an age range of 48 to 71 years, with a mean of 57.44. The average preoperative duration of 20 surgical patients was 5.3 days (range 1 to 12). The average length of stay for surgical patients in the SICU was 3.25 days (range 1 to 9). Most patients were observed on the 4th postoperative day. All of the 5 medical patients with myocardial infarction were directly admitted in MICU. The average length of stay for the medical patients in MICU was 6.4 days (range 4 to 9). The medical patients were observed on a day between the fifth and tenth days following myocardial infarction.

Most medical patients did not take analgesics for pain whereas most surgical patients had mild to severe pain during the observation period. Five surgical patients took one usual dose of intramuscular Demerol (I.M.) or by mouth (P.O.) for pain relief within 12 hours prior to the observation. Patients were on 13 different types of medications—antianginal, antiarrhythmic, digitalis, antihypertensive, diuretic, anticoagulant, bronchodilator, dietary supplement, antibiotic, GI preparation, analgesic, tranquilizer, and hypnotic-sedative. Some of these medications may have contributed to a patient's sleep pattern disturbance, fatigue, lethargy, lassitude, drowsiness, weakness, agitation, or restlessness. However, the extent of the adverse actions of the drugs in the development of sleep pattern disturbance was hard to determine.

Vital signs and blood chemistry values (for example, SMA-6 and arterial blood gases) of the patients remained relatively stable during the observation period. The coefficient alpha for the total score obtained from clinical assessment was 0.821, with a grand mean and standard deviation of 2.957 and 1.297. The average interitem correlation was 0.171, and this was statistically significant ($p < 0.05$). Most corrected item-total correlations were 0.30 or above, except for Items 1, 8, 25, and 28 (see Box 3). However, deleting these items did not increase the coefficient alpha for the total score. Corrected item-total correlation and alpha values for Items 6, 22, 26, 27, 31, 32, and 33 were not obtained since none of these were present (SD = O). On the other hand, similar values for Item 11 were not obtained because it was always present (SD = O).

The data from the two phases (II and III) were combined in order to determine the essential defining characteristics for SPD. The coefficient alpha for the total score was 0.838, with a grand mean and standard deviation of 2.526 and 0.968. The average interitem correlation was 0.144, which was significant ($p < 0.05$). The majority of corrected item-total correlations were 0.30 above, except for Items 8, 11, 12, 25, and 26 (see Box 4).

The average of the medians (2.530) from the latter two phases was designated as the cutoff point for selection of essential defining characteristics. Fifteen defining characteristics met the criteria and were subsequently retained:

1. Difficulty falling asleep
2. Awaking earlier or later than desired
3. Interrupted sleep
4. Not feeling well rested
5. Malaise
6. Tiredness
7. Lethargy
8. Restlessness
9. Irritability
10. Sensitivity to pain and discomfort
11. Listlessness
12. Apathy
13. Slow reaction
14. Feeling of floating
15. Disturbed bodily sensation

BOX 4　　　**Construct validity of 33 defining characteristics (phases II and III combined)**

Grand mean	Standard deviation	Coefficient alpha	Interitem correlation
2.526	0.968	0.838	0.144

Item	Corrected item-total correlation	Alpha if item deleted
* 1	0.272	0.836
* 2	0.288	0.835
* 3	0.239	0.837
* 4	0.507	0.829
* 5	0.488	0.829
* 6	0.426	0.832
* 7	0.432	0.831
8	0.122	0.838
9	0.376	0.833
10	0.357	0.823
11	0.104	0.842
12	0.130	0.842
13	0.299	0.835
14	0.571	0.829
15	0.517	0.829
16	0.446	0.832
*17	0.535	0.827
*18	0.411	0.832
*19	0.374	0.833
*20	0.529	0.827
*21	0.522	0.828
22	0.204	0.838
*23	0.631	0.823
24	0.351	0.833
25	0.054	0.841
26	0.088	0.840
27	0.306	0.835
28	0.335	0.834
*29	0.267	0.838
*30	0.331	0.835
31	0.284	0.836
32	0.235	0.837
33	0.231	0.837

*Essential defining characteristics.

BOX 5   **Construct validity of 15 essential defining characteristics**

Grand mean	Standard deviation	Coefficient alpha	Interitem correlation
3.467	0.504	0.902	0.375

Item	Corrected item-total correlation	Alpha if item deleted
1	0.247	0.908
2	0.588	0.895
3	0.343	0.903
4	0.619	0.894
5	0.822	0.886
6	0.757	0.891
7	0.629	0.894
8	0.413	0.901
9	0.244	0.906
10	0.479	0.899
11	0.852	0.884
12	0.593	0.895
13	0.722	0.890
14	0.704	0.891
15	0.749	0.888

Finally, the internal consistency of these 15 defining characteristics was ascertained. The coefficient alpha for the total score of 15 defining characteristics was 0.902 with a grand mean and standard deviation of 3.467 and 0.504. The average interitem correlation was 0.375, and this was significant ($p < 0.05$). All corrected item-total correlations of 15 essential defining characteristics were 0.30 or above except for Items 1 and 9 (see Box 5).

DISCUSSION

Although a number of defining characteristics of SPD were identified by the National Conference Group on Classification of Nursing Diagnoses and the literature, construct validity of the SPD has not been tested in the clinical setting. This paper presents a method and statistical analysis by which the construct validity of a nursing diagnosis can be established. This approach may be useful for establishing the validity of other nursing diagnoses.

Two inductive approaches were utilized in this method in order to validate a nursing diagnosis: one based on knowledge and clinical experience of qualified nurse raters, and the other by actual clinical assessment of patients by the investigator. The combination of expert knowledge and prior clinical experience anchored in direct clinical assessment was thought to be a comprehensive approach which would yield valid results.

The three phases that were employed in the study merit further attention. The comprehensive literature review during phase I is essential and is as critical as the subsequent phases. Nursing, being an applied science, draws its elements from other sciences and can benefit from previous studies in the field. Patients' sleep pattern disturbance is not a problem exclusive to nursing practice. It affects medical as well as other health professionals who are involved in patient care. However, the problem impinges on nursing practice more so than others since nurses deal with the problem every day, around the clock. From this standpoint, synthesis of available knowledge on SPD is the very first step that needs to be taken in order to guide nursing practice.

The nurse raters who participated in the study had medical-surgical background at the post-baccalaureate level. However, selection of clinical nurse specialists in medical-surgical nursing would have been better since they are considered clinical experts in nursing.

Clinical assessment by the investigator was limited in terms of time (2 hours per assessment) but served as an anchoring point for the data to be clinically relevant. Reassessment on randomly selected patients by a master's-prepared clinical nurse specialist following the investigator's assessment would have reaffirmed the validity and established the reliability of the data. This was initially planned, but lack of time on the part of the clinical specialist prevented its implementation.

This study employed Cronbach's alpha, interitem correlations, and item-total correlations to test the homogeneity of items and the quality of items. The results showed that all alphas were greater than 0.80, all average interitem correlations were significant ($p < 0.05$), and the majority of corrected item-total correlations were at least 0.30, which suggests that the selected items share a common core. It should be noted that Cronbach's alpha is the average of all possible split-half correlations whereas the average interitem correlation is the average of the correlations between individual items. Thus, seemingly low interitem correlations can result in an acceptable Cronbach's alpha, particularly when the number of items is greater than 10 (Zeller and Carmines, 1978).

The alpha of 0.902 of 15 selected items suggests homogeneity; hence these items can be considered the essential defining characteristics of SPD. The median score of 2.53 was used rather than the mean score for selection of 15 essential defining characteristics, because normal distribution of data could not be assumed with the small sample in the study.

In order to establish external validity, a follow-up study is planned in which a large nationwide sample of nurses with heterogeneous backgrounds will be asked to rate the defining characteristics that emerged from this study. The final outcome of such a study would facilitate the process of identifying key characteristics of the nursing diagnosis, sleep pattern disturbance, which can provide direction for relevant nursing therapy.

REFERENCES

Fabijan, L., and Grosselin, M.D.: How to recognize sleep deprivation in your ICU patient and what to do about it, Can. Nurse 78(4):20-23, 1982.

Hayter, J.: The rhythm of sleep, Am. J. Nurs. **80:**457-461, 1980.

Helton, M.C., Gordon, S.H., and Nunnery, S.L.: The correlation between sleep deprivation and the intensive care unit syndrome, Heart Lung **9**(3):464-468, 1980.

Hemenway, J.A.: Sleep and the cardiac patient, Heart Lung **9**(3):453-463, 1980.

McFadden, E.H., and Giblin, E.C.: Sleep deprivation in patients having open-heart surgery, Nurs. Res. **20:**249-253, 1971.

Nunnally, J.C.: Psychometric theory, ed. 2, New York, 1978, McGraw-Hill Book Co.

Walker, B.: The postsurgery heart patient: amount of uninterrupted time for sleep and rest during the first, second, and third postoperative days in a teaching hospital, Nurs. Res. **21:**164-169, 1972.

Woods, N.: Pattern of sleep in postcardiotomy patients, Nurs. Res. **21:**347-352, 1972.

Zeller, R.A., and Carmines, E.G.: Measurement in the social sciences, Cambridge, England, 1980, Cambridge University Press.

The validation of a nursing diagnosis: a nurse-consensus survey*

KAREN G. VINCENT, M.S., R.N.

The professional literature in the late 1970s and early 1980s has reflected an increasing interest in nursing diagnosis. Articles by Roy (1975), McKay (1977), and Kritek (1979) emphasized the importance of formalizing the diagnostic phase of the nursing process. *The Nursing Clinics of North America* and *Advances in Nursing Science* (1979) each devoted an issue to the concept of a nursing taxonomy. The clinical and academic articles presented in those symposia addressed the task of documenting the profession's unique role within the health care system. In 1983 the American Nurses Association began to assess the impact of cost containment legislation on the progression of nursing science. The current movement to limit health care costs mandates that the profession document the nature and cost effectiveness of nursing actions (American Nurse, 1983; Feild, 1979; Gordon, 1980; Roy, 1976; Weber, 1979). The nursing diagnosis taxonomy is being considered for this task because it attempts to classify nursing actions.

Gordon (1976) defined nursing diagnosis as "actual or potential health problems which, by virtue of their education and experience, nurses are capable and licensed to treat." The signs and symptoms representative of these diagnoses have been identified by five National Conferences for the Classification of Nursing Diagnoses. No published research studies have described how frequently clinicians use the specific defining characteristics when formulating a diagnosis. Several research studies were used to identify the signs and symptoms of the diagnostic categories "Rape trauma syndrome" (Burgess and Holmstrom, 1975) and "Ineffective coping" (Guzzetta and Forsyth, 1979). These studies were used to define the diagnosis, and no further research has been published to describe how frequently these signs and symptoms are used in practice. Clinical and nurse consensus research is needed to empirically support the diagnostic categories (Gordon and Sweeney, 1979).

The signs and symptoms for the nursing diagnosis, ineffective coping (individual), were chosen by the National Conference Group on Nursing Diagnoses in 1980 (Kim and Moritz, 1982). Those 11 defining characteristics were

---

*Study conducted as partial fulfillment of the Master's of Science degree at Boston College School of Nursing. The author was funded by Department of Health and Human Services, Public Health Services, ADAMHA, Clinical Training Program 5T01MH07872-21. Research Advisement was provided by Miriam-Gayle Wardle, R.N., Ph.D., Professor, Boston College School of Nursing.

believed to represent the behaviors of a client with coping difficulties. Two behaviors were added to the list for the purposes of this study: anxiety and reported life stress. Bell (1977), Burgess and Holmstrom (1976), Guzzetta and Forsyth (1979), and Pearlin and Scholar (1978), have shown in their studies on coping that individuals exhibit some form of anxiety when faced with both daily and major (death, divorce, rape) life events. The significant relationships between anxiety, life stress events, and an individual's coping skills presented in these studies supported the inclusion of these behaviors to the list of officially accepted defining characteristics.

Since ineffective coping (individual) became an official diagnosis, no research reports have been published to document the presence of these behaviors in a clinical setting. The purpose of this study was to describe how frequently clinical specialists identified that the defining characteristics occurred when the diagnosis was present in their clinical practice.

METHODS
Definition of terms

Validation: to confirm that the defining characteristics of ineffective coping (individual) are nearly always or frequently present when clinicians make this diagnosis in a practical setting.

Clinical specialist: a clinical specialist has a master's or doctorate degree in a specialty area of nursing and supervised experience at a graduate level (ANA, 1980).

Defining characteristics: signs and symptoms of the health problems of patients.

Ineffective coping (individual): impairment of adaptive behaviors and problem solving abilities of a person in meeting life's demands and roles (Kim and Moritz, 1982).

Subjects

A sample of 1183 clinical specialists in the United States was obtained from the American Nurses Association. The pen and paper surveys were sent to a random selection of 1000 participants. These professionals were chosen as the population of study because of their advanced training in nursing.

Instrument

A graphic rating scale was designed in which each defining characteristic of the diagnosis, ineffective coping (individual), were listed. The two additional behaviors, life stress events and anxiety, were also included on the list. Finally, there was an open-ended question for participants to write in other criteria they used when making the diagnosis in practice. The clinical specialists were instructed to consider a hypothetical sample of 100 clients with ineffective coping. They were asked to indicate how frequently this population exhibited the specific signs and symptoms of the diagnosis. A five-point scale was used, ranging from 1 (rarely present) to 5 (nearly always present). A pilot test was conducted with graduate students in psychiatric/mental health nursing at Boston College.

Data analysis

Each participant was sent a questionnaire. After the surveys were returned, they were coded using ordinal level measurement. A frequency distribution and the median for each defining characteristic from the survey list was obtained using the SPSS (Nie and associates, 1975). The categories of the scale were collapsed and the frequencies grouped to facilitate interpretation of the findings. The data were analyzed as to the frequency of clinical specialists who identified that the defining characteristics were nearly always to frequently present (60% to 100%), sometimes present (40% to 59%), or seldom to rarely present (0% to 39%) in their clients with the diagnosis.

RESULTS
Characteristics of the sample

There was a 51.3% return rate on the survey. The final sample consisted of 513 clinical specialists. The age range of the participants was from 26 to 45 years (388, or 76%); the respondents had from 5 to 16 years of experience in nursing (305, or 60%); and 366 (71%) of the specialists had extensive experience with clients who exhibited ineffective coping behaviors. The majority of specialists (351, or 68%) indicated a master's in psychiatric/mental health nursing as their specialty training, 107 (21%) had a master's in nursing, and 29 (6%) a master's degree in counseling and guidance. All of the specialists had a master's degree, and 13 (2.5%) also had reached the doctoral level of preparation. There was representation in the study by clinical specialists from all 50 states. (See Box 1.)

Frequency distribution

The frequency distribution and median for each defining characteristic were used to illustrate how frequently clinical specialists identified the signs and symptoms in their clients with the ineffective coping diagnosis. The median score for each defining characteristic was located first to document the central tendency of scores on the graphic rating scale. This measurement divided the distribution exactly in half to describe the score above which and below which 50% of the frequencies fell. The behaviors, anxiety and life stress, had the highest median score of 5 (see Table 1).

The frequency distribution documented how often the clinical specialists observed the signs and symptoms when formulating the diagnosis, ineffective

BOX 1   **Demographics**

Master's degree: 513 (100%); doctoral degree: 13 (2.5%)
Discipline of master's degree:

Psychiatric/mental health nursing	351 (68%)
Nursing	107 (21%)
Counseling and guidance	29 (6%)
Psychology	9 (2%)
Medical-surgical nursing	7 (1%)

Age			
	26 to 35	205	(40%)
	36 to 45	183	(36%)
	46 to 55	96	(19%)
	56 to 65	22	(4%)
	Over 65	4	(1%)
	Under 25	1	(0.2%)

Years of experiences in nursing

11 to 16	169 (33%)
5 to 10	136 (27%)
17 to 22	106 (21%)
23 to 28	45 (9%)
Over 28	47 (9%)

Experience with clients having ineffective coping

None	2 (0.4%)	Moderate	128 (25%)
Limited	13 (3%)	Extensive	366 (71%)

coping (individual). A client's inability to problem solve was identified as being nearly always to frequently present when 422 (83%) of the clinicians made the diagnosis. This officially accepted characteristic was identified as appearing in clinical practice by the highest percentage of clinicians. Four hundred and six (79%) of the clinical specialists identified that an alteration in social participation was also nearly always to frequently present. The client's inability to meet role expectations was observed to be nearly always to frequently present by 387 (76%) of the clinicians. Two additional behaviors identified as occurring with high frequency were verbalization of inability to cope (341, 66%), and change in usual communication patterns (275, 53%); 228 (44%) of the clinical specialists indicated that verbal manipulation was sometimes present. Finally, verbalization of inability to ask for help was identified by 181 (35%) of participants as being seldom to rarely present in clients with coping difficulties.

Those characteristics added to the list by the researcher were observed frequently by the clinicians. Anxiety was identified by 482 (94%) of the respondents as being nearly always to frequently present in clients with inef-

TABLE 1   **Median scores**

Defining characteristics	5 Nearly always present (80% to 100%)	4 Frequently present (60% to 79%)	3 Sometimes present (40% to 59%)	2 Seldom present (20% to 39%)	1 Rarely present (0% to 19%)
1. Verbalization of inability to cope		4			
2. Verbalization of inability to ask for help		3			
3. Inability to meet role expectations		4			
4. Inability to meet basic needs		3			
5. Alteration in social participation		4			
6. Inability to problem solve		4			
7. Alteration in social participation		4			
8. Change in usual communication patterns		4			
9. Destructive behavior toward self or others		3			
10. Verbal manipulation		3			
11. High illness or accident rate		3			
12. Anxiety		5			
13. Reported life stress		5			
14. Other		4			

fective coping (individual). Similarly 457 (84%) of the participants observed that clients nearly always or frequently report life stress when experiencing coping problems. Only 14 (4%) of the clinicians reported that these behaviors were seldom to rarely present (see Table 2).

One hundred and thirteen clinical specialists answered the open-ended question on the list. They wrote in an additional 90 behaviors used as criteria in making their diagnoses. These behaviors have been classified under anxiety and life stress events in Table 3. Depression was a common behavior identified by 13 (12%) of the specialists in clients with ineffective coping. Inability to sleep or eat properly was also a common characteristic observed by 8 (7%) of

TABLE 2   Frequency distribution

Defining characteristics	Nearly always to frequently present (60% to 100%)	Sometimes present (40% to 59%)	Seldom to rarely present (0% to 39%)
1. Verbalization of inability to cope	341 (66)	113 (22)	59 (11)
2. Verbalization of inability to ask for help	117 (23)	210 (41)	181 (35)
3. Inability to meet role expectations	387 (76)	99 (19)	24 (4)
4. Inability to meet basic needs	145 (29)	187 (36)	178 (34)
5. Alteration in social participation	406 (79)	90 (18)	15 (3)
6. Inability to problem solve	422 (83)	67 (13)	20 (4)
7. Inappropriate use of defense mechanisms	363 (71)	110 (21)	28 (6)
8. Change in usual communication patterns	275 (53)	175 (34)	60 (12)
9. Destructive behavior toward self or others	158 (31)	215 (42)	139 (27)
10. Verbal manipulation	178 (34)	228 (44)	92 (18)
11. High illness or accident rate	242 (47)	179 (35)	88 (18)
12. Anxiety	482 (94)	23 (5)	5 (1)
13. Reported life stress	457 (89)	42 (8)	9 (3)
14. Other (113 answered)	92 (82)	13 (12)	7 (6)

TABLE 3   Additional behaviors

Anxiety	Reported life stress
Depression (13)	Inability to eat or sleep properly (8)
Poor self-image (7)	Drugs, alcohol (5)
Psychotic thought processes	Poor support systems (5)
Unable to express own anger	Physical illness or hospitalization (5)
Moodiness, irritability, affective distress	Significant life-style changes (3)
Fear of change	Lack of support systems (2)
Poor judgment or impulse control	Noncompliance with medical regimen (2)
Alterations in school or job performance	Family history of alcohol or sexual abuse

the specialists. These written-in behaviors were identified by 92 (82%) of the clinicians as occurring nearly always to frequently in clients with coping problems.

DISCUSSION

The reliability of the instrument with the final study population was 0.740, using Cronbach's alpha reliability coefficient. The magnitude of this coefficient supports the strength of the findings in the study. It was not anticipated that the specialists would identify that 100% of the clients exhibited the behaviors because the diagnostic categories were general guides to clarify client concerns. However, two findings from the study did suggest that the list of defining signs and symptoms for this diagnosis is incomplete. It was significant that the two symptoms added to the list by the researcher were identified as occurring with higher frequency by more clinical specialists than the official characteristics. The 90 signs and symptoms written in by the specialists also suggest that perhaps the list is incomplete.

Over 50% (257) participants did identify that the official defining characteristics were exhibited at least sometimes (40% to 59%) by their clients with ineffective coping. Therefore, these data suggest that, rather than eliminating any currently accepted behaviors from the category, the list can be expanded. Another implication from these results is the possibility of labeling certain symptoms as "critical" defining characteristics. It may be suggested that those signs and symptoms identified as nearly always to frequently present by over 50% of the clinicians surveyed are critical to formulating the diagnosis.

The study demonstrated how frequently the defining characteristics are found in the clinical practice of clinical nurse specialists. However, differences may exist in the practice settings of clinicians in specialty groups, that is, community health or maternal-child health nursing. An acknowledged weakness also exists in the study instrument design because it has not been used in research over time and with different nursing specialties. This limitation will be corrected when the instrument is used again with different populations and even different nursing diagnoses.

RESEARCH RECOMMENDATIONS

Further research needs to be conducted before the diagnostic categories can serve as a useful guide for nursing practice. The diagnosis, ineffective coping (individual), can be studied again by surveying other specialty groups and staff nurses. It may also be useful to use this same survey and add the written in behaviors to the list. The validation of the diagnostic categories is a large endeavor. Yet it is an essential task as nursing strives to establish its unique and professional domain within the health care system.

REFERENCES

American Nurses' Association: Nursing: a social policy statement, Kansas City, Mo., 1980, The Association.

Bell, J.: Stressful life events and coping methods in mental-illness and -wellness behavior, Nurs. Res. **26:**136-140, 1977.

Burgess, A., and Holmstrom, L.: Coping behaviors of the rape victim, Am. J. Psychiatry **133:**413-417, 1976.

Feild, L.: The implementation of nursing diagnosis in clinical practice, Nurs. Clin. North Am. **14:**497-507, 1979.

Gordon, M.: Nursing diagnoses and the diagnostic process, Am. J. Nurs. **8:**1298-1300, 1976.

Gordon, M.: Determining study topics, Nurs. Res. **29:**83-86, 1980.

Gordon, M., and Sweeney, M.A.: Methodological problems and issues in identifying and standardizing nursing diagnoses, Adv. Nurs. Sci. **1:**1-15, 1979.

Guzzetta, C., and Forsyth, G.: Nursing diagnostic pilot study: psychophysiological stress, Adv. Nurs. Sci. **2:**27-44, 1979.

Kim, M.J., and Moritz, D.A., editors: Classification of nursing diagnoses—Proceedings of the Third and Fourth National Conferences, New York, 1982, McGraw-Hill Book Co.

Kritek, P.: The development of nursing diagnosis and theory, Adv. Nurs. Sci. **2:**73-79, 1979.

Massachusetts Governor sued for bargaining interference, Am. Nurse, April 1983.

McKay, R.: What is the relationship between the development and utilization of a taxonomy and nursing theory? Nurs. Res. **26:**222-224, 1977.

Nie, N., and others: Statistical package for the social sciences, ed. 2, New York, 1975, McGraw-Hill Book Co.

Pearlin, L., and Schoolar, C.: The structure of coping, J. Health Social Behav. **19:**2-21, 1978.

Roy, C., Sr.: A diagnostic classification system for nursing, Nurs. Outlook **23:**90-95, 1975.

Weber, S.: Nursing diagnosis in private practice, Nurs. Clin. North Am. **14:**533-539, 1979.

CHAPTER 8

Process

The PES system: a time for change

MARGARET LUNNEY, M.S.N., R.N.

The framework of problem, etiology, signs and symptoms (PES) is currently being suggested and used to guide the thinking of nurses as they diagnose (Gordon, 1982; Shoemaker, 1984). Up to now it has served its purpose well, judging by the increased use of nursing diagnosis over the last ten years. But the perspective of nursing is changing so that the utility of this framework for the future is questionable. Ten years after the first conference is an ideal time to evaluate the extent of its usefulness and to make any changes that are indicated.

The purpose of a framework like PES is to standardize a way of thinking and a way of communicating. Yet even though it probably has achieved that specific purpose—for example, Shoemaker (1984) reported at the last conference that expert nurses were using it to organize their thinking and recording—the PES system does not help to achieve another important purpose of nursing, that is, the purpose of portraying the essence of nursing in diagnostic labels. The structure and function of the PES system is incongruent with essential aspects of nursing philosophy and practice. According to the literature, the focus of nursing is the wholeness of the person and the health of the person (Donaldson and Crowley, 1978; Flaskerud and Halloran, 1980; Riehl and Roy, 1980). Nurses believe that health is more than the absence of problems. In fact, the two models of health that nurses primarily use are (1) health is the process of achieving optimum potential, or self-fulfullment, throughout the life process and (2) health is the successful adaptation to life stresses (Smith, 1981). In addition, the ANA social policy statement clearly defines human responses as the focus of nursing (American Nurses' Association, 1980). These distinctive concerns of the profession—(a) people and how they are achieving health and (b) a view of health that is more comprehensive than that which is inherent in the medical model—are not reflected in, nor are they served by, the PES format for nursing diagnosis.

ANALYSIS OF THE CONCEPT OF PROBLEM

To begin with, the concept of problem is too broad and simultaneously too narrow to generate accurate descriptions of nursing phenomena. It is too broad in that it is a generic term used by every discipline, every group, and every individual when describing both discipline-specific phenomena and common happenings of everyday life. For this reason it is correct but not accurate to say that nurses diagnose and treat actual or potential problems. The term *problem* encompasses so much of human existence that it could hardly be considered as incorrect.

Evidence that the term is too broad can be noted in the list of categories that have been accepted over the past five national conferences. The word *problem* has generated diagnostic concepts at all levels of abstraction, from broad categories like coping, which could theoretically depict the whole adaptive model of health (Smith, 1981), to specific categories like cardiac output, which, as Hurley (1984) has shown, represents only a number (stroke volume times heart rate). The lack of consistency or organization within the list can be attributed to the absence of specificity of the word *problem.*

In addition, it can be expected that the term *problem* will not provide direction for future growth of this list of diagnostic labels. Any problem that nurses diagnose and treat, regardless of its level of agreement with nursing science, could fit within this frame of reference. Two examples of diagnoses which have been proposed but may not fit the purpose of nursing are Reluctance to donate blood and Sexual deviance. All that an interested nurse would need to do is to show by research data that these phenomena are being diagnosed and treated in clinical practice for them to be considered for approval by NANDA. This is an unrealistic method of describing nursing phenomena because nurses have always used and continue to use the models of other disciplines in practice, education and research (Munhall, 1982; Phillips, 1977). It is expected, then, that many of the problems nurses diagnose and treat reflect the perspectives of these other disciplines and are not necessarily nursing phenomena.

And yet it has always been a significant goal of the diagnostic movement to tease out the differences between nursing and other disciplines (Gebbie and Lavin, 1974). More recently a commitment to this goal was reflected in the landmark document of the social policy statement (American Nurses' Association, 1980) when it referred to the phenomena of nursing as human responses to health problems, the core of nursing as those phenomena that nurses are responsible to treat, and the boundaries of nursing as fluid and overlapping. Awareness of the goal to differentiate the focus of nursing from that of other disciplines raises the question, can the word *problem* help to achieve this goal or purpose? I propose that it is too broad, or generic, a term to be useful toward this end.

Although it may seem paradoxical, even though it is too broad it can also be considered too narrow. The implication of using *problem* as a primary reference point is that the purpose of nursing is to look for problems. The term is inaccurate because it specifies only a part of nurses' frame of reference and ignores those two major aspects of nursing that the discipline has been trying to portray, wholeness and health (Donaldson and Crowley, 1978; Ellis, 1982; Fawcett, 1984; Flaskerud and Halloran, 1980; Riehl and Roy, 1980). Since these two concerns, which often make the difference in delineating nursing from other disciplines, are not incorporated into the PES framework, they fail to influence the development of diagnostic labels in any consistent way. In the current list only some of the diagnostic concepts are indicative of wholeness and health (for instance, nutrition, coping, and self-concept). From other diagnostic concepts, however, it would seem that a nursing focus is the parts of the biological system, such as the skin or the heart. Other diagnostic concepts on the list refer to problems of the whole person but do not indicate a concern for the promotion, maintenance, and restoration of health (for example, powerlessness, fear, rape trauma).

The narrow approach of choosing labels for *problems* instead of choosing labels that show nursing's interest in the health of the whole person leads to an inability to portray the essence or core of nursing. A consumer who looks at the list of approved diagnoses from the five national conferences would not be able to interpret from this list that a major aspect of nursing is an interest in the person as opposed to an interest in problems or illnesses.

There are legitimate questions that consumers might ask—Why do people need their problems labeled by nurses? Aren't these problems labeled already by other disciplines? Do we really need more labels? It is very possible that the answer to this last question would be, No! Labels tend to encourage stereotypic responses to people rather than an individualized "real" response. Labels can also be stigmatizing. Yet the word *problem* encourages lists of labels; if the person has the problem it is listed. Some people that nurses work with have multiple problems (like, the client with emphysema who may have ineffective gas exchange, activity intolerance, potential for injury [infection], plus many others). If these problems exist in conjunction with the disease, they may never resolve or change in any way. They just exist, and with this approach to nursing diagnosis the person carries these labels through life like excess baggage.

If instead a perspective that is uniquely nursing is evident in diagnostic statements it would overcome the aforementioned limitations. Diagnoses would be assessed and decided on with clients (Williamson, 1981). Decisions about whether phenomena should be treated or not would be the key to diagnosing. With this approach, even if the person had an intolerance for activity, it would not be a nursing diagnosis unless the nurse and client agreed to perform some action in relation to it and agreed that there would be some worth in communicating it to others. The focus would be on whether the response is optimum for this client, not on whether it is a problem. In those cases when a client is not able to participate in this process the nurse may have to make decisions independently, for instance, when the client is experiencing decreased levels of consciousness. The same approach would prevail: the nurse diagnoses those situations which need to be treated and avoids labeling patient situations just because they are problems.

ANALYSIS OF THE CONCEPT OF ETIOLOGY

Two conflicting interpretations of the term *etiology* have been reported by Gordon and Forsyth. Gordon (1982) described the meaning of etiology which underlies current use of the term for nursing diagnosis. She showed that the process of identifying the etiology is considered as "very important" since therapeutic modalities differ according to the cause of the problem. Forsyth (1984) articulated the uneasiness that many nurses had been expressing about this concept. She outlined philosophical positions that are incongruent with using etiology for a nursing diagnosis framework. Two of her conclusions were that (1) the multidimensional nature of nursing phenomena does not lend itself to drawing conclusions about etiology and (2) etiology, or cause, "can never be demonstrated empirically," (in other words, the practicing nurse who is making clinical decisions cannot identify the cause of the problem). According to Forsyth, cause(s) can be identified only by advanced experimental research.

A major difference between Gordon's explanation of the concept of etiology and that of Forsyth is the assumptions which underlie each interpretation about levels of probability. Gordon assumes that "etiological factors are probable causes. They are treated as hypotheses not facts." Forsyth assumes that there is a degree of certainty inherent in the concept of *etiology*.

The fact that these two scholars of nursing diagnosis differ in their view of etiology is not surprising. Their differences are consistent with differences expressed in other sciences. Cook and Campbell (1979), specialists in experimental research design, have illustrated the complexity of these philosophic issues in a discussion of the various views. One conclusion which they draw is "logical analyses by philosophers show that there is a hodgepodge of nearly contradictory essences in the cause-effect relationship."

Practically speaking, for purposes of nursing diagnosis, it should be questioned, then, whether this concept will continue to be useful. Even though practicing nurses may not be aware of conflicting philosophic views, the common sense notions of etiology that they do use are just as varied. Because nurses are exposed to conflicting common sense notions through teachers and other role models, they do not have a common meaning of the term *etiology*.

This lack of clarity in the meaning of etiology suggests that the term should not be used in a framework for nursing diagnoses.

The following clinical example will illustrate the potential for lack of consistency among nurses in operationalizing this concept:

Consider a 23-year-old female who has nutritional habits that are dangerous to her health and for whom the nurse diagnoses an Alteration in nutrition. Some of the explanations or reasons why this woman has an altered nutrition are as follows:

She works the evening shift so she does not have the same eating hours as others in her family; she does not like to cook; she tends not to be independent in the planning and carrying out of meals; she is a philosophy major and would much rather sit and think than take care of a concrete task such as managing food; she smokes heavily and loves coffee, so she often prefers to sit with cigarettes and coffee instead of eating a meal; she does not believe that good nutrition is essential to her health; she likes simple sugars and convenience foods rather than complex sugars and proteins; she does not like to eat alone; she does not like to exercise.

All of these factors, plus others which have not been identified, are part of the reasons why this female has an Alteration in nutrition. Whether all of them, or even more than one of them, would be identified by nurses who work with her is unknown. From common sense notions of etiology it is logical that some nurses would identify factors which existed previous to the alteration, others would identify factors that were observable at the same time as the alteration, others would identify ones which they felt able to manipulate, etc. There is no way of ascertaining, either, which of these factors, or methods of conceptualizing etiology, are better explanations for her Alteration in nutrition than the others, so there is no way of knowing which approach is better. In addition, if all of them are known etiological factors, then, with the PES format, all of them should be listed with the diagnosis, especially since it is possible to manipulate all of them in one way or the other.

Another common-sense notion is that etiology is relatively simple to identify; the diagnostician just has to observe the situation. With this approach the nurse who is able to identify known etiological factor(s) will terminate the assessment phase and begin treating the problem. In assessing a client who has a speech impairment, for example, a logical diagnosis might be Alteration in communication related to stroke 2 months ago. This is certainly the most obvious of the causative factors. Yet it is not the most useful in guiding nursing treatment of this Alteration in communication. The nurse cannot change the client's history—she had a stroke 2 months ago. To avoid this notion of simplicity, authors who teach others how to diagnose (Carpenito, 1983; Gordon, 1982; Price, 1980) tell them to identify the etiology that can be treated, changed, or mitigated in some way; for example, in this case it might be knowledge deficits regarding alternative methods of communication, perceptions of powerlessness, feelings of rejection, or low self-esteem.

Knowing the many ways that etiology can be interpreted requires qualifications and explanations in regard to the most useful interpretation of the concept. These explanations may be diluting the concept of etiology so that the concept itself is not providing the framework as much as the explanations regarding its use. Explanations and illustrations of how etiology should be interpreted by proponents of the NANDA system seem to be more consistent with a two-part diagnostic system (Mundinger and Jauron, 1975) than they are of *problem* and *etiology.* For example, Carpenito (1983) states, "The more specific the second part of the statement, the more specialized the interventions can be. The linking of the diagnostic category with contributing factors also helps the nurse in validating the category." Nurses are being advised to decide which aspects, factors, or dimensions of the problem can be treated for improvement of the problem. In other words, they are being told to *diagnose* the specific dimensions of the problem that can be changed. This is consistent with Forsyth's idea that, perhaps, it is not etiology that nurses are identifying but indicators that further validate the problem.

In addition to the confusion about meaning and use, the concept of etiology is also philosophically inconsistent with the way that some nurses view people and their relationship with the environment. For example, Rogers' conceptual system (1970) has had a significant impact on the profession such that many nurses have difficulty accepting the term *etiology* and its causal implications. They think of human and environmental relationships as reciprocal. With this view, human and environmental factors occur together, not necessarily for particular reasons. The term *etiology* may be preventing nurses who have this type of world view from using the NANDA system. Most likely NANDA would not want to intentionally exclude that group from using its system.

ANALYSIS OF THE CONCEPT OF SIGNS AND SYMPTOMS

The assumption that every nursing diagnosis has signs and symptoms that should be reported by the diagnostician is a valid one. A practical concern, which will be addressed briefly, is whether the signs and symptoms should be listed with the diagnostic statement as suggested by the PES format? If NANDA decides to examine the feasibility of its framework, perhaps it will consider this question.

One disadvantage of listing signs and symptoms with the diagnosis is that it encourages only brief descriptions of data. A system which rewards brevity in reporting data may be fostering sloppy diagnosing (that is, inadequate collection of data).

Another disadvantage of listing signs and symptoms with the diagnosis is that it penalizes nurses who have already done a comprehensive data collection by requiring them to rewrite parts of it. When so many positive and negative impressions are part of the final interpretation that is validated with the client, it seems incongruous that only a few selected pieces of that impression should be cited with the diagnostic statement. If this information, that is, the signs and symptoms, is needed for research and evaluation of nursing diagnosis, then researchers should be required to solicit the cooperation of nurses and should not expect this extra work as routine practice. In this age of cost effectiveness it does not make sense to use valuable time to write data in more than one place on the client's chart.

FROM A MEDICAL MODEL TO A NURSING MODEL

The PES system was developed at a time when nurses were still enmeshed within the medical model. Though nursing science was developing, it did not have widespread support (Jacob and Heuther, 1978) and nurses were more aware of differences than of similarities in the various nursing perspectives. It was a natural step for the first ten-year period of developing a structure for diagnostic statements to use a format that was consistent with familiar ways of thinking, the medical model of diagnosis, etiology, signs and symptoms.

The medical model has also influenced assumptions that underlie use of nursing diagnosis. For example, the assumption that the problem statement should be as specific as possible is reflective of the decision-making process of physicians. While diagnosing, physicians move from broad categories like respiratory, cardiovascular, and neurological to specific categories like infection, malignancy, and chemical disorders and then to specific subcategories in each of these. The goal of diagnosing in medicine is to be as specific as possible; and after achieving this goal, the broad categories are of little use. In medical science, for example, it is obvious that pneumococcal pneumonia is a subcategory of the respiratory system. This assumption does not fit, however, with nursing science. Specific problems are understood in the context of how they affect the whole person's (or group's) achievement of health. Specific problems have the potential to affect many different categories of health functioning and thus are not purely derived as they are with medicine (see Fig. 1).

Since nursing science has matured significantly in the last 6 years, it is possible to examine these issues in light of current knowledge. The basic commonalities that represent a nursing perspective have been recognized and valued (Donaldson and Crowley, 1978; Ellis, 1982; Flaskerud and Halloran, 1980). As Feild and Winslow (1983) have suggested in a paper developed for the Division on Medical-Surgical Nursing Practice, it is time for full implementation of a nursing model by practicing nurses. In conjunction with the mandate contained in that paper and the mandate in the Social Policy Statement (American Nurses' Association, 1980), it seems appropriate to move on to the next step. NANDA has the resources to make this move by developing a structure that is more consistent with a nursing model than is PES, a new structure which illustrates clearly to ourselves and others the holistic nature

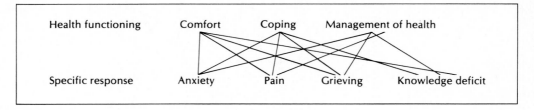

FIGURE 1

of nursing work as well as nursing's focus on health. It should be exquisitely clear in all statements that are labeled as nursing diagnoses that nurses focus on the whole person in interaction with the environment and that nurses assist people with their unique responses to help them be more healthy.

ALTERNATIVES TO PES

If members of NANDA accept the validity of this position, then decisions have to be made about a framework for the future. A survey of members would give NANDA the data it needs.

Although a change in structure is suggested in this paper, the change does not have to differ that much from the previous method. One possibility, for example, is the format that I have been using (Lunney, 1982, 1984). With this format, instead of a NANDA diagnosis being structured as *problem related to etiology*, it would be changed to a two-part diagnosis, with the first part always indicative of the nurse's focus on person and health and the second part indicating a more specific level of diagnosing (see Fig. 2). The two-part diagnosis satisfies the goal of being specific (second part) as well as of identifying the effect of the specific response on the overall response (first part)—for example, alteration in nutrition related to knowledge deficits with regard to food groups and alteration in protection related to infectious process. With the two-part statement it is evident that not only do nurses treat specific problems (e.g., knowledge deficits, infectious processes) but they also assist the person to optimize health behaviors (e.g., nutrition, protection).

The tools to facilitate change are already available. One tool is the work that the taxonomy group did at the last national conference. This group began to sort diagnostic categories by levels of abstraction (Kritek, 1984). Those concepts that the group classified as Level 1 abstraction are more holistic and health-oriented than those of Levels 2, 3, and 4. Level 1 concepts would be appropriate, then, for the first part of the diagnosis and the other levels would be used for the second part of the diagnosis. For the second part the level of specificity would depend on the nature of the client problem, the nurse-client relationship, and the expertise of the nurse. It might be expected, for example,

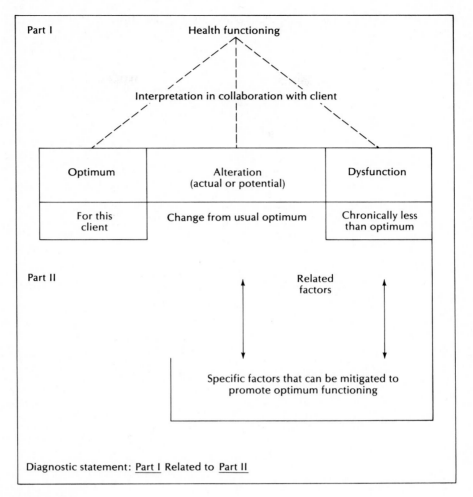

FIGURE 2

that experts would be more specific than novices in diagnosing the contributing factors.

To further clarify the Level 1 concepts, NANDA could examine and compare concepts from other systems (see Table 1). Similarities and differences could be noted and philosophical decisions could be made respecting which terminology best reflects a nursing perspective, such as activity versus the balance of activity/rest. This position is based on the assumption that the inductive method of identifying diagnoses should be combined with the deductive method, as was first suggested by Gebbie and Lavin (1974).

Another tool to accomplish consistent congruent change is the ANA Social Policy Statement. The availability of this statement makes it possible to change

TABLE 1   Comparison of major concepts in three classification systems

NANDA (Level 1)	Gordon	Lunney
Activity ('82) mobility*	Activity-exercise	Activity/rest
Comfort	Self-perception/self-concept	Comfort
Communication		Communication
Coping, individual, family	Coping-stress tolerance	Coping
Elimination	Elimination	Elimination
		Growth and development
		Independence/dependence
Knowledge		Learning
		Life-style
Health maintenance ('82)*	Health perception/health management	Management of health
		Management of illness
Nutrition	Nutritional-metabolic	Nutrition
		Oxygenation
	Role-relationship	Parenting
		Protection
Role performance†	Role-relationship	Relationships
Self-concept	Self-perception/self-concept	Self-concept
	Sexuality-reproductive	Sexuality
Sleep†		Sleep/wake
Thought processes	Cognitive-perceptual	Thought
Spiritual	Value-belief	

*Approved as diagnostic concepts in 1982, consistent with Level 1 abstraction.
†Not chosen as Level 1 concept by taxonomy group.

problem and *etiology*, whenever NANDA is ready, to the term *human response*. This term goes back as far as 1972 with the inception of New York State's Nurse Practice Act, so that many nurses are familiar with it from general usage if not through the ANA statement. The framework for a two-part diagnosis could be human response, overall related to specific. (This idea evolved from discussions with P. Hageman, former president of New York State Nurses' Association and with P. Munhall, faculty member of Hunter-Bellevue School of Nursing.) In the future other terms that represent a nursing perspective and that generate descriptions for wholeness and health might be considered.

Since a major goal of the nursing diagnosis movement is to describe the phenomena of nursing, the PES format was evaluated in this paper for its ability to organize the process. Even though PES has been useful thus far, it may need to be changed so that NANDA's classification system will be consistent with a nursing model for practice.

REFERENCES

American Nurses' Association. Nursing: a social policy statement, Kansas City, Mo., 1980, The Association.

Carpenito, L.J.: Nursing diagnosis: application to clinical practice, Philadelphia, 1983, J.B. Lippincott Co.

Cook, T.D., and Campbell, D.T.: Quasi-experimentation: design and analysis issues for field settings, Boston 1979, Houghton-Mifflin Co.

Donaldson, S.K., and Crowley, D.M.: The discipline of nursing, Nurs. Outlook **26:**113-120, 1978.

Ellis, R.: Conceptual issues in nursing, Nurs. Outlook **30:**406-410, 1982.

Fawcett, J.: Analysis and evaluation of conceptual models of nursing, Philadelphia, 1984, F.A. Davis Co.

Feild, L., and Winslow, E.H.: Transition to a nursing model for practice: an opportunity to clarify, control and improve nursing practice, Kansas City, Mo., 1983, American Nurses' Association.

Flaskerud, J.H., and Holloran, E.J.: Areas of agreement in nursing theory development, Adv. Nurs. Sci. **3:**1-7, 1980.

Forsyth, G.L.: Etiology: In what sense and of what value? In Kim, M.J., McFarland, G., and McLane, A., editors: Classification of nursing diagnoses—Proceedings of the Fifth National Conference, St. Louis, 1984, The C.V. Mosby Co.

Gebbie, K., and Lavin, M.A.: Classifying nursing diagnoses, Am. J. Nurs. **74:**250-253, 1974.

Gordon, M.: Nursing diagnosis: process and application, New York, 1982, McGraw-Hill Book Co.

Hurley, M.: Nursing diagnosis in the critical care setting. Paper presented at Nursing Diagnosis in Critical Care. Conference of the New York City Chapter of the American Association of Critical Care Nurses, New York, February 1984.

Jacobs, M.K., and Heuther, S.E.: Nursing science: the theory-practice linkage, Adv. Nurs. Sci. **1:**63-73, 1978.

Kritek, P.B.: Report of the group work on taxonomies. In Kim, M.J., McFarland, G., and McLane, A., editors: Classification of nursing diagnoses—Proceedings of the Fifth National Conference, St. Louis, 1984, The C.V. Mosby Co.

Lunney, M.: Nursing diagnosis: refining the system, Am. J. Nurs. **82:**456-459, 1982.

Lunney, M.: A framework to analyze a taxonomy of nursing diagnosis. In Kim, M.J., McFarland, G., and McLane, A., editors: Classification of nursing diagnoses—Proceedings of the Fifth National Conference, St. Louis, 1984, The C.V. Mosby Co.

Mundinger, M.O., and Jauron, G.: Developing a nursing diagnosis, Nurs. Outlook **23:**94-98, 1975.

Munhall, P.L.: Nursing philosophy and nursing research: in apposition or opposition, Nurs. Res. **31:**176-177, 1982.

Phillips, J.R.: Nursing systems and nursing models, Image, **9:**4-7, 1977.

Price, M.R.: Nursing diagnosis: making a concept come alive, Am. J. Nurs. **80:**668-671, 1980.

Riehl, J.R., and Roy, Sr. C.: Conceptual models for nursing practice, ed. 2, New York, 1980, Appleton-Century-Crofts.

Rogers, M.E.: An introduction to the theoretical basis of nursing, Philadelphia, 1970, F.A. Davis Co.

Shoemaker, J.A.: A research study on the definition of nursing diagnosis. In Kim, M.J., McFarland, G., and McLane, A., editors: Classification of nursing diagnoses—Proceedings of the Fifth National Conference, St. Louis, 1984, The C.V. Mosby Co.

Smith, J.A.: The idea of health, Adv. Nurs. Sci. **3:**43-50, 1981.

Williamson, J.A.: Mutual interaction: a model of nursing practice, Nurs. Outlook **29:**104-107, 1981.

The influence of practice on students' abilities to assess a pediatric case study and formulate nursing diagnoses

RENE CLARK, Ed.D., R.N.

In a panel discussion at the Third National Conference on Classification of Nursing Diagnoses, nurse educators agreed that baccalaureate students are not receiving adequate instruction in the process of formulating nursing diagnoses (Kim and Moritz, 1982). Baccalaureate schools of nursing have a responsibility to provide students with the knowledge and skill they will need as professional licensed nurses. While it is important to graduate students with measurable skills and knowledge, another goal of baccalaureate education is to produce graduates who can analyze data about a patient and formulate an accurate nursing diagnosis so that appropriate action can be taken. Specific skills such as history-taking, physical assessment, and technical procedures are commonly taught in baccalaureate schools of nursing. In addition to presentation of theory and facts, most nursing schools provide laboratory practice of these skills prior to their use with patients. However, performing the steps of the nursing process involves the use of cognitive strategies, and these are often neglected as a focus of attention in nursing instruction (Aspinall, 1976; Matthews and Gaul, 1979).

There is a need for nursing education to look at how nursing diagnosis, as a step in the nursing process, is taught (Gordon, 1982a; Tanner, 1979). College faculty often assume that students possess adequate problem-solving skills; consequently information is presented and the nursing student is expected to apply independently the information to patient situations. Practice sessions in applying critical thinking skills to patient situations may not be provided (Dincher and Stidger, 1976; Matthews and Gaul, 1979; Tanner, 1979).

Arriving at a nursing diagnosis is a cognitive process, and the concern of this research was how to guide students in use of the necessary thought processes when applying knowledge to a patient situation. In order to make an accurate diagnosis, the nurse must apply theoretical knowledge to a patient situation, discriminate the meaning of cues assessed during contact with the patient, categorize cues into previously learned groupings, and finally make a judgment as to the presence of a specific problem that can be resolved through nursing intervention (Gordon, 1982a; Matthews and Gaul, 1979).

This process is representative of Bruner and associates' (1967) theory of concept attainment. According to these researchers, humans form concepts of categories in order to organize the vast amount of information in their environment. The categories enable one to mentally group objects or information according to attributes recognized. In forming a concept a person makes a decision about what attributes belong in what categories. If memory of similar categories exists and is recalled, one is able to attach meaning in the form of a concept. Thus the nurse with a number of attributes collected during assessment begins to mentally process the attributes or pieces of information into categories. Once categories are recognized, the nurse's memory bank searches for previously learned concepts that contain the attributes. If a concept is identified, the final step is a judgment on whether or not the existence of these attributes constitutes a problem for the patient.

Bircher (1982) refers to nursing diagnosis as a complex concept that is a "tripartite relationship" consisting of the named nursing diagnosis, the concept it represents, and the facts or attributes that cluster within the concept. Bircher recognizes, however, that nursing diagnosis is really a judgment of the nurse based on sound knowledge, good observations, and the ability to combine through thought processes what one knows and what one perceives. Bircher supports the need for students to have guided learning experiences in the critical thinking aspects of nursing. Gordon (1982ab) reviewed strategies used by nurses to formulate categories and diagnoses. She found that nurses used forms of concept attainment and inferential reasoning as well as clinical judgment based on experience. Gordon emphasizes the need for diagnostic strategies to be taught in educational programs.

PURPOSE OF THE STUDY

The purpose of this study was to examine the impact of providing baccalaureate nursing students with practice in the cognitive skill of formulating nursing diagnoses for specific patient situations. Evaluation was accomplished by comparing the relative influences of two forms of practice, one teacher guided and one independent study, on nursing students' performances on a case study test. The research question was: Do nursing students exposed to different forms of practice in formulating nursing diagnoses perform differently on a case study test of their ability to formulate nursing diagnoses?

METHOD
Subjects

The subjects for this study were 59 baccalaureate nursing students enrolled in a pediatric nursing course at a midwestern university. Homogeneity between the subjects and the other half of the junior nursing class was demonstrated by nonsignificant t-tests on ages, admitting grade point averages, and American College Testing Program scores. Some differences in background and experience existed in the subjects that could influence their performance on the case study test. Therefore, these differences which included assignment to a pediatric nursing unit during the principles of nursing course, completion of the maternity nursing course, and work experience of at least seven days on a pediatric nursing unit were treated as independent variables.

Procedure and instruments

The procedure and instruments for this research were designed to integrate the study into an already existing course in pediatric nursing. The goals of instruction included that students would demonstrate knowledge of the psychosocial effects of hospitalization and that they would be able to apply knowledge to nursing practice by recognizing cues presented by pediatric patients and their families and to formulate related nursing diagnoses.

For the instructional portion of the design, students were required to view independently in the audiovisual lab five slide tape programs from the series *Pediatrics: Psychosocial Implications* (Concept Media, 1982). This series presents content on the psychosocial effects of hospitalization on children and families. Students' achievement of knowledge of the concepts presented in the slide tape series was measured with the Effects of Hospitalization Test. This 16-item, multiple choice test, was developed by experienced faculty members and had been pilot tested with two previous groups of students. Reliability of the 28-item pilot test was 0.85 using Cronbach's alpha; reliability of the 16 items selected for the final test was 0.89. Content validity was determined by a panel of three judges, among whom there was 100% agreement on the validity of each of the 16 items.

Within the same week as the objective test, subjects were assigned randomly to one of two treatment groups or the control group. Treatment conditions were based on the assumption that students need teacher contact in addition to independent audiovisual instruction when they are expected to apply content to patient situations. It was also assumed that students needed teacher guidance and feedback in learning to identify appropriate patient cues and formulate nursing diagnoses. Group I (teacher-guided, treatment) met in a class session for approximately 1½ hours with an experienced pediatric nursing faculty member. During this session, subjects were provided with five written pediatric patient case studies. After reading each case study, subjects participated in discussion of each case. The discussion was facilitated by the instructor, who focused on identifying relevant data in the cases and formulating actual and potential nursing diagnoses. Group II (independent study, treatment) subjects were given the same five written case studies and asked to practice independently on the cases by identifying the relevant data and formulating actual and potential diagnoses. Group III (no practice, control) did not receive any form of practice or exposure to the case studies.

During regularly scheduled conference time the week following the treatments, all subjects took the Case Study Test. The Case Study Test was designed by the researcher to evaluate students' ability to apply nursing assessment and diagnosis formulation skills to a simulated patient situation. For the Case Study Test students first viewed a 30-minute videotape of a 3-year-old child's first day in the hospital *(Darryl, On the Day of Admission,* Center for Television Studies, Ltd., Prince Edward Island, Canada). While viewing the video-tape, subjects were asked to list data they observed which were relevant to the psychosocial effects of hospitalization on the child and his family. Then subjects were asked to interpret and analyze the data collected and formulate a list of nursing diagnoses or problems related to the psychosocial effects of hospitalization for the child and for the family. This procedure simulated the approach a nurse is expected to use in actual patient situations. Content validity of the Case Study Test was determined by three pediatric faculty members who agreed 100% that the test was a sample of behaviors and situations presented in the slide tape series and that the test simulated the activities of data collection and diagnosing that are expected of students.

A method of content analysis as described by Polit and Hungler (1978) was used by a jury of four practicing pediatric nurses to determine categories for correct answers to the Case Study Test. The jury agreed on 11 data categories, five categories of nursing diagnoses for Darryl, and six categories of diagnoses for the family. Reliability of a problem-solving test such as this using free responses is difficult to determine, as usual methods of statistically estimating reliability cannot be used appropriately; test/retest methods may result in low estimates of reliability as a result of test experience (Tanner, 1979). Internal consistency was evaluated by determining that 100% of the problems identified by the jury of registered nurses had relevant data presented in the videotape.

A scoring system for the Case Study Test was chosen on the basis of simplicity and ease of application. One point was given to each category for which the student was able to list data or a nursing diagnosis; one point was subtracted for incorrect or inaccurate responses. Scores were subdivided into total Case Study Test score, data score, total diagnosis score, Darryl diagnosis score, and family diagnosis score. Scoring was performed by the same four RN judges who developed the categories. Consensus was used to determine each subject's score. Reliability of the scoring system was determined by randomly selecting 40% of the tests to be scored a second time. Judges were unaware of the insertion of duplicate tests. Percentage of agreement between the first and second scorings was as follows: data score, 83%; Darryl score, 78%; and family score, 70%.

RESULTS

The major hypothesis tested in this study was:

No significant differences will be found among mean Case Study Test Scores for the three treatment groups, after adjustment for scores on the Effects of Hospitalization Test and demographic data.

Analysis of covariance revealed no significant differences in performance on the Case Study Test regardless of treatment group, assignment to a pediatric nursing unit, completion of the maternity course, and work experience in pediatrics or covariates of age, objective test score, grade point average, and ACT scores. Therefore the null hypothesis was not rejected. Neither teacher-guided nor independent study practice made a difference in subjects' scores.

DISCUSSION

This study supports the need for further exploration into the ways in which nursing students acquire the skills of formulating nursing diagnoses and into developing valid means of evaluating diagnostic skills. Findings supported DeBack's (1981) conclusion that there was no correlation between teaching strategies used in the schools she surveyed and students' ability to make a nursing diagnosis. Tanner (1982) also found no significant difference in teaching methods and she cited as reasons: (1) the novice states of the learners as compared to the criterion group of expert nurses, and (2) the lack of differentiating ability of the scoring procedure.

It is believed that a memory bank of categories is a prerequisite to the ability to sort and understand new information. The subjects for this study were junior nursing students who were faced for the first time with pediatric patients with psychosocial needs which are unique and different from the more familiar adult patient. It is likely that these students did not have an adequate number of remembered diagnostic categories into which data could be organized.

A noteworthy point is that this study measured the ability to formulate only psychosocial diagnoses, and student subjects were able, following instruction, to formulate a variety of psychosocial diagnoses. Aspinall's (1979) subjects who were RNs had the most difficulty identifying a psychosocial problem. It may be that formulating psychosocial diagnoses is a higher level skill than formulating more concrete physical diagnoses.

The Case Study Test challenged subjects to collect data that they recognized as relevant without a data collection tool. This task might be too advanced for the junior nursing student. Also, it is possible that more than one practice session was needed to significantly influence subjects' performance on the Case Study Test.

The Case Study Test developed for this study possessed inherent limitations of no interaction between learner and client, scoring methodology, and limited means of assuring validity and reliability. Student performance on the Case Study Test was lower than expected with a mean for all subjects of only 43.59% correct (Table 1). Subjects did better on formulating diagnoses (m = 47.64%) than on data recognition (m = 39.64%). In retrospect, this is not surprising, as the data task expected may have been vague and abstract to the subjects.

Subjects' mean scores for total nursing diagnoses identified represented a 48% correct response rate, which was consistent with Matthew and Gaul's (1979) finding that undergraduate students were able to identify 50% of all

TABLE 1 **Summary of Case Study Test scores showing means, standard deviations, and ranges for all subjects combined (n = 59)**

Case Study Test scores	Mean score	SD	Range of observed scores
Total Case Study score (22.0)*	9.59(43.59)†	2.27	5-15
Data score (11.0)	4.36(39.64)	1.27	2-8
Diagnosis score (11.0)	5.24(47.64)	1.47	2-9
Darryl score (5.0)	2.76(55.20)	0.88	1-5
Family score (6.0)	2.48(41.33)	0.94	1-4

*Total possible points.
†Percent of total possible points.

possible nursing diagnoses. DeBack (1981) found not only that teaching strategies did not correlate with the ability to formulate nursing diagnoses, but that only 28% of her student sample met the criteria for identifying correct diagnoses; 35% met none of the criteria. Registered nurses in Aspinall's (1979) study averaged 45% correct diagnoses.

From the literature come additional explanations for low scores on the Case Study Test. Aspinall (1979) cited Simon's concept of "bounded rationality" as a factor in inaccurate diagnosis identification. "Bounded rationality" refers to "limitation of complete objective rationality in making decisions," that is, limitation in the number of alternatives considered due to "inadequate deliberation and judgment." Aspinall concluded that nurses were unable to use theoretical knowledge to make a nursing diagnosis. Tanner (1979) recognized "premature closure" on the consideration of possible diagnoses and lack of time spent on the task as factors in nursing students difficulty with making diagnoses. Tanner also identified failure to gather pertinent information as a contributing factor.

The scoring procedure for the Case Study Test had several limitations. First, scoring was a subjective process done by a panel of RN judges rather than by an objective process. This was necessitated by the open-ended responses allowed on the test. The responses ranged from clear statements to vague, poorly stated data or problems that could not be categorized. Second, the panel achieved agreement (reliability) on 70% to 83% of the tests scored a second time. The lack of higher reliability scores represents the subjective and imprecise nature of the scoring decisions made by the judges. In addition, the panel was reluctant to count any responses as wrong.

This study differentiated between teacher-guided practice, independent practice, and no practice in applying assessment and diagnostic skills. With a limited sample in a specific situation, the results showed that practice sessions did not make a difference. It is, in reality, unlikely that there is no benefit from practice in learning to assess clients and formulate diagnoses. It is important for nurse researchers to continue to explore the cognitive processes involved in formulating nursing diagnoses, the effectiveness of methods used to teach diagnostic skills, and methods of evaluating diagnostic skills.

With respect to current teaching practices, it is important for nursing faculty to pay attention to how students formulate nursing diagnoses and to explore with them the thought processes used in determining a diagnosis. Students need to be taught the importance of an accurate and adequate data base for each diagnosis. Emphasis also should be placed on exploring alternative diagnoses and including psychosocial as well as physical diagnoses for all patients.

Simulations can be used in nursing education for formative and summative evaluation of students' diagnostic skills. Types include written and computerized case studies, audiovisual simulations, and simulated live patients. An objective, well-designed test can reduce many of the uncontrollable variables inherent in actual patient situations. Tanner (1979) states that the ideal test will "simulate reality, assess multiple components of the nursing process, allow for a high degree of interaction, minimize the effect of cuing, and be easy to administer and score." There is a need to continue to develop and evaluate simulations as tools for assessing clinical competence in students.

REFERENCES

Aspinall, M.J.: Nursing diagnosis—the weak link, Nurs. Outlook **24**(7):433-437, 1976.

Aspinall, M.J.: Use of a decision tree to improve accuracy of diagnosis, Nurs. Res. **28**(3):182-185, 1979.

Bircher, A.U.: The concept of nursing diagnosis. In Kim, M.J. and Moritz, D.A., editors: Classification of nursing diagnoses—Proceedings of the Third and Fourth National Conferences, New York, 1982, McGraw-Hill Book Co.

Bruner, J., Goodnow, J.J., and Austin, G.A.: A study of thinking, New York, 1967, Science Editions, Inc.

DeBack, V.: The relationship between senior nursing students' ability to formulate nursing diagnoses and the curriculum model, Adv. Nurs. Sci. **3**(3):51-66, 1981.

Dincher, J.R., and Stidger, S.L.: Evaluation of a written simulation format for clinical nursing judgment, Nurs. Res. **25**(4):280-285, 1976.

Gordon, M.: The diagnostic process. In Kim, M.J., and Moritz, D.A., editors: Classification of nursing diagnoses—Proceedings of the Third and Fourth National Conferences, New York, 1982a, McGraw-Hill Book Co.

Gordon, M.: Nursing diagnosis: process and application, New York, 1982b, McGraw-Hill Book Co.

Kim, M.J., and Moritz, D.A.: Classification of nursing diagnoses—Proceedings of the Third and Fourth National Conferences, New York, 1982, McGraw-Hill Book Co.

Matthews, C.A., and Gaul, A.L.: Nursing diagnosis from the perspective of concept attainment and critical thinking, Adv. Nurs. Sci. **2**(1):17-26, 1979.

Polit, D., and Hungler, B.: Nursing research: principles and methods, Philadelphia, 1978, J.B. Lippincott Co.

Tanner, C.A.: Testing for process: stimulation and other alternative modes of evaluation. In Developing tests to evaluate student achievement in baccalaureate nursing programs, New York, 1979, National League for Nursing.

Tanner, C.A.: Instruction on the diagnostic process: an experimental study. In Kim, M.J., and Moritz, D.A., editors: Classification of nursing diagnoses—Proceedings of the Third and Fourth National Conferences, New York, 1982, McGraw-Hill Book Co.

Baccalaureate nursing education: teaching pathophysiology with a nursing diagnosis framework

MARITA TITLER, M.A., R.N.

Nurses are emerging as visible and distinct health care professionals with a special expertise and perspective to offer their clients. Nursing diagnosis has been an integral part of this evolvement. Nurses are realizing that nursing diagnoses are the pivotal points upon which nursing interventions are planned and implemented. Educators, researchers, and practitioners are accepting nursing diagnosis as a part of their professional role.

In formulating nursing diagnoses, nurses use their knowledge base to synthesize incoming cues. Within this knowledge base is the understanding of a variety of pathophysiological concepts. Understanding these concepts is necessary to formulate diagnostic statements (Carnevali, 1983). Some nursing diagnoses reflect the pathological process in the problem portion (for instance, impaired gas exchange related to excessive secretions), while others have the pathological process in the etiology portion (for instance, decreased activity tolerance related to decreased cardiac output). It is evident that nurses need to understand the relationship between pathophysiological processes and nursing diagnoses. Therefore, the focus of this paper is to describe a methodology for teaching pathophysiology to baccalaureate nursing students using the nursing diagnostic framework of unitary humans.

RELATIONSHIP TO THE CURRICULUM

The pathophysiology course is offered within a baccalaureate nursing curriculum at Coe College, a private liberal arts college with a full-time enrollment of 1058 students. The nursing program is in its infancy; the first class graduated in May, 1985. The nursing curriculum is based on the belief that a strong liberal arts education provides a rich foundation for professional education in nursing. Furthermore, it is the belief of the faculty that nurses require a strong knowledge base from the humanities and sciences in the application of nursing roles. For the curricular framework in nursing, the faculty selected Rogers' (1970) view of humans as open systems always in a state of becoming. Unique among creation, humans possess the ability for thought, feeling, and emotion. Humans have the capacity to experience, perceive, interpret, and assign meaning to oneself and their realities. The basic characteristic of humans is the forward movement of all life processes in the direction of creative, constructive, productive, personal and community life. Human responses occur as a component of the life process and include physiological, emotional, cognitive, and social reactions to developmental and environmental changes encountered throughout life (Loomis and Wood, 1983). The life process encompasses developmental life changes, which include physiological evolvement, and cognitive, emotional, and social growth. The uniqueness of beings is manifested in human responses to life processes which are exhibited through behaviors and affect one's health. Human responses are categorized according to the nine human environment interactional patterns of exchanging, communicating, relating, valuing, choosing, moving, perceiving, knowing, and feeling (Roy, 1984).

Nursing is concerned with assisting humans to attain and maintain their maximum health potential. Health is defined as a dynamic process that is subject to self-regulatory control and influenced by energy supply and demand. Nursing practice centers on the diagnosis and treatment of human responses observed in the behaviors of individuals, groups, and communities. Thus the

TABLE 1   **Courses in the Coe College nursing curriculum**

Fall term	Winter term	Spring term
Freshman year		
Introduction to Modern Culture	Elective	The Nature of Science
General Biology I		Introduction to Health Care Systems
Introductory Chemistry		Introduction to Organic and Biological Chemistry
Introductory Psychology		Introductory Sociology
Sophomore year		
Human Anatomy and Kinesiology	Nutrition (or Elective)	Human Physiology
Introduction to Nursing Process and Skills I		Introduction to Nursing Process and Skills II
Microbiology		Nutrition (or Elective)
Human Life-span Development		Pharmacology
Junior year		
Nursing Care of Adults (two credits)	Elective	Nursing Care of Childbearing-Childrearing Families (two credits)
Pathophysiology		Mental Health Nursing
Elective		Elective
Senior year		
Advanced Application of the Nursing Process (two credits)	Elective	Community Health Nursing
Introduction to Nursing Research		Nursing Leadership and Issues (two credits)
Elective		Elective

purpose of the pathophysiology course in the Coe nursing curriculum is to provide students with a knowledge base necessary to diagnose and treat human responses encountered in the life process. It provides the basis for the integration and application of pathophysiological concepts in formulating nursing diagnoses and appropriate nursing interventions. By consensus of the nursing faculty, this course emphasizes the altered physiological processes and does not focus on psychopathology. Students in the course examine the effects that altered physiological functioning have on one's ability to achieve or maintain their maximum health potential. Guided by the unitary human framework (Roy, 1984), students explore how various pathophysiological processes influence human responses. Etiological factors, pathogenetic mechanisms, and manifestations of altered physiological functioning are emphasized.

Placement of pathophysiology in the curriculum is presented in Table 1. When students enroll in pathophysiology, they are familiar with the steps of the nursing process and have focused on the assessment phase. They are novices in diagnostic reasoning, but they have experienced the formulation of nursing diagnoses with regard to mobility, self-care, and skin integrity.

COURSE CONTENT

The unitary human environment interaction patterns emphasized in pathophysiology are exchanging, knowing, communicating, feeling, perceiving, and moving. These particular patterns were selected to reflect the emphasis on the course; the student is able to

1. Understand humans as open systems acted upon by stressors in the environment
2. Explain the biological responses of humans experiencing altered physiological processes
3. Identify the relationship between the unitary human framework and the pathological processes
4. Determine the effects that altered physiological functioning have on one's ability to maintain a dynamic equilibrium with regard to the human patterns of exchanging, moving, knowing, feeling, communicating, and perceiving
5. Describe the etiological factors, pathogenic mechanisms, and manifestations of the following pathological processes:
   5.1 Alterations in physical integrity
   5.2 Alterations in fluid and electrolyte balance
   5.3 Altered immune responses
   5.4 Altered cell growth
   5.5 Alterations in oxygenation
   5.6 Alterations in circulation

5.7   Alterations in nutrition
5.8   Alterations in elimination
5.9   Alterations in self-concept
5.10 Sensory/perceptual alterations
5.11 Altered thought processes
5.12 Alterations in comfort: pain
5.13 Alterations in physical mobility
5.14 Altered communication among bodily systems
6. Use the pathophysiological concepts as a basis for making nursing diagnoses with selected clients

ORGANIZATION OF CONTENT

At the Fifth National Conference on Classification of Nursing Diagnoses, the taxonomy group classified each of the existing nursing diagnoses under one of the nine patterns of unitary humans (Kritek, 1984). This taxonomy system is built on a hierarchical relationship of general to specific and thereby can be used to organize course content. The patterns of human environment interaction are the major category headings. Selected diagnostic categories (human responses) are the subcategory headings and delineate the content areas. (See Box 1.)

BOX 1   **Hierarchical relationship**

I. Exchanging
   A. Alterations in circulation: systemic
      1. Altered tissue perfusion
      2. Altered venous flow
      3. Fluid volume deficit
   B. Alterations in circulation: cardiac
      1. Altered tissue perfusion
      2. Decreased cardiac output

This course begins with an overview of the unitary human framework. During the overview, students study the concepts of human, environment, open systems, energy, health, and illness. Time is spent discussing the purpose of the course as well as the relationship between pathology and nursing diagnosis.

The first major unit in the course is exchanging. It is defined as "mutual giving and receiving" (Roy, 1984). The content for this unit is reflected in Box 2. Alterations in fluid and electrolyte balance, alterations in acid-base balance, altered immune response, and altered cell growth are not currently classified

BOX 2   **Content outline for exchanging**

A. Alterations in physical integrity
   1. Cellular response to attack: compensations, cell injury, cell death
   2. Inflammatory response
   3. Infection
B. Alterations in fluid and electrolyte balance
   1. Fluid volume deficit
   2. Fluid volume excess
   3. Serum electrolyte imbalance
C. Alterations in acid-base balance
   1. Acidosis
   2. Alkalosis
D. Altered immune responses
   1. Hypersensitivity reactions
   2. Autoimmune diseases
   3. Immunodeficiency
E. Altered cell growth
   1. Neoplasms
   2. Altered growth of WBC, lymph nodes, plasma cells, and related structures
   3. Congenital defects
F. Alterations in oxygenation: respiration
   1. Restrictive lung disorders
   2. Obstructive lung disorders
   3. Neoplasms
   4. Impaired gas exchange
   5. Ineffective airway clearance
   6. Ineffective breathing patterns
G. Alterations in oxygenation: anemias
H. Alterations in circulation: systemic
   1. Altered tissue perfusion
   2. Altered venous flow
   3. Fluid volume deficit
I. Alterations in circulation: cardiac
   1. Altered tissue perfusion
   2. Decreased cardiac output
J. Alterations in nutrition
   1. Carbohydrate imbalance
   2. Alterations in ingestion and digestion
   3. Alterations in absorption
K. Alterations in elimination: bowel
   1. Constipation
   2. Diarrhea
   3. Inflammation
   4. Neoplasms
L. Alterations in elimination: urine
   1. Inflammation and infection
   2. Obstruction
   3. Familial diseases
   4. Neoplasms
   5. Nephropathies
   6. Renal insufficiency
   7. Renal failure

as diagnostic categories by the taxonomy group (Kritek, 1984). However, these human responses can be conceptualized as mutual giving and receiving. Thus they are classified as exchanging processes.

The second major unit is organized according to the human pattern of perceiving. Major human responses studied in this unit are alterations in self-concept and sensory-perceptual alterations. Perceiving is "reception of information" (Roy, 1984). Box 3 illustrates the organization of content in this unit. Altered level of awareness is used as a diagnostic classification under sensory/ perceptual alterations because this phenomenon includes more than the alteration of sensory organs. Sensory/perceptual alterations are defined by Carpenito (1983) as "a state in which the individual experiences or is at risk of experiencing a change in the amount, pattern, or interpretation of incoming stimuli." Thus metabolic and neurological alterations are taught with regard to the impact that these states have on levels of awareness and ultimately upon the processing of incoming stimuli.

The third major unit involves the pattern of knowing. The definition of knowing is "meaning associated with information" (Roy, 1984). The major human response addressed is altered thought processes. Students study the relationship between organic brain syndromes, such as Alzheimer's disease and dementia, and altered thought processes.

BOX 3   **Content outline for perceiving**

A. Alterations in self-concept
   1. Alterations in sexuality and sexual functioning
B. Sensory/perceptual alterations
   1. Alterations in sensory organs
   2. Altered levels of awareness
      a. Increased intracranial pressure
      b. Metabolic changes
      c. Seizures

Feeling is the next major unit and is defined as "the subjective awareness of information" (Roy, 1984). Alterations in comfort, pain, is the human response studied within this unit.

Moving is the fifth major unit heading. It is defined as "activity" (Roy, 1984). Alterations in physical mobility is the focus of this unit. Box 4 illustrates the structure within this unit. It becomes apparent that there is potential for overlap between sensory-perceptual alteration and altered physical mobility. For example, should spinal cord injury be taught with altered physical mobility or with sensory-perceptual alteration? I chose to teach spinal cord injury as a

BOX 4	Content outline for moving

A. Alterations in physical mobility
   1. Neurological impairment
   2. Musculoskeletal impairment
   3. Fatigue
   4. Complications of immobility

major pathologic alteration contributing to altered physical mobility. At the same time students learn about sensory/perceptual alterations that are precipitated by spinal cord injuries.

The last major unit is communicating. It is defined as "sending messages" (Roy, 1984). Hormonal imbalances are studied with regard to the changes that occur in communication among the bodily systems. This unit emphasizes how hormonal imbalances contribute to alterations in (1) growth, (2) self-concept, (3) cellular metabolism, (4) fluid balance, and (5) the stress response.

Thus the unitary human framework serves as a hierarchical structure for organizing course content. Each subcategory (human response) is a diagnostic concept title. Students begin each subcategory by defining the human response and then describe the etiologies, pathogenesis, and manifestations of the response. It is within this context that students learn about the pathophysiological processes of specific disorders. They study the impact that these processes have on human responses in the life process. From this knowledge base, students generate several nursing diagnoses which are applicable for clients with the pathophysiological processes discussed. Defining characteristics are identified for each nursing diagnosis and critical cues are selected. This provides students with the cross-linkage between pathophysiological concepts and nursing diagnoses as recommended by Carnevali (1983, 1984b) and Tanner (1984).

The diagnostic classification alterations in oxygenation: respiration will serve as a model to illustrate the cross-linkage between pathophysiological concepts and nursing diagnosis within this course (see Box 5). The unit begins by defining alterations in oxygenation, specifically respiration. Students describe the processes which interfere with ventilation, perfusion, and diffusion. They identify people at risk for developing alterations in oxygenation: respiration as well as describing manifestations of this phenomenon. They learn the etiology, pathogenesis, manifestations, and complications of restrictive lung disorders, obstructive lung disorders, and lung neoplasms. They then study the impact that these lung disorders have on various human responses. Specifically, they explain how the pathological processes of the lung can result in ineffective breathing patterns, impaired gas exchange, and ineffective airway

BOX 5   **Alterations in oxygenation: respiration**

1. Definition
2. Etiologies and risk factors
   a. Alterations in ventilation
   b. Alterations in perfusion
   c. Alterations in diffusion
3. Manifestations of altered respiration
4. Restrictive lung disorders
   a. Extrapulmonary
   b. Diseases of the pleura
   c. Diseases of lung parenchyma
5. Obstructive disorders
   a. Chronic obstructive pulmonary disease
   b. Bronchial obstruction
6. Neoplasms
7. Ineffective breathing patterns
   a. Etiology
   b. Defining characteristics
8. Impaired gas exchange
   a. Etiology
   b. Defining characteristics
9. Ineffective airway clearance
   a. Etiology
   b. Defining characteristics
10. Additional nursing diagnoses

clearance. Students are then guided in formulating additional nursing diagnoses which could occur as a result of these lung pathologies (for example, activity intolerance, self-care deficit.)

TEACHING METHODOLOGIES

Teaching methodologies used in the course are lecture, films, and seminars. Case studies are used for analyzing possible nursing diagnoses related to selected pathophysiological processes. Each case study includes the client's history, manifestations of specific pathologies, and coping mechanisms used by the client to live with the disorder. From the case study, students (1) identify all possible nursing diagnoses and the defining characteristics for each, (2) identify the pathophysiological processes operant in the client, and (3) explain how the pathophysiological processes influence the human response inherent in the nursing diagnosis. These case studies provide the basis for seminars and worksheet assignments.

Thus it is evident that students are provided with a cross-linkage between pathophysiological concepts and nursing diagnoses. It is necessary that nurses understand the dynamics of pathology as a basis for many nursing diagnoses and treatment plans. Nurses cannot diagnose what they do not understand (Carnevali, 1984c). This necessitates that nurses are knowledgeable of the etiologies, pathogenesis, and manifestations of pathophysiological processes. In order to use this knowledge in the nursing domain, it is important that nurses link the pathophysiological concepts with altered human responses (Carnevali, 1983). This pathophysiology course offers the methodology for developing such a cross-linkage. Carnevali (1984a) proposes that it is the responsibility of nursing education to develop this type of cross-linkage "in both nursing-to-nursing, nursing-to-biomedical, and biomedical-to-nursing concepts."

ISSUES

A major issue in offering a pathophysiology course which links pathological concepts with nursing diagnoses is that the resulting diagnostic label implies collaboration between nurses and physicians. Some authors suggest that nursing diagnoses are applicable only for the phenomena which nurses can diagnose and treat independently of other health care professionals (Bircher, 1975; Gordon, 1976; Moritz, 1982). For a number of reasons, this author disagrees with placing that constraint on nursing diagnoses. First, it is reality that nurses do engage in collaborative interventions when they diagnose and treat clients. "It is a fact of life that nurses must diagnose regularly in both the biomedical and nursing domains as a part of their professional role" (Carnevali, 1984b). To ignore those problems which necessitate collaborative and dependent nursing interventions, or to label them as clinical problems, only fragments the diagnostic reasoning process. Nursing offers the unique perspective of viewing humans as whole open systems in constant exchange with their environment. Therefore, one cannot limit nursing diagnoses or the diagnostic process to only those phenomena which nurses can treat independently. Nurses must also assume the responsibility for diagnosing and treating those problems which evolve from a pathophysiological base.

Second, the purposes for designing a nursing taxonomy include (1) development of a scientific knowledge base for nursing, (2) retrieval of nursing data, (3) provision of a reimbursement mechanism for nursing services, and (4) guidance and direction for nursing research activities (Carpenito, 1983; Gordon, 1982). If the nursing taxonomy is to fulfill these expectations, the profession must include those diagnoses which require the collaborative and dependent nursing interventions.

Third, and most important, nurses are demonstrating through research that nursing diagnoses which have a pathophysiological base (for example, decreased cardiac output, ineffective breathing pattern, impaired gas exchange) do require independent nursing interventions. Individual nursing research studies by Dougherty (1983) and by Wessel (1981) have demonstrated that the majority of nursing interventions for clients with decreased cardiac output are independent in nature. Dougherty (1983) found that 77% of the nursing interventions for decreased cardiac output are independent, 18% are collaborative, and 0% are dependent as classified by both nurses and physicians. These findings are in agreement with Wessel's (1981) research findings.

McDonald (1983) demonstrated that the nursing diagnoses of ineffective airway clearance, ineffective breathing pattern, and impaired gas exchange were associated with independent nursing interventions. The nursing interventions used most frequently for adult patients with these diagnostic labels were patient-family teaching (74%), coughing and deep breathing (74%), encouraging ambulation (63%), elevating the head of the bed (63%), ensuring adequate intake of oral fluids (53%), and using the Triflo (53%). These interventions can all be classified as independent nursing functions. The most frequently used interventions for the infant group were chest physical therapy (82%), environmental manipulation (77%), patient-family teaching (77%), suctioning (73%), organization of care (68%), elevating the head of the bed (64%), monitoring vital signs and arterial blood gases (50%), and psychological support (50%). The majority of these interventions are also independent nursing functions.

ADVANTAGES

The advantage of using the unitary human framework to design a pathophysiology course is that it provides students with a framework for information storage which facilitates the diagnostic reasoning process. This framework is organized in a hierarchical relationship of general to specific with linkages among the categories within each unit. This type of organizational structure (1) allows for a more economical storage of cues, (2) facilitates categorization of incoming data from the client, thereby reducing cognitive strain, (3) enhances learning by improving the categorization process of new information, (4) permits a more efficient storage of information from episodic memory, such as previous client situation, and (5) facilitates retrieval of categorical information associated with the presenting cues (Carnevali, 1984b; Tanner, 1984).

POTENTIAL PROBLEMS

A potential problem in offering a separate pathophysiology course is that students tend to focus only on the disease process. One advantage of the methodology used in this course is that the course content is organized, presented, and linked with nursing diagnoses, thereby offering a solution to that problem. As a result of this methodology, sound diagnostic reasoning patterns for nurses should be expedited. A cross-linkage between the dynamics of pathophysiology and nursing diagnoses should develop (Carnevali, 1984a). One cannot teach pathophysiology using a medical model and then realistically expect students to retrieve this information without first creating a new mental framework. "When the knowledge and experience are deliberately stored with diagnostic strategies in mind, the access routes are also incorporated so that when particular cues (signs, symptoms, risk factors, etc.) are perceived in the presenting situation, the appropriate packets of knowledge are retrieved" (Carnevali, 1984b). Hence students enrolled in subsequent nursing courses have begun developing a long-term memory storage based on this hierarchical framework and have linked this knowledge with nursing diagnoses.

In offering a separate pathophysiology course, it is imperative that coordination occurs among nursing courses. Coordination can be enhanced by using the unitary human framework as the organizing outline for all nursing courses. More importantly, faculty need to commit themselves to a type of course content outline that promotes the diagnostic reasoning process (Carnevali, 1984a). Nursing educators must also assist students in developing linkages between diagnostic concepts. "Modeling this cross-linkage is important, not only in the presentation of theory, but in the clinical situation" (Carnevali, 1984a).

SUMMARY

In summary, nurses must be cognizant of pathophysiological processes and the influence these processes have on human responses in the life process. Teaching pathophysiology using the methodology described assists students in developing a relationship between pathophysiological concepts and the human environment interactional patterns of exchanging, moving, perceiving, knowing, feeling, and communicating. Within this context, students develop a mind-set for analyzing cues based on a nursing diagnostic framework rather than a disease-oriented model. This should enhance diagnostic reasoning and result in more accurate and complete nursing diagnoses.

REFERENCES

Bircher, A.: On the development and classification of nursing diagnoses, Nurs. Forum, **14**:10-29, 1975.

Carnevali, D.L.: Nursing care planning: diagnosis and management, Philadelphia, 1983, J.B. Lippincott Co.

Carnevali, D.L.: Development of diagnostic reasoning skills: Implications for nursing practice, education, management, nursing literature, and research. In Carnevali, D., Mitchell, P., Woods, N., and Tanner, C., editors: Diagnostic reasoning in nursing, Philadelphia, 1984a, J.B. Lippincott Co.

Carnevali, D.L.: The diagnostic reasoning process. In Carnevali, D., Mitchell, P., Woods, N., and Tanner, C., editors: Diagnostic reasoning in nursing, Philadelphia, 1984b, J.B. Lippincott Co.

Carnevali, D.L.: The nursing domain for diagnostic reasoning. In Carnevali, D., Mitchell, P., Woods, N., and Tanner, C., editors: Diagnostic reasoning in nursing, Philadelphia, 1984c, J.B. Lippincott Co.

Carpenito, L.J.: Nursing diagnosis application to clinical practice, Philadelphia, 1983, J.B. Lippincott Co.

Dougherty, C.M.: Defining the characteristics and interventions for the nursing diagnosis of decreased cardiac output. Unpublished master's thesis, University of Iowa, 1983.

Gordon, M.: Nursing diagnosis and the diagnostic process, Am. J. Nurs. **76:**1298-1300, 1976.

Gordon, M.: Nursing diagnosis process and application, New York, 1982, McGraw-Hill Book Co.

Kritek, P.: Report of the taxonomy group. In Kim, M.J., McFarland, G., and McLane, A., editors: Classification of nursing diagnoses—Proceedings of the Fifth National Conference, St. Louis, 1984, The C.V. Mosby Co.

Loomis, M.E., and Wood, D.J.: Cure: the potential outcome of nursing care, Image **15:**4-7, 1983.

McDonald, B.: Validation of defining characteristics of three nursing diagnoses and associated nursing interventions. Unpublished master's thesis, University of Iowa, 1983.

Moritz, D.A.: Nursing diagnoses in relation to the nursing process. In Kim, M.J., Moritz, D.A., editors: Classification of nursing diagnoses—Proceedings of the Third and Fourth National Conferences, New York, 1982, McGraw-Hill Book Co.

Rogers, M.E.: An introduction to the theoretical basis of nursing, Philadelphia, 1970, F.A. Davis Co.

Roy, C.: Framework for classification systems development: progress and issues. In Kim, M.J., McFarland, G., and McLane, A., editors: Classification of nursing diagnoses—Proceedings of the Fifth National Conference, St. Louis, 1984, The C.V. Mosby Co.

Tanner, C.A.: Factors influencing the diagnostic process. In Carnevali, D., Mitchell, P., Woods, N., and Tanner, C.A., editors: Diagnostic reasoning in nursing, Philadelphia, 1984, J.B. Lippincott Co.

Wessel, S.L.: Nursing functions related to the nursing diagnosis "decreased cardiac output." Unpublished master's thesis, University of Illinois, 1981.

Types of statements made by nurses as first impressions of patient problems*

JENNIFER L. CRAIG, Ph.D., R.N.

Why is it that registered nurses have difficulty in stating the patient problems that they as nurses are accountable to treat independently (Fatzer, 1979; Silver and associates, 1982)? Failure to articulate nursing diagnoses may be a function of a lack of a vocabulary of summary diagnostic statements, or the result of a faulty clinical reasoning process used to arrive at a diagnosis. The purpose of this study was to describe one aspect of the clinical reasoning process: statements of initial impressions of patient problems (hypotheses) by nurses who varied in length of education and experience.

Studies of clinical reasoning or the diagnostic process may be classified into one of three general paradigms (Bordage, 1982). The decision-making approach examines how clinicians ought to make optimal decisions under uncertainty and is rooted in Bayesian theory. Studies in nursing using this paradigm include one by Aspinsall (1979). The judgment paradigm asks how clinicians use information available to them and with what accuracy. It attempts to capture policy and may use Brunswick's lens model. Hammond (1966) and Gordon (1980) used this paradigm. The information processing approach asks how clinicians actually solve problems and with what cognitive processes. A current study by Tanner and associates (1983) falls within this paradigm, whereas the major work within this paradigm was conducted by Elstein and colleagues (1978).

The theory of medical problem-solving proposed by Elstein and co-workers (1978) describes four major components in the cognitive process used to arrive at a diagnostic decision:

1. *Cue acquisition.* The process begins with attention to initial cues (information) from, or about, the patient.
2. *Hypothesis generation.* Prompted by as few as two cues, the clinician generates tentative hypotheses about the cause of the problem.
3. *Cue interpretation.* Guided by the mental list of hypotheses, the clinician gathers more data and interprets them as supporting or refuting existing hypotheses or suggesting new ones.
4. *Diagnostic decision.* Step 3 is continued until a decision is reached about which is the most likely problem. Decisions about intervention are then made.

*Research supported in part by the National Health Research and Development Program (Canada) through a National Health Fellowship to Jennifer L. Craig.

Although physicians were subjects in this and other studies which support this description (Feltovich, 1982; Kassirer and Gorry, 1978), current work by Tanner and associates (1983) demonstrates that a similar model operates in nurses.

Central to the clinical reasoning process is the early generation of first impressions of patients problems (hypotheses). These hypotheses are important for a number of reasons. First, they reduce the boundless set of possible problems to a manageable number (Elstein and associates, 1978; Tanner, 1978). Second, they guide the collection and interpretation of data. The percentage of "hypothesis driven" questions was found to be 60% to 80% by Kassirer and Gorry (1978), 50% by Neufeld and co-workers (1981). Third, there is evidence to suggest that the content of the hypothesis list generated early in the encounter is a major determinant of a successful diagnostic outcome (Neufeld and co-workers, 1981; Tanner, 1978).

Several studies of clinical reasoning have examined differences between expert and novice diagnosticians. One established characteristic of an expert problem-solver is the ability to recognize relevant information in the environment and disregard irrelevant information (Lesgold and associates, 1981; Simon and Chase, 1973). Although the quantity of hypotheses generated by experts and novices has been found to be similar (Hassebrock and Johnson, 1983) the differences lie in the quality. Experts tend to consider a broader range of possibilities which are more problem-specific (Lesgold and co-workers, 1981; Neufeld and co-workers, 1981).

The questions asked in this study were that, given a limited number of cues (pieces of information), (1) how many hypotheses were generated, (2) what types of hypotheses were generated, (3) how many cues were used, and (4) what type of cues were selected by nurses (who varied in length of education and of experience)? Furthermore, it was asked whether directions to suggest only nursing diagnoses affected the number of medical diagnoses generated.

METHOD
Subjects

Groups of nurses who spanned a variety of education and experience were chosen. The groups were as follows:

DIP-A	Students who had completed their diploma program except for the 4-month internship
DIP-B	Students who were ready to graduate from their diploma program, including the internship experience
RN	Registered Nurses with a diploma who had practiced for at least 1 year
RN-BSN	Baccalaureate students in their final year who had entered with experience as RNs
BSN	Basic baccalaureate students who were in their final year
MSN-0	Masters of Science in Nursing (MSN) students who entered with a degree in something other than nursing in their first year

MSN-1   MSN students who entered as nurses in their first year
MSN-2   MSN students who entered as nurses in their second year
MS-NDX   MSN students who entered as nurses and who were specifically taught
         the diagnostic process and the use of a standard list of nursing diagnoses

The total number participating was 243.

The MS-NDX group comprised students who had been taught a specific course in nursing diagnosis by an expert in nursing diagnosis and had studied texts on the subject (Gordon, 1982ab). They were considered the standard, and against them other groups were compared.

The task

Six tasks, each consisting of nine cues, were prepared. The nine cues were such that

4 together suggested a specific nursing diagnosis (NDX) (individually they could suggest other problems)
1 gave demographic data such as gender, age, religion (DEMO)
1 gave the medical diagnosis or reason for seeking medical help (MDX)
2 were "doctors' orders" or medical regimen (REGIMEN)
1 was a physical finding or laboratory or x-ray result (PX)

These cues were chosen because they were the type of information found in nurses' notes, Kardexes, or patient charts and were therefore read. An attempt was made to select common cues that did not require extensive knowledge or specialty training to interpret.

The six specific nursing diagnoses were
• Alteration in nutrition
• Potential skin integrity impairment
• Sleep pattern disturbance
• Impaired communication
• Self-care deficit
• Lack of knowledge

The first five were chosen because (1) they appear in the list of 13 most frequently reported nursing diagnoses in a study designed to discover and document the terms used by nurses to describe the human conditions for which they care (Jones and Jakob, 1982) and (2) they are included in the list of diagnoses accepted by the North American Nursing Diagnosis Association (NANDA) and are sufficiently developed that defining characteristics can be listed. As patient teaching is an important nursing function, the sixth, knowledge deficit, was chosen by the investigator because, although it is on the NANDA list, it was conspicuous by its absence from the Jones and Jakob list.

The nine cues of each task were randomly ordered once so that the resulting order was the same for all subjects. The tasks were submitted to a panel of experts who were asked to judge whether the four cues were characteristic of

BOX 1   **Example of task based on the nursing diagnosis "Potential skin integrity impairment"**

			I	I	S
1	2	3	4	5	6

1. Becomes very uncomfortable when lying on side   1
2. Considerable restriction of motion in hands, knees, and ankle joints   2
3. Female (age 70 yr, married, Jehovah's Witness)   3
4. Reddened area over coccyx   4
5. Rheumatoid arthritis   5
6. White blood cell count 13,000 per cu mm   6
7. High calorie–high protein–high vitamin diet   7
8. Prednisone 2.5 mg a.c. and h.s.   8
9. Skin tight and shiny over bony prominences   9

Possible problem(s)	Cue(s) used	For office use
1. _____		
_____	7 8 9 10	11 12
2. _____		
_____	13 14 15 16	17 18
3. _____		
_____	19 20 21 22	23 24
4. _____		
_____	25 26 27 28	29 30
5. _____		
_____	31 32 33 34	35 36

the task nursing diagnosis, whether the cues were familiar to any registered nurse (RN) and whether the task fell within the capabilities of any RN.

An example of a task is shown in Box 1. Subjects were asked to read the cues and write down the patient problems or potential problems that occurred to them and the identification number of the cue(s) that suggested the problem. Half the subjects received directions to ignore problems they would refer to a physician.

The tasks were ordered in six different sequences. The order in which the subjects received tasks and the type of directions given were randomly determined.

Coding

Each patient problem was coded into one of 13 categories by two coders. The coding scheme, shown in Table 1, was developed from the work of Silver and co-workers (1982). Half of each group's questionnaires were coded by each coder and 10% by both. Interrater simple percentage agreement averaged 91%. Intrarater agreement was 94% in one case, 93% in the other.

Vocabulary which differed from the NANDA list was accepted if the meaning was judged to be similar. For example, skin breakdown, decubitus ulcers, or bedsores were considered equivalent to potential skin integrity impairment. Furthermore, statements coded 01 (Nursing diagnosis) did not include etiology; a complete nursing diagnosis was impossible given the partial data provided.

Results

The number of hypotheses generated was 4199. The range of average number per subject in each group was 14.8 to 19.5 over six tasks. The difference between groups was significant ($F8234 = 2.84$, $p < 0.01$). The differences lay in the RN-BSN group, who generated fewer than average, and the MSN-2 group, who generated more.

Types of hypotheses as percentages of each group's total are illustrated in Fig. 1. For easier interpretation the 13 categories have been compressed into six so that

01 + 02	Nursing
04	Concept
11 + 12 + 13	Data
08 + 09	Care plan
03 + 05 + 14	Medical
07 + 15	Miscellaneous

Table 2 displays the types of hypotheses as frequencies both observed and expected (in italics). The difference between groups is so large that the value of χ^2 is significant far beyond the 0.001 level.

TABLE 1   **Short version of the hypothesis coding scheme**

Code	Category	Definition	Examples
01	Nursing diagnosis	Label for a cluster of signs and symptoms describing an actual or potential health problem which nurses, by virtue of their education, are capable, licensed, and accountable to treat	Those accepted by NANDA. Those listed in Gordon's manual plus others, e.g., incontinence
02	Task nursing diagnosis	Label for 4 cues of each of the 6 tasks which, clustered, suggest a specific nursing diagnosis	Knowledge deficit. Impaired communication
03	Medical diagnosis	Label for a cluster of signs and symptoms describing a condition which a nurse is not licensed to treat independently and for a condition that would be referred to a physician	Cancer. Congestive heart failure. Mononucleosis
04	Concept label	Label describing a functional pattern, biological system, developmental stage, category of a conceptual framework, or unrefined problem	Aging process. Support systems. Behavior problems. Stress
05	Medical pathology	Label describing an actual or potential generalized physiological deviation	Electrolyte imbalance. Paralysis. Increased intracranial Pressure
07	Multiple labels	Labels describing more than one problem or sign or symptom	Sad, depressed, withdrawn, anxious
08	Intervention	Label describing an action implemented to help meet a patient/family goal	Assist with parenting skills. Hygiene care
09	Goal	Label describing an intended expectation of the patient/family health status by a certain time	Regulation of pain. Rehabilitation
11	Sign or symptom	Label describing a subjective or objective indicator of a patient/family health status	Loss of appetite. Nausea. High blood pressure
12	Repeat cue	Label describing information given as a whole or partial cue (takes precedence over other codes)	Feeling of inadequacy. Cancer. Tired
13	Risk factor/etiology	Label describing a factor, circumstance, pattern of behavior, or emotional state which may produce an alteration in patient/family health status for which nursing intervention is needed but which is not itself a problem	Poor fluid intake. Change in life-style. Lack of exercise. Role conflict
14	Side effect/complication	Label describing an actual or potential undesirable result of a therapeutic intervention	Reaction to chemotherapy. Fluid overload
15	Miscellaneous	Jargon word, abbreviation or statement that does not qualify for the above categories	Organic brain. Feeding baby. Urine precautions

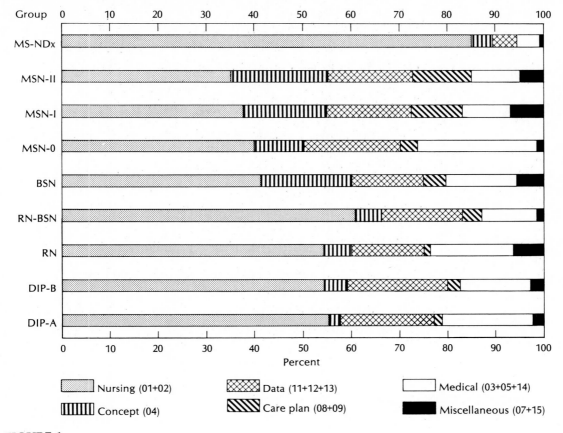

Legend:
- Nursing (01+02)
- Data (11+12+13)
- Medical (03+05+14)
- Concept (04)
- Care plan (08+09)
- Miscellaneous (07+15)

FIGURE 1

TABLE 2   Types of hypotheses: observed and expected frequencies, all groups

Group	n	01	02	Nursing	Concept	Data	Care plan	Medical	Miscellaneous
DIP-A	27	*177.6*	*86.2*	*263.8*	*36.9*	*72.9*	*17.0*	*60.1*	*15.9*
		164	91	255	10	88	6	87	12
DIP-B	43	*282.7*	*137.3*	*420.1*	*58.7*	*116.1*	*27.1*	*95.7*	*25.3*
		311	117	428	25	174	20	118	19
RN	23	*151.3*	*73.4*	*224.7*	*31.4*	*62.1*	*14.5*	*51.2*	*13.5*
		165	69	218	24	66	7	70	29
RN-BSN	24	*157.8*	*76.6*	*234.5*	*32.8*	*64.8*	*15.1*	*53.4*	*14.1*
		148	70	218	18	59	14	43	3
BSN	34	*223.6*	*108.6*	*332.2*	*46.5*	*91.8*	*21.4*	*75.7*	*20.0*
		159	86	245	103	89	26	91	32
MSN-0	6	*39.5*	*19.2*	*58.6*	*8.2*	*16.2*	*3.8*	*13.4*	*3.5*
		29	16	45	12	22	4	29	2
MSN-1	21	*138.1*	*67.1*	*205.2*	*28.7*	*56.7*	*13.2*	*46.8*	*12.4*
		103	35	138	60	65	42	35	25
MSN-2	14	*92.1*	*44.7*	*136.8*	*19.1*	*37.8*	*8.8*	*31.2*	*8.2*
		67	30	97	55	47	33	29	12
MS-NDX	52	*335.4*	*162.9*	*498.2*	*69.7*	*137.7*	*32.1*	*113.5*	*30.0*
		452	262	714	25	46	1	39	9
	243	1598	776	2374	332	656	153	541	143

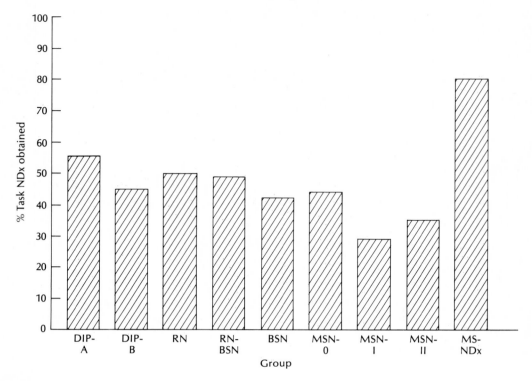

FIGURE 2

The number of task nursing diagnoses that were offered by each group is illustrated in Fig. 2. The numbers are reported as a percentage of the total number possible, that is, one per subject per task. Omitting the MS-NDX group from the calculation, the differences in frequencies of obtained task nursing diagnoses is not significant $(\chi^2_7 = 16.07, p > 0.01)$.

Cues

The total number of cues used was 12,209. Of those, the following could be said of them:

4 were used for 36.3% of the hypotheses
3 were used for 31.6% of the hypotheses
2 were used for 20.9% of the hypotheses
1 was used for 11.1% of the hypotheses

The range between groups of the average number of cues used per subject over six tasks was 44.0 to 58.4%.

When the hypothesis was the task nursing diagnosis, 90.4% of the cues used were NDX cues.

When the hypothesis was a nursing diagnosis other than the task one,

59.7% of the cues chosen were NDX
16.2% of the cues chosen were MDX
18.3% of the cues chosen were PX and REGIMEN
When the hypothesis was a medical diagnosis,
52.2% of the cues chosen were PX and REGIMEN
17.0% of the cues chosen were MDX
30.0% of the cues chosen were NDX
In all cases demographic cues were relatively insignificant.

Directions

Ninety-seven subjects generated medical diagnoses when no special directions were given, compared to 77 subjects who received special directions. This difference is significant ($\chi^2_1 = 7.87$, p<0.01).

DISCUSSION

The quantity of hypotheses generated by the groups is of little importance compared to the quality. The numbers cannot be related to previous findings from "think aloud" protocols: those hypotheses were a product of short-term memory whereas the subjects in this study had the benefit of paper and pencil and time to reflect. The numbers may have varied in relation to education and, therefore, knowledge had the task not been designed to present little difficulty to any RN.

With the exception of the MS-NDX group, the types of hypotheses did not vary as one might expect. The percentage of nursing diagnoses offered tended to decrease with increasing levels of education. The code 04 (Concept) was used for statements such as "nutrition," "emotional problems," or other general statements which could be interpreted as consideration of an area of interest to nursing, albeit nonspecific. Expert clinicians tend to generate specific hypotheses. In this study the reverse was demonstrated: the percentage of Concept category increased with level of education or experience. Whether the eventual diagnosis would be specific is an interesting question for further study.

If NDX and Concept are considered desirable hypotheses, then in all groups they exceeded 50%. Although these figures compared unfavorably with the MS-NDX figure of 88.6%, they exceeded the findings of Silver and associates (1982), where 28% of problems on problem oriented records were nursing diagnoses.

The other types of hypotheses are in need of attention by nursing educators. The Data category included statements that repeated information given in the task or other signs or symptoms suggesting minimal information processing by the subject. The notion that a sign or a symptom meant exactly that, the sign or symptom of a problem, was missing. The Care Plan category incorporated statements which indicated that subjects could not distinguish between a patient problem and the interventions or goals planned to alleviate the problem. Stating Medical problems suggested that those subjects who did so could not differentiate between medical and nursing practice. All subjects were asked to state problems that they as nurses treat. Half the subjects received directions which reinforced the original by a request to ignore problems that they would refer to a physician. Despite the significant difference these directions made, 77 of 121 subjects suggested medical problems when asked to ignore them.

With the exception of the MS-NDX group, the number of hypotheses stating the task NDX was not significantly different between groups. Four cues were clustered to suggest these diagnoses. That 90% of the cues used for the task NDX were NDX cues confirmed their validity. The task NDX with the highest percentage of subjects suggesting it was Potential skin integrity impairment, with 80.9% (that is, the task illustrated in Box 1). Excluding the percentages obtained by the MX-NDX group, the remaining task scores were

Knowledge deficit	49.3%
Impaired communication	44.6%
Self-care deficit	39.1%
Alteration in nutrition	34.5%
Sleep pattern disturbance	15.9%

Given that Knowledge deficit was not included in the list of most commonly used diagnoses in the Jones and Jakob study, it is interesting that the percentage of subjects suggesting it was relatively high. Indeed, it was suggested by 100% of the MS-NDX group.

Turning now to the cues, we see that nurses, like physicians, do suggest patient problems on the basis of few cues. Thirty percent of the total number of hypotheses were prompted by only one or two cues. Nursing educators may find it a rewarding exercise to ask students what this information suggests to them, give three or four pieces of information, and analyze their responses. Clarification of their hypotheses may help students become better diagnosticians.

When a nursing diagnosis other than the task 1 was offered, 60% of the chosen cues were NDX, with MDX assuming importance. However, when a medical diagnosis was suggested, the NDX cues were ignored in favor of PX and REGIMEN cues. This finding suggests that, if the objective of nurse educators is to have students make nursing diagnoses, then they must assess the type of information that students consider relevant.

Further research is needed to confirm the relationship between the initial hypotheses generated on the basis of a small amount of information and the final set of nursing diagnoses made following unlimited information. It would also be worthwhile to describe the extent to which hypotheses direct the questions nurses ask and the observations they make.

REFERENCES

Aspinall, M.J.: Use of a decision tree to improve accuracy of diagnosis, Nurs. Res. **28**:182-185, 1979.

Bordage, G.: The psychology of clinical reasoning. Paper presented at the Kellogg Centre for Advanced Studies in Primary Care, Montreal, October 1982.

Elstein, A.S., Shulman, L.S., and Sprafka, S.A.: Medical problem solving. An analysis of clinical reasoning, Boston, 1978, Harvard University Press.

Fatzer, C.: The relationship between logical reasoning and nursing diagnosis, Monograph (Fall 1979) Nursing diagnosis, Denton, Tex., College of Nursing.

Feltovich, P.J.: Knowledge based components of expertise in medical diagnosis. Pittsburgh, 1982, University of Pittsburgh Learning Research and Development Center.

Gordon, M.: Predictive strategies in diagnostic tasks, Nurs. Res. **29**:39-45, 1980.

Gordon, M.: Manual of nursing diagnosis, New York, 1982, McGraw-Hill Book Co.

Gordon, M.: Nursing diagnosis: process and application, New York, 1982, McGraw-Hill Book Co.

Hammond, K.: Clinical inference in nursing, Nurs. Res. **15**:27-38, 1966.

Jones, P.E., and Jakob, D.F.: The definition of nursing diagnoses: Phase 3 and final report, Toronto, 1982, University of Toronto Faculty of Nursing.

Kassirer, J.P., and Gorry, G.A.: Clinical problem solving: a behavioral analysis, Ann. Intern. Med. **89**:245-255, 1978.

Lesgold, A.M., Feltovich, P.J., Glaser, R., and Wang, Y.: The acquisition of perceptual diagnostic skill in radiology, Pittsburgh, 1981, University of Pittsburgh Learning Research and Development Center.

Neufeld, V.R., Norman, G.R., Feightner, J.W., and Barrows, H.S.: Clinical problem-solving by medical students: a cross-sectional and longitudinal analysis, Med. Educ. **15**:315-322, 1981.

Silver, S.M., Halfmann, T.M., McShane, R.E., Hunt, C.A., and Nowak, C.A.: The identification of clinically recorded nursing diagnoses and indicators. In Kim, M.J., McFarland, G., and McLane, A., editors: Classification of nursing diagnoses—Proceedings of the Fifth National Conference, St. Louis, 1984, The C.V. Mosby Co.

Simon, H.A., and Chase, W.G.: Skill in chess, Am. Sci. **61**:394-403, 1973.

Tanner, C.: Instruction on the diagnostic process: an experimental study. In Kim, M.J., and Moritz, D.J., editors: Classification of nursing diagnoses—Proceedings of the Third and Fourth National Conferences, New York, 1982, McGraw-Hill Book Co.

Tanner, C., Putzier, D., Westfall, U.B., and Padrick, K.: Diagnosis—more than just a label. Paper presented at the Third Northwest Regional Conference on Nursing Diagnosis, Portland, October 1983.

Outcome criteria generation: a process and product

UNA E. (BETH) WESTFALL, M.S.N., R.N.

I would like to ask you to put yourselves into this picture. You are assigned to care for a group of patients. One of the patients with whom you will be working this shift is a 62-year-old man on the eighth day of his continuous hepatic arterial chemotherapy infusion. The catheter is threaded through his femoral artery. To minimize the risk of displacing the catheter, he has been on bedrest with his leg restrained since the catheter was inserted. He has 2 more days of infusion before the treatment is complete. You are also working with his roommate, who had the left lower lobe of his lung removed yesterday. He is attached to a commercial, three-bottle, closed chest drainage setup and is reluctantly looking forward to his first walk after surgery.

Both patients have been diagnosed by their primary nurses as having "impaired physical mobility." You shape your plans of care for the shift to address this diagnosis. But how will you know if you are successful? What will the patients look like, or act like, if good nursing care is given? Do any of the following statements assist in answering these questions? "Will be ambulating without assistance"; "skin will remain intact"; "will have good muscle tone with isometrics"; "prevent pulmonary complications." Each of these statements is an outcome criterion for the nursing diagnosis of impaired physical mobility that was found during the chart review portion of a recent clinical practice project. The project had as its purpose to develop example screening outcome criteria for selected nursing diagnoses that are in use.

Today I would like to tell you about this project: first, by highlighting the importance of nurse-developed outcome criteria; second, by describing the process that was used; and third, by providing some specific examples of the screening criteria that were generated.

Major efforts in the nursing community are currently directed toward changes in the health status of a person receiving nursing care, because nursing is all, or part, of that care. Our professional challenge is to seek out and validate those differences that nursing makes to the well-being of the consumer.

The use of diagnostic labels by nurses to describe those areas that are significant to nursing is, I believe, a giant step into the world of professional nursing practice. Our pioneering efforts have been documented in the nursing literature, with the most detailed accounting found in the reports of these National Conferences, the first of which was held in 1973. (Gebbie and Lavin, 1975; Gebbie, 1976; Gordon, 1982; Kim and Moritz, 1982). One of the most exciting trends evident when reviewing the short history of nursing diagnoses is the placement of this crucial labeling activity within the larger perspectives of nursing practice and quality assurance.

There are three major approaches to evaluating nursing care. These are (1) evaluations of resources (structure), (2) activities by the clinician (process), and (3) impact or the health status of clients following nursing actions (outcome).

The least well developed, but often most understandable, perspective is that of outcome-focused statements. Outcome criteria for selected target populations provide an important way to look at the effectiveness of health care, as these criteria ask only whether actions taken were successful. Because nursing is a large part of that care, it is appropriate and responsible for nurses to generate and use outcome criteria when planning, delivering, and evaluating nursing care.

Few guides or examples exist to assist nurses in the development of clear, precise, measurable outcome criteria that reflect the intent of good nursing care. It was this challenge that stimulated my clinical practice project. It has as its focus generating example screening outcome criteria for target populations. The task of selecting target populations that enable us as nurses to examine care from our unique perspective is met, at least in part, through the use of nursing diagnostic labels (Gordon, 1980).

Shortly after joining the faculty at a western university school of nursing, clinical nurses within the institution started using accepted diagnostic labels from the National Conference Group (Kim and Moritz, 1982) and the problem-oriented charting format for documentation of care. Each nursing diagnosis recorded was to have specific outcome criteria included in the care plan as well as current nursing orders. Thus nursing diagnostic labels accepted at the Fourth National Conference on Classification of Nursing Diagnoses were being used by the clinicians and became the target populations for this clinical project.

I used the definition of criteria by Donabedian (1981). He states that criteria are " . . . set(s) of discrete, clearly definable, and precisely measurable phenomena . . . that in some specifiable way are relevant to the definition of quality." In other words, criteria are statements that are measurable and reflect an agreed upon level of excellence.

The project was designed to take full advantage of the work to date by both nurses within the institution and other nurse groups that have struggled to develop and refine pertinent nursing-influenced outcome criteria. It was anticipated that the time-consuming work by individual clinicians to derive these criteria from scratch could be reduced.

The steps used in generating the example outcome criteria are as follows:
- Select records
- Complete forms
- Evaluate OC (outcome criteria) for each diagnosis
- Refine OC
- Examine refined OC
- Ratify OC

The plan was based on prior work by the VNA of Omaha nursing staff (1980). The process began with charting of clinical nurses found in the problem-oriented care plan. The first step was to select patient records to be reviewed for nursing diagnoses and their accompanying outcome criteria. The names of patients admitted and discharged from the unit that had been using the problem-oriented record (POR) format for at least 6 months were collected for a 2-month period. Records were requested for every tenth patient.

A demographic information form and a form for recording the nursing diagnoses and developed expected outcome criteria were completed for the first 16 patient records obtained. Ten of the patients were male. Eleven of the 16 were married. The patients ranged in age from 17 to 77, with half the patients 60 years of age or older. Fourteen of the 16 patients had more than one active medical diagnosis. The body systems most frequently involved were the cardiovascular and gastrointestinal. Ten of the patients had a definite diagnosis of cancer. Fifteen of the 16 patients reported either recent, or multiple previous, hospitalizations.

These 16 patients had 26 admissions in which the POR format was used by nurses. The 26 hospitalizations provided the project data (see Box 1).

BOX 1　　**Sample data**

n = 16 (records which contained 26 admissions)
Age range: 17 to 77 yr (50% were 60 and over)
Major systems involved
　　Cardiovascular
　　Gastrointestinal
Major medical diagnosis: cancer (62%)

Examination of the data took many forms. Initially the number and variety of nursing diagnoses present were screened. The intent of this activity was to decide if further data gathering would likely result in new information. The conclusion was that pulling of additional records would probably not add substantially to the diagnoses already obtained. An analysis was also done to determine if the etiology of the problem influenced the outcome criteria statements. With this sample of 16 patients over 26 hospitalizations, the etiology of the problem did not alter the outcome criteria, although it did, as expected, influence the nursing actions.

Nurses recorded 16 different diagnostic labels. There were a total of 55 diagnoses with accompanying outcome criteria. An additional 27 diagnoses were labeled as temporary problems. They were almost all written as signs or symptoms (such as temperature spike, vomiting, or nausea) and did not have outcome criteria. They were not included in the sample.

TABLE 1   **Distribution of nursing diagnoses by frequency**

Nursing diagnostic label	Frequency
Alteration in comfort	15
Knowledge deficit	6
Ineffective airway clearance	5
Alterations in nutrition	5
Impairment of skin integrity	3
Alterations in coping	3
Disturbance in thought processes	3
Impaired mobility	3
Alterations in cardiac output	2
Sensory input disturbances	2
Sleep deprivation	2
Disturbance in self-concept	2
Impaired gas exchange	1
Constipation	1
Alterations in communication	1
Self-care deficit	1
TOTAL	55

Of the 16 different diagnostic labels, *Alteration in comfort: pain* occurred most often—15 times. *Knowledge deficit* occurred next in frequency—6 times. Four diagnoses occurred 3 times, 2 times, and once respectively (see Table 1).

Dossey and Tucker (1981) presented a categorization for accepted diagnoses that had six general headings. This classification system was used both in examining the data and later in the project. Using these headings, recorded labels appeared in five of the six categories. The highest percentages were in the areas of physiological (64%), activity (60%), and orientation (100%). These all have a strong physical emphasis. Considerably fewer problems were identified that related to emotional status and psychosocial concerns. Forty-six percent of the approved diagnoses were found in the chart review. These data from the 16 labels were the foundation for the remainder of the project (see Table 2).

The outcome criteria that had been developed for each nursing diagnosis were then examined. A total of 133 criteria accompanied the 55 diagnoses. Almost all these criteria focused on the health status of the client. There was evidence of repetition in some outcome criteria when the statements were grouped under the 16 diagnostic labels. The total number of outcome criteria for the diagnoses ranged from 43 to 1. Of the 43 found with the *Alteration in comfort: pain* label, only 15 different behaviors were identified. The next most

TABLE 2   **Frequency and percentage score for used nursing diagnoses by category**

Diagnostic category	Total possible	Percentage score
Physiological	11	0.64
Activity	5	0.60
Orientation	3	1.00
Emotional status	2	0
Psychosocial	10	0.20
Health maintenance	3	0.33
TOTAL	35	0.46

commonly used diagnosis—*Knowledge deficit*—had a total of 13 criteria identified. Each of these was a different behavior. As you can see from Table 3, 11 of the 16 labels (or 69%) show no duplication of patient behaviors in the outcome criteria present.

The outcome criteria were also clustered according to the six general categories mentioned earlier (see Table 4). All but four of the duplicative criteria

TABLE 3   **Distribution of nursing diagnoses by number of outcome criteria present**

Nursing diagnostic label	Outcome criteria	
	Total	Different
Alteration in comfort	43	15
Knowledge deficit	13	13
Ineffective airway clearance	13	7
Alterations in nutrition	10	10
Impairment of skin integrity	6	6
Alterations in coping	6	6
Disturbance in thought processes	7	6
Impaired mobility	8	7
Alterations in cardiac output	6	6
Sensory input disturbances	5	3
Sleep deprivation	5	5
Disturbance in self-concept	4	4
Impaired gas exchange	3	3
Constipation	2	2
Alterations in communication	1	1
Self-care deficit	1	1
TOTAL	133	95

TABLE 4   Distribution of outcome criteria by diagnostic category

	Outcome criteria	
Diagnostic category	Total	Different
Physiological	83	49
Activity	14	13
Orientation	13	10
Emotional status	0	0
Psychosocial	10	10
Health maintenance	13	13
TOTAL	133	95

were found in the physiological area. Possible explanations for this finding may be that (1) there is more agreement among staff regarding behaviors expected with physiological problems, or (2) there is increased difficulty in achieving precision with criteria that are not physiological in nature, or (3) there is lack of clarity with some labels when more than one specific diagnosis may be included within a single label.

After the outcome criteria from the chart review were clustered by diagnostic label, the statements were examined individually and as part of the cluster. Each statement was examined to validate an outcome focus. The characteristics of well-written criteria were then used to screen the individual statements. Was the statement accurate, clear, measurable, singular in focus, pertinent to the diagnostic label, and important to or significant for nursing? Because the intent of the project was to develop screening criteria, the characteristic "possible to achieve" was less important at this time. It would be necessary for the staff nurses to consider this aspect when selecting criteria for given clients. This critique of phrases concluded the evaluation of the outcome criteria statements from the chart review.

These empirical data and analyses provided direction for the next step—refining the outcome criteria phrases. Source of nurse-generated outcome criteria were limited at the time of this project. Four useful resources I found were the following:

Guidelines for Review of Nursing Care at the Local Level (ANA, 1976)

Manual for Instrument of Health Status Measures, Vol. 2 of *Development of Criterion Measures of Nursing Care* (Horn and Swain, 1978)

Final Report: Field Testing of a Problem Classification Scheme and Development and Field Testing of Expected Outcome-Criterion Measure Schemes with a Methodology for Use (VNA of Omaha, 1980)

Manual: Nursing Quality Assurance (Zimmer, 1976)

These resources were used to compare and modify the empirical criteria and to generate example screening criteria for diagnostic labels not found in the chart review. These activities concentrated primarily on making the statements more measurable and precise. Outcome criteria were drafted for each of the labels, with the exception of those related to family coping. The differences among these labels were unclear, and none of these labels had been used by the clinicians. Further clarification about these labels would be sought before proceeding to work with them.

The questions that were asked earlier to critique the criteria were also used as guides for refining and deriving criterion statements. Every effort was made to have the criteria reflect positive patient states and to have only one behavior per criterion.

After refining the criterion statements, staff nurse participation was essential in the form of critiquing the refined criteria. This activity should move fairly quickly, if the criteria are clear, because such criteria appear deceptively simple.

Staff nurses from the pilot unit and a second unit were asked to respond to the criteria for each diagnostic label. This was a lot to ask. The nurses were to consider the same set of questions identified earlier for criterion statements. (Box 2 contains the instructions attached to the materials.) The nursing diagnoses and accompanying example screening criteria were grouped into the six general categories mentioned earlier. The labels were clustered in this way to make the revised criteria more manageable for staff to review and comment on. At the end of a 2-week period, completed forms were collected. All comments from clinicians were carefully considered and revisions and deletions were made.

The actual ratification of the criteria occurs by the clinicians as the criteria are used and further refined. As with all criteria, these must be viewed as "pencil and eraser" endeavors subject to revisions and adaptations that con-

---

BOX 2   **Outcome criteria for review**

Please look at the outcome criteria, considering
1. Clarity
2. Accuracy
3. Significance or importance for nursing
4. Measurability
5. Pertinence to diagnostic label
When looking at the group of criteria under each label, please consider
1. Aspects that are missing (add thoughts in space after each grouping)
2. Preferred statement, if duplication

---

tribute to their accuracy and usability as nursing's knowledge base grows in content and focus.

This process could be used as the labels in the current list are expanded or modified and become more precise.

Having described the process used, I would like to now present the results of this process for three different labels: (1) Alterations in nutrition: less than body requirements; (2) Alterations in thought processes; and (3) Impaired physical mobility (Boxes 3 to 5). The outcome criteria from the chart review are listed on the left and the refined example screening criteria from the project are listed on the right.

The label *Alterations in nutrition* was used by nurses exclusively for "less than body requirements." The 10 outcome criteria phrases from the chart review provide examples of ways to make important areas measurable, such as body weight or the percentage of meats eaten. Other statements identify areas that are important but, as stated, are less clearly defined. The screening criteria attempted to include not only the objective measures of body weight

---

BOX 3　　**Diagnostic label:** *Nutrition, alterations in (less than body requirement)*

Outcome criterion statements

Chart review	*Sample screening*
Will eat at least 50% of each meal	Ingests food without pain or discomfort
Weight will stabilize at 10 pound gain by discharge	Reports improved appetite
Resolution of nausea and vomiting	Expresses satisfaction with meals
Improvement in energy level in order to perform ADLs with minimal assistance	Demonstrates improving (improved) calorie-balanced intake
Will demonstrate use of jejunostomy tube	OVERWEIGHT
Will maintain or increase admission weight	Loses weight to specific goal (may include time frame)
Will take in adequate amounts of protein to facilitate healing	Ingests _____ calories/day
Able to tolerate soft food with minimal discomfort	May specify calories/day
Will regain 5 pounds of lost weight before discharge	UNDERWEIGHT
Will express satisfaction with meals at least once a day	Gains weight to specific goal
	Ingests _____ calories/day
	May specify calories/day

BOX 4   **Diagnostic label:** *Thought processes, alterations in*

Outcome criterion statements

Chart review	*Sample screening*
Will remain oriented ×3	Demonstrates orientation to time, place, and person
Alert	Recalls accurately
Appropriate affect and statements	Demonstrates increased concentration on task and conversation(s)
Neurological signs within normal limits	Stays on topic of conversation or interaction
Steady on feet	Avoids distractions and interruptions
Laboratory values within normal limits	Gives responses that indicate attention to other's statements or questions, or both
	Reports coping with confusion
	Emotions appropriate to situation

---

and calorie counts, but also subjective attributes such as appetite and satisfaction with food.

For the label *Alterations in thought processes* the importance of orientation is carried through in the example screening criteria. Other behaviors that would indicate attention span and attention to the environment have been included in the screening criteria.

The final label, *Impaired physical mobility,* provides interesting perspectives on the use of this label in clinical practice. The outcome criteria from the chart review reflected different interpretations of the label. The largest number of criteria addressed hazards of immobility—"skin will remain intact" and "free from rales." In these situations the label was being used to describe the etiology of an integumentary or pulmonary problem. It was also this perspective that was used in the first clinical example at the beginning of this paper—the man on his eighth day of forced bedrest.

A second group of criteria addressed, indirectly, maintenance of current musculoskeletal status with reference to "muscle tone." A single criterion reflected desired ambulatory status following temporary immobility. (This phrase relates directly to the second clinical example at the start of this presentation, the man who was 1 day postoperative.) Because of the multiple ways that this label had been used, guidelines were written rather than a cluster of screening outcome criterion statements. These guidelines identify three major areas for which the label may be used—problems with temporary or long-term

BOX 5   **Diagnostic label:** *Mobility, impaired physical*

Outcome criterion statements

Chart review

Will be ambulating without assistance

Skin will remain intact

Will do ROM exercises to other extremities (other than leg with femoral arterial catheter)

Will have good muscle tone with isometrics

Avoid constipation by having bowel movement at least once a day

Prevent pulmonary complications—be free of rales and have good breath sounds

Edema will be absent in patient's legs

Sample screening—guidelines

Outcome criteria: may be written to describe different aspects of this broad category; outcomes may be classified under the following headings

TEMPORARY IMMOBILITY

Outcome criterion: Ambulates without assistance (may specify distance(s) and frequency)

LONG-TERM OR PERMANENT IMMOBILITY

Outcome criteria: May be written to reflect such concerns as
1. Preventing further immobility (may specify body areas)
2. Improving what mobility is present (may specify body areas)

HAZARDS OF IMMOBILITY

Outcome criteria: Refer to the appropriate physiologic label for sample criteria, e.g., skin integrity, impaired gas exchange

When developed using this focus, caution should be used to determine if impaired mobility is the problem or a cause for problems such as skin breakdown or atelectasis

---

immobility, or hazards of immobility. Clinical usefulness may be the critical determinant in how to consistently apply this label.

SUMMARY

The steps of the process used in this project have provided insights about the interpretation and use of selected diagnoses in the clinical setting. Review of the outcome statements from the chart has made it clear that some diagnostic labels do not mean the same thing to all nurses using them. Physiologically based labels are much more frequently used than those describing psychosocial concerns. Labels for these areas reflect many personal, or sensitive, perspectives. As an aside, when observing the nursing care administered to clients by nurses on the pilot unit project, such areas as self-concept alterations, fear, and anticipatory grief, are handled sensitively by the nurses. However, these diagnoses have not been made explicit in the nursing care plan. Several factors that may influence inclusion of these more sensitive diagnoses in a plan may include (1) difficulty in articulating measurable outcome criteria for selected diagnoses, (2) lack of research-based nursing interventions to use with given nursing diagnoses, (3) ambiguity in interpreting some nursing diagnostic labels, (4) cultural values of patients and families, (5) placement of nursing care plans and records in patient rooms, and (6) lack of precision about nursing's domain and its full impact on patient care.

REFERENCES

American Nurses' Association: Guidelines for review of nursing care at the local level, Kansas City, Mo., 1976, The Association.

Donabedian, A.: Criteria, norms, and standards of quality: what do they mean? Am. J. Public Health **71:**409-12, 1981.

Dossey, B., and Tucker, D.: The use of nursing diagnoses in a critical setting, Nurs. Diagn. Newsletter **8:**2-7, 1981.

Gebbie, K., and Lavin, M., editors: Classification of nursing diagnoses—proceedings of the First National Conference, St. Louis, 1975, The C.V. Mosby Co.

Gebbie, K.: Classification of nursing diagnoses—summary of the Second National Conference, St. Louis, 1976, National Group for Classification of Nursing Diagnoses.

Gordon, M.: Determining study topics, Nurs. Res. **29:**83-87, 1980.

Gordon, M.: Nursing diagnosis: process and application, New York, 1982, McGraw-Hill Book Co.

Horn, B., and Swain, M.: Manual for instrument of health status measures. Vol. 2, Development of criterion measures of nursing care (NTIS no. PB 267005), Springfield, Va., 1978, National Technical Information Service.

Kim, M., and Moritz, D., editors: Classification of nursing diagnoses—Proceedings of the Third and Fourth National Conferences, New York, 1982, McGraw-Hill Book Co.

Visiting Nurse Association of Omaha: A classification scheme for client problems in community health nursing. Nurse planning information series no. 14, (DHHS Pub. no. HRA 80-16), Hyattsville Md., 1980a, Division of Nursing.

Visiting Nurse Association of Omaha: Field testing of a problem classification scheme and development and field testing of expected outcome-criterion measure schemes with a methodology for use. Final report, Springfield, Va., 1980b, National Technical Information Service, Division of Nursing, (Contract no. 231-77-0068.)

Zimmer, M.: Manual: nursing quality assurance, Madison, Wisc., 1976, University Hospital and Clinics.

CHAPTER 9

Implementation

Symposium on implementation of nursing diagnosis: *overview*

MI JA KIM, Ph.D., R.N., F.A.A.N.

This symposium presents the problems and successes of implementing nursing diagnoses in the clinical setting and educational arena from three different perspectives: (1) head nurse and hospital administrator, (2) clinical specialist, and (3) educators in undergraduate and graduate programs. Factors which facilitate implementation of nursing diagnoses in the hospital setting are discussed by an administrator who is in charge of clinical specialists. Common concerns expressed by staff nurses in using nursing diagnoses are discussed, with pragmatic solutions that would enable the hospital to continue to use these diagnoses. A clinical specialist discusses her role as an expert clinician and teacher in implementing nursing diagnoses in the hospital setting and emphasizes the importance of having a collegial relationship with staff nurses for successful integration of nursing diagnoses into daily practice. Additionally, an educator shares insights gained from working with both undergraduate students and staff nurses to implement nursing diagnoses. The discrepancy and possible incompatibility between academic teaching and actual clinical practice are elucidated from the vantage point of a faculty with joint appointment in both a college of nursing and a hospital. Major difficulties encountered in incorporating nursing diagnoses in curricula are also shared, with some suggestions by faculty members of undergraduate and graduate programs.

The viewpoints expressed in this symposium are intended to facilitate the implementation of nursing diagnoses in academic and clinical settings.

Implementing nursing diagnosis: administrative/staff nurse perspectives

JOAN McMAHON DUSLAK, M.S.N., R.N.
LUNA COLLADO, B.S.N., R.N.

This paper describes from an administrative and staff development perspective the process followed in the past 6 months in one university-affiliated VA medical center to implement nursing diagnosis in the intensive care units. Issues to be addressed include the nursing climate in which the effort is occurring, resources which support it, observations on the process and outcomes to date, and future plans and issues for consideration by the nursing community. The intent is to describe the gradual approach chosen to introduce this change and relate some of the practical considerations involved in making the decision to proceed in this manner.

THE NURSING CLIMATE
Service level

The question of promoting nursing diagnosis among our nurses through workshops, policies, etc. had been discussed in the 2 years preceding the start of our current project, but no commitment had been made. It was the belief of the nursing leadership that other maintenance needs of the service such as staffing were of higher priority and that some prior developmental work organizationally and with staff was necessary before we would be ready to initiate nursing diagnosis. We were aware too of the relative infancy of the concept, the lack of sufficient research in some categories, and the controversies surrounding the issue.

In the 2-year period before our effort was initiated, several phenomena occurred which contributed to staff professional growth. Subsequently there was a desire awakened in the staff to devote time and energy to efforts to increase accountability and to advance the quality of professional nursing in our Medical Center.

1. The team-oriented management philosophy of the chief nurse brought more staff participation to policy decisions affecting clinical nursing practice.
2. Preparation for a JCAH visit focused staff's attention on professional nursing practice and quality-assurance issues.
3. Financial incentive to seek professional certification enhanced the growth of professional values.
4. Standards of nursing practice were developed for the service by a group of nurses representing each unit. Utilization of ANA Standard II in our own standards reinforced the concept of nursing diagnosis to the staff.

5. Relative staff stability allowed head nurses to develop their clinical and managerial skills and to engage themselves and their staffs in educational and other professional activities to promote staff growth.
6. Clinical and teaching skills of relatively new clinical nurse specialists were refined. These people were already knowledgeable about nursing diagnosis and had solidified their role (and their credibility) as clinical resources to staff and head nurses.
7. Nursing process review in the form of a workshop with a follow-up clinical component was conducted for all RN staff to address deficiencies noted on monthly audits. We introduced the term *nursing diagnosis* at this workshop and distributed the list of diagnoses approved at the 1982 National Conference, but no attempt was made to teach the total concept at this time.

All of these phenomena contributed to the development of the degree of readiness in our staff that was necessary before we could consider it wise to support such a change.

Unit level

The request for assistance to provide RN continuing education in use of nursing diagnosis came initially from the head nurse and staff of the medical and coronary intensive care unit (MICU). That unit has known relative staff stability for 2 years and has a strong team spirit, which is supported by the midlevel nursing manager.

Characteristics of the MICU include visible *esprit de corps* among the nursing staff and comfortable interdisciplinary professional relationships, strong administrative and peer support for learning, and administrative support to test out new ideas. The head nurse also values documentation and uses it as a valid criterion in evaluation of individual staff nurse performance.

The staff in the MICU had a variety of exposures to nursing diagnosis before developing the confidence to consider adopting it as the professional model in their unit. Most exposures were directly unit based—such as feedback from the head nurse and two staff nurses who attended the 1983 Nursing Diagnosis in Critical Care conference in Milwaukee, development of a nursing diagnosis manual by one of the staff who attended the conference, role modeling by the head nurse in the development of a care plan using nursing diagnosis, and a unit journal club where articles on the topic were included for discussion.

RESOURCES TO SUPPORT THE EFFORT
Administrative supports

The decision to implement nursing diagnosis was made by the unit staff, and the role of the upper level administrative staff became that of facilitators. From the standpoint of introducing change we were in an excellent position, with the desire to change having originated in the involved staff. As facilitators several policy decisions were made and included the following:

Scope of the project. The options were to limit to MICU, extend to the other two special care units, or extend to all the units. The decision was to extend to the other special care units if they wished to be included. There were differences between MICU and the other two units in climate and levels of readiness, but there were factors, such as clinical specialists with direct unit responsibilities, present in the other units which added strength and seemed to enhance the potential for success. The head nurses of the SICU and respiratory care unit indicated their desire to be included by making a commitment to follow through with implementation activities after an initial workshop.

Level of expectation for performance. Nurses were given the latitude to develop skills at their own pace under the guidance of the head nurses, who would monitor performance, coach, and call in resource persons as needed. It was recognized that some nurses would require more time than others to become proficient. Because it was felt important to avoid administrative pressure while encouraging peer support and collegial relationships, no policy was written to require use. Guidelines for the use of nursing diagnosis will be developed in the future.

Administrative support for learning. This support was demonstrated in a variety of ways. We received funding by our Regional Medical Education Center to bring experts in for a workshop. Attendance at the workshop was strongly encouraged by the Chief Nurse, who also attended. Enthusiastic head nurses worked absolute magic with scheduling and sparked a zest in their staff to be part of this activity. Many staff nurses agreed to work their full tour plus attend the all-day workshop while others came on days off without expectation of repayment in time or money.

Other supports

Peer support for learning. Peer support has been highly visible and has greatly strengthened this project. Staff nurses, particularly in MICU, where the momentum has had a longer time to build, are involved in a variety of individual and group activities where nursing diagnosis is either the focal point or an integral part of the content. An "article of the week" discussion program reinforces the concept, as does the reference manual developed by a staff nurse. Unit coleaders on each tour, who are CCRNs, also act as resources for clinical follow-up.

Support in workshop development. Assistance to develop a workshop, formal teaching, and group leadership at the workshop and ongoing clinical follow-up was provided by nursing instructors and clinical specialists.

OBSERVATIONS OF THE PROCESS AND OUTCOMES TO DATE

During the past 6 months we have experienced some problems as well as seen positive outcomes.

Nursing process issues

Data base. Our experience supports the need cited by Bruce (1979) and Guzzetta and Dossey (1983) for a comprehensive nursing data base. Ours was deficient when we implemented our program. We found that, without an organized framework, nurses tended to resort to a quasi–systems review to gather data. Usually only one nursing diagnosis was made from a group of unrelated symptoms and observations, leaving many other areas of potential nursing diagnosis unexplored. Although, in retrospective analysis, the diagnosis made was usually an appropriate one, it was often made without sufficient data to support it. In effect the right diagnosis was made for the wrong reasons. As a result an improved data base assessment form was developed by our Standards of Nursing Practice Committee. A limited pilot test of this form has demonstrated that there are still problems, however, with organized collection of data subsequent to the initial data base. We have found that a majority of nurses still have some degree of difficulty with the assessment process, despite its having been reviewed in our nursing process and nursing diagnosis workshops. The nursing diagnosis, with its defining characteristics, should prove helpful to provide a more organized framework for ongoing collection of data throughout the period of hospitalization, but staff will need to be taught to use the defining characteristics in this manner.

Nursing care plans. Hospital-based staff nurses have traditionally been reluctant to fully utilize the nursing care plan as a tool in accomplishing the daily work of patient care. However, if nursing diagnosis is to be more than an exercise, the diagnosis must be written along with outcomes and interventions planned, and periodic notes in the patient record must describe the patient's progress toward resolution. Although some progress has been made in incorporating use of the care plan into daily work routines, there is still much to be done. A comprehensive care plan that will become a part of the patient's permanent record at discharge is presently being pilot tested. Daily charting on the patient's progress note will reflect the nursing diagnosis, interventions, outcomes, and rationale for alterations in the nursing plan as well as the data reflecting nursing activity in carrying out aspects of the medical treatment plan. Regular audits by the staff and head nurses who comprise the evaluation arm of the Standards of Nursing Practice committee will provide quantitative and qualitative data to help us evaluate our patient care as well as our developing skill in use of these concepts. Summaries of audit findings will be reported in such a way that each unit can see its compliance level in relation to others.

Clinical follow-up. Our experience tells us that a mechanism for follow-up and coaching in the clinical setting is critical after an educational program such as nursing diagnosis. We sometimes overlook the follow-up aspect in staff development activities, forgetting that students in the basic nursing programs have many more opportunities to reinforce what they have learned through examinations, clinical conferences, additional courses, etc. Nurses, as adult learners, need reinforcement also, but it is best given as part of their work, and in ways that do not threaten self-esteem or appear to threaten job security. Strong head nurses and staff nurses providing administrative and peer support are essential but may not be enough, especially given the time contraints they function under in most hospital settings. Other devices such as discussion at change of shift report, weekly case presentations by staff nurses, or care plan/charting clinics may help by setting up conditions where all staff nurses will have an opportunity to present actual case data to an audience of peers and clinical resource persons—in essence, a clinical consultation program.

Some of the approaches suggested call for building what has traditionally been considered "educational activity" into the daily work routine. To accomplish it, administrative support is essential. Most will interpret that as support from the top, and that is essential, but we believe the most critical support must come at the level of the head nurse, since it is that individual who is responsible for the day-to-day planning and scheduling of the work activities and who can best interpret to the nursing director the needs for staffing based on overall unit needs which include programs such as these.

Repeated use of some diagnostic categories. Analysis of the diagnoses most commonly used reveals a tendency to select the same few repeatedly, related to the patient's physiological problem. Several factors may contribute to this: the fact that much of the work in critical care units focuses on primary physiological and safety needs; the traditional orientation toward medical diagnosis persists despite the fact that a nursing diagnosis has been listed; difficulty with the assessment process; the tendency of many nurses, especially critical care nurses, to be less comfortable with the psychosocial aspects of nursing; and the fact that some nurses feel the present diagnostic categories do not adequately meet their patients' diagnostic needs. We believe all to be true in our setting. We plan to address this problem in a variety of ways. Initially our resource staff will work more closely with unit staff to facilitate better use of the currently approved list of diagnoses. We also plan clinical case conferences and possibly an intermediate level nursing diagnosis workshop next year which will focus on psychosocial aspects of nursing. We will provide time and consultation support to a staff member who will be willing to conduct research in this area and will make it known to the community of nurse researchers that our facilities are available to support research activity if our staff can be involved in the research process.

Peer support. Peer support for learning and peer role modeling have been extremely important. Several staff nurses are more skilled than others in use of the concept and are open in sharing and coaching. Staff may independently seek out these nurses or the head nurses may refer them. Nurses, particularly in the MICU, attend many outside educational programs together, often at their own time and expense. Nurses have readily changed their work schedules to accommodate a colleague who wishes to attend an educational program. The fact that this kind of collegial interchange occurs has been most important.

Constructive competitiveness. The interunit competitiveness we have observed has been constructive. Head nurses of other units have requested similar assistance to introduce the concept on their units, and some have begun informal initiatives in this direction. Staff on the project units who are less skilled in the concept do not seem threatened by those who are more expert. The use of administrative support rather than pressure has allowed the staff to develop skill at their own pace.

Computer. The computerized patient data monitoring system has proven to be an excellent tool to facilitate clinical teaching and follow-up. Nurses enter progress notes at the computer terminal, and these notes are displayed visually on the monitor for review and analysis by one or groups of nurses. Printouts are readily available if desired. Memory capabilities allow the total hospitalization to be reviewed. Head nurses are finding this a valuable tool in identifying the nurses who need greater support to carry out the nursing process. Eventually the computer will be programmed with the approved nursing diagnoses and defining characteristics of each.

Staff in non–special care areas. Staff on general units have felt themselves at a disadvantage and unable to be consistent in use of the diagnosis when patients were transferred from special care areas. We did not consider this to be a major problem and, in fact, believe it has contributed to creating the demand by the general unit staff for continuing education of the topic. This issue will soon be addressed by offering a basic workshop on Nursing Diagnosis to that staff. Additional ongoing reinforcement will be provided by including some content related to nursing diagnosis in each edition of the quarterly *Nursing Education Newsletter* published by our instructors.

The staff in the non–special care areas will also require direct reinforcement in the clinical area, but several work team characteristics will make it more difficult to provide. Variances in value placed on professional nursing issues are more observable on those units than in special care areas; priority assigned to care planning and documentation is also lower.

Medical versus nursing diagnosis. The controversy in the national movement regarding the place in the care plan for medical diagnosis and orders has surfaced in our setting as well. Our resource staff are encouraging nurses to limit their diagnoses to problems nurses can diagnosis and treat, and to integrate nursing and medical interventions into the plan of care. We do not foresee changing those guidelines in the future without consensus from the national group. Meanwhile those of us in practice settings are responsible for finding creative ways to assist staff long accustomed to organizing daily work around a medical diagnosis to make the transition to organizing their thoughts and efforts around nursing diagnosis. The development of nursing standard care plans using nursing diagnosis might be one way to encourage this transition. It would be exciting if these standard plans could be jointly developed by cooperating service and educational agencies, so staff and the students affiliating for clinical experiences could use the same tools and see the patient in the same way. Students would be faced with less dissonance as they went from classroom to clinical site, and staff would see more relevance in the professional nursing concepts being taught to students.

CONCLUSIONS

Our findings after 6 months of effort reveal both problems yet to be resolved and strengths on which to build. The approach to change that we followed—supporting professional staff in their desire to improve professional skills—has been effective in our setting. Much of the original level of interest and enthusiasm has been sustained on the project units, while head nurses on other units are requesting assistance to begin. Our resource persons are more knowledgeable about the problems, more skilled in guidance of staff. Some staff nurses have emerged as peer role models and will be valuable resources for future efforts. Our activities for the next 6 months will focus on educational activity in the form of a nursing diagnosis workshop with a clinical follow-up component for remaining staff; establishment of nursing diagnoses clinical conferences, initially on the day tour of duty but eventually on all three tours to aid staff in refining skill with the diagnostic process; ongoing monitoring of outcomes of our educational activities, utilizing a tool developed for the purpose as well as data from our standards of practice evaluations; and enlargement of our support team to include the staff nurses who are especially proficient. As we carry out these activities, we can never afford to forget that, to ensure success, the staff must see the relevancy of this concept to their daily work of providing patient care.

ISSUES FOR FUTURE CONSIDERATION

As the nursing diagnosis concept is further researched, developed, and refined, some issues will emerge for consideration by nursing administrators and educators:

1. How will skill with the nursing diagnostic and treatment process be recognized in evaluations of RN performance as contrasted with skill in activities that support and maintain the organization?
2. Will we say at some point that professional nurses must be skilled with

this diagnostic process in order to practice? What parameters will help us decide that question? What about practicing nurses who are not successful in making the transition?

3. Can we say with certainty that a patient cared for using the nursing diagnosis framework will receive better care than one cared for in the traditional way?

4. Is the individual accountability inherent in the use of nursing diagnosis compatible with the team and functional organizational strategies currently used in many inpatient nursing settings?

5. What mechanisms will hospital nursing services need to develop to ensure that patients are not discharged without adequate resolution of nursing diagnosis? How will we know what is adequate resolution, particularly in some of the psychosocial diagnoses in which resolution may occur only after a process of maturation, often involving family or significant others and often extending into the community?

REFERENCES

Bruce, J.A.: Implementation of nursing diagnosis, Nurs. Clin. North Am. **14**:509-515, 1979.
Guzzetta, C.E., and Dossey, B.M.: Nursing diagnosis: framework, process, and problems, Heart Lung **12**:281-291, 1983.

Implementation of nursing diagnosis: the role of the clinical nurse specialist

KATHRYN HUBALIK CZURYLO, M.S., R.N.
ROSEMARIE SUHAYDA, M.S.N., R.N.

The clinical nurse specialist is a highly skilled practitioner of nursing who is responsible for ensuring high-quality care to a select group of patients. Rendering high-quality nursing care has been fostered with the advent of the nursing diagnosis concept. Nursing diagnoses are currently the best vehicle for providing continuity of care between nurses and between care settings (Gordon, 1979). Nursing diagnoses provide a good communication system (Bircher, 1975; Dodge, 1975; Gebbie, 1976; Weber, 1979) and help place the emphasis on the patient's human response to his illness, to his life experience, and to his coping abilities (Bircher, 1975; Dodge, 1975; Komorita, 1963; Rothberg, 1967; Roy, 1976; Shoemaker, 1979; Weber, 1979). This is congruent with the definition of nursing as stated in the social policy statement by the American Nurses' Association: "Nursing is the diagnosis and treatment of human responses to actual or potential health problems" (ANA, 1980). The use of nursing diagnoses also increases accountability (Komorita, 1963; Lash, 1978; Roy, 1976; Weber, 1979). Practitioners are realizing that they must perform the diagnostic process accurately and initiate appropriate action in accordance with the diagnosis (Fortin and Rabinow, 1979). It is clear that if quality patient care is the outcome nursing diagnoses should be included among the responsibilities of every staff nurse. Since clinical nurse specialists work along with staff nurses, we can be instrumental in the implementation of the nursing diagnosis concept. Yet the literature provides little support in identifying how this role can be implemented.

This paper outlines the role of clinical nurse specialists in the implementation of nursing diagnoses in the hospital setting, as defined by four major responsibilities: (1) clinical practice, (2) education, (3) administration, and (4) research (West Side VA Medical Center, 1983).

CLINICAL PRACTICE

One of the responsibilities associated with clinical practice is that of role modeling excellence in nursing practice by providing comprehensive nursing care to a select group of patients. Since this comprehensive care includes patient assessment and problem identification, clinical nurse specialists can use nursing diagnoses during direct patient care to role model. Using the nursing diagnosis labels appropriately in care plan writing and charting in progress notes is one way to foster the use of nursing diagnoses in the clinical setting. The staff can learn about the use of nursing diagnoses from clinical nurse specialists' examples, and also learn the value of the process (Feild, 1979). They must not only be taught about nursing diagnoses but must see its use consistently. Nursing diagnosis implementation can be extended to include use during patient care conferences, nursing grand rounds, and end-of-shift reports. It cannot be emphasized enough that this should be started and continued with the clinical nurse specialists present. We can facilitate the excellent use of nursing diagnoses in clinical practice, as well as assessing further learning needs and either intervening immediately, or making a referral to the staff development department. Because of our availability and ability to troubleshoot, clinical nurse specialists can continue what the educational process starts by working with staff nurses on a day-to-day basis.

Finally, since clinical nurse specialists usually follow patients throughout the many phases of their illness, it can be illustrated to staff nurses how nursing diagnoses change as patients' responses to illness change. Following the various diagnoses made throughout a patient's diagnostic workup, acute care and recovery can help staff nurses realize that priorities change and nursing care changes as well. Excellent use of nursing diagnoses can illustrate that care can become more organized, communication among health care professionals made easier, and nursing can indeed make a significant contribution to patient wellness.

Clinical nurse specialists' major goal is to ensure the quality of patient care; however, they cannot accomplish this goal alone. As clinical nurse specialists role-model the use of nursing diagnoses and staff nurses begin to imitate these behaviors, we begin to see the following: (1) improved quality of documentation, (2) increased use of logic in the diagnostic process, (3) increased quality and quantity of nursing orders, and (4) increased ability to prioritize patient problems. These developments, in turn, are making a direct impact on quality of patient care.

EDUCATION

Although the primary target of educational responsibilities of clinical nurse specialists is the patient, we also have responsibility for the education of staff nurses. Depending on the setting the responsibility for the major educational workshop on the concept of nursing diagnosis may or may not rest with clinical nurse specialists. If it is our responsibility, we can use our skills and make the program focus on information that is practical and relevant to the clinical setting. Background theory is extremely important when a new concept is introduced. However, examples and strategies shared with staff nurses in the beginning can prevent frustration during initial use when proficiency has not yet been developed.

Once the initial training program has been completed, the job of clinical nurse specialists in the implementation process has just begun. Because of varying levels of readiness and different educational backgrounds among staff nurses, clinical nurse specialists must work individually with staff nurses, so that strengths can be fostered and weaknesses eliminated. Basic to the nursing diagnosis concept is a working knowledge of the nursing process. Staff nurses may need a review of the diagnostic process before they can be expected to use nursing diagnoses well. Since clinical nurse specialists are experts at identifying learning needs, we can determine if the diagnostic process needs to be reviewed before introduction of the nursing diagnosis concept.

Clinical nurse specialists also act as resource people once the nursing diagnoses are being used on a day-to-day basis. We should provide assistance, support, and validation in the identification of nursing diagnoses for specific patients (Feild, 1979). Being a resource person depends on availability. Staff nurses should feel they can call upon clinical nurse specialists any time to help them problem solve, not only during inservice times or at the clinical nurse specialist's convenience. This availability should extend to all three shifts.

Since the diagnostic labels along with their etiologies, defining characteristics, and nursing interventions are still evolving, the clinical nurse specialist must establish a climate in which we and the staff nurses can work together and learn together. It is crucial that a collegial relationship be developed between clinical nurse specialists and staff nurses initially. As clinical nurse specialists work with patients, giving direct care, we establish our credibility and become an "insider," not an outsider or intruder. Since we all have one goal in mind, that of giving the best patient care possible, the methods used to reach this goal can be established together.

One of the major challenges facing clinical nurse specialists is that of orienting staff nurses to a concept which has not yet been accepted by the entire nursing community. Unless nurses internalize the value of nursing diagnoses, their commitment to the application of the concept will be limited. Clinical nurse specialists are instrumental in facilitating professional nursing forums where issues and feelings about nursing diagnoses can be discussed.

Clinical nurse specialists may also be asked to educate other health care providers about the concept of nursing diagnoses, including physicians, dietitians, physical therapists, and hospital administrators. As health practitioners who function interdependently it may benefit nurses in some settings to share their method of problem solving and documentation of patient responses.

ADMINISTRATION

Clinical nurse specialists in staff positions lack administrative authority, although we may have responsibility for policies and procedures related to our specialty area and may participate on nursing or hospital committees. Developing interest and fostering healthy competition are ways to involve staff nurses in using nursing diagnoses, but they do not replace administrative support and expectations. The most difficult task for clinical nurse specialists may be to "sell" the concept to a reluctant administration.

When clinical nurse specialists act as consultants, we may introduce nursing diagnosis at that time. For example, there may be the following problems on a particular unit or in the nursing service as a whole: insufficient amount of organized documentation, nursing care plans which are not patient-nurse oriented, or lack of staff nurse accountability. As a problem solver clinical nurse specialists after entry into the consultation process and diagnosis of the problem, can assume several different roles (Blake, 1977). As advocate and change agent we may try to convince the administration that the use of nursing diagnoses can solve the problem and collaborate with them to revise existing practice. Clinical nurse specialists, however, must realize that consultation has a "take-it-or-leave-it" quality. In the instances where the initiation of nursing diagnosis is blocked by administration it is important to determine the reason. There may be organizational problems which the administration needs to solve before the concept is introduced. If the administration remains reluctant, then we can use our expertise to present proof stated in research studies, many of which still need to be done, that the use of nursing diagnosis does improve the quality of patient care.

RESEARCH

Clinical nurse specialists should maintain knowledge of the status of current research studies involving nursing diagnosis. Participation in research studies is expected. Clinical nurse specialists may be involved in studies on the diagnostic process, finding strategies for the staff nurse to improve diagnostic accuracy. We should also participate in studies involving identification and validation of nursing diagnoses in our specialties. As experts with one particular group of patients we are instrumental in the determination of appropriate and clinically relevant nursing diagnoses, etiologies, defining characteristics, and nursing interventions.

Research being done on nursing diagnoses should be disseminated by clinical nurse specialists to staff nurses. Clinical nurse specialists should assist staff to interpret and implement relevant research findings when appropriate. This can be done by the initiation of a journal club or an article of the week program, so that research is a familiar presence. The proceedings of the North American Nursing Diagnosis Association (NANDA) conferences should be shared with the staff, as should the newsletters of NANDA.

While working with staff nurses, clinical nurse specialists must keep an open mind. Many topics leading to possible research studies come from discussions with nurses who use the diagnostic labels on a day-to-day basis. Addition of new nursing diagnoses, appropriateness of the critical defining characteristics, and determination of appropriate nursing interventions are all possible research questions that may be addressed by a group of staff nurses with the guidance of clinical nurse specialists. Participating in a research study and getting actively involved in the research process is increasingly appropriate for staff nurses and must be fostered. In fact, one of the goals of clinical nurse specialists may be to have staff nurses at their institution present their research at a national nursing diagnosis conference.

In addition to research studies on the diagnostic process and the nursing diagnosis nomenclature (Kim, 1981), clinical nurse specialists must do research to ensure that staff nurses are using nursing diagnosis and are using it appropriately. Audit tools should be developed, including checklists to determine that nursing diagnoses are derived from health assessment data and to determine appropriateness of patient outcomes and nursing interventions. Clinical nurse specialists may begin using the audits, but the responsibility may eventually be given to the staff nurses, to establish a peer review environment. This may be an ideal way to foster accountability, and develop staff nurses, thus allowing clinical nurse specialists to move on to other areas requiring our skills.

Finally, it cannot be stressed enough that clinical nurse specialists should become expert diagnosticians and retain that status. The gap between service and education can indeed be bridged by clinical nurse specialists as we bring expertise to the practice setting and make several educational concepts come alive. By role modeling, problem solving, and availability to staff nurses, clinical nurse specialists can be instrumental in helping nurses to successfully implement the nursing diagnosis concept as an aid in the delivery of high-quality patient care.

REFERENCES

American Nurses' Association: Nursing: a social policy statement, Kansas City, Mo., 1980, The Association.

Bircher, A.U.: On the development and classification of diagnoses, Nurs Forum **14:**11-29, 1975.

Blake, P.: The clinical specialist as nurse consultant, J. Nurs. Admin. **7**(10):33-36, 1977.

Dodge, G.H.: Forces influence move toward nursing diagnosis, AORN J **22:**327-328, 1975.

Feild, L.: The implementation of nursing diagnosis in clinical practice, Nurs. Clin. North Am. **4:**497-508, 1979.

Fortin, J.D., and Rabinow, J.: Legal implications of nursing diagnosis, Nurs. Clin. North Am. **14:**553-561, 1979.

Gebbie, K.: Classification of nursing diagnoses—summary of the Second National Conference, St. Louis, 1976, National Group for Classification of Nursing Diagnoses.

Gordon, M.: The concept of nursing diagnosis, Nurs. Clin. North Am. **14:**487-496, 1979.

Kim, M.J.: Issues related to research on the classification of nursing diagnosis. In Kim, M.J., and Moritz, D.A., editors: Classification of nursing diagnoses: Proceedings of the Third and Fourth National Conferences, New York, 1982, McGraw-Hill Book Co.

Komorita, N.I.: Nursing diagnosis, Am. J. Nurs. **63**:83-86, 1963.

Lash, A.A.: A re-examination of nursing diagnosis, Nurs. Forum **17**:332-343, 1978.

Rothberg, J.: Why nursing diagnosis? Am. J. Nurs. **67**:1040-1042, 1967.

Roy, Sr. C.: The impact of nursing diagnosis, Nurs. Digest **4**(3):67-69, 1976.

Shoemaker, J.: How nursing diagnosis helps focus your care, RN **42**(8):56-61, 1979.

VA West Side Medical Center: Position description: cardiovascular clinical specialist. Chicago, 1983.

Weber, S.: Nursing diagnosis in private practice, Nurs. Clin. North Am. **14**:533-539, 1979.

Implementing nursing diagnosis: faculty perspective

ROSEMARIE SUHAYDA, M.S.N., R.N.
MI JA KIM, Ph.D., R.N.

Faculty involved in teaching nursing diagnoses at various levels of both formal and informal courses have found inconsistency and incongruence in the ways nursing diagnoses are introduced and taught. One source of variability lies among faculty themselves. Another comes from differences in understanding of the concept and its use by faculty and practicing nurses at clinical sites. Still another lies within curricular structure. While research studies indicate that faculty are incorporating nursing diagnoses into their educational programs, successful methods of integrating diagnoses throughout the various levels are not clearly identified, nor is the relationship between graduate and undergraduate levels in their organization of nursing diagnoses evident (Gaines and McFarland, 1984; McLane, 1982). Perhaps expecting such a relationship is too premature at this time.

This paper addresses three major factors which impact the implementation of nursing diagnoses in undergraduate and graduate curricula: (1) faculty influences, (2) curricular influences, and (3) the current status of clinical practice. In addition, this paper proposes a conceptual approach which integrates nursing diagnoses throughout the undergraduate and graduate levels. Problems associated with the implementation of nursing diagnoses in the educational and clinical settings from the perspective of a faculty holding a joint appointment will also be discussed.

FACULTY INFLUENCES

One of the major influences impacting implementation of nursing diagnoses within a curriculum is the philosophy of individual faculty. Divergent philosophical views regarding the taxonomy and its conceptual framework or lack of framework in general and the proposed North American Nursing Diagnosis Association (NANDA) list in specific have sparked resistance to accepting the concept. Arguments against the use of nursing diagnoses include that they have not been clinically tested and that introducing them into course content or using them as an organizational theme is premature. Some espouse opinions that students would be wasting their time on short-lived conceptual models and that the NANDA list is too constrictive, locking students into incomplete structures.

Certainly the most advantageous conditions for teaching nursing diagnoses would be a fully developed taxonomy as well as a sound and tested conceptual framework. The taxonomy, however, is not yet established; it is evolving, as is the science of nursing. Discouraging the use of nursing diagnoses until an ideal taxonomy and conceptual framework upon which everyone agrees are developed is asking for something that is next to impossible and intellectually counterproductive, especially since nursing diagnoses are already being introduced into clinical practice. Students need to learn about nursing diagnosis and be sensitized to the issues facing nursing practice. They need to be aware of the theoretical underpinning of a nursing taxonomy in order that they might better respond to their own professional responsibilities.

Faculty's understanding of and familiarity with the concept also influence implementation. Personal experience can attest to the fact that not all faculty within the same clinical course, let alone within the same program, share common interpretations of how the diagnostic label is developed and applied, or how it is incorporated into the structure of a care plan. Some faculty, for example, accept general nondescriptive labels such as Alterations in gastrointestinal function while others accept medical diagnoses as either problem or etiology. Still others accept multiple problem and etiological combinations within the same statement.

Such labels obliterate the unique focus of nursing and give little direction to students in their internalization of professional nursing values. Students progress through their courses trying to meet the expectations of different faculty members while unlearning and relearning yet other new specifications imposed by the clinical setting. Hence, nursing diagnoses and care plans tend to become educational tools and academic exercises that have little actual relevance to practice.

Faculty, too, must be educated in the development and use of nursing diagnoses in order that greater consistency may exist within a curriculum. Faculty forums, workshops, and curricular review sessions may offer opportunities for faculty to discuss issues and curricular strategies as well as to develop their skills.

Also crucial is faculty's skill in teaching clinical reasoning. The premise that nursing is the identification of those patient health problems which nurses diagnose and treat includes the assumption that diagnostic competence is of major importance to the practice of nursing. Nevertheless, studies have shown that both students and practicing nurses are neither comfortable nor competent in execution of this activity (Aspinall, 1976; Feild, 1979; Matthews and Gaul, 1979). DeBack (1981) reported that senior nursing students did not demonstrate competency in the formulation of nursing diagnoses on nursing care plans. Tanner (1982), in her study of the cognitive processes used in diagnostic problem solving, found that students had difficulty deriving possible nursing diagnoses if the correct diagnosis was not one of those originally hypothesized. Mallick (1983) contends that the difficulties with nursing diagnosis are due to the way in which the concept is being taught. Whereas medical students and practicing physicians spend much of their time learning and perfecting the art of diagnosing, nursing students focus on too many diverse roles such as caregiver, teacher, and patient advocate. The role of diagnostician in nursing tends to become secondary.

Socialization of the student into the role of diagnostician is a function of both the teaching strategies and the curricular model. Brenner (1984) suggests that teaching strategies differ between the novice and the expert diagnostician. Whereas the novice requires concrete information with specific rules to guide actions, the experienced diagnostician operationalizes diagnoses intuitively, with the major difficulty in analyzing and narrowing the search field to identify the clusters of homogeneous signs and symptoms.

Teaching diagnostic reasoning based on hypothesis-driven iterative methods may facilitate diagnostic competency in both the novice and the expert. The iterative method is a guided tour through the diagnostic process: identifying a problem, establishing a hypothesis to explain the problem, accumulating pertinent data to refine the hypothesis, becoming satisfied that the hypothesis explains all the findings, and using the hypothesis in a predictive mode (Kassirer, 1983).

Kassirer (1983) describes the process as it applies to one clinical faculty and eight or nine students. The student who is to present the case serves as the data repository and is the only one who has information regarding the client. Other students ask questions to produce data. Any student asking a question must identify the projected diagnostic hypothesis, the purpose of the question, expected outcome, and whether or not the question can be expected to evoke information with diagnostic impact. After data are obtained, the questioner is asked to interpret the information and to explain how it influences earlier diagnostic hypotheses. Did it change the working diagnosis? Refine it? Did the piece of data suggest some immediate need to take action? Did it make some previously unexplained finding understandable? In the iterative method the serial questioning, justification, and interpretation continue until all relevant data have been identified, until all of the diagnostic management issues have been discussed, or until time runs out. With the instructor's guidance the group participants assess the validity of a questioner's hypothesis, discuss the reasons for seeking particular information, or consider the appropriateness of identifying more cues. Throughout the process the hypotheses are eliminated or confirmed; those that remain are made progressively more specific. Student learning occurs as the information is being processed and the nursing diagnosis confirmed.

CURRICULAR INFLUENCES

In developing a curricular model which supports development of diagnostic competency as well as the integration of nursing diagnoses, one must give consideration to both the requisite cognates and the curricular schema.

Particularly important is the early introduction of cognates which foster logic and mathematical reasoning. Cognates in computer science which require students to develop and test algorithms in high-level educational languages such as PASCAL expose students to data organization and mathematical logic as well as develop computer literacy. Introductory nursing courses would include core content on the nursing process with clinical simulations which incorporated branching logic and decision trees. Aspinall (1979) suggests that the use of decision trees may be a valid strategy in teaching novices the skills of nursing diagnoses.

Organizational schemata for integrating and threading nursing diagnoses throughout the various horizontal and vertical curricular levels may vary. Diagnoses may serve to structure courses or may be incorporated within an established conceptual schema.

Consider a schema utilized in teaching medical-surgical nursing content which embodies aspects of general systems theory. Within this schema man is viewed as a complex of dynamically interacting systems, each having the capacity for self-regulation to maintain orderly balance within and between systems. Individual units of content might focus on specific regulatory imbalances. Nursing diagnoses could be introduced when discussing responses to the imbalanced states. For example, consider *Respiratory Dysfunction* as a unit of study. Nursing diagnoses reflecting the imbalance states might include *Gas exchange* related to *ineffective breathing patterns, ineffective airway clearance,* or *alveolar capillary membrane changes.* Nursing focus would include identifying critical assessment parameters and developing decision strategies which prevented the imbalance or supported return to a balanced state.

Selected nursing diagnoses could be introduced into the curriculum according to increasing levels of complexity and abstraction. At Level I, for example, the focus might be on elementary concepts and concrete tasks. Discussion might center on univariate assessment parameters and simple branching logic. In Level II, nursing diagnoses involving multivariate assessment parameters and more complex branching logic and decision strategies could be introduced. Concurrently, some of the diagnoses introduced at Level I could be reintroduced at higher levels of abstraction and complexity in Level II depending on content focus. The graduate program could focus on factor isolation and perhaps factor relating stages of theory development by which validity, reliability, sensitivity, and relevance of nursing diagnoses could be studied, and interrelations among nursing diagnoses could be depicted (Dickoff and associates, 1968). This would enhance clinical testing of a particular set of nursing interventions on the basis of nursing diagnoses. Findings obtained in graduate study would serve to refocus and refine the content at the undergraduate level.

CLINICAL SETTING INFLUENCES AND JOINT APPOINTMENT

While the educational foundation helps students formulate their own philosophy of nursing, a crucial adjunct for the internalization of professional values is the philosophy of nursing at clinical agencies in which students' practicum occurs. And yet, quite frequently affiliating agencies do not embrace the philosophy of the educational institution. Students caught in between the expectations of faculty and the clinical agency attempt to comprehend what should be done versus what is done. Many students quickly learn the artificiality of care plans for patient care when working in agencies which do not support or value such activities. Some become disillusioned about the values promoted throughout their education. The gap between education and practice is not contrived; it is real. Furthermore, personal experience indicates that it is not narrowing as rapidly as we would expect. The reality shock of educators returning to the clinical arena is that of seeing new graduates practice nursing at levels inconsistent with that promoted throughout their educational experience. The reality of practice can either promote or undermine educational goals and ideals, and nurture or break the spirit of the novice practitioner.

Faculty must assume responsibility and accountability for not only developing students and promoting quality educational programs but also developing experienced practitioners and promoting high-quality patient care. Joint appointment models of faculty practice are an alternative for facing this challenge.

However, assuming joint appointment roles is not without problems or challenges. Problems are more serious when faculty practice in agencies which do not support nursing judgments and decisions.

One of these problems involves *stabilizing practice* which has an ill-defined level of entry. Educational preparation of staff nurses varies; yet patient responsibilities are basically the same. Sensitivities often emerge surrounding the issue of who is given responsibility to make nursing diagnoses and develop patient care plans. Since the distinction in practice is not clear, all must be given the skills to satisfy this expectation. Programs set up to meet the various educational needs should include specific content on techniques of patient assessment, the diagnostic process and problem identification, development of patient care plans including writing the diagnostic statement and developing expected outcomes, theoretical background required or development of decision strategies, documentation formats, and patient teaching techniques. Additional programs could include establishing nursing forums for discussion of nursing issues and trends in the literature and research.

Another challenge facing faculty entering practice is that of *promoting a patient care model* which supports high-level quality care. Frequently this involves all of the intricacies, skills, and energy required of change theory. Crucial is the establishment of support and an influential power base, since ascribed power may not be an inherent component of the role. Furthermore, not all administrators support or recognize the need for change. In order for change to be effective, the ownership of the process and the outcomes must belong to the participating nurses. The faculty role is that of engineering the change.

A third important challenge facing faculty in joint appointment roles is that of *establishing clinical credibility*. Role modeling through direct patient care, collaboration with staff, and contributing to the care plan are critical if the faculty are to provide any impetus for change. Working at the bedside with staff nurses offers insights into the realities and issues facing nursing practice as well as an opportunity for teaching and problem identification. Additionally, faculty can be instrumental in identifying and developing capable preceptors who later can become involved in helping students learn bedside skills. Such preceptors, in turn, can free faculty to promote cognitive competencies of both staff nurses and students through iterative methods.

While frustrations coexist with satisfactions in bringing academic ideals to a seemingly different world in the practice setting, the joint appointment model can be an effective mechanism for closing, not merely bridging, the gap between education and practice. Faculty in this joint role can help make the world of practice a nursing laboratory in which students and practitioners pursue their inquiries and test hypotheses and interventions to bring the best possible nursing care to patients. At the same time faculty in this role will bring the actual clinical perspective of nursing to other faculty so that research questions and our conceptual base are sensitized by the reality of today's practice. In this manner faculty's attempt to build tomorrow's nursing science can be firmly grounded in the real world.

In conclusion, faculty play a pivotal role in implementing nursing diagnoses in curricula development and in the clinical setting. Fostering students' internalization of professional values and philosophy of nursing via the concept of nursing diagnosis throughout undergraduate and graduate programs and serving as a role model in the clinical setting as a faculty with joint appointment are some of the ways to achieve successful implementation of nursing diagnoses in academia and in practice.

REFERENCES

Aspinall, M.J.: Nursing diagnosis: the weak link, Nurs. Outlook **24**(3):433-347, 1976.

Aspinall, M.J.: Use of decision tree to improve accuracy of diagnosis, Nurs. Res. **28**(3):182-185, 1979.

Brenner, P.: Characteristics of novice and expert performance: implications for teaching the experienced nurse. Researching second step nursing education. Rohnert Park, Calif., 1981, Sonoma State University.

DeBack, V.: The relationship between senior nursing students' ability to formulate nursing diagnoses and the curriculum model, Adv. Nurs. Sci. **3**(3):51-66, 1981.

Dickoff, J., James, P., and Wiedenbach, E.: Theory in a practice discipline. I. Practice oriented theory, Nurs. Res. **17**(5):415-435, 1968.

Feild, L.: The implementation of nursing diagnosis in clinical practice, Nurs. Clin. North Am. **14**(3):553-561, 1979.

Gaines, B., and McFarland, M.: Nursing diagnosis: its relationship to and use in nursing education, Top. Clin. Nurs. **5**(4):39-49, 1984.

Kassirer, J.P.: Teaching clinical medicine by iterative hypothesis testing, N. Engl. J. Med. **309**:921-923, 1983.

Kassirer, J.P., and Gorry, G.A.: Clinical problem solving: a behavioral analysis, Ann. Intern. Med. **89**:244-55, 1978.

Mallick, J.: Nursing diagnosis and the novice student, Nurs. Health **8**:455, 1983.

Matthews, C., and Gaul, A.: Nursing diagnosis from the perspective of concept attainment and critical thinking, Adv. Nurs. Sci. **2**(1):17-26, 1979.

McLane, A.: Nursing diagnosis in baccalaureate and graduate education. In Kim, M.J., and Moritz, D.A., editors: Classification of nursing diagnoses—Proceedings of the Third and Fourth National Conferences, New York, 1982, McGraw-Hill Book Co.

Tanner, C.: Instruction on the diagnostic process: an experimental study. In Kim, M.J., and Moritz, D.A., editors: Classification of nursing diagnoses—Proceedings of the Third and Fourth National Conferences, New York, 1982, McGraw-Hill Book Co.

CHAPTER 10

Utilization

Computerized nursing care planning utilizing nursing diagnosis

JOAN M. CROSLEY, M.S., R.N.

Impetus for this project came from the advent of computerized information systems. These systems have the potential for the provision, documentation, review, and development of high-quality nursing care through the storage of vast amounts of care-planning information. There is a need to create and accept an organized method of naming and coding patients' responses which nurses treat. Computers, with their potential for managing information, "have something to offer nursing, beleaguered with problems of documentation, quality control, cost containment, and the explosion of knowledge related to patient care" (Zielstorff, 1980).

The crucial element in any nursing information system is the description of the patient. Two methods currently available to describe patients are patient classification systems and nursing diagnoses. Patient classifications address the amount and mix of nursing staffing. Nursing diagnoses not only have the potential for indicating the mix and the amount of staffing resources needed but also base the need for these resources on the type of nursing interventions prescribed. Nursing diagnoses provide for the measurement of patient outcomes achieved through the use of these resources. It should be recognized that the purpose of a patient classification system is the collection of information in order to predict staffing levels, while the emphasis of nursing diagnoses is to provide guidelines for care planning rather than care-giving allocation. Although beginning studies in consensual validation are currently taking place, it must be noted also that nursing diagnostic nomenclature has not been thoroughly tested for consensus. Not all diagnoses have been labeled (Guzzetta, 1979; Kim, 1982; Kritek, 1979). Computerization offers the promise of aiding the consensus process through the storage of large amounts of data needed for reliability and validity testing. The Patient Care System (PCS), the information system used in our institution, is a comprehensive online hospital information system as well as a set of tools which may be used to tailor information and develop new applications (Patient Care System application development system, 1983).

In an effort to build a theoretical base for this project, the review of the literature focused on concept attainment, nursing diagnoses and computerized information systems. The literature review of the cognitive theory of concept attainment indicates that categorization is an active, decision-making process. Human subjects selectively attend to environmental cues, choose hypotheses to test, and arrive at a judgment about the correct concept (Bruner, 1956, 1962; Gordon, 1973, 1979; Kramer, 1970; Norris, 1970, 1982; Piaget, 1951, 1963, 1973).

According to Battista (1978) knowledge exists in relationships rather than in the objective world or in subjective experience. Our knowledge of the relationship comes from our interaction with it. The system is a process and we are part of that process. Concepts of uncertainty, organization, probability, and entropy are utilized. Battista defines information, in information theory, in terms of a relationship between an input and a receiving device. Processes for generating information are described by both the analytic and holographic model.

Analytical models separate the whole into its parts in order to determine the nature, proportion, function, and relationship of each part. The analytical model bears some semblance to the mechanistic energy-drive models utilized in Newtonian physics. However, according to Battista, the analytical model is actually holistic. A holistic model considers the entire universe to be interconnected and hierarchically organized (Bohm, 1976). The analytic model utilizes concepts of information: uncertainty, organization, probability, and entropy, rather than: energy-drive, force, mass, and determination (Battista, 1982). Holographic models attempt to maintain the whole. The holographic model (Pribram, 1976) stresses the interdependent, parallel, and simultaneous processing of information. Nevertheless, the theory of holograms lies in information theory which is needed to explain and predict "what is happening." Both holographic and analytical models are needed to explain "how" something is occurring. The conceptual framework for the development of the computerization of nursing care planning utilizing nursing diagnosis is based on the belief that the analytical and holographic models are complementary rather than competitive. Examination of the basic assumptions which underlie both leads one to conclude that information system theory is a theoretical structure capable of integrating analytical and holographic models. In information theory our knowledge of the system comes from our interaction with it. This system is a process and we are part of the process.

The search of the literature on nursing diagnosis reveals qualitative and quantitative work reported by the National Conferences for the Classification of Nursing Diagnoses, a method of inquiry which has been both inductive and deductive, a model which reflects what nursing has known intuitively (that man is holistic), and a framework which is consistent with modern scientific theories and with the author's own value systems (Carpenito, 1983; Gebbie, 1976; Gebbie and Lavin, 1975; Gordon, 1982; Kim and Moritz, 1982; Kim and associates, 1984).

Computerized information systems support communication as well as the synthesis and development of patient data through all phases of hospitalization. Its application in nursing is designed to improve the efficiency with which clerical tasks are completed, to present data in formats which facilitate clinical decision making, and to provide the means for planning, documenting, and evaluating patient care (Edmunds, 1984). Computerized information systems sustain the concept of holism. They allow the nurse-user to utilize bits of information, synthesize these pieces into an organized whole, and reflect the process in a nursing care plan founded on nursing diagnoses.

THE PROJECT: Phase I

This project's task included the introduction of a computerized information system to the nursing staff of a tertiary care hospital and the introduction of computerized nursing care planning utilizing nursing diagnosis.

The computerization of nursing care planning utilizing nursing diagnosis is based on the premise that cueing influences the phenomena to which nurses attend. For the purposes of this project the terms nursing diagnosis, cueing, and computerized information system have been defined as follows:

> *Nursing diagnosis* is a statement that describes an actual or potential altered interaction pattern of an individual, family, or community to life processes (physiological, psychological, sociocultural, developmental, and spiritual).
> *Cueing* is the signal to begin a specific vein of thought.
> *Computerized information system* is the IBM patient care system.

The Patient Care System (PCS) is a software package developed at Duke University and announced by IBM in early 1978. It is an automated information system designed to assist in the management of the complex information processing needs of hospital organizations. It can be modified, with user involvement, to meet the information requirements of a particular hospital (Patient Care System, application development system, 1983). Participants in the development process are nurses and other health care personnel within the organization, who know *what* work must be done, and data processing personnel, who know *how* to accomplish the job. Although some typing is required to use the system, most work can be facilitated by the use of a light pen to select items from a list on the cathode ray tube (CRT) screen. Confidentiality of data is maintained by a combination of individual security codes and limited access. IBM's nursing care plan (NCP) package is a separate application module.

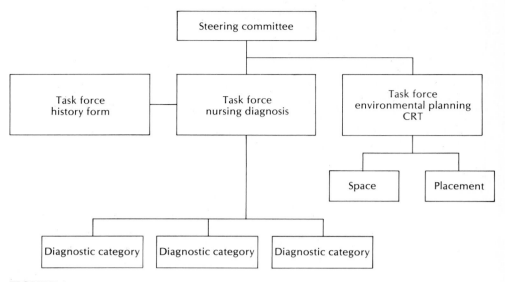

FIGURE 1

The content was recreated to reflect our beliefs regarding the notion of nursing diagnoses.

THE PROJECT: Phase II

In the creative process of diagnosing and treating human responses, the nurse utilizes perception, memory, analog, and regrouping. For this reason the design of the computerized nursing care plans utilizing nursing diagnosis had to overcome the constraints of the linear, tree-branching model utilized in currently available computer software. In the NCP many small pieces act almost independently and interact without determination. It was projected that the nursing care plan would be realistic and flexible rather than ideological and programmatic.

To facilitate the implementation of this project the director of nursing organized a steering committee. Its membership comprised representatives from nursing administration, nursing research, the nursing care coordinator council, and nursing education. The focus of this committee was twofold: the logistics of placing the hardware on existing patient care units, and the revision and implementation of the system in nursing. Task forces were set up, one for each of these purposes. Each task force then formed small groups involving staff level nurses (see Fig. 1). There was a decided effort to build from the bottom up, which is consistent with the trend to reverse centralization. In a small way it demonstrates the validity of Naisbitt's analysis of megatrends.

The remainder of this paper will address the work of the task force which

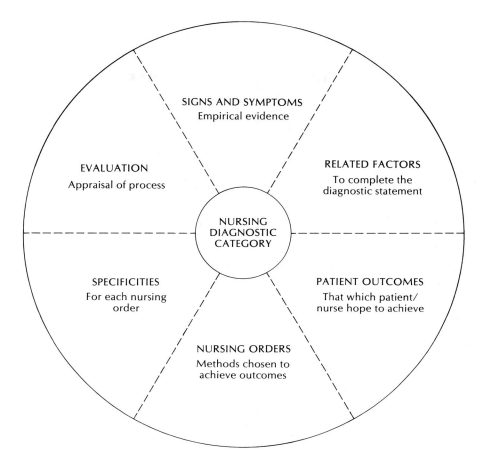

FIGURE 2

was responsible for the design and implementation of the computerized nursing care planning utilizing nursing diagnosis.

The IBM software was recreated. Seven sets of screens were designed and developed: Nursing Diagnostic Categories, Signs and Symptoms, Related Factors, Expected Patient Outcomes, Nursing Orders (based on outcomes), Specificities for each Nursing Order, and Evaluation (see Fig. 2). The content of each set of screens relating to each nursing diagnostic category was developed inductively and from descriptions found in the literature. Concepts of content analysis were utilized in the selection of items for each set of screens. These items serve as cues for the nurse-user, who has the opportunity to select cues and/or type in other indicators. (See Boxes 1 and 2.) The content of each set of screens relating to each of the diagnostic categories was validated by consensus of nurse experts.

BOX 1   **Nursing diagnostic categories**

? Anxiety
? Breathing: ineffective
? Cardiac status, alterations in: decreased
? Comfort, alterations in: pain
? Communication, impaired: verbal
? Coping: ineffective individual
? Elimination, alterations in bowel: constipation
? Elimination, alterations in bowel: diarrhea
? Elimination, alterations in bowel: incontinence
? Fluid volume: excess
? Grieving
? Mobility, impaired physical
? Nutrition, alterations in: less than body requirements
? Parenting
? Parenting, alterations in: actual/potential
? Powerlessness
? Rape trauma syndrome
? Self-care: deficit
? Self-concept, disturbance in: body image
? Self-concept, disturbance in: self-esteem
? Self-concept, disturbance in: role performance
? Self-concept, disturbance in: personal identity
? Sexuality/reproductive, alteration in: actual/potential
? Skin integrity, impairment of: actual
? Sleeping pattern, disturbance
? Thought processes, alteration of
? Trauma, potential for: fall
? Violence, potential for

Policies governing identification and passwords, access, plans for inservicing, and a proposal for staging the advent of computers onto the patient care areas were developed. Strategies for inservicing included creating a 22-minute videotape, "Introduction to the CRT and Computerized Nursing Care Planning," writing a manual on computerized nursing care planning utilizing nursing diagnosis, and 15 to 20-minute hands-on learning situations followed by individual practice. After 2 weeks of on-unit orientation to the CRT and computerized nursing care planning, we went "on line" with a real patient census on two pilot units. The race to keep ahead of software bugs and user errors ensued. The staff nurses achieved competency in the use of NCPs within a short time. (There is no way to avoid the growing pains involved when a technologically complicated computer system is installed in an institution as organizationally complex as a hospital.) Following the advice of Edmunds (1983), during the transition from manual to automated procedures on the pilot

BOX 2   **Screens for a specific nursing diagnostic category**

1. Nursing diagnostic category
   Impaired home maintenance
2. Signs and symptoms
   ? Significant other requests assistance with finances
   ? Significant other requests assistance with personal care
   ? Significant other requests assistance with meal preparation
   ? Significant other requests assistance with lodging
   ? Significant other requests assistance with cleaning
   ? Significant other requests assistance with medication compliance
   ? Significant other requests placement
   ? Patient requests assistance with finances
   ? Patient requests assistance with personal care
   ? Patient requests assistance with meal preparation
   ? Patient requests assistance with lodging
   ? Patient requests assistance with cleaning
   ? Patient requests assistance with medication compliance
   ? Patient requests placement
   ? Inaccessible facilities within home (i.e.; steps, bathroom, stairs)
   ? Inadequate hearing
   ? Inadequate cooking facilities
   ? Inadequate plumbing
   ? Unsanitary living conditions
   ? Lack of electricity
   ? Presence of rodents
   ? Infestation
   ? Need for environmental safety measures (hand rails, grab bars, etc.)
   ? Inability to safely maintain self
   ? Confusion
   ? Exhausted family members
   ? Other _____
3. Related factors
   ? Inadequate support systems
   ? Patient rejects family/community support
   ? Individual/family member disease/injury
   ? Change in roles within family structure
   ? Impaired cognitive/emotional function
   ? Insufficient finances
   ? Knowledge deficit
   ? Other _____
4. Patient outcomes
   ? Placement
   ? Home with home attendant (Medicaid)
   ? Home with home care program (physical therapist, social worker, home health aide)
   ? Home with private help (RN, LPN, attendant, housekeeper)
   ? Home with direct referral
   ? Other _____

BOX 2   **Screens for a specific nursing diagnostic category—cont'd**

5. Nursing orders
   (Placement)
   ? Referral to social worker
   ? Complete DMS-1
   ? Update DMS-1
   ? Other _____
   (Home with home attendant—Medicaid)
   ? Referral to social worker
   ? Complete M 11 Q
   ? Other _____
   (Home with home care program)
   ? Referral to home care coordinator
   ? Complete inter-agency referral (home care form)
   ? Other _____
   (Home with private help)
   ? Give patient/family private agency resource information sheet
   ? Other _____
   (Home with direct referral)
   ? Complete interagency referral (home care form)
   ? Call referral into community nursing agency
   ? Other _____

---

units particular attention was paid to the informal interpersonal communications network that already existed among hospital staff. Problems could thus be addressed immediately and solved with good humor.

In summary, the NCP package is in its early stages of implementation. The process is, by nature, dynamic and ever evolving. The content must be updated periodically. Guidelines (protocols) will be programmed for the nursing management of clinical problems. Data for correlation of medical diagnosis, nursing diagnosis (with the related factors and signs and symptoms), and nursing orders will be collected. They may then be correlated with DRGs.

Computerized nursing care planning utilizing nursing diagnoses has implications for practice, education, administration, and research. It assists in the clarification of the domain of responsibility and accountability of the nurse; identification of a focus for clinical studies (for example, the critical elements of specific nursing diagnoses); identification of a focus for the development of expertise in assessment and nursing diagnoses for researchers, students, and practitioners; and costing out of nursing care within a prospective reimbursement system. The application of computer technology appears to be of great value in improving patient care. However, no hard evidence has been presented to support this thesis. The reliability and validity of information collected by

BOX 3   **NCP printout**

Long Island Jewish-Hillside Medical Center Nursing Care Plan

DATE: 10/05/83

PATIENT: Ross, Betsy   MEDICAL RECORD NO. 999999999930
AGE/SEX: 029/F   STAT-RM-BED: L5NS-506-MED   ATT MED: Aspirin, Bayer

NURSING DIAGNOSIS
    HOME MAINTENANCE: IMPAIRED   001

RELATED SYMPTOMS
    LEFT-SIDED PARALYSIS   001 A
    EXHAUSTED FAMILY MEMBERS   001 A

RELATED FACTORS
    CHANGES IN ROLES WITHIN FAMILY STRUCTURE   001 A

EVALUATION CODING LEGEND
A, OUTCOME MET. PROBLEM RESOLVED. DISCONTINUE CARE PLAN
B, OUTCOME MET. PROBLEM ONGOING. CONTINUE CARE PLAN
C, OUTCOME MET. OTHER PERTINENT OUTCOMES STILL TO BE ACHIEVED
D, OUTCOME MET. ADDITIONAL OUTCOME CRITERIA SELECTED
E, OUTCOME MET, ADDITIONAL OUTCOME FORMULATED. CARE PLAN REVISED
F, OUTCOME NOT MET. CONTINUE CARE PLAN
G, OUTCOME NOT MET. NURSING ORDERS REVISED
H, OUTCOME NOT MET. UNACHIEVABLE. CARE PLAN REVISED

OUTCOMES/NURSING ORDERS/SPECIFICITIES/EVALUATIONS
  HOME WITH HOME ATTENDANT   001 A
    REFER TO SOCIAL WORKER   001 A
      AT PT. CARE ROUNDS, 11:00 AM TODAY   001 A
    COMPLETE M 11 Q   001 A
      TODAY   001 A

  HOME WITH HOME-CARE PROGRAM   001
    REFER TO HOME CARE COORDINATOR   001 A
      AT PT. CARE ROUNDS, 11:00 AM TODAY   001 A
    COMPLETE INTERAGENCY REFERRAL   001 A
      TODAY   001 A
— — — — — — — — — EVALUATIONS — — — — — — — — — —
AUDIT TRAIL:
001   10/04/83   14:19   FINK, RN
002   10/05/83   9:30   MOLLOY, RN

computer-based patient interfaces have been demonstrated, but it has not been demonstrated that providers can make better or less costly decisions because of this information. The project introduces new technology and begins to build the foundation for examining its effects on nursing practice and patient care.

REFERENCES

Aspinall, M.J., and Tanner, C.A.: Decision making for patient care, New York, 1981, Appleton-Century-Crofts.

Battista, J.: The holistic paradigm and general systems theory, Gen. Systems **22**:65-71, 1977.

Battista, J.: The holographic model, holistic paradigm information theory and consciousness, Re-Vision **1**:3-4, 1978.

Birckhead, L.M.: Nursing and the technetronic age, J Nurs Admin. **8**(2):16-19, 1978.

Bohm, S.: Wholeness and the implicate order, London, 1980, Routledge and Kegan Paul.

Bruner, J.S., Goodnow, J.J., and Austin, G.A.: A study of thinking, New York, 1956, John Wiley & Sons, Inc.

Bruner, J.: On knowing—Essays for the left hand, Cambridge, Mass., 1962, Harvard University Press.

Carpenito, L.: Nursing diagnosis, application to clinical practice, Philadelphia, 1983, J.B. Lippincott Co.

Edmunds, L.: Computer-assisted nursing care, Am. J. Nurs. **82**(7):1076-1079, 1982.

Edmunds, L.: Teaching nurses to use computers, Nurse Educ. **7**:32-38, 1982.

Edmunds, L.: A computer assisted quality assurance model, J. Nurs. Admin. **13**(30):36-43, 1983.

Edmunds, L.: Computers in patient care, a complete system, AORN J. **39**(2):176-182, 1984.

Gordon, M.: (1973). Strategies in probabilistic concept attainment. Unpublished doctoral dissertation, Boston College, 1972. University microfilms, Ann Arbor, University of Michigan.

Gordon, M., and Sweeney, N.A.: Methodological problems and issues in identifying and standardizing nursing diagnosis, Adv. Nurs. Sci. **2**:3-15, 1979.

Gebbie, K.M., and Lavin, M.A., editors: Classification of nursing diagnoses—Proceedings of the First National Conference, St. Louis, 1975, The C.V. Mosby Co.

IBM: Patient Cue System application development system, IBM, 1983.

Kiley, M., Halloran, E., Weston, J., and others: Nurs. Manage. **14**(7):26-29, 1983.

Kim, M., MacFarland, G., and McLane, A., editors: Classification of nursing diagnoses—Proceedings of the Fifth National Conference, St. Louis, 1984, The C.V. Mosby Co.

Kim, M.J., and Moritz, D., editors: Classification of nursing diagnoses—Proceedings of the Third and Fourth National Conferences, New York, 1982, McGraw-Hill Book Co.

Kramer, M.: Concept formation. In Batey, N.V., editor: Communicating nursing research. Boulder, Colo., 1970, Western Interstate Commission for Higher Education.

Kritek, P.: Commentary: the development of nursing diagnosis and theory, Adv. Nurs. Sci. **2**(1):73-79, 1979.

Naisbitt, I.: Megatrends for new directions transforming our lives, New York, 1982, Warner Books.

Norris, C.M., editor: Proceedings of nursing theory conference, Kansas City, 1970, University of Kansas, Department of Nursing Education.

Norris, C.: Concept clarification in nursing, Rockville, Md., 1982, Aspen Corp.

Peplau, H.: Automation: will it change nurses, nursing, or both? ANA clinical sessions, New York, 1962, American Nurses' Association.

Piaget, J.: Plays, dreams, and imitation in childhood (translated by R.M. Hougson and C. Gattengo), New York, 1951, W.W. Norton & Co.

Piaget, J.: The child's conception of the world (translated by Joan and Andrew Tomlinson), Totowa, N.J., 1963, Littlefield, Adam & Co.

Piaget, J.: The psychology of intelligence (translated by N. Piercy and D.E. Berlyne, Totowa, N.J., 1973, Littlefield, Adam & Co.

Pribram, K.: Languages of the brain, Englewood Cliffs, N.J., 1971, Prentice-Hall, Inc.

Rees, R.: Understanding computers, J. Nurs. Admin. **8**(2):47, 1978.

Zielstorff, R.: Computers in nursing, Wakefield, Mass., 1980, Nursing Resources, Inc.

Nursing diagnosis for identification of severity of condition and resource use

EDWARD J. HALLORAN, Ph.D., R.N.
MARYLOU KILEY, Ph.D., R.N.
DEBORAH NADZAM, M.S.N., R.N.

The advent of nursing theory constructs, the use of medical diagnosis-related groups (DRGs) as a means to reimburse by case for all hospital resources, including nursing and cost overruns in health care have all created an opportunity and an imperative to make more rapid progress in development of nursing knowledge, practice, and management. Information about patients receiving care and nurses giving care is essential if progress is to be accomplished.

Nurses have collected, used, transmitted, stored, and retrieved information for decades. The absence of a means for accumulating, manipulating, and timely retrieval of large amounts of data as well as delayed agreement on a uniform data base have prevented nurses from organizing their extensive data in a systematic way (Kiley and associates, 1983; Study Group on Nursing Information Systems, 1983). The elements to create a valid information system for nursing practice and management are available now—technology (automation) to process the volume of information necessary to allow generalizations about nursing process, and terminology (nursing diagnoses) to standardize the data base.

Nurses need a clinical management control mechanism that is meaningful to nurses, one that enables us to look first at our patients and then at ourselves, and finally to relate how our work articulates with medical patient care systems and economic reality. To achieve the status in a nursing data base comparable to the medical data bases upon which decisions about health care delivery are currently being made, nurses need large samples across different settings. Uniformity in data base is the important factor in developing comparability of data. Nursing diagnoses offer comparability of patient/client descriptions.

The Department of Nursing at University Hospitals of Cleveland is engaged in a study that is twofold in purpose: (1) to develop a valid nursing information system in order to improve clinical management and resource allocation and (2) to enable research on patterns of nursing condition during a hospital stay. Pilot data were obtained March to July, 1983. Nursing diagnoses were used as a theoretically sound, meaningful method available to describe patient demand for nursing care (NANDA, 1982). The nurse/patient summary used in this study offers a means of implementing nursing diagnoses in nurse assessments (Box 1). The system has the potential for serving as a fully integrated nursing management program and a complement to the DRG medical management

BOX 1   **Nurse/patient summary**

Nursing staff assigned:

	RN code no.	Other code no.
Today		
Last night		
Last evening		

Check the items below if present or *must be considered:*

Health perception-management
___ 1. Injury, potential for
___ 2. Noncompliance
Nutritional-metabolic
Fluid/electrolyte imbalance:
___ 3. Excess volume
___ 4. Volume deficit
___ 5. Electrolyte
Nutrition:
___ 6. Excess
___ 7. Potential for excess
___ 8. Depletion
Impaired skin integrity:
___ 9. Surgical wound
___10. Decubitus
___11. Trauma
___12. Burn
___13. Rash or irritation
___14. Oral mucous memb. imprd.
Elimination
Bladder function:
___15. Retention
___16. Frequency
___17. Incontinence
GI motility/function
___18. Constipation
___19. Impaction
___20. Nausea
___21. Vomiting
___22. Diarrhea
___23. Incontinence
___24. Distention
Activity-exercise
___25. Activity intolerance
___26. Airway impaired
___27. Secretions
___28. Tracheostomy
___29. Breathing pattern disturb.
___30. Gas exchange impaired

Blood pressure:
___31. Hypertension
___32. Hypotension
___33. Tissue perfusion (alternation)
___34. Shock
Cardiac status:
___35. Arrhythmia
___36. Decreased cardiac output
___37. Diversional activity defctv.
___38. Health maintenance (altrn.)
___39. Home maintenance mgmt.
Mobility impaired:
___40. Turning
___41. Positioning
___42. ROM
___43. Gait
___44. Traction
___45. Ambulation
___46. Paresis
Self-care deficit:
___47. Feeding
___48. Bathing/hygiene
___49. Toileting
___50. Dressing/grooming
Temperature:
___51. Hyperthermia
___52. Hypothermia
Cognition-perception
Comfort, alteration in:
___53. Pain
___54. Discomfort
___55. Itching
Consciousness level:
___56. Lethargic
___57. Stuporous
___58. Semicomatose
___59. Comatose
___60. Delusions

___61. Hallucinations
Hearing deficit (uncorrected):
___62. Hard of hearing
___63. Deaf
___64. Knowledge deficit
___65. Memory deficit (short term)
___66. Psychosis
Seizures:
___67. History of
___68. Occurred this hospital
Sight (uncorrected):
___69. Reads with difficulty
___70. Blurred vision
___71. Sees shadows only
___72. Blind
___73. Smell deprivation
___74. Touch deprivation
___75. Thought processes (altrn.)
Sleep-rest
___76. Sleep disturbance
Self-perception–self-concept
Anxiety:
___77. Acute
___78. Chronic
___79. Situational
___80. Depression
___81. Disturbance in body image
___82. Disturbance in self-esteem
___83. Fear
___84. Personal identity confusion
___85. Powerlessness
Role relationships
___86. Anger
___87. Family process alteration
___88. Grieving
___89. Parenting, alteration in
___90. Social isolation
___91. Suspiciousness
___92. Verbal communication impaired

BOX 1 Nurse/patient summary—cont'd

___ 93. Language barrier
___ 94. Does not speak
___ 95. Aphasic
___ 96. Cannot speak
___ 97. Violence
Sexuality-reproduction
Sexual dysfunction:
___ 98. Physiological
___ 99. Psychological
Coping-stress tolerance
___100. Coping, family, potential growth
___101. Coping, ineffective: patient
___102. Family, disabling
___103. Family, compromised

Value-belief
___104. Spiritual distress
Additional:
___105. ADL assistive devices
Bleeding:
___106. Internal
___107. External
___108. Oozing from wound
___109. Hemorrhage
___110. Contagion
___111. Susceptible to infection
___112. Cultural considerations
___113. Socioeconomic considerations
___114. Disability, prolonged

___115. Disease, prolonged
___116. Hormonal influences
___117. Instability (physio/psycho)
Medical treatment includes:
___118. Elect. monitors
___119. Dialysis
___120. Hyperalimentation
___121. Respirator
___122. Pregnancy
___123. Reaction to medication, blood, etc.
___124. Substance abuse
___125. Suicidal
___126. Terminal illness
___127. Triple last 24 hours

system. The basic elements are patient and nurse descriptors that have meaning and relevance to the least well-trained or most experienced registered nurse. First, the implications of the system for clinical management are described. Second, some results from this beginning effort to characterize population commonalities by severity of nursing need are summarized.

CLINICAL MANAGEMENT

The basis for sound professional nursing practice has been identified by individual nurse theorists and supported by nursing organizations (American Nurses' Association, 1980; Fitzpatrick, 1982). Nursing practice, however, has been operationally described using either medical terminology or procedures to characterize nursing. Neither the patient's medical condition nor procedures done sufficiently explain the performance of nursing practice (Halloran, 1980; Halloran and Kiley, 1983).

The nursing care a patient receives depends on the person who gives it as well as on the nursing condition of the patient. Resource allocation encompasses aspects of both nurse and patient. The assignment of a nurse to a patient is the basic operational unit regarding the quality and the cost of nursing care.

The patient data base currently consists of 1294 hospital cases. It includes (1) uniform and comparable patient descriptions and (2) a record of the nurse responsible for each patient each shift. Nurses assessed patients daily on four wards using the 127 item nurse/patient summary checklist, in which 84 items represent nursing diagnoses and 43 reflect additional patient circumstances thought to affect need for nursing. The nursing diagnoses are arranged on the list according to Gordon's (1982) patterns. The data base provides an improved

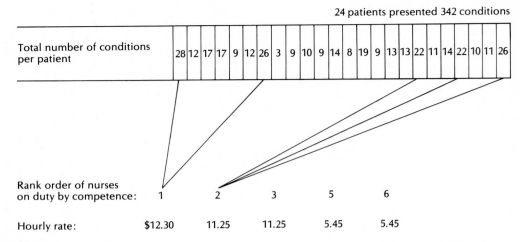

24 patients presented 342 conditions

Total number of conditions per patient: 28 12 17 17 9 12 26 3 9 10 9 14 8 19 9 13 13 22 11 14 22 10 11 26

Rank order of nurses on duty by competence: 1   2   3   5   6

Hourly rate: $12.30   11.25   11.25   5.45   5.45

FIGURE 1

method of explaining what nurses do for patients. The uniform and comparable nurse data include (1) the nurse's educational preparation, experience, skill evaluation by the head nurse,* and hourly rate of pay; and (2) a retrievable record of each nurse's patient assignment over specified time periods. The data base developed using nursing diagnoses helps nurses manage clinical practice at the nurse-patient, ward, and department levels (Halloran and Kiley, 1984).

At the *nurse-patient* level the information system assists the nurse to determine how she/he will allocate her/his own time to assigned patients, thus assisting the nurse to make resource allocations at the bedside.

At the *ward* level the determination of the capability of the nurse to meet a patient's demand in an assignment is made. The optimal decision assigns the most competent nurse to the most complex patient. The nursing information system (NIS) to support the assignment process provides nurse data, patient data, and a report format that allows rapid synthesis of information. Nurse productivity may be monitored with assignment data. No previous attempt to determine the allocation of groups of nurses to groups of patients has used an approach describing patient need in nursing terms and nurse competence. Thus far no valid measure of nurse productivity has been developed (Jelinek and Dennis, 1976).

Retrospectively an ideal evening shift assignment pattern was written for one of the pilot study wards. All nursing conditions present that day were

---

*Knowledge base; depth of work experience; assessment, technical, teaching, psychosocial, and comfort skills.

TABLE 1   Cost algorithm using nurse-patient assignment

Nurse	Hourly rate ($)	Nurse rate per shift ($)	Number of conditions of patients assigned	Patient cost/weight	Distribution of nurse cost* by patient ($)
1	12.30	98.40	28	28/54	51.00
			26	24/54	47.40
2	11.25	90.00	26	26/70	33.50
			22	22/70	28.25
			22	22/70	28.25
3	11.25	90.00	19	19/53	33.00
			17	17/53	28.50
			17	17/53	28.50
4	11.25	90.00	14	14/51	24.70
			13	13/51	22.90
			12	12/51	21.20
			12	12/51	21.20
5	5.45	43.60	12	12/56	9.50
			12	12/56	9.50
			11	11/56	8.60
			11	11/56	8.60
			10	10/56	7.40
6	5.45	43.60	10	19/39	11.20
			9	9/39	10.00
			9	9/39	10.00
			8	8/39	8.90
			3	3/39	3.50

TOTAL COST $455.60

*Assumes that the assignment is based on the degree of patient complexity and nurse competence. Fringe benefit costs are not included.

tabulated for each of the 24 patients. Skill indices were determined for each of the six nurses working. Fig. 1 demonstrates the principle of assigning nurses with higher skill indices to the most complex patients. Nurses ranked 1 and 2 had skill indices of 61.4 and 52.7 respectively. Nurse 1 is assigned to the two most complex patients (number of nursing conditions 28 and 26). Nurse 2 is assigned to the next most complex (number of conditions 22, 22, and 26). Comparing this ideal assignment to the actual assignments revealed that nurse-patient assignments often were not based on nurse competence and patient complexity.

Based on the ideal assignment pattern, a direct cost algorithm for the shift is suggested in Table 1. The algorithm assumes use of a problem identification that the assigned nurse uses to exercise judgment about whether or not to treat before initiating treatment. Complex patients demand a highly skilled nurse and more time. Therefore, in the algorithm, their cost for nursing care is higher than in the case of patients with fewer nursing care needs. Cost reimbursement

TABLE 2   **Rank order of incidence of occurrence of top 20 nursing conditions with corresponding nursing diagnoses (n = 1294)**

Rank	Condition	n	Occurrence per patient	Nursing Diagnosis
1	Discomfort	982	4.6	Alteration in comfort
2	Surgical wound	784	7.2	Impaired skin integrity
3	Pain	782	5.2	Alteration in comfort
4	Knowledge deficit	714	3.6	Knowledge deficit
5	Anxiety, situational	707	3.7	Anxiety
6	Activity intolerance	672	4.7	Activity intolerance
7	Injury, potential for	653	4.7	Injury, potential for
8	Susceptible to infection	643	5.1	Impaired skin integrity
9	Diversional activity deficit	641	4.0	Diversional activity deficit
10	Ambulation, impaired	627	5.4	Mobility, impaired physical
11	Bathing/hygiene deficit	625	6.4	Self-care deficit: bathing
12	Nutrition depletion	523	5.6	Nutrition alteration: less than body requirements
13	Electrolyte imbalance	521	4.9	Fluid volume, alteration in
14	Home maintenance management impaired	509	3.9	Home maintenance management impaired
15	Toileting deficit	504	6.1	Self-care deficit: toileting
16	Health maintenance alteration	478	3.7	Health maintenance, alteration in
17	Dressing/grooming deficit	472	5.8	Self-care deficit: dressing/grooming
18	Disturbance in body image	458	4.1	Disturbance in body image
19	Depression	349	4.9	Self-esteem disturbance
20	Disease, prolonged	319	6.2	

for nursing care by case must consider the nurse provider and the complexity of the patient demand.

The major impact of *departmental* decisions on the ward is allocation of resources in the form of manpower and equipment. Resource allocation and cost control by the department of nursing will be assisted by the data base from the ward that describes patient conditions, nurse competence, and nurse assignments. The case demand differs by patient. The patient demand placed on wards differs and the cumulated patient demand by ward must be determined more differentially than is possible with traditional patient classification systems. All of these clinical decision levels—nurse/patient, ward, department—are assisted by the same data base that contains the patient descriptors, the nurse descriptors, and the nurse assigned to each patient each shift (Halloran and Kiley, 1984).

SUMMARY OF BEGINNING ANALYSIS OF SEVERITY OF NURSING NEED

Initial analysis of patient data was both descriptive and analytical. The mean length of stay was 8.4 days, with a range of 1 to 89 days. The total number

TABLE 3   **Similarities in identification of nursing diagnoses from two series of cases**

	Percent of cases	
Nursing diagnoses	1978 n = 2560	1983 n = 1294
1. Discomfort	83.5	79.9
2. Pain	45.9	60.4
3. Nutrition depletion	35.2	40.3
4. Disturbance in body image	28.9	35.4
5. Sleep disturbance	28.2	20.0
6. Bowel elimination: constipation	26.3	31.4
7. Decreased cardiac output	23.9	9.4
8. Excess nutrition	19.1	11.3
9. Fluid volume deficit	16.7	31.8
10. Excess fluid volume	13.2	24.1
11. Bowel elimination: diarrhea	13.2	21.6
12. Thought process alteration	8.6	12.6
13. Urinary elimination: retention	8.3	21.9
14. Urinary elimination: incontinence	4.6	13.8
15. Bowel elimination: incontinence	3.4	9.7
16. Bowel elimination: impaction	1.3	3.9

$r = 0.909$; significant at $<<0.01$.

of patient days was 10,870; the total number of nursing conditions was 88,047. The mean number of nursing conditions per patient day was 8.1, a figure consistent with those of previous studies (Castles, 1975; Halloran, 1980).

In keeping with the concept of case mix, the rank order of the presence of a nursing condition during a patient/client hospitalization was tabulated. Table 2 shows the incidence of occurrence of the 20 nursing conditions identified most often, and the corresponding nursing diagnoses identified by NANDA (1982). These nursing conditions are reflective of the predominantly surgical patient sample (75%).

The sample of 1294 cases in this investigation is the second series of cases to be described by incidence of nursing diagnoses. In 1978 Halloran obtained data on nurse assessments of 2560 cases in a community general hospital employing the 37 nursing diagnoses that were available. Sixteen of the diagnoses were common to both samples and were found to occur in similar proportions in each sample. The result of a correlation between the proportions of these diagnoses is $r = 0.909$ ($p<<0.01$). The diagnoses are shown in Table 3. The results prognosticate beginning ability to describe nursing needs of patient populations using specific characteristics. Furthermore, the observation of these phenomena in highly correlated proportions indicates development of elements of reliability (efficiency of estimators of population parameters). But many more cases are needed before any conclusions can be drawn.

Although the 1983 sample of patients was predominantly surgical, nurses identified self-care, comfort, and cognitive-emotional needs (n_{tot} = 23,568) almost as frequently as physiological needs (n_{tot} = 26,454). The frequent observation of psychosocial and unprescribed treatment for physiological needs supports that medical diagnoses (i.e., DRGs) do not give a complete description of patients' health care needs in acute care settings. In addition, these observations demonstrate that the domain of nursing practice encompasses much more than prescriptions guided by medical diagnosis. Nursing conditions of patients cut across medical diagnostic lines. A patient with a CVA may be unable to feed, dress, or bathe himself, just as a person in orthopedic traction for multiple fractures is unable to perform self-care activities. Nursing conditions are not necessarily the result of one physiological medical diagnosis.

A comparison of two linear regressions demonstrates this point further. In each regression, the dependent variable was length of stay (LOS) and the independent variables were 54 nursing conditions from Box 1. The first regression was on a subset of 225 surgical cases, representing the 12 most frequently occurring surgical DRGs. The second regression was on a subset of 156 medical cases, representing the 8 most frequently occurring medical DRGs. The model for the regressions of LOS on nursing conditions was

$$Y = b_0 + b_1 x_1 + b_2 x_2 + \ldots + b_n x_n + e$$

where

$$x_i = 0 \text{ if } x_i = 0 \qquad x_i = 1 \text{ if } x_i > 0 \qquad i = 1, 2, \ldots, 54$$

Table 4 lists eight variables which were common to the first 20 variables entered into the equations in both regressions. In addition, each list contained two (different) self-care deficits. The percent of cases presenting each nursing diagnosis also differed, with medical cases showing the greater proportion in every term. In essence, then, half of the first 20 nursing conditions explaining LOS in surgical cases, also explained LOS in medical cases, supporting the position that many nursing care needs are independent of physician's diagnosis.

The question of the effect of nursing conditions on length of stay (LOS) comes to mind again. If there is agreement that the practice of nursing in acute care settings concerns itself with the care of the whole person, and the effect of illness on this person, then we must take a closer look at the variables which reflect effect of illness on the whole person, that is, the psychosocial variables. Still referring to the regression analyses of surgical and medical cases, over half of the first 20 variables entered into each of the two regression equations were psychosocial conditions: 11 in the surgical cases, 12 in the medical. Not only are many of them represented, but they contribute greatly to R^2 (the multiple correlation coefficient squared). In the surgical cases, the first two variables entered are both psychosocial ones, producing R^2 = 0.5183;

TABLE 4   **Comparison of linear regressions of LOS in 54 nursing conditions from two subsets of cases: 12 surgical DRGs and 8 medical DRGs**

Surgical (n = 225 cases)*	Medical (n = 156 cases)*
1. Coping, ineffective (family disabling)	1. Self-care deficit: feeding
2. Coping, ineffective (family compromised)	2. Disturbance in self-esteem
3. Fluid/electrolyte imbalance: volume deficit	†3. Decubitus
†4. Decubitus	†4. Spiritual distress
5. Airway impaired	5. Hypertension
†6. Fluid/electrolyte imbalance: excess volume	†6. Acute anxiety
7. Sexual dysfunction, physiological	7. Family process alteration
8. Self-care deficit: bathing/hygiene	†8. Gas exchange impaired
9. Fear	9. Verbal communication impaired
10. Coping, ineffective (patient)	†10. Personal identity confusion
11. Powerlessness	11. Sexual dysfunction, psychological
†12. Gas exchange impaired	12. Knowledge deficit
†13. Suspiciousness	†13. Sleep disturbance
†14. Sleep disturbance	14. Surgical wound
†15. Anxiety	15. Social isolation
†16. Personal identity confusion	†16. Suspiciousness
17. Health maintenance alteration	17. Coping, family (potential growth)
18. Self-care deficit: dressing/grooming	18. Self-care deficit: toileting
†19. Spiritual distress	†19. Fluid/electrolyte imbalance: excess volume
20. Sight impaired	20. Depression

*Rank order of variables entered into equation.
†Independent variables (nursing diagnoses) common to both surgical and medical cases.

the next 18 variables contribute another 0.3202 to the R^2, and half of those were psychosocial variables (Fig. 2). The nursing diagnoses explained over 83% of the variance in LOS for surgical DRGs. In the medical cases, the first variable is physiological, but certainly within nursing's domain of practice; it explains 28.23% of the variation in length of stay. The second variable entered is psychosocial, and contributes almost 10% to the R^2, giving a total $R^2 = 0.3809$ for these two variables (Fig. 3). The next 18 variables then provided 26.1% explanation of the variance in length of stay; eleven of these 18 were psychosocial variables. In medical DRGs over 64% of variance in LOS was explained by nursing diagnoses. So not only are many nursing needs independent of medical diagnosis, but they also have significant explanatory power regarding length of stay.

To compare the nursing conditions' explanatory power with that of medical diagnoses, two more regression analyses were done, again using the two subsets of surgical and medical DRGs. Length of stay was the dependent variable and DRG the independent variables in both of these regressions.

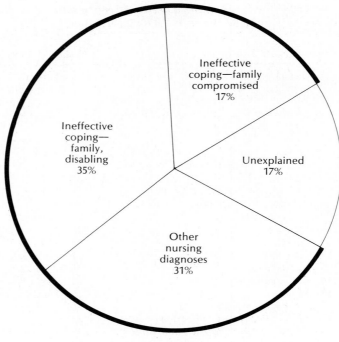

Total R^2 = 83.8%

FIGURE 2

The regression models were similar to those used with nursing conditions:

$$Y = b_0 + b_1 x_1 + \ldots + b_n x_n + e$$

where

$$x_i = 0 \text{ if } x_i = 0 \qquad x_i = 1 \text{ if } x_i > 0$$
$$n = 12 \text{ for surgical DRGs} \qquad n = 8 \text{ for medical DRGs}$$
$$i = 1, 2, \ldots, n$$

In the surgical regression cases nursing diagnoses explained 83.8% of the variation in LOS whereas surgical DRGs explained only 38.4%. In the medical regression cases nursing conditions explained 64.2% of the variation while the associated DRGs explained 20.8%.

Summarizing the implication of these four regressions, we find that (1) many nursing conditions are independent of medical diagnosis; (2) psychosocial needs of patients contribute significantly to the R^2 when explaining variation in LOS; and (3) nursing diagnoses have more explanatory power for hospital resource consumption than do medical diagnoses. Although the number of cases is relatively small, there is clearly an indication that nursing diagnoses

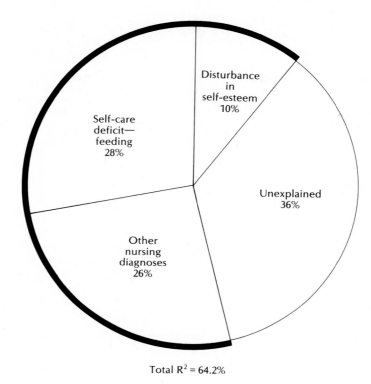

Total $R^2 = 64.2\%$

FIGURE 3

not only describe patients differently from medical diagnoses but have significant explanatory power as well. Therefore further research on larger data bases is imperative, with the results called to the attention of health care reimbursement agencies.

The relationship between patients' LOS in hospital, their need, and their treatment must be brought into better focus for justification of reimbursement. This preliminary examination of a sample of 1294 patients shows that nursing diagnoses explain length of stay as well as or better than medical diagnoses. However, more research on explanatory power is needed. The nurse's daily assessment of patient demand using the nurse/patient summary and the data storage and retrieval capability outlined in this project (aside from its other benefits regarding resource allocation) has the considerable potential for reflecting severity of illness within DRGs.

An enlarged data base of patients will be required. A test of the nursing diagnosis as a severity of illness measure could be achieved with approximately 60,000 patient cases from more than one hospital. This is based upon experience with the data base developed at university Hospitals of Cleveland where the DRG yield from 1300 cases was 16 DRGs of 15 or more cases. Investigation of the 127 individual variables obtained in the nurse's daily assessment of the patient and a sufficient number of DRGs necessitates that the DRGs with 15 cases be increased to, say 750, a sample 50 times the magnitude of the present sample. To acquire a large enough data base within 1 year, multiple hospital participation should be obtained. With the use of nursing diagnoses, the consumption of resources during hospitalization will be better explained and more informed decisions regarding patient need for care and the limits placed on resource use will be made.

REFERENCES

American Nurses' Association: Nursing a social policy statement, Kansas City, Mo., 1980, The Association.

Castles, M.: Nursing diagnosis research report. Newsletter of the Clearinghouse for the Classification of Nursing Diagnoses, 1975.

Fitzpatrick, J.J., and Whall, A.L.: Conceptual models of nursing: analysis and application, Bowie, Md., 1983, Robert J. Brady Co.

Gordon, M.: Nursing diagnosis: process and application, New York, 1982, McGraw-Hill Book Co.

Halloran, E.J.: Analysis of variation in nursing workload by patient medical and nursing condition. Doctoral dissertation, University of Illinois at the Medical Center, 1980. Dissertation Abstracts International, 41-09B. (University Microfilms no. 8106567.)

Halloran, E., and Kiley, M.: Case mix management for nurses, Nurs. Manage. 15(2):39-45, 1984.

Jelinek, R.C., and Dennis, L.C.: A review and evaluation of nurse productivity, DHEW Publication no. (HRA)77-15, Washington, D.C., 1976, Government Printing Office.

Kiley, M.L., and others: Computerized nursing information systems, Nurs. Manage. 14(7):26-29, 1983.

North American Nursing Diagnosis Association: Nursing diagnoses accepted for testing, St. Louis, 1982, The Association.

Study Group on Nursing Information Systems: Computerized nursing information systems—An urgent need, Res. Nurs. Health 6(3):101-105, 1983.

Nursing diagnosis among adolescents

SYBLE OLDAKER, Ph.D., R.N.

Adolescents have attracted recent attention and concern not only because of increases in the population of this age group, but also because of recent startling statistics. Today Americans aged 15 to 24 years have a higher death rate than 20 years ago (*Healthy People*, 1979; Holinger, 1979, 1980). Increasing trends in violent, self-destructive, and risk-taking behaviors among adolescents have created new concern for the health of this age group (Holinger, 1979, 1980). Deaths among adolescents, the majority of which have been attributed to maladaptive behavior patterns, raise questions about the psychological health of young persons (*Healthy People*, 1979).

Formal conceptualizations of adolescence and research of adolescent phenomena are relatively recent endeavors, with explanations of adolescent behavior and development proceeding within general expectations for "deviance." The adolescent has been viewed within the context of inherent emotional instability with psychological symptoms and problem behavior minimized as normal developmental phenomena. Negative views of the adolescent experience have led to confusion in estimates of the psychological problems and needs of this age group.

Psychological symptoms among adolescents have been underestimated (Weiner, 1970, 1980). True estimates of the psychological health of adolescents are often obscured by the lack of nosological consensus, lack of specificity, and reliance on clinical populations. Hypotheses formulated on the best evidence available suggest that clinical maladaptation among school children is likely to be 12% of any representative community in the general population (Dohrenwend and associates, 1980). Estimates of the nation's psychological health reflect that at least 10% (Kiefer, 1979) to 15% (Dohrenwend and coworkers, 1980) of the general population is in need of psychological services. There are few precise data on the mental health of adolescents in the general population, and consequently a need exists for studies of nonclinical adolescent populations to determine the needs of this age group.

PURPOSE

Concern for the increasing incidence of self-destructive and risk-taking behaviors among relatively healthy young people prompted questions regarding psychological symptoms among adolescents and their relationship to healthy adolescent development. This research investigated psychological health and symptomology among a group of adolescents within the general population. The study focused on a population of secondary school adolescents in north central Texas. Research questions concerned: (1) the prevalence of psychological symptoms among adolescents in the general population and (2) the identification of predictive relationships among sets of personality, demographic, and symptom variables. This paper presents those research findings, which have implications for nursing diagnosis among adolescents. Kiefer (1979) has emphasized that America's mental health cannot be defined in terms of disabling mental illness or psychiatric disorder. The diagnoses of developmental difficulty among adolescents and nursing intervention, which support the resolution of developmental problems, represent primary prevention for mental health in adolescence and for later stages of development.

THEORETICAL FRAMEWORK

Erikson's (1964, 1965, 1968, 1975) formulation of adolescent personality development as a process of psychosocial development provides a useful model for considerations of adolescents for several reasons: (1) it is comprehensive in the incorporation of biological, sociocultural, and individual factors as constituents of the developmental process; (2) the theoretical emphasis is healthy development; and (3) it provides a more optimistic view of human development as a process of psychosocial growth which neither begins nor ends with each developmental period. Erikson describes personality development in terms of the assumption of a psychosocial identity which evolves from the continuous interaction of biological, social, and individual events (Erikson, 1964, 1965, 1968, 1975). Central to her conceptualizations of personality formation and psychological health is the concept of identity. An optimal sense of identity is associated with a sense of psychosocial well-being. The most obvious concomitants are a feeling of "being at home in one's body" with a sense of "knowing where one is going," and an inner assuredness of anticipated recognition from others who count (Erikson, 1968).

The nuclear conflict of the stage of adolescence is the crisis of "identity" versus "identity confusion" (Erikson, 1968). Hogan (1976) observed that Erikson considers the identity conflict to be the prototype of neurosis among the young in modern society. The prime danger of the adolescent period is identity confusion—a state containing both subjective and objective aspects. Identity confusion exists on a continuum, with "mild" confusion at one end and "aggravated" and "malignant" confusion at the other. Identity confusion is not considered a diagnostic entity but rather is seen as a description of a developmental crisis which becomes a part of any diagnostic picture. Acute identity confusion usually becomes manifested when the individual is exposed to a combination of experiences which demand simultaneous commitment to physical intimacy, to decisive occupational choice, to energetic competition, and to psychosocial self-definition (Erikson, 1968). Four symptom areas of identity confusion have been cited by Erikson (1968): (1) the problem of intimacy, (2) diffusion of time perspective, (3) diffusion of industry, and (4) the choice of negative identity.

METHOD

A cross-sectional analytical survey of 138 white secondary school adolescents (35% male, 65% female) aged 14 to 18 years was conducted. Descriptive and predictive relationships between personality variables, variables of age, sex, level of achievement, and 20 psychological symptoms were analyzed using nonparametric and multivariate statistical techniques. Data were analyzed using the statistical package for the social sciences (SSPS, version M, Release 9.1, 1982). Validity and reliability of the Symptom Scales for adolescents were assessed by Chronbach's coefficient alpha reliability. Principle axis factor analysis, using varimax rotation, was used to examine symptom dimensions among the 20 symptom scale variables. Significance was accepted at the 0.05 level or less.

INSTRUMENTS

Participants completed a biographic questionnaire, the *Comrey Personality Scales* (CPS), and the *Psychiatric Epidemiological Research Interview* (PERI) *Symptom Scales*, which were modified for adolescents. The PERI symptom scales is an instrument designed to measure symptoms of psychopathology in the general population. Written in a fixed-alternative format, the instrument contains 25 symptom scales designed for use among adults. The scales have been assessed as reliable and valid by major studies utilizing samples of 200 and 705 subjects respectively (Dohrenwend and associates, 1980; Vernon and Roberts, 1981). In this study five of the symptom subscales within the original instrument were deleted for reasons of ethical responsibility inherent in anonymously reported data and for unsuitability of content for adolescent experience. Changes were also made in two subscales to accommodate to adolescent vocabulary and experience.

The *Comrey Personality Scales*, for assessing eight major personality dimensions among adolescents, represents a theoretically derived instrument developed by factor-analytical investigation (Comrey, 1970). Correspondence between the factorially derived personality dimensions and Erikson's stages of psychosocial development makes it useful for application within frameworks of psychosocial health. Intended for use among individuals whose social functioning is "normal" the Comrey personality dimensions are held to underlie the everyday behavior of individuals (Comrey, 1970). A substantial body of research supports the validity and reliability of the instrument (Comrey, 1979, 1980). The biographical instrument requests information of subject's age (in years and months), nationality, and self-reported school achievement.

FINDINGS
Symptom factors

Principal axis factor analysis of symptom scales, using Varimax rotations, yielded four independent symptom dimensions. A symptom was accepted as a component of a factor if the obtained factor score coefficient was at least as large as ±0.40. Individual factors and their symptom components were analyzed for descriptive commonalities and given designations which most characterized the symptom clusters.

The study subjects reported symptoms which obtained high correlations with personality variables associated with Erikson's stages of psychosocial development. Supportive evidence was supplied for Erikson's notions of the relationships and interrelationships between symptoms and personality constructs of psychosocial theory. The descriptive commonalities of symptom clusters associated with anxiety, antisocial behavior, and depression and confusion were consistent with theory descriptors of adolescent identity confusion.

Evidence confirming construct congruence for the present study factors and Erikson's constructs of identity confusion follows.

Factor I was defined by eight symptoms that accounted for 58.4% of the total variance. Highest loadings were obtained on anxiety with moderate loadings on the remainder of the contributing variables. The factor is descriptive of individuals who are anxious, sad, and somewhat fearful and rigid. They perceive their health as poor, and they experience psychophysiological symptoms and sleep problems. This symptom dimension denotes individuals who are "anxious fearful worriers."

The problem of intimacy is related to the young person's seeking of experiences in friendships, competition, sex play, and love. When identity is insecure, the youngster is apt to experience the anxiety and fear of an "interpersonal fusion," amounting to a further loss of identity and requiring a tense inner reservation and caution in commitment. Symptomatically, this may be experienced and expressed as interpersonal isolation and withdrawal. There may be attempts toward intimacy by stereotyped and formalized relationships or an overall shame and inability to derive a sense of accomplishment from any kind of activity. Erikson's construct of intimacy and the study factor of "anxious fearful worrier" shows

Intimacy	Factor I
Anxiety	Anxiety
	Psychophysiological symptoms
	Insomnia
	Perceived poor health
	Dread
Interpersonal isolation	Perceived hostility from others
	Sadness
Stereotyped behaviors	Rigidity

Factor II comprised five symptoms and accounted for 16.6% of the total symptom variance. Variable loadings were high on reasons for drinking and active expressions of hostility with close loadings on antisocial history, distrust, and drinking problems. The factor is descriptive of actively hostile, distrusting, and antisocial individuals who use alcohol for many reasons and for whom drinking alcohol presents problems. These individuals are characterized as "hostile antisocial drinkers."

Negative identity or role fixation is often expressed in scornful and snobbish hostility toward the roles offered as appropriate and desirable by family or community. Any or all roles of masculinity, femininity, nationality, or class membership may become the focus of disdain. Negative identity is described as "an identity perversely based on all those identification and roles which, at critical stages of development, have been presented to (the adolescent) as most undesirable or dangerous and yet also as most real" (Erikson, 1968). Erikson's construct of negative identity and the study factor "hostile antisocial drinker" is

Negative identity	**Factor II**
Scornful hostility to acceptable social roles	High reasons for drinking
	Active expressions of hostility
	Distrust
	Drinking problems

Four variables accounted for 8% of the total variance in *Factor III*. Symptoms of low self-esteem, hopelessness-helpnessness, sadness, and confused thinking were incorporated in the dimensions. Descriptive of individuals experiencing symptoms associated with depressive states, this factor was designated as "depressive."

A diffusion of time perspective is characterized by a sense of great urgency and yet a loss of consideration of time as a dimension of living. The young person may feel very young and babylike and simultaneously old beyond rejuvenation. This contradiction is often expressed in a general slowing of movement and behavior. These youngsters face difficulties in going to bed and facing sleep and also difficulties getting up and facing the day. Complaints, such as "I don't know," "I give up," and "I quit," are often expressions of the kind of despair on the part of the ego "to let itself die" (Erikson, 1968). Erikson's construct of diffusion of time perspective and the study factor "depressive" is as follows:

Diffusion of time perspective	**Factor III**
Despair and depressive behavior	Low self-esteem
	Hopelessness-helplessness
	Sadness
	Confused thinking

Factor IV yielded five variables and accounted for 6.7% of the variance among symptom scores. This factor portrays confused somewhat fearful individuals with low energy levels who perceive their health as poor, and who experience psychophysiological symptoms. The factor was denoted as "low energy fearfully confused."

A diffusion of industry is accompanied by an upset in the sense of workmanship with an inability to concentrate. It may occur in self-destructive preoccupation with some one-sided activity. Youngsters who are confused with their identities may be fearful of competition, afraid to fail, and skeptical about succeeding. In situations where they are compelled to prove themselves, they may be stricken with an inability to concentrate or apply themselves. Erikson's construct of diffusion of industry and the study factor "low energy, fearfully confused" is

Diffusion of industry	Factor IV
Upset in workmanship, with difficulty concentrating, fearfulness of competition, and ambivalence with success and failure	Low energy Confused thinking Psychophysiological symptoms Perceived poor health Dread

Significance to nursing diagnosis

The relationship of theory to nursing practice has become axiomatic. Gast (1979) summarized the present state of nursing diagnosis as "still largely ambiguous in regards to parameters, disordered in regards to classification, and isolated in regards to theories which might serve as a basis for deduction." While theoretical models of nursing serve as frameworks for diagnostic focus and for the delineation of nursing goals, nursing diagnoses are needed which are derived from those theories which serve nursing practice and which have application to a wide range of nursing models. If nursing diagnoses are abstractions which summarize a cluster of signs, symptoms, and inferences to form a diagnostic concept, and if nursing is an empirical science which derives its practice from the development and utilization of testable theory, then diagnostic abstractions (whether derived by induction or deduction) must have theoretical relevance. Though it is evident that a theory is not needed to determine that an ineffective airway clearance or an alteration in bowel elimination is dysfunctional, the explanations which guide interventions and practice lie in the application of existing acceptable theory. Often what is called "intuitive knowing" or "tacit inference" as a clinical model of inferential reasoning results from our "tacit knowing" of paradigms of explanations which are derived from theoretical models of knowledge.

Developmental phenomena and patterns of developmental growth have long been implicated in nursing practice and nursing education. Developmental patterns are included as a focus of concern, either tacitly or explicitly, in models of nursing. Carnevali and associates (1984) have identified two discipline-specific domains for diagnostic reasoning as those of daily living and functional health status. Gordon (1982) has derived a taxonomy of diagnostic classification related to functional health patterns. Both authors acknowledge the importance of developmental variables in health and illness. Developmental patterns among adolescents may constitute actual or potential dysfunctional health patterns of immediate or long-range consequences to individuals and to groups of individuals. Though frameworks for classifying diagnoses incorporate notions of developmental phenomena, specific developmental dysfunction or difficulty has not been addressed diagnostically. Developmental phenomena have many theoretical explanations—biological, psychological, and sociocultural. Theories of development are the basis for developmental explanations. Nursing diagnosis of developmental difficulty can be derived from theories of development and can be tested empirically. This paper presents four nursing diagnoses derived from Erikson's notions of identity confusion among adolescents (see Table 1).

TABLE 1   **Nursing diagnosis of identity confusion among adolescents**

Diagnostic concepts	Diagnostic criteria
Identity confusion related to problems of intimacy	
Anxiety	Increased anxiety
	Psychophysiological symptoms
	Dread
	Insomnia
	Perceived poor health
Interpersonal isolation	Perceived hostility from others
	Sadness
Stereotyped behaviors	High needs for order
	Rigidity
	Compulsiveness
Identity confusion related to problems of negative identity	
Scornful	High reasons for drinking
Snobbish hostility	Active expressions of hostility
Rejection of acceptable social roles	Distrust
	Drinking problems
	Antisocial history
Identity confusion related to problems of time perspective	
Depression	Low self-esteem
Despair	Hopelessness-helplessness
	Sadness
	Confused thinking
Identity confusion related to diffusion of industry	
Concentration difficulties	Low energy
Fearfulness of competition	Confused thinking
Success and failure ambivalence	Psychophysiological symptoms
	Perceived poor health
	Dread

Further testing and confirmation are needed to validate and refine the diagnoses. Concept analyses of the diagnostic entities and the generation of empirical indicators are needed to provide greater descriptive specificity. Further investigation of diagnostic criteria for inclusiveness and for application to a wider range of instrumentation is called for. Research utilizing criterion groups representative of clinical disturbance might provide evidence for determining functional and dysfunctional limits, leading to more accurate and refined diagnoses and greater predictive potential. Finally, research utilizing the diagnoses within models of nursing is needed to test their usefulness and application to nursing practice.

REFERENCES

Carnevali, D., Mitchell, P., Woods, N., and Tanner, C.: Diagnostic reasoning in nursing, Philadelphia, 1984, J.B. Lippincott Co.

Comrey, A.L.: EDITS manual: Comrey personality scales, San Diego, 1970, EDITS Publishers.

Comrey, A.L.: Handbook of interpretations for the Comrey Personality Scales, San Diego, 1980, EDITS Publishers.

Dohrenwend, B.P., and others: Mental illness in the United States: epidemiological estimates, New York, 1980, Praeger Co.

Dohrenwend, B.P., Shrout, P.E., Egri, G., and Mendelsohn, F.S.: Nonspecific psychological distress and other dimensions of psychopathology, Arch. Gen. Psychiatry **37:**1229-1236, 1980.

Erikson, E.H.: Youth: fidelity and diversity. In Erikson, E.H., editor: The challenge of youth, ed. 2, New York, 1956, Doubleday & Co., Inc.

Erikson, E.H.: Childhood and society, ed. 2, New York, 1964, W.W. Norton and Co., Inc.

Erikson, E.H.: Identity youth and crisis, New York, 1968, W.W. Norton and Co., Inc.

Erikson, E.H.: Life history and the historical moment, New York, 1975, W.W. Norton & Co., Inc.

Gast, H.L.: A review of some recent studies of nursing diagnoses. In Monograph: nursing diagnosis, pp. 1-6, Denton, Tex., 1979, College of Nursing, Texas Woman's University.

Gordon, M.: Nursing diagnosis, process and application, New York, 1982, McGraw-Hill Book Co.

Healthy people: The Surgeon General's report on health promotion and disease prevention, Department of Health, Education, and Welfare, Public Health Service, DHEW (PHS) Publication no. 79055071, Washington, D. C., 1979, Government Printing Office.

Holinger, P.C.: Violent deaths among the youth: recent trends in suicide, homicide, and accidents, Am J. Psychiatry **136**(9):1144-1147, 1979.

Keifer, H.C., editor: Sourcebook on mental health, Chicago, 1979, Marquis Academic Media.

Nie, N.H., and others: Statistical package for the social sciences, New York, 1982, McGraw-Hill Book Co.

Vernon, S.W., and Roberts, R.E.: Measuring nonspecific psychological distress and other dimensions of psychopathology, Arch. Gen. Psychiatry **38:**1239-1247, 1981.

Weiner, I.B.: Psychological disturbance in adolescence, New York, 1970, John Wiley & Sons, Inc.

Weiner, I.B.: Psychopathology in adolescence. In Adelson, J., editor: Handbook of adolescent psychology, New York, 1980, John Wiley & Sons, Inc.

Nursing diagnosis in the chronically ill

LOIS M. HOSKINS, Ph.D., R.N.
ELIZABETH A. McFARLANE, D.N.Sc., R.N.
M. GAIE RUBENFELD, M.S., R.N.
ANN M. SCHREIER, Ph.D., R.N.
MARY B. WALSH, M.S.N., R.N.

The purpose of this study was to determine the nursing diagnoses in a population of chronically ill persons. The sample consisted of 169 subjects, 25 years of age and older, with a medical diagnosis of chronic illness, who attended a medical outpatient clinic in a 900-bed hospital serving a large eastern metropolitan area.

Human need and motivation theories provided the framework for health assessment of the subjects and for the formation of the nursing diagnoses. Diagnostic labels were generated that were based upon significant clusters of data that indicated the absence of fulfillment or alteration in fulfillment of a human need.

A research questionnaire was developed by the investigators to obtain data from subjects about the human needs for

Air	Safety and security
Nutrition	Sexual integrity
Elimination	Love and belonging
Activity/mobility	Self-esteem
Sleep and rest	Self-actualization

Data from the demographic physical examination and laboratory reports were obtained from the subject's health record. Content validity for the questionnaire was obtained through a review by eight experts.

Selection and interviews of the subjects were conducted over a 4-month period by five master's prepared nurses. These nurses were doctoral candidates who were trained for the data collecting. Interrater reliability in the interview procedure was an average of 91% agreement. The data which they collected were subsequently analyzed by a panel of five judges, the research associates listed as authors of this study. The panel of judges did not participate in the data collection.

The methodology of the study can be described in two phases, a clinical phase and a validation phase (Table 1). Gordon and Sweeney (1979) described the *clinical phase* of a study as involving direct observation of patient behaviors

*Research supported by a grant from Nursing Research Branch, Division of Nursing, Department of Health and Human Services, Public Health Services, Grant no. 1R21 NU-00824.

TABLE 1   Summary of methodology

	n	Statistical test
Clinical phase		
Judges made diagnoses	50	t = Test (NS)*
Validation phase		
Computer made diagnoses	108	Chi square analysis (NS)*
	158	

*If nonsignificant (NS), the two groups were not different from each other.

as the source of information for forming diagnostic labels and the *validation phase* as determining the presence of pre-identified clusters of defining characteristics in a sufficient number of cases to be considered valid diagnoses.

In this study data were collected on all 169 subjects during one 4-month period. The first 11 subjects interviewed were used as a test of the interrater reliability. The data from these 11 were excluded from all further analysis leaving a sample of 158.

From the 158, 50 subjects were randomly selected (constituting Group I), and the data from these subjects were analyzed independently by each of the five judges; the five then met to arrive at consensual validation. The results of this phase were the formation of the nursing diagnoses and the identification of their defining characteristics and critical indicators. These criteria established for the diagnoses were then computerized.

In the validation phase the data from the remaining 108 subjects (constituting Group II) were analyzed via computer. This resulted in a comparison of the frequency of occurrence of given diagnoses in each sample. As defined for this study critical indicators were those defining characteristics (signs or symptoms), or combinations thereof, that had to be present for a specific diagnosis to be assigned.

Fifty-one diagnoses were identified. The mean number of diagnoses in the 50 subjects in Group I was 11.56 and the mean number in the 108 subjects in Group II was 11.43. A t-test for differences in the means resulted in a nonsignificant value (t, 156 df = 0.16, p = 0.876), indicating that the two groups were not different in terms of the average number of diagnoses in the subjects in each group. A chi square analysis was done to compare the frequencies of subjects in each group for each diagnosis. There were no significant differences in the percentage of subjects in Group I compared to the percentage in Group II who had the diagnosis, with one exception. The occurrence of the diagnosis Loneliness was significantly different in the two groups; one other diagnosis, Impaired circulation, uncontrolled hypertension, approached significance. These two tests validated that 50 of the 51 diagnoses derived in Group I were present in the same proportion in Group II.

TABLE 2   **Major characteristics of the sample (n = 158)**

	No.	%
Age (yr)		
Range (24-90)		80% (n = 127) were between the ages
Median (66)		of 55 and 80
Sex*		
Female	117	75
Male	40	25
Race		
Black	153	97
Education*		
Less than 8th grade	74	47
8th grade	52	33
More than 8th grade	31	20
Income		
Less than $10,000	137	87
Living arrangements		
Alone	61	39
With others	97	61
Closest relative		
Children	54	34
Spouse	29	19
Brothers, sisters, grandparents	32	20
Other	33	21
Medical diagnoses†		
Hypertension	113	72
Heart/circulatory	88	56
Arthritis	88	56
Diabetes mellitus	66	42
Pulmonary	29	18
Renal	22	14
Other	110	70

*One missing.
†Majority had been diagnosed for longer than 2 years.

Selected characteristics from the total sample (n = 158) are reported in Table 2. The age range was 24 to 90 years, with the median being 66 years. Eighty percent (n = 127) were between 55 and 80 years of age; 10 subjects were over 80, and 18 were less than 55. Seventy-five percent of the sample were female, and 97% were black. The socioeconomic status was low; 47% had less than an eighth-grade education, and 87% had an annual income of less than $10,000. With respect to living arrangements, 39% lived alone and 61% lived with others. The closest related persons for 34% were their children; 19% had spouses, 20% listed brothers, sisters, grandparents, and 21% included "others."

TABLE 3   **Number of subjects and diagnoses by need**

		Subjects with	
	Diagnoses	**At least one diagnosis**[*]	**No diagnoses in this need**
Lower-level needs			
Air	5	103	55
Nutrition	9	144	14
Elimination	5	64	94
Sleep and rest	2	126	32
Activity and mobility	5	118	40
Safety and security	12	152	6
	38		
Higher-level needs			
Love and belonging	3	49	109
Sexual integrity	3	44	114
Self-esteem	3	61	97
Self-actualization	4	17	141
	13		

[*]Subjects could have more than one diagnosis in each need.

The medical diagnoses were taken from the subject's health record and placed in the broad categories of Table 2. The diagnosis of hypertension occurred most frequently (72%), significant in a primarily black and female population. Heart/circulatory problems, arthritis, and diabetes occupied the next three most prominent categories.

Nursing diagnoses were established based upon an absence of, or an alteration in, need fulfillment. Subjects' responses to interview items were analyzed and were considered significant if they indicated abnormal behavior in comparison to an accepted standard or normative value, a change from the subjects' usual behavior, or risk factors. These abnormal responses were clustered within each need. There was no limit on the number of clusters that could be defined, but to be considered a cluster, at least two responses were required. Information about one need could be used to support a problem in another need. In this manner clusters of items were formed and were labeled within each need. For interest we categorized the needs into higher level and lower level needs and compared the numbers of diagnoses and the numbers of subjects in each (see Table 3). There were 13 diagnoses within the higher level needs and 38 diagnoses within the lower-level needs, with a far greater number of subjects having problems in fulfilling lower level needs. Human need and motivation theories indicate that lower-level needs become predominant under adverse living conditions. The findings from this study provide support to these theories. It is interesting to note that 17 subjects were able to identify the need for self-actualization and problems in meeting this need. Although relatively few in

BOX 1   **Nursing diagnoses categorized within the needs**

Air
  Alteration in tissue perfusion
  Impaired circulation, uncontrolled hypertension
  Altered breathing pattern: respiratory difficulty
  Health management deficit: respiratory self-care
  Potential decreased tissue oxygenation

Nutrition
  Obesity
  Nonadherence to prescribed diet
  Inconsistency in data reporting
  Potential for uncontrolled diabetes
  Knowledge deficit: diet
  Overweight
  Potential for nutritional deficiency
  Dysphagia
  Dysfunctional digestion pattern

Elimination
  Constipation
  Perceived constipation
  Potential fluid imbalance
  Perceived urinary pattern problem
  Diarrhea

Sleep and rest
  Impaired sleep/rest pattern
  Potential sleep/rest pattern

Activity and mobility
  Impaired mobility
  Potential for social isolation
  Inadequate physical activity
  Interference with activity/mobility: pain
  Decreased tolerance for physical activity

Safety and security
  Potential for eye/vision alteration
  Limited health care follow-up
  Inadequate dental care
  At risk for illness: stress, grief
  Potential health management deficit: financial insecurity
  Potential for injury: sensorimotor alterations
  Potential for communication deficit: hearing loss
  Threatened safety: noise
  Threatened safety: crime

BOX 1   **Nursing diagnoses categorized within the needs—cont'd**

Safety and security—cont'd
  Threatened safety: rats, roaches, pests
  Threatened safety: structural hazards
  Threatened safety: quality of air

Love and belonging
  Potential for loneliness
  Loneliness
  Lack of spiritual support

Sexual integrity
  Illness imposed changes in sexual activity
  Threat to sexual integrity
  Impotence

Self-esteem
  Threat to self-esteem: loss of control
  Low self-esteem
  Threat to self-esteem: body image disturbance

Self-actualization
  Imbalance of inner- and outer-directed self
  Lack of purpose in life
  Self-management deficit: medications
  Self-management deficit: diet, exercise

---

number compared to the lower-level needs, these problems have implications for nursing.

Safety and security had the greatest number of diagnoses and it was a conclusion of the judges that this category is too broad, encompassing such problems as skin conditions, sensory limitations, and threats to safety due to crime. The next largest category of problems fell in the need for nutrition, with 144 subjects having at least one of the 9 diagnoses. Subjects could have more than one diagnosis in each need. Sleep and rest had only two diagnoses, but 126 subjects had problems meeting this need. Of least importance with respect to problems in lower-level needs was the need for elimination. Box 1 lists the diagnoses by need.

Table 4 presents the major findings in nursing diagnoses for the total sample. There were 51 diagnoses, with a mean number of 11 per subject. Although only 50 of the diagnoses were validated, all 51 are listed in this table according to their frequency of occurrence in the total sample. Those marked with a

TABLE 4   **Major findings in nursing diagnoses, total sample**

	n	%
No. *(n)* of diagnoses 51		
Mean n per subject 11		

CODE: Number preceding diagnosis indicates need category

1 Love and belonging	6 Nutrition
2 Sexual integrity	7 Elimination
3 Self-esteem	8 Sleep and rest
4 Self-actualization	9 Activity and mobility
5 Air	10 Safety and security

	n	%
Occurring in greater than 50% of sample		
6 Potential for nutritional deficiency	125	79
9 Interference with activity/mobility: pain	101	64
* 6 Obesity	92	58
* 10 Threatened safety: rats, roaches, pests	87	55
* 8 Impaired sleep pattern	86	54
* 10 Potential for eye or vision alteration	86	54
Occurring in 40% to 49% of sample		
* 9 Impaired mobility	66	42
Occurring in 30% to 39% of sample		
9 Decreased tolerance for physical activity	61	39
* 5 Altered breathing pattern: respiratory difficulty	61	39
* 10 Threatened safety: crime	59	37
6 Inconsistency in data reporting: nutrition	58	37
* 10 Threatened safety: noise	50	32
* 5 Alteration in tissue perfusion	49	31
10 Inadequate dental care	48	30
Occurring in 20% to 29% of sample		
6 Potential for uncontrolled diabetes	46	29
9 Inadequate physical activity	45	29
* 5 Potential decreased tissue oxygenation	44	28
8 Potential sleep impairment	40	25
1 Potential for loneliness	38	24
2 Illness imposed changes in sexual activity	38	24
* 3 Threat to self esteem: loss of self-control	37	23
* 10 At risk for illness: stress, grief	34	22
* 3 Threat to self-esteem: body image disturbance	33	21
Occurring in less than 20% of sample		
6 Dysfunctional digestion pattern	28	18
5 Health management deficit: respiratory self-care	27	17
* 7 Constipation	26	17
10 Potential health management deficit: financial insecurity	26	17
6 Knowledge deficit: diet	25	16
* 10 Threatened safety: structural hazards	24	15
5 Impaired circulation, uncontrolled hypertension	23	15
* 10 Potential for communication deficit: hearing loss	22	14

*Similar to Fourth National Conference list.   *Continued.*
†Groups significantly different on this diagnosis were not validated.

TABLE 4   Major findings in nursing diagnoses, total sample—cont'd

	n	%
Occurring in less than 20% of sample—cont'd		
* 7 Perceived urinary pattern problem	22	14
10 Limited health care follow-up	21	13
* 10 Potential for injury: sensorimotor alteration	21	13
9 Potential for social isolation	20	13
* 3 Low self-esteem	19	12
7 Perceived constipation	16	10
* 6 Overweight	16	10
1 Loneliness†	13	8
6 Nonadherence to prescribed diet	12	8
6 Dysphagia	10	6
2 Threat to sexual integrity	10	6
* 4 Self-management deficit: diet, exercise	10	6
* 7 Potential fluid imbalance	9	6
4 Imbalance of inner- and outer-directed self	7	4
4 Lack of purpose in life	7	4
* 7 Diarrhea	5	3
* 4 Self-management deficit: medications	5	3
* 10 Threatened safety: quality of air	5	3
* 2 Impotence	4	3
1 Lack of spiritual support	2	1

*Similar to Fourth National Conference list.
†Groups significantly different on this diagnosis were not validated.

TABLE 5   Interference with activity/mobility: pain, (n = 101 or 64% of sample)

	n	%
Critical indicator		
Physical symptoms with activity	101	100
Other defining characteristics		
Mobility restrictions due to disease	66	65
Arthritis	63	62
Gets as much activity as thinks is needed	49	49
Illness affects leisure activities	42	41.5

single asterisk have the same or a similar label as those appearing in the list accepted at the Fourth National Conference. Six diagnoses occurred in greater than 50% of the sample, with the most frequently occurring one being "potential for nutritional deficiency" (79%). The next four, in descending order of occurrence, were Interference with activity/mobility: pain, 64%; Obesity, 58%: Threatened safety: rats, roaches, pests, 55%; Impaired sleep pattern, 54%; and Potential for eye/vision alterations, 54%.

TABLE 6   **Obesity (n = 92 or 58% of sample)**

	n	%
Critical indicator		
20% above ideal weight	92	100
Other defining characteristics		
Bodily appearance overweight by rater	74	80
Sees self as overweight	64	70
Physical examination: general appearance obese	—	—
Physical examination: abdomen and inguinal area abnormal	—	—

TABLE 7   **Threatened safety: rats, roaches, pests (n = 87 or 55% of sample)**

	n	%
Critical indicators		
Neighborhood (rats, roaches, pests)	75	95
Home (rats, roaches, pests)	68	86

TABLE 8   **Impaired sleep/rest pattern (n = 86 or 54% of sample)**

	n	%
Critical indicators		
Feels well rested (sometimes, never)	57	66
Does not fall asleep easily	49	56
Wakes more than 3 times a night	23	27
Other defining characteristics		
Nocturia disturbs sleep	74	86
Restlessness	68	79
Lethargy	62	72
Worries disturb sleep	55	64
Listlessness	51	59
Dreams disturb sleep	38	44
Five or fewer hours of sleep per night	35	41
Irritability	35	41
Noise disturbs sleep	35	41
Hand tremor	33	38
Cough disturbs sleep	31	36
Pain disturbs sleep	30	35
Yawning	28	33
Dark circles around eyes	22	26
Shortness of breath disturbs sleep	21	24
Disorientation	19	22
Change in life-style disturbs sleep	18	21
Takes medication to fall asleep	12	14
Takes food to fall asleep	2	2

TABLE 9   Defining characteristics of potential for eye/vision alterations

Item	Characteristic	Group I (n = 30)	Group II (n = 56)	Total (n = 86)
		Subjects having diagnosis		
7	Hypertension	21 (70.0%)	36* (65.5%)	57 (67.1%)
9	Diabetes mellitus	14 (46.7%)	24 (42.9%)	38 (44.2%)
260	Wears glasses, contacts (always or just for reading)	25 (83.3%)	44 (78.5%)	69 (80.2%)
261§	Other problems with eyes	30 (100%)	56 (100%)	86 (100%)
429	Physical examination: eyes, abnormal	2† (33.3%)	8‡ (80.0%)	10 (62.5%)

*Missing data, 1 of 56.
†Missing data, 24 of 30.
‡Missing data, 46 of 56.
§Critical indicator.

TABLE 10   Defining characteristics at risk for illness: stress, grief

Item	Characteristic	Group I (n = 14)	Group II (n = 20)	Total (n = 34)
		Subjects having diagnosis		
20	Marital staital status, widowed	6 (42.9%)	8 (40.0%)	14 (41.2%)
21	Duration of marital status 12 mo	3 (21.4%)	1 (5.0%)	4 (11.8%)
127	Budget for food inadequate	6 (42.9%)	10 (50.0%)	16 (47.1%)
206	Worries, concerns affect sleep (always, sometimes)	12 (85.7%)	18 (90.0%)	30 (88.2%)
211	Changes in life-style presently affect sleep	8 (57.1%)	8 (40.0%)	16 (47.1%)
276*	Experiencing emotional stress now	14 (100%)	20 (100%)	34 (100%)
278	Good job taking care of self	3 (21.4%)	2 (10.0%)	5 (14.7%)
339	Feel lonely (frequently or always)	5 (35.7%)	1 (5.0%)	6 (17.6%)

*Critical indicator.

Impaired mobility was the only diagnosis in the 40% range of the sample. Seven diagnoses occurred in the 30% range, nine in the 20% range, and 28 in the less than 20% range.

Each of the nursing diagnoses in the need for elimination occurred in fewer than 20% of the sample. Activity/mobility had a diagnosis in each of the given percentage ranges. The three diagnoses about threatened safety related to rats, roaches, and/or pests, noise, and crime were found in 32% to 55% of the population. Each of the diagnoses related to self-actualization occurred in less than 20% of the population. Of the nine diagnoses in nutrition, two occurred in 50% or greater but five occurred in less than 20%. The greatest occurrence of diagnoses in higher-level needs was in the 20% range, with five diagnoses falling there.

Tables 5 to 8 present examples of diagnoses, their frequencies of occurrence in the total sample, their critical indicators, and other defining characteristics. Tables 9 and 10 demonstrate the comparison of frequency of occurrence of a diagnosis and its defining characteristics in Group I (50 subjects) and Group II (108 subjects).

Data from this study are still being analyzed for relationships; the questionnaire is being revised to eliminate those items that did not identify defining characteristics. Analysis of the data comparing the defining characteristics of this study to those listed in the Proceedings of the National Conference is being done. It is recommended that this work be validated among other populations of chronically ill in different settings.

REFERENCE

Gordon, M., and Sweeney, M.A.: Methodological problems and issues in identifying and standardizing nursing diagnoses, Adv. Nurs. Sci. 2(1):1-15, 1979.

Use of nursing diagnosis in community health agencies using the PORS

KATHLEEN A. BALDWIN, M.S.N., R.N.
ANNETTE G. LUECKENOTTE, M.S., R.N.

Nursing diagnosis provides the nurse with a tool for documenting health problems and the nursing process in a comprehensive client-focused manner. The problem-oriented records system (PORS), as a charting form used by many community health agencies, requires the nurse to note the subjective (symptoms) and objective (signs) data for each problem. This form of charting thus requires the nurse to specify the cues used to diagnose the problem. As Gordon (1982) noted, the PORS arrived on the scene about the same time that nurses began to think about practice in terms of nursing diagnosis. The blending of nursing diagnosis and the PORS reinforces the concepts of nursing process and nursing diagnosis.

The problem-oriented recording system (PORS) was developed by Weed (1969) to organize a method of recording health data and provide for ongoing audit of services rendered. Although originally conceived as a method for educating medical students, this record system was found to have applicability to many health-related disciplines, including nursing (Aradine and Guthneck, 1974; Larkin and Backer, 1977; Niland and Bentz, 1974; Schell and Campbell, 1972; Woody and Mallison, 1973).

The manner in which the PORS system operates may be briefly summarized. A defined data base is collected, from which the problems are identified, and each problem is given a number. An initial plan of care is developed for each problem and given the same number as the corresponding problem. Actual outcomes of care are noted in the progress notes, which are also numbered and titled according to the problem.

This system gained popularity in nursing during the 1970s because its component parts—data base, problem list, initial plans, and progress notes—closely correlated with the steps of the nursing process, particularly assessment, nursing diagnosis, planning, implementation, and evaluation. In addition to being useful as a framework for record-keeping, the problem-oriented record system provided an orderly and logical methodology for the application of the nursing process.

Community health agencies use a wide variety of recording systems to document the provision of services, one of which is the PORS (Bonkowsky, 1972; Kelly, 1974; Reines, 1979; Schell and Campbell, 1972). Modifications of the Weed problem-oriented record system have appeared in many agencies, including the Indian Health Service, the VNA of Omaha, and the VNS of

Burlington (Vermont) (Freeman and Heinrich, 1981). Simmons (1980) identified that the implementation of this record system can facilitate the development of a classification scheme for nursing. Specifically, the problem list is that component of the record which relates directly to nursing diagnoses, which in turn are derived from any number of classification systems.

Simmons (1980) and her colleagues developed such a classification scheme of 45 client health problems diagnosed by nurses in a community health setting. A study by Jones (1981) attempted to discover what terms are used by nurses to label the client-patient problems for which they care. The nurses sampled were from a wide range of clinical settings, including nonhospital community health care settings. The research culminated in a taxonomy of nursing diagnoses useful for care planning. Gottlieb (1981) developed a health-related category system to describe and differentiate nursing practice in a variety of settings, including community health. Finally, the efforts of the National Conference since 1973 have been directed toward the development of a taxonomy of nursing diagnoses for all of nursing.

Gordon (1976) proposed that the problem/etiology/signs/symptoms (PES) format could be adapted to the problem-oriented record system. Dalton (1979) further described that home health agencies using the problem-oriented records system provide " . . . an optimal climate and setting for the implementation of nursing diagnosis within the concept of nursing process." However, Shamansky and Yanni (1983), in an opposing view, asserted " . . . there are a variety of patient problems in the community health nursing setting that are unsuitable for a taxonomy of nursing labels." Because of the varied and diverse points of view related to standardization of the nomenclature and use of diagnoses in community health clinical practice, study is indicated to determine applicability and use of the developed classification system.

STUDY DESIGN

This paper reports the findings of a study of community health nurses' use of problem statements in local health departments. The authors conducted a descriptive survey of open client records at three county health departments which were using the problem oriented record system. The study was designed to answer two questions: (1) What are the problem statements community health nurses use on the problem oriented record? (2) Are those problem statements synonymous with the nursing diagnosis classification system developed by the National Conference Group for Classification of Nursing Diagnoses?

The three central Illinois county health departments where the study was conducted provided both skilled home care and health promotion nursing services. One agency served a predominantly rural population of 120,000. Its staff made approximately 6000 home visits per year, half home care and half health promotion. The second agency, serving an urban population of approx-

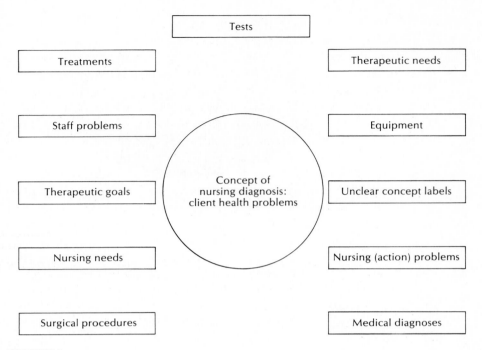

FIGURE 1

imately 200,000, reported nearly 12,000 home care visits and 9000 health promotion visits annually. The third agency served a primarily suburban population of 130,000 and conducted over 6000 home care visits and 3000 health promotion visits per year.

METHOD AND DATA ANALYSIS

A record review of 25 skilled home care and 25 health promotion records from each of the three health departments yielded a total of 150 records and 472 problem statements. Fifty records were randomly selected from active client files at each agency. The problem statements were transcribed from the records and categorized according to traditional and current conceptions of client situations requiring nursing intervention. The typology developed by Gordon (1982) was used for the content analysis (see Fig. 1). This typology consists of terms which have historically been considered the legitimate focus of nursing but are viewed as incongruent with the current concept of nursing diagnosis. These terms are operationally defined in Table 1.

The researchers separately reviewed and classified each problem statement according to the above typology. To determine the degree of interrater reliability a Pearson r was calculated. No significant difference between raters was found ($r = +0.96$).

TABLE 1   **Definitions of terms excluded from the concept of nursing diagnosis**

Terms	Definitions	Examples
Tests	Examinations or tools which yield objective information about the client; each such examination or tool has a normal/abnormal range that establishes area within which client is considered or not considered to have a pathological condition	Denver Developmental Screen Test (DDST), cardiac catheterization, physical assessment
Treatments	Activities of care prescribed by physician or dentist	Catheterization, medication administration, 1200 American Diabetes Association diet
Staff problems	Health care providers' difficulties in coping with clients	Uncooperative, hostile, foreign language, demanding
Therapeutic goals	Statements of desirable, measurable, and attainable outcomes given client's current condition and circumstances	To prevent postoperative wound infection, to maintain independent home living, to self-administer insulin
Nursing needs	Tangible or intangible requisites common to all human beings for attainment or maintenance of homeostasis	Nutritional needs, nurturing needs
Therapeutic needs	Generally stated determinations of nursing actions; use of therapeutic needs as diagnoses bypasses problem formulation step in nursing care planning	Needs prenatal education, needs emergency plan, needs diversional activities
Surgical procedures	Operations performed by physicians to correct physical defects, repair injuries, or diagnose and treat disease	Vasectomy, cesarean section, cholecystectomy, circumcision
Signs and symptoms	Isolated subjective and objective data descriptive of client's condition and circumstances	Dyspnea, elevated blood lead level, epigastric distress, vaginal bleeding
Medical diagnoses	Disease labels derived from physician analysis of client's presenting signs and symptoms	Emphysema, urinary tract infection, ectopic pregnancy, diabetes mellitus
Nursing (action) problems	Nurse's difficulty in prescribing, initiating, and evaluating nursing care	How to prevent infection, how to determine adherence to medical regime, how to assure adequate nutritional intake
Unclear concept, labels	Abstractions, which by definition are intrinsic, and thus provide little direction for nursing care	Pain, maternal-infant bonding, nutrition, growth and development
Equipment	Paraphernalia, supplies	Foley catheter, dressing, apnea monitor

TABLE 2   **Frequency and percentage distribution of problem statements classified according to Gordon's typology**

Terms included in Gordon's typology	*n*	%
Unclear concept labels	159	34
Therapeutic needs	80	17
Signs and symptoms	74	16
Medical diagnoses	59	13
Treatments	30	6
Therapeutic goals	25	5
Tests	21	5
Nursing diagnoses	9	2
Staff problems	5	1
Nursing (action) problems	4	1
Nursing needs	3	1
Surgical procedures	2	1
Equipment	1	1
TOTAL	472	100

RESULTS

The combined problem statements from all three agencies (n = 472) were classified into the following most frequently used terms: unclear concept label (n = 159), 34%; therapeutic needs (n = 80), 17%; and signs and symptoms (n = 74), 16%. The frequency of use of all other terms was less than 15%. Only 2% of problem statements were classified as nursing diagnoses as defined by the National Conference Group (see Table 2).

Further analysis was done after dividing the records into two groups, skilled home care (n = 251) and health promotion (n = 221). Unclear concept label, therapeutic needs, and signs and symptoms were the three most frequent types of problem statements used on each of the two types of records (see Tables 3 and 4). This result is similar to that found when these records were analyzed as a total group (n = 472).

Few of the problem statements were used more than once. Emergency plan, hypertension, health maintenance, diabetes, and parenting skills were exceptions. Table 5 displays those diagnoses with frequencies greater than 1% of the total.

CONCLUSIONS

The above findings suggest that community health nurses are using a wide variety of problem statements in their practice. Many of these statements

TABLE 3   **Frequency and percentage distribution of skilled home care record problem statements classified according to Gordon's typology**

Terms	*n*	%
Unclear concept labels	56	22
Therapeutic needs	54	22
Signs and symptoms	40	16
Medical diagnoses	35	14
Treatments	24	10
Tests	15	6
Therapeutic goals	13	5
Nursing diagnoses	6	2
Staff problems	4	2
Surgical procedures	2	1
Equipment	1	1
Nursing needs	1	1
Nursing (action) problems	0	0
TOTAL	251	100

TABLE 4   **Frequency and percentage distribution of health promotion record problem statements classified according to Gordon's typology**

Terms	*n*	%
Unclear concept labels	103	47
Signs and symptoms	34	15
Therapeutic needs	26	12
Medical diagnoses	24	11
Therapeutic goals	12	5
Tests	6	3
Treatments	6	3
Nursing (action) problems	4	2
Nursing diagnoses	3	1
Nursing needs	2	1
Staff problems	1	1
Equipment	0	0
Surgical procedures	0	0
TOTAL	221	100

TABLE 5   **Frequency and percentage distribution of five most *frequently* reported problem statements**

	n	%
Emergency plan	12	2.5
Hypertension	10	2.1
Health maintenance	9	1.9
Diabetes	8	1.7
Parenting skills	5	1.1
All others	428	90.7
TOTAL	472	100.0

would seem to provide little guidance to actual nursing care. Use of the National Conference Group taxonomy was extremely limited in records sampled. However, this variety and use exemplifies the profession's development and application of the concept of nursing diagnosis. Findings cannot be indiscriminantly generalized to community health practice throughout the country because of the study's limited sample size.

RECOMMENDATIONS

The outcome of this study demonstrates the need for a standardized diagnostic system in community health nursing. Such a system would reduce the wide variety of client problem statements and benefit both community health agencies and their clients.

A standardized system of diagnosis could be an enormous problem-solving aid. Nurses would be directed toward analysis of clusters of data rather than labeling as problems single, isolated signs and symptoms. Continuity of care would be enhanced as communication among staff members improved. Using clearly defined nursing diagnoses, agencies would be better able to demonstrate the need for third-party pay to insurance companies.

With these benefits in mind, it is time community health agencies begin using a classification system such as that developed by the North American Nursing Diagnosis Association.

REFERENCES

Aradine, C.R., and Guthneck, M.: The problem-oriented record in a family health service, Am. J. Nurs. **74**(6):1108-1112, 1974.

Bonkowsky, M.L.: Adapting the POMR to community child health care, Nurs. Outlook **20**(8):515-518, 1972.

Dalton, J.M.: Nursing diagnosis in a community health setting, Nurs. Clin. North Am. **14**(3):525-531, 1979.

Freeman, R.B., and Heinrich, J.: Community health nursing practice, Philadelphia, 1981, W.B. Saunders Co.

Gordon, M.: Nursing diagnosis and the diagnostic process, Am. J. Nurs. **76**(8):1298-1300, 1976.

Gordon, M.: Nursing diagnosis: Process and application, New York, 1982, McGraw-Hill Book Co.

Gottlieb, L.N.: Small steps toward the development of a health classification system in nursing. In Kim, M.J., and Moritz, D.A., editors: Classification of nursing diagnoses—Proceedings of the Third and Fourth National Conferences, New York, 1982, McGraw-Hill Book Co.

Jones, P.E.: Developing terminology: a University of Toronto experience. In Kim, M.J., and Moritz, D.A., editors: Classification of nursing diagnoses—Proceedings of the Third and Fourth National Conferences, New York, 1982, McGraw-Hill Book Co.

Kelly, M.E., and McNutt, H.: Implementation of problem-oriented charting in a public health agency, Nurs. Clin. North Am. **9**(2):281-287, 1974.

Larkin, P.D., and Backer, B.A.: Problem-oriented nursing assessment, New York, 1977, McGraw-Hill Book Co.

Niland, M.B., and Bentz, P.M.: A problem-oriented approach to planning nursing care, Nurs. Clin. North Am. **9**(2):235-245, 1974.

Schell, P.L., and Campbell, A.T.: POMR—not just another way to chart, Nurs. Outlook **20**(8):510-514, 1972.

Shamansky, S.L., and Yanni, C.R.: In opposition to nursing diagnosis: a minority opinion, Image **15**(2):47-50, 1983.

Simmons, D.A.: A classification scheme for client problems in community health nursing, Publication no. HRA 80-16, Hyattsville, Md., 1980, Department of Health and Human Services.

Woody, M., and Mallison, M.: The problem-oriented system for patient-centered care, Am. J. Nurs. **73**(7):1168-1175, 1973.

CHAPTER 11

Evaluation

Evaluation of a predictive model of diabetic compliance

JEAN JENNY, M.Ed., M.S.N., R.N.

A review of diabetes studies suggests that there is room for improvement in patients' management of their therapeutic regimen (Berkowitz and associates, 1963; Donabedian and Rosenfeld, 1964; Halloner, 1968; Watkins and associates, 1967). The demanding self-care regimen for diabetes offers many opportunities for noncompliance. Since self-regulation offers the best chance for disease control and delay of progression (Skyler, 1979), facilitating compliance is an important goal for clinicians. The purpose of this study was to test the validity of a theoretical model of diabetic compliance in a clinical setting.

The model emerged from three different sources in the literature: patient teaching theory, studies of behavioral management of diabetes, and compliance studies. Patient teaching sources stressed the importance of knowledge about the health problem and its management for effective patient self-care. The need for appropriate client motivation and learning set is endorsed, and several strategies are offered (Jenny, 1979). Redman (1981) suggests the need for a broader model for patient teaching than that used traditionally in the school setting, one incorporating more contextual variables and the patient's frame of reference.

The burgeoning literature on compliance identifies more than 200 associated factors (Sackett and Haynes, 1976), suggesting that patient compliance has become the best documented but least understood health-related behavior (Becker and Maiman, 1975). Factors associated with the patient, the disease,

Acknowledgments

Study supported by grants from the National Health Research Development Program, Health and Welfare, Ottawa, and the Ottawa Civic Hospital Foundation, Ottawa, Canada. The help of Thomas Goss, Ph.D., Ottawa, and John Bell, the Health Research Unit of University of Ottawa, in data processing and interpretation is most gratefully acknowledged.

and the treatment have all received exhaustive exploration, but few have shown consistency in their relationships with compliance across the studied spectrum of health and disease-related behaviors. Knowledge of therapy and disease, so frequently the sole dimension addressed in patient teaching, is a good starting point, but has repeatedly proved to be a necessary but not sufficient condition for adherence (Becker, 1979). The gap between knowledge and behavior has given rise to a search for a set of intervening variables or specific motivating components of health-related behaviors. The most consistently successful group of variables to predict compliance in both preventive health and therapeutic situations has been the health belief model (HBM) (Rosenstock, 1974), and a sizable body of findings now exists to document this success (Becker and associates, 1977). As originally conceived, the HBM hypothesized that persons would generally not seek preventive care or health screening unless they possessed minimal levels of relevant health motivation and knowledge, viewed themselves as potentially vulnerable and the condition threatening, were convinced of the efficacy of intervention, and saw few difficulties in undertaking the recommended action (Rosenstock, 1974).

Organized instruction to patients is the theme of many studies in the diabetes literature (Bowen and associates, 1961; Tagliacozzo and associates, 1974). Improvement in knowledge, skill, and attitudes is demonstrated, but no significant changes in adherence behaviors, and no relation is demonstrated between increased patient knowledge and diabetes control. Williams and co-workers (1967) suggested a model of diabetes control incorporating the patient's biological and disease characteristics, psychic influences such as stress, the appropriateness of the medical therapy, and the degree to which the patient performed the recommended therapy. Results showed that relatively good control was possible without much knowledge of diabetes, that knowledge of diabetes was inversely correlated with control, and that the biological nature of the disease was an important factor in control.

From her observations of clinic patients, Backscheider (1974) concluded that four types of capacities were required to follow a diabetic regimen: cognitive, physical, motivational, and orientational, that is, concern with health in the daily activities. Cerkony and Hart (1980) tested the relationship between the HBM elements and compliance in 30 people treated with insulin, and accounted for 25% of the variance in compliance behavior.

Study variables

From the foregoing review, a theoretical model of compliance was adopted and is described in detail elsewhere (Jenny, 1983). The independent variables for the study were defined as follows:

- Belief in diagnosis: belief that the information received satisfactorily explains the health problem and supports the symptoms experienced

- Perceptions of severity: belief that the condition is serious and chronic and can cause further health problems
- Benefits of the regimen: perception that each aspect of the treatment prescribed is useful in controlling the condition
- Instruction: indication, yes or no, that instruction has been received about the condition, medication, diet, exercise, daily urine or blood monitoring, footcare, diabetic identification, and balancing aspects of the regimen
- Health motivation: the degree to which behavior supports one's health and degree of concern about health
- Social support: a composite of the number of people perceived as helpful in managing self-care, the number in the household, and the number of days of the teaching program attended
- Satisfaction with clinician: the degree to which the clinical staff was perceived as friendly, helpful, informative, and empathic
- Health problems: the number and kind of physical and functional problems with which the person must contend
- Family problems: perception of the degree to which problems within the family interfere with diabetes management
- Barriers: the sum of eight negative factors which might affect compliance with each aspect of the self-care regimen
- Special concerns: the degree to which eight specified negative perceptions contribute to the general burden of being diabetic

In addition, Green's (1970) three-factor formula was used to derive an index of the socioeconomic status. Years of education, range of income, and type of occupation all were considered. The dependent variables were *compliance*, the stated degree to which the person carried out the seven aspects of the therapeutic regimen, and *control*, a single number derived from a mean of the last six values for the fasting plasma glucose (FPG) on the person's clinical record.

METHOD
Setting and subjects

The study was conducted in a regional diabetic day center located in a large university-affiliated teaching hospital. Patients were accepted into the study if they were current members of the clinic, over age 16, had been following diabetic treatment for at least 6 months, and were able to read and write English sufficiently well to complete the testing instrument. The sample consisted of 245 adults with diabetes, from a total of roughly 3000 current files, ranging in age from 16 to 88 years of age. The average age was 54, with 73% of the sample over 45. Average age of onset was 45, and the mean number of years diagnosed was 9. Men comprised 48% of the sample, 56% were insulin dependent, and 10% took no medication. Patients saw the same physician at each clinic visit, and completed the self-report questionnaire during their visit. Data collection

TABLE 1   Correlation matrix of index scores

Index	1	2	3	4	5	6	7	8	9	10	11	12
1. Belief in diagnosis	1.0											
2. Perception of severity	0.14*	1.0										
3. Instruction	0.20‡	0.29§	1.0									
4. Regimen benefits	0.29§	0.26§	0.56§	1.0								
5. Satisfaction with clinicians	0.34§	0.05	0.03	0.24§	1.0							
6. Social support	0.07	0.12	0.18‡	0.21§	-0.06	1.0						
7. Health motivation	0.08	0.22§	0.07	0.19‡	0.17†	-0.04	1.0					
8. Health problems	-0.05	0.18‡	0.09	0.05	0.00	-0.15*	0.8	1.0				
9. Family problems	-0.08	0.07	0.12	0.02	-0.17†	0.04	0.10	0.21§	1.0			
10. Barriers	-0.07	0.02	0.10	-0.09	-0.25§	0.07	-0.12	0.14*	0.24§	1.0		
11. Special concerns	0.03	0.24§	0.15*	0.11	-0.11	0.05	0.12	0.15*	0.28§	0.34§	1.0	
12. Compliance	0.12*	0.19†	0.25§	0.48§	0.10	0.14*	0.18‡	-0.05	-0.06	-0.39§	-0.03	1.0
13. Control (FPG)	0.04	0.06	0.16†	0.04	-0.07	-0.06	-0.02	0.16†	0.15*	0.15*	0.14*	-0.02
Standard alpha	0.59	0.61	0.48	0.50	0.76	0.30	0.74	0.63	0.73	0.77	0.82	0.57

* p ≤ 0.05
† p ≤ 0.01
‡ p ≤ 0.005
§ p ≤ 0.001

occurred over a period of 5 weeks, and visits were made over rotating days of the week to obtain a representative sample of physician clients. All subjects were advised of the study objectives and signed an informed consent.

Instrument and data analysis

An original 10-page self-report questionnaire was used to operationalize the study variables. Several questions could be answered yes or no, but most used a five-point Likert scale of graduated agreement to disagreement. The demographic and clinical descriptors were checked with the subject's clinic record. No discrepancies were found.

In determining face validity, a panel of four clinicians was asked to identify the model element which each test item attempted to sample. The source of the majority of each item was correctly identified; the few presenting problems were dropped. Another factor considered was the distinctiveness of each construct representation. An index might be considered redundant if it correlated too closely with other indices. Kerlinger (1978) has suggested that an interscale correlation of 0.2 to 0.3 would indicate the distinctiveness of the areas sampled. Table 1 reveals only two coefficients higher than 0.3, which confirms the independence of the indices. A pilot study was conducted with 35 subjects, resulting in revision of the format and the dropping of two problem questions.

Questionnaire items were combined on the basis of manifest content to construct twelve index measures for the study variables. An index score was derived by summing its item scores. Indices did not contain the same number of questions or the same total score. Questionnaire data were coded and analyzed using selected programs for computer from the statistical package for the social sciences (Nie and associates, 1975).

A reliability test for internal consistency of each index using Cronbach's alpha (1951) standardized form revealed modest to moderate coefficients, with a mean of 0.63 (Table 1). Nunnally (1978) suggests that in the early stages of research on predictor tests an instrument with only modest reliability, between $r = \leq 0.5$ or ≤ 0.6, will suffice.

FINDINGS AND DISCUSSION

The predictive validity coefficients, determined by the correlation of the predictor test scores with scores on the criterion variable, are shown on Table 1. Seven of the eleven predictor variables are significantly associated with Compliance. The strongest indicators are Regimen benefits ($r = 0.48$, $p \leq 0.001$), Barriers ($r = 0.39$, $p \leq 0.001$), Instruction ($r = 0.25$, $p \leq 0.001$), Perceived severity ($r = 0.19$, $p \leq 0.005$), and health motivation ($r = 0.18$, $p \leq 0.005$), variables derived from the HBM. Although four variables showed nonsignificance (satisfaction, health and family problems, and concerns), all variables showed an association in the hypothesized direction. Instruction, the core construct

TABLE 2   Association between severity of diabetes and compliance

Medication	Levels of compliance		Row total
	Low	High	
Insulin	49 (35.5%)	89 (64.5%)	138 (56.1%)
Oral	37 (45.1%)	45 (54.9%)	82 (33.3%)
None	19 (73.1%)	7 (26.9%)	26 (10.6%)
TOTAL	105 (42.7%)	141 (57.3%)	246 (100%)

$\chi^2 (2) = 12.92$; $p \leq 0.002$.

of patient education, was positively associated with all the cognitive elements of the model.

Of the five variables associated with Control, none was below 0.01 level of significance. Only the negative variables, with Instruction, showed any relationship to Control (Table 1). There was no demonstrated association between Compliance and Control, a fact frequently remarked upon in the literature. Investigating disease severity effect on compliance, two levels of compliance were identified by dichotomizing the compliance scores into low and high groups. Table 2 depicts insulin-dependent subjects (64% of the high compliance group), resulting in a $\chi^2 (2) = 12.92$, $p \leq 0.002$. For this sample insulin-dependent subjects were characterized by better compliance and poorer control.

Construct validity demonstrates a relationship between the test instrument and the theoretically relevant variables: Do the supposed measures of the constructs behave as expected? Do they indicate the hypothesized direction and strength in their relationships with the criterion variables and the other model elements? Table 1 shows a clustering of variables around the two poles of the model, the positive (enabling) and the negative (modifying) elements. Positive variables, the first seven identified on the matrix, are all related to each other, as are the negative factors at the bottom of the matrix.

To demonstrate that the model can discriminate between groups of subjects, the sample was divided into two groups characterized by the only "hard" indicator available, FPG levels. The lower and upper thirds of the FPG continuum of scores contained two groups of equal numbers, n = 85, 86. It was hypothesized that the more severely affected (high FPG) group would display higher scores on the negative or modifier variables and on those reflecting the severity of the condition. Table 3 indicates a comparison of index scores between the two groups. The scores for each index reflect the hypothesized direction of variance. Scores for the four negative indices, Health Problems, Family Problems, Barriers, and Special Concerns, are all significantly higher for the High FPG group. It also shows higher Instruction scores. This corroborates Williams and associates' findings (1976), who suggest that those in poor

TABLE 3   Comparison of index means between high and low FPG groups

	High FPG ≥200 mg/dl (11.0 mmol/L)	Low FPG ≤150 mg/dl (8.3 mmol/L)	f Ratio
Belief in diagnosis	9.07	8.83	1.26
Perceived severity	13.93	13.52	1.41
Instruction	24.19	22.76	1.23
Benefits of regimen	20.47	19.88	1.04
Satisfaction with clinician	14.49	14.91	1.41
Social support	6.32	6.64	1.15
Health motivation	18.71	18.93	1.03
Health problems	4.33	3.25	2.05
Family problems	1.69	1.30	1.63
Barriers	2.24	1.67	2.28
Special concerns	9.24	6.93	1.49

df = 167.

control have more experience with problems and more attention paid to them, resulting in greater knowledge of the disease and regimen. Although not significant, the high FPG group also showed more acceptance of the diagnosis and greater perceived severity, less clinician satisfaction, and greater perceived regimen benefits. Possibly the continued inability to demonstrate improved control (as evidenced by a high FPG) elecits negative attitudes toward the care provider.

The model as a whole

It was assumed that a set of determinants, rather than a single factor, influenced subjects' decision to conform. To test how well the combination of model elements predicted compliance, multiple regression analyses were performed, employing three approaches; simple, hierarchical, and stepwise procedures. Table 4, with the variables entered in no predetermined order, displays the best results obtained. Four model elements combine to account for 40% of the variance. In the simple regression Clinician satisfaction and Concerns represent a negligible contribution yet have a significant correlation with other model elements. Presumably, their influence is subsumed into the territory of the others yet is necessary as a mediating influence on the significant variables.

Demographic variables

Only disease severity (as measured by type of medication) was significantly associated with compliance (χ^2 (2) = 12.93; $p \leq 0.002$). Age, income, and so-

TABLE 4   Regression of model elements on compliance

Variable	Multiple r	r Square	rsq Change	Beta	f
Age	0.02703	0.00073	0.00073	0.04857	0.447
Socioeconomic status	0.06545	0.00428	0.00355	−0.05942	1.016
FPG	0.07165	0.00513	0.00085	−0.05907	0.995
Medication	0.32383	0.10487	0.09973	−0.19686	9.119*
Belief in diagnosis	0.34466	0.11879	0.01392	−0.00148	0.001
Perceived severity	0.38656	0.14943	0.03064	−0.09233	2.467*
Instruction	0.41181	0.16959	0.02016	0.01996	0.084
Regimen benefits	0.52004	0.27044	0.10085	0.34534	23.029*
Health motivation	0.52598	0.27666	0.00622	0.06499	1.326
Clinician satisfaction	0.52602	0.27669	0.00004	−0.06337	1.037
Social support	0.53070	0.28164	0.00495	0.06540	1.081
Health problems	0.54237	0.29417	0.01253	−0.05909	1.011
Family problems	0.54309	0.29417	0.00078	0.01671	0.082
Barriers	0.62620	0.39213	0.09718	−0.35074	32.491*
Concerns	0.62621	0.39214	0.00002	0.00500	0.007

Multiple r = 0.62621.
r Square = 0.39214.
*p = ≤ 0.01
df = 15,218
f = 9.38*

cioeconomic status were all negatively associated with compliance. Teaching was positively though weakly associated (χ^2 (2) = 3.6; p ≤ 0.1). Subjects claiming no instruction were almost evenly divided between the high and low compliance cells, but of the group claiming 4 days of instruction, twice as many were in the high compliance cell.

Disease severity was the only descriptor associated significantly with control. Age, income, and socioeconomic status were all negatively associated, but not at significant levels. These findings are consistent with conclusions reached in the compliance literature, which fails to demonstrate a consistent predictive demographic characteristic (Haynes, 1976).

Limitations of the study

Limitations of the study, including a nonstandardized instrument of modest reliability, a convenience sample of compliance-oriented clinic patients (their presence at the clinic implies a certain level of compliance with regard to their health problem), and the use of self-report limit the applicability of the study findings. Repeating the study with a questionnaire of increased reliability, a broader subject sampling, and utilizing additional measures of compliance to complement the self-report would be desirable.

Implications for practice

Better patient teaching can result from knowledge of factors affecting patients' decision to conform to prescribed regimes of self-care. To assist with diagnosis of patients' educational needs, a brief list of questions employing the study variables could help identify patients' perceptions of their situation. Variables with a poor response would indicate areas for clinician assistance, perhaps additional instruction or referral to other care providers. Since disease severity was a significant predictor of patient variance, separate instructional groups might facilitate counselling directed to specific topics or levels of need. Elements of the model could profile differences in the needs of older versus youthful patients (Jenny, in press). Since three elements accounted for nearly 40% of patient variance, teaching strategies in any diabetes program should emphasize topics of perceived severity of diabetes, the regimen benefits, and specific methods for overcoming perceived barriers to self-care.

REFERENCES

Backsheider, J.E.: Self-care requirements, self-care capabilities, and nursing systems in the diabetic nurse management clinic, Am. J. Public Health **64**:1138-1146, 1974.

Becker, M.H.: Understanding patient compliance: The contribution of attitudes and other psychosocial factors. In Cohen, S.J., editor: New directions in patient compliance, Lexington, Mass., 1979, Lexington Books.

Becker, M.H., and others: Selected psychosocial models and correlates of individual health-related behavior, Med. Care **15**:27-46, 1977.

Becker, M.H., and Maiman, L.A.: Sociobehavioral determinants of compliance with health and medical care recommendations, Med. Care **13**:10-20, 1975.

Berkowitz, N.H., Malone, M.F., Klein, M.M., and Eaton, A.: Patient follow-up in the out-patient department, Nurs. Res. **12**:16-23, 1963.

Bowen, R.G., Rich, R.R., and Schlotfeldt, R.M.: Effects of organized instruction for patients with the diagnosis of diabetes mellitus, Nurs. Res. **10**:151-159, 1961.

Cerkony, K.A., and Hart, L.K.: Relationship between the health belief model and compliance of patients with diabetes mellitus, Diabetes Care **3**:594-598, 1980.

Cronbach, L.J.: Coefficient alpha and the internal structure of tests, Psychometrika **16**:297-335, 1951.

Donabedian, A., and Rosenfeld, L.S.: Follow-up study of chronically ill patients discharged from hospital, J. Chron. Dis. **17**:847-862, 1964.

Green, L.O.: A manual for scoring socioeconomic status for research on health behavior, Public Health Rep. **85**:815-827, 1970.

Halloner, W.M.: The diabetic supplement of the National Health Survey, III. The patient reports on his diet, J. Am. Diet. Assoc. **52**:387-396, 1968.

Haynes, R.B.: A critical review of the determinants of patient compliance with the regimen, In Sackett, D.L., and Haynes, R.B., editors: Compliance with therapeutic regimens, Baltimore, 1976, The Johns Hopkins University Press.

Jenny, J.: A humanistic strategy for patient teaching, Health Values **3**:175-180, 1979.

Jenny, J.: A compliance model for diabetic instruction, Rehabil. Lit. **44**:258-263, 1983.

Jenny, J.: A comparison of four age groups' adaptation to diabetes. Can. J. Public Health **75:**237-244, 1984.

Kerlinger, F.N.: Foundations of behavioral research, New York, 1978, Holt, Rinehart & Winston.

Nie, N.H., Hull, C.H., Jenkins, J., Steinbrenner, K., and Bent, D.H.: Statistical package for the social sciences, New York, 1975, McGraw-Hill Book Co.

Nunnally, J.: Psychometric theory, New York, 1978, McGraw-Hill Book Co.

Redman, B.K.: Issues and concepts in patient education, New York, 1981, Appleton-Century-Crofts.

Rosenstock, I.M.: The historical origins of the health belief model, Health Educ. Monogr. **2:**325-336, 1974.

Sackett, D.H., and Haynes, R.B.: Compliance with therapeutic regimens, Baltimore, 1976, The Johns Hopkins University Press.

Skyler, J.S.: Complications of diabetes mellitus: relationships to metabolic dysfunction, Diabetes Care **2:**457-535, 1979.

Tagliacozzo, D.M., Lushkin, D.B., Lashof, J.C., and Ima, K.: Nurse intervention and patient behavior, Am. J. Public Health **64:**596-603, 1974.

Watkins, J., and others: A study of diabetic patients at home, Am. J. Public Health **57:**452-457, 1967.

Williams, T.F., and others: The clinical picture of diabetes control, studied in four clinical settings, Am. J. Public Health **57:**441-451, 1976.

Development of an instrument to measure altered levels of awareness in significant others who have experienced psychological impact

KAREN LAWSON, M.N., R.N.
NANCY R. LACKEY, Ph.D., R.N.

A nursing diagnosis is described as an existing or potential health problem that nurses are qualified and licensed to treat. Nursing diagnosis suggests an etiology requiring interventions within the realm of nursing. Nursing interventions are centered around the client and his family. The Third National Conference on the Classification of Nursing Diagnoses accepted approximately 37 broad diagnostic category areas that nurses can use to state the client's actual or potential health problem. Altered levels of consciousness is one of these diagnoses (Price, 1980). This investigator believes this diagnostic category to be too general to depict clearly the client's health problem.

Gatschet (1982) summarized nursing diagnosis by stating that it is an essential component within the nursing process. It is the concept on which the unique body of nursing knowledge is being built. She pointed out that nurses might choose to develop a new nursing diagnosis. The need to observe and describe in detail certain nursing diagnoses is essential to expand and develop this unique body of nursing knowledge.

PURPOSE

This study was designed to identify the defining characteristics for the nursing diagnosis of altered levels of awareness of significant others who have experienced psychological impact due to an injury or illness of a loved one and to develop an instrument which would measure these levels. Defining characteristics needed to be identified so these levels could be diagnosed and appropriate nursing interventions instituted.

BACKGROUND

The review of literature contained citations which alluded to this phenomenon of altered levels of awareness due to psychological impact. The review of literature failed to substantiate the defining characteristics of altered levels of awareness of significant others who have experienced psychological impact. Nursing needs a well-documented definition of altered levels of awareness due to psychological impact which has predictive validity across a variety of personality types and nursing situations.

The literature review centered on induced states of consciousness which occur during hypnosis, ingestion of alcohol and/or drugs, and near-death experiences (Hine, 1978; Ludwig and Levine, 1966; Tart, 1972). Characteristics were identified which were present in most altered states of consciousness.

Ludwig and Levine (1966) were able to demonstrate the presence of many features in alterations of consciousness induced by hypnosis and LSD. According to Ludwig and Levine, similar features, in greater or lesser degree, tend to be characteristic of most altered states of consciousness. The characteristics identified were alterations in thinking, disturbed time sense, loss of control, change in emotional expression, body image change, perceptual distortions, change in meaning or significance, sense of the ineffable, feelings of rejuvenation, and hypersuggestibility.

Noyes and Kletti (1976) conducted a descriptive analysis of near-death experiences. A variety of life-threatening circumstances were responsible for the experiences reported such as falls, near-drownings, automobile accidents, serious illnesses, battlefield explosions, cardiac arrests, allergic reactions, and miscellaneous accidents. The subjective phenomena reported through the analysis were: altered passage of time, unusually vivid thoughts, increased speed of thoughts, sense of detachment, feeling of unreality, automatic movements, lack of emotion, detachment from body, sharper vision or hearing, revival of memories, great understanding, a variety of colors or sharper vision, sense of harmony or unity, control by external force, objects small or far away, vivid mental images and hearing voices, music, or sounds.

Watson and Wyatt (1981) used Ludwig's and Levine's characteristics in formulating a behavioral definition for altered levels of awareness. They identified alterations in the sensory-perceptual environment, body chemistry, and neurophysiological processes as the three major causes or antecedents of altered levels of awareness and generalized one behavioral definition for these altered levels of awareness. The objective behaviors were described as alterations in thought processes, change in the individual's attention span, and lability in emotional expressions. Subjective feelings were: feelings of loss of control, change in the meaning and significance of what is being observed and experienced, a sense of rejuvenation, ineffability, and expressions of altered body image. Neither specific examples nor validated research were reported to establish these behavioral characteristics.

A pilot study was conducted by Lawson (1980) to identify the defining characteristics of altered states of consciousness of significant others due to psychological impact. The characteristics identified by Ludwig and Levine (1966) were used as a basis for this study. All of the characteristics described by Ludwig and Levine were found to be applicable except for perceptual distortions.

An altered level of awareness can result from a variety of stressors. The altered level of awareness can be present in the significant others as well as in the client. Practicing nurses are confronted with altered levels of awareness due to acute illness and trauma in a variety of settings such as emergency rooms, intensive care units, surgery units, community health centers, and clinics. Many times altered levels of awareness of significant others who have experienced psychological impact are not diagnosed. Altered levels of awareness of significant others must be identified and assessed in order for nurses to intervene appropriately. This investigator believes the proper assessment of altered levels of awareness has implications for nursing. This seems especially important when nurses instruct the significant other regarding the care and prognosis of the client. If these levels remain undiagnosed and appropriate adaptive measures are not employed, the person's emotional state may deteriorate and he may not carry out the instructions given by the health personnel. As a result, he may have to come back to the hospital or he may misinterpret the prognosis. Failure of the nurse to identify an altered level of awareness may lead to miscommunication that later could be grounds for a liability suit of negligence and malpractice. Thus, it seemed imperative to conduct an empirical study of this nursing diagnosis.

DEFINITION OF TERMS

The following terms were defined to assist in limiting this analysis and attaining comprehension. Common language was retained for terms not defined here.

An altered state of awareness is "different from the state of awareness in which one spends the majority of time" (Armstrong, 1977). For the purpose of this study, the terms *altered states of awareness, altered levels of awareness,* and *altered states of consciousness* were used interchangeably. For consistency in this study, the phenomenon was referred to as altered levels of awareness.

An altered state of consciousness is a "qualitative alteration in the overall pattern of mental functioning, such that the experiencer feels his consciousness is radically different from the way it functions ordinarily" (Tart, 1972). An altered state of consciousness is on a continuum from blissful states to unconsciousness.

Psychological impact is the mental process which follows the sudden accident or acute or chronic illness of a close friend or family member.

A significant other is a family member or friend emotionally involved with the victim who is present during the event or immediately thereafter.

Perception of the event is the significant other's interpretation of the event.

Trauma is any physical injury great enough to cause a psychological impact in a significant other and great enough to send the client to the hospital on an emergency basis.

Sense of the ineffable is an "inability to communicate the nature of an experience to someone who has not undergone a similar experience; the tendency of people to develop varying degrees of amnesias for their experiences during profound alterations in consciousness" (Ludwig, 1966).

ASSUMPTIONS

The assumptions of this study were that

1. Persons experiencing altered levels of awareness are able to recall their behaviors and feelings experienced as a result of psychological impact once they return to a normal level of awareness.

2. There are common characteristics of altered levels of awareness in everyone which can be identified and assessed.

3. After the altered level of awareness has been resolved, the person returns to a "normal" level of awareness.

4. Altered levels of awareness may be verbally and/or nonverbally communicated.

5. Once the loved ones are out of danger, their significant other returns to his normal or usual way of thinking and feeling (Jones, 1982).

LIMITATIONS

1. Some of the behavioral manifestations of anxiety are similar to those of altered levels of awareness, but the literature did not differentiate between the two. The purpose of this study was to identify the defining characteristics of altered levels of awareness, but this investigator did not attempt to differentiate between altered levels of awareness and anxiety.

2. The data were as reliable and valid as the subjects utilized were willing to share their true thoughts and feelings.

DELIMITATION

This study focused only on a continuum of altered levels of awareness of significant others who have experienced psychological impact due to an injury or illness of a loved one.

METHOD
Subjects

There were two groups of subjects used in developing the instrument. For further references they will be referred to as Group A and Group B. Demographic data were collected for members of both groups.

Group A (panel of experts) comprised five professionals with expertise in the area of altered levels of awareness. Each member has conducted research with either near-death situations or out-of-body experiences, which are both considered as altered levels of awareness.

Group B consisted of 30 persons known to this investigator. The following criteria had to have been met in Group B:

1. Subject was an adult (18 years of age or older).
2. Subject was a family member or close friend who was emotionally involved with a patient who had been involved in an emergency situation.
3. Subject was available to complete the instrument two times in a 4-week period.
4. The emergency situation did not result in the death of the patient.
5. Subject stated the crisis situation had been resolved.
6. Subject was able to read, write, and understand English.

Each of the persons in Group B had been emotionally involved with a patient in a situation within the past 12 months. In all of the emergency situations, the crisis had been resolved; however, four had residual deficits. Examples of factors which precipitated the emergency situations were: mitral valve prolapses, gunshot wounds, asthma attacks, viral encephalitis, GI bleed, brain stem injury, third degree burns, stroke, fractured pelvis, fractured hip, fractured leg, and seizure. The purpose of this group was to establish the reliability of the instrument as a whole by the test-retest procedure.

Instrument

An instrument was developed on the basis of a review of the literature, experiences of the investigator, and study Groups A and B. Content validity was used to identify those behaviors and feelings believed to be indicative of altered levels of awareness due to psychological impact. Test reliability was established by the test-retest procedure.

Study Group A established content validity by the Q-sort methodology. A list of 102 behaviors and feelings were derived from characteristics identified by Ludwig and Levine (1966), research completed by Noyes and Kletti (1976), and personal experiences of this investigator. These behaviors and feelings were believed to be indicative of altered levels of awareness due to psychological impact. Examples of some of these behaviors and feelings were increased speed of thoughts; seeing things happen in slow motion; calm, automatic movements; feeling that one's body is not a part of one, and feeling that the world is unreal.

The panel of experts (Group A) were mailed the 102 cards to Q-sort. Each member was instructed to rank from the most to the least important the behaviors and feelings which they perceived to be significant in determining altered levels of awareness due to psychological impact. Each member was given the opportunity to add other behaviors or feelings which he/she believed to be important but were not included in the data. However, any additions by any panel member were not included in the first Q-sort. One panel member added four behaviors of feelings which he believed also to be indicative of altered levels of awareness due to psychological impact. They were as follows:

103. Peace
104. Awareness of nonphysical being present
105. Awareness of things going on elsewhere, as if by ESP
106. Entering some other, unearthly world

Seventy of the 102 behaviors and feelings which were sorted the first time by Group A had a mean rank of 60 or below, with number 1 being most indicative of altered levels of awareness. Behaviors and feelings receiving a mean rank above 60 were deleted before the second Q-sort. The 70 remaining behaviors and feelings were changed to items which were indicative of altered levels of awareness due to psychological impact. For example, the behavior and feeling of "Went blank" was changed to "Everything seemed to go blank." "Loss of control" was changed to, "I felt as though I had lost control." Each of these 70 items plus the four identified by one panel member was printed on a 3 × 5 card and returned to each member of Group A. The member was instructed to rank again the items as to how well he/she measured the behaviors and feelings indicative of altered levels of awareness from the most to the least important. Items from the list that yielded a mean rank of less than 40 were utilized to develop the instrument. There were 38 items remaining. The 38 were randomly placed upon a four-point Likert-type scale with a separate column to indicate if an item could not be recalled. Thirteen of these items were negatively stated, and 25 were positively stated to avoid response set bias.

Once the instrument was devised, the reliability of the test as a whole was established by the test-retest procedure. A description of the study, a return envelope, and the instrument were mailed to each member of Group B. Each member of Group B was instructed to recall his emergency situation with a loved one and to complete the instrument regarding his feelings at the time of the incident. Upon returning the first instrument, each subject was sent an identical copy of the instrument to complete again regarding his feelings at the time of the emergency incident. A minimum of 1 week elapsed from the first administration of the instrument before the second instrument was mailed. After the 30 instruments were returned the second time, a correlation coefficient was calculated to determine reliability of the instrument, and coefficient alpha was calculated to determine internal consistency of the instrument.

RESULTS

The total scores for the first and second administration of the instrument for each subject were analyzed by the Pearson product-moment correlation coefficient. The correlation coefficient obtained was 0.77. The range of the sum of the scores for each subject on the first administration of the instrument was from 102 to 144. The range of the sum of the scores for each subject on the second administration of the instrument was from 101 to 148. Means, standard deviations, and standard error of mean were also computed for each of the 38 items on the post-test.

Polit and Hungler (1983) stated that the coefficient alpha (or Cronbach's alpha) is a method of testing internal consistency. It produces a reliability coefficient which can be interpreted by the same means as other reliability coefficients. Coefficient alpha is not really a necessary statistical measure for this study since a test-retest was conducted. However, due to the experimental nature of these data, a coefficient alpha was completed. The internal consistency as measured by the coefficient alpha was .85. This finding, too, according to Nunnally (1978), demonstrates a high degree of instrument reliability.

DISCUSSION OF THE FINDINGS
Defining characteristics

The defining characteristics of altered levels of awareness due to psychological impact were identified in this study. The defining characteristics may be divided into nine of the 10 categories identified by Ludwig and Levine (1966). The nine categories identified in this study were alteration in thinking, disturbed time sense, loss of control, change in emotional expression, body image changes, perceptual distortions, change in meaning or significance, sense of the ineffable, and hypersuggestibility. The majority of the defining characteristics were concerned with alteration in thinking, disturbed time sense, changes in emotional expressions, perceptual distortions, and body image changes. Of the four characteristics added by one of the expert panel members, only one, peace, was retained by the panel of experts for the development of the instrument.

The criteria which were validated in this study were also the same as described by Ludwig and Levine (1966). However, Ludwig and Levine identified the feeling of rejuvenation, which was not validated by this study. Similar characteristics were also identified by Noyes and Kletti (1976) in their research with near-death experiences and by Watson and Wyatt (1981) in their behavioral definition of altered levels of awareness.

It may not be feasible for nurses during an emergency incident to administer the developed instrument to identify altered levels of awareness of significant others due to psychological impact. Therefore, it will be necessary for nurses to assess the significant others for the presence of behaviors which might indicate that an altered level of awareness exists. Both verbal and nonverbal cues must be assessed. Behaviors which the nurse might observe are extreme calmness, excessive talking, pacing back and forth, frequently watching the clock, or frequently asking the time. The significant others might have a blank look on their faces and have to be touched or spoken to in order to gain their attention. Others may be hyperacute and jump at every little noise or interruption. Quite frequently the significant other is heard to say, "I can't believe this is happening to me." Thus, it is imperative for nurses to assess the significant others for behaviors which might indicate altered levels of awareness. These behaviors which are observable need to be validated.

Instrument

In this study an instrument was developed to measure altered levels of awareness of significant others who have experienced psychological impact due to an injury or illness of a loved one. It is called the Lawson's scale to assess altered levels of awareness. As evidenced by a correlation coefficient of 0.77 and a coefficient alpha of 0.85, reliability for the instrument has been established. As manifested by these findings, it is evident that persons experiencing altered levels of awareness are able to recall their behaviors and feelings which they experienced as a result of psychological impact once they return to a normal level of awareness.

Many of the characteristics included for the panel of experts (Group A) to Q-sort the first time were similar. There were many which were concerned with alteration in thinking, disturbed time sense, and alteration in body image. Due to the similarity and large number of these characteristics, the ranking of these characteristics was difficult. There was one characteristic which was omitted on the first Q sort by Group A which this investigator believes to be indicative of altered levels of awareness due to psychological impact. This was "open to suggestions or decisions made by others," which indicates hyper-suggestibility. This phenomenon has been witnessed by this investigator several times.

There were 15 items which were omitted by the second Q-sort with a ranking of between 40 and 45. This rank was very close to the cutoff point of below 40. These items should be considered for future research. Some of the items were

35. I would like to have done things differently.
36. I felt as though I was controlled or influenced by some outside force.
50. I was afraid.
53. I did not believe what was happening.

There needs to be more research completed to refine this instrument.

IMPLICATIONS FOR NURSING PRACTICE

According to Gatschet (1982) the identification and description of a nursing diagnosis is the means by which nursing knowledge can be further compiled, supplemented, and researched. The nursing diagnosis identification is the reason for nursing care, and from the nursing diagnosis flows the plan of interventions individually designed for each client. She emphasized the need to observe and describe in detail certain nursing diagnoses in order to expand and develop a unique body of nursing knowledge. This study endeavored to contribute to this body of nursing knowledge by the description of the nursing diagnosis Altered levels of awareness due to psychological impact.

This study should make nurses aware of the existence of the important nursing diagnosis Altered levels of awareness due to psychological impact. It can be identified in many different client populations. Nurses need to be able to identify and assess it. The assessment of this nursing diagnosis can indicate the need for the nurse to provide psychological support for the significant other, even though the significant other's actions may not reflect his inner turmoil. At this point the type of psychological support needed for the significant other has not been ascertained. Further research should be done to determine what nursing interventions are necessary.

The instrument can be used by nurses to assess the significant other's level of awareness in many different settings. It may be administered before the prognosis of the client is given, before home instructions are given, and before the significant others are asked to make important decisions. It may be necessary for the nurse to repeat the same things time and time again. The significant other should be asked to repeat to the nurse the prognosis of the loved one, home instructions, or his interpretation of what has been explained to him. These repetitions will help the nurse to determine whether or not the significant other is cognating effectively. Also the significant other should be given the opportunity to phone the nurse at any time he might have a question regarding instructions he has been given. It may also be necessary for the nurse to write on paper the prognosis or home instructions. If it is determined by the administration of the instrument that the significant other is indeed in an altered level of awareness, interventions should be taken to alleviate or further assess this state before further nursing interventions are implemented.

The identification and assessment of this nursing diagnosis are necessary to enhance the communication process between client and family, client and the health-care providers, and family and the health-care providers. If the significant other is in an altered level of awareness, he will not be cognating effectively to communicate with the loved one. This altered level of awareness may be perceived by the loved one and heighten his fears and concerns. The needed psychological support may not be given to the loved one by the significant other when an altered level of awareness exists. The significant other also needs to be able to convey to the health-care providers his feelings and concerns. In addition, the significant other needs to be aware and able to comprehend instructions given by the health care providers.

In summary, the assessment of this important nursing diagnosis of altered levels of awareness of significant others due to psychological impact enhances the nursing process and improves client-family care. The nursing diagnosis identification is the reason for the nursing care; from the nursing diagnosis flows the plan of interventions individually designed for each client and family. Since altered levels of awareness is a psychosocial state, it must be assessed by subjective validation by the client. Thus, the need to administer this instrument seems to be imperative.

RECOMMENDATIONS FOR FUTURE RESEARCH

There has been little nursing research done which is concerned with the significant others of patients who become ill suddenly or are involved in accidents. Now that this instrument has been developed, more research can proceed in this area. The following are recommendations for future studies:

1. The developed instrument should be given to a group of significant others of clients who are involved in an emergency-type situation in order to establish construct validity of the instrument.

2. Item analysis should be completed on the instrument to establish the validity of each item included in the instrument.

3. Since the relationship between altered levels of awareness and anxiety is unknown, a study should be designed to differentiate between the two by using the developed instrument and Spielberger's *State-Trait Anxiety Inventory.*

4. A study should be done to determine whether a correlation exists between the responses of the significant others that indicate altered levels of awareness and the degree of seriousness of an injury or acute illness.

5. A study should be conducted to validate the verbal and nonverbal behaviors of altered levels of awareness due to psychological impact.

6. After refinement of the instrument, a study should be done utilizing the instrument to examine sudden-death producing incidents whereby decision making was necessary by the significant other during an altered level of awareness. An example is the client with a massive head injury which resulted in brain death. How can family members be expected to make decisions regarding life-preservation means under these circumstances?

REFERENCES

Armstrong, M.E.: Use of altered states of awareness in nursing practice, AORN J. **25**(1):49-53, 1977.

Gatschet, C.: Nursing diagnosis. A term whose time has come, Kansas Nurse **57**(1):8-9, 1982.

Hine, V.H.: Altered states of consciousness: a form of death education? Death Educ. **1**:377-396, 1978.

Jones, F.: Personal interview, Kansas City, Kans., July 1982.

Lawson, K.S.: Altered states of consciousness due to psychological impact. Unpublished paper prepared for "The nursing process: nursing diagnosis as a directive for care of the chronically ill adult patient," 1980, Pittsburg, Kansas, through The University of Kansas.

Ludwig, A.M.: Altered states of consciousness, Arch. Gen. Psychiatry **15:**225-233, 1966.

Noyes, R., and Kletti, R.: Depersonalization in the face of life-threatening danger: a description, Psychiatry **39:**19-27, 1976.

Nunnally, J.C.: Psychometric theory, ed. 2, New York, 1978, McGraw-Hill Book Co.

Polit, D., and Hungler, B.: Nursing research: principles and methods, ed. 2, Philadelphia, 1983, J.B. Lippincott Co.

Price, M.R.: Nursing diagnosis: making a concept come alive, Am. J. Nurs. **80**(4):668-671, 1980.

Tart, C., editor: Altered states of consciousness, ed. 2, New York, 1982, Doubleday & Co., Inc.

Watson, C.A., and Wyatt, N.N.: Altered levels of awareness. In Hart, L.K., Reese, J.L., and Fearing, M.O., editors: Concepts common to acute illness, St. Louis, 1981, The C.V. Mosby Co.

Diagnosing altered comfort states: analysis of pain expression styles of blacks and whites

JUDITH FITZGERALD MILLER, M.S.N., R.N.

While there is disagreement about the nature of nursing and nursing's specific phenomena of concern for research and intervention, there is general agreement that diagnosing and treating altered comfort states is a priority for nursing intervention and continued study. Diagnosing and treating pain is also congruent with social expectation for nurses' care; that is, patients and prospective clients expect and trust nurses to have competence to provide comfort. Developing the competence expected of nurses in diagnosing and treating pain is dependent on research on these aspects of pain management.

In specific acute care settings, the nursing diagnosis, altered comfort states is the diagnosis which occurs with the highest frequency. This is confirmed in hospital areas such as surgical, orthopedic, rheumatology, and emergency rooms as well as in hospice settings. Patients in these settings are challenged with accomplishing pain tasks of pain expression, pain endurance, and obtaining pain relief (Fagerhaugh and Strauss, 1977; Strauss and associates, 1974). Pain tasks of the nurse, on the other hand, include diagnosing pain, preventing pain, and providing pain relief. Diagnosing pain states by analyzing the patient task of pain expression is the focus of this research. It is hoped that specific qualities of pain expression identified will be reflected in the defining characteristics of the nursing diagnosis Altered comfort states.

Cultural differences in the manifestation of various nursing diagnoses have not been addressed in published studies on nursing diagnoses to date. Specifically cultural differences in verbal reports of pain have not been addressed by the current classification system.

A common characteristic of altered comfort states is the patient's verbal report describing the pain (Carpenito, 1983; Kim and Moritz, 1982). Gordon's (1982) definition of alteration in comfort states that pain is "verbal report and presence of indicators of severe discomfort." The patient's verbal report of pain is viewed by some as the most reliable indicator for diagnosing an altered comfort state (Hilgard, 1969; Jacox, 1979; McCaffery, 1979). Despite the importance of patients' verbal communication regarding their pain state for accurate diagnosis of pain, reported studies have not systematically examined the content of patient self-disclosure to determine the nature of pain expression styles of individuals in pain.

The purpose of this study was to determine the effects of race, sex, and age on pain expression styles of hospitalized patients in acute pain. *Pain expression style* refers to (1) willingness of the patient to use pain disclosure statements,

(2) the variety and number of pain descriptors used, and (3) the variety and number of pain intensifiers used. *Pain descriptors* refers to types of descriptive words patients use to convey the nature of the pain (i.e., sore, tender, spasm). *Pain intensifiers* refers to types of descriptive words patients use to convey the intensity of their pain (i.e., unbearable, severe, mild). *Pain disclosure statements* are the number of entire phrases patients use to disclose the nature and/or intensity of their pain (Shuter and Miller, 1982). The literature review reported here will be limited to pain and communication and pain and culture.

PAIN AND COMMUNICATION

Early studies on pain and communication focused on development of word lists or typologies of pain descriptors so that physicians could associate patients' selected terminology with a tentative medical diagnosis (Dana, 1911). Melzack and Torgersen (1971) devised a detailed word list categorizing 102 pain descriptors into three categories of complaints: sensory, affective, and evaluative. The purpose of their work was to develop a means for patients to accurately describe a pain sensation and for professionals to accurately interpret the patient's expression. Melzack and Torgersen hoped that the pain descriptors could be used to develop a questionnaire for evaluating the effectiveness of anesthetics and analgesics. A modified form of this tool (McGill-Melzack Pain Questionnaire) has been used as a nursing pain assessment tool (Meissner, 1980). Agnew and Merskey (1976) interviewed 128 ambulatory patients with chronic pain to determine the types of word descriptors used for pain of organic and psychiatric origins. Forty-six patients with organic diagnoses used sensory-thermal (hot, burning) words more frequently than the psychiatric patients. The sixty-three psychiatric patients used sensory-tempered descriptors (throbbing, beating, pounding) but used fewer descriptive words in total than patients in the organic group. The 19 patients with mixed diagnoses (both organic and psychiatric) used affective-tension words (nagging, tiring).

The need for verbal expression of an individual's pain state in order for the patient to obtain relief was noted in a study by Bond and Pilowsky (1966). Forty-seven patients with advanced cancer were studied to determine the relationship between the patient's subjective assessment of pain (recorded in a diary), communication of pain and the reaction of the nursing staff in terms of the treatment given for pain relief. Although 38 of the 47 subjects recorded that they did have pain, thirteen of the subjects experiencing pain did not verbally request pain relief and did not receive any pain intervention from the nurse. Although women made fewer requests for pain medication than men, women received more powerful analgesics than men. Besides the gender differences, a profound finding of the study was, if the patient did not speak up, pain intervention was not provided (Bond and Pilowsky, 1966).

Baer and associates (1970) studied inferences of physical pain and psychological distress in relation to verbal and nonverbal patient communication. Twenty-five social workers, 25 nurses, and 24 physicians reviewed 16 paired vignettes: one in which the patients verbalized discomfort and the other in which discomfort was expressed through patient nonverbal behavior. The professionals rated the amount of physical pain and psychological distress they noted in the patients. All three groups of professionals inferred greater pain for subjects with verbal indicators. The social workers inferred the greatest amount of pain, followed by nurses, and physicians inferred the least pain. Verbalization of the pain state was important for the nurse to recognize pain and therefore initiate a pain relief strategy.

Jacox (1979) interviewed 443 nurses to determine what nurses used as a basis for pain assessment. Despite verbal communication being described as the most reliable indicator of the degree of pain a patient is suffering, nurses reported that physiologic signs were more frequently used as an indicator of pain than the patient's verbal communication.

PAIN AND CULTURE

Mark Zborowski's (1952) conclusions about four different cultural groups and pain pervades almost all literature on pain response and cultural differences. Zborowski studied 26 "Old Americans," 24 Italians, 31 Jews, and 11 Irish subjects using retrospective interviews with the patients (after the pain episode), observations of patients' behavior, discussion of "individual cases" with doctors, nurses, and other people directly or indirectly involved in the pain experience of the individual. Healthy family members were interviewed to determine their attitudes toward pain. The results of his qualitative study are summarized according to each cultural group. Jews and Italians were very emotional in their response to pain (exaggerated their pain experience, being very sensitive to pain). They freely expressed feelings and emotions by words, sounds, and gestures, complained about pain, manifested their sufferings by groaning, moaning, and crying. They willingly admitted they were in pain and expected sympathy and assistance from others. This uninhibited display of expression provokes distrust in helpers instead of provoking sympathy. The Italians were concerned with the immediacy of the pain experience and were disturbed by the actual pain sensation which they experienced at the present. Once the pain was relieved, the Italians were no longer distressed. The Jews, on the other hand, focused on the symptomatic meaning of pain, significance of pain in relation to future functioning, future health and welfare. The Jews were reluctant to display complete relief. The Old Americans displayed a role of a detached, unemotional observer during their pain experience. Patients who did not fall into the category of quiet suffering were viewed by the staff as deviants, hypochondriacal, and neurotic. Old Americans viewed emotionality as purposeless and hindering in the situation which calls for knowledge, skill and efficiency. Irish Americans were stoical, and afraid to "act like babies" by displaying discomfort (Zborowski, 1952).

Sternbach and Tursky (1965) studied pain perception thresholds and pain tolerance in 60 women of Jewish, Italian, Irish, and Yankee origin by use of an electric shock to the forearm. Yankee women tended to have a "matter of fact attitude" toward pain. Italians showed a present time-orientation focusing on the immediacy of the pain. Jewish subjects were future oriented and were not dismayed by the experimental pain. Irish were undemonstrative. The pain tolerance (in this laboratory setting using experimental pain) was greatest for Yankees, followed by Jews, then Irish, and Italians having the least pain tolerance.

Similar to the above research, studies involving blacks examined pain tolerance, pain attitudes, and pain anxiety without analysis of explicit documentation about how the subjects expressed the nature and intensity of pain. Chapman and Jones (1944) concluded that differences in pain sensitivity and tolerance exist due to "ethnic factors." A pain stimulus of radiant heat to the forehead was used to compare pain tolerance in 18 blacks with 18 Americans of Northern European ancestry. They found that blacks had a lower pain perception threshold and were able to tolerate less pain than the Northern Europeans. Chapman and Jones also studied a total of 30 individuals divided into groups of Russian, Jewish, and Italian subjects. These subjects had pain perception and reaction thresholds similar to the blacks. Of particular interest was that the subjects of Mediterranean descent complained loudly, whereas the blacks did not complain similarly. McCabe's (1960) qualitative observations of hospitalized black Americans concluded blacks were hesitant to ask for relief of pain.

To determine differences in response to obstetrical pain between blacks and whites, Winsberg and Greenlich (1967) studied 207 white and 158 black women immediately after childbirth. The patients and staff (physician, nurse, and aide) independently evaluated the patient's degree of pain and response on a five point scale. No differences were found between blacks' and whites' rating of their pain intensity. However, the subjects uniformly rated their pain as being more severe than was judged by the staff.

Anxiety and pain attitudes of blacks, whites, and Puerto Rican patients in an outpatient dental emergency clinic were studied using the *State-Trait Anxiety Inventory*, palmar sweat prints, interviews, dental anxiety scales, and posttreatment dentist rating of fear, pain reaction, discomfort, and cooperation (Weisenberg, Kreindler, Schachat, and Werboff, 1975). Puerto Rican subjects were the most anxious, followed by blacks, with whites being least anxious. Puerto Rican subjects were "interested in denying, getting rid of the pain and not dealing with it." Whites were the most willing to confront and deal with the pain, whereas blacks seemed to fall in the middle in relation to their attitude about pain.

Pain tolerance was measured in 41,119 subjects using the automated multiphasic screening test and found that (1) tolerance to pain decreased with age; (2) men tolerated more pain than women; and (3) whites tolerated more pain than Orientals, while blacks occupied an intermediate pain tolerance between whites and Orientals (Woodrow and associates, 1975).

These studies indicate there is a difference in pain tolerance, sensitivity, and response by various cultural groups. However, the nature of the expression of pain and requests for pain relief have not been systematically studied. Since persons of different race, sex, and age appear to differ in pain tolerance, it was thought that there would be differences in styles of verbal expression about pain as well.

Research questions used to explore the willingness of patients to disclose information describing qualities of their pain were

1. Do blacks and whites, males and females, and older (>40) and younger (<40) patients differ significantly on frequency of pain descriptors and pain intensifiers?
2. Do blacks and whites, males and females, and older (>40) and younger (<40) patients differ significantly on frequency of pain disclosure statements? (Shuter and Miller, 1982).

METHOD

A convenience sample of 60 middle class subjects, 34 whites and 26 blacks, 31 females and 29 males ranging in age from 20 to 60, participated in the study. (See Table 1.) All subjects were experiencing acute postoperative pain. Subjects on their second postoperative day who were receiving analgesics every 4 to 6 hours and had not received analgesics 3 hours prior to the interview were included in the study. No efforts were made to examine patients with only one type of abdominal surgery, since Copp (1974) concluded that patients' reported pain intensity varies from minimal to severe regardless of the type of surgery.

TABLE 1   **Age and sex characteristics of black and white subjects (N = 60)**[*]

	White (34)		Black (26)	
	Male (16)	**Female (18)**	**Male (13)**	**Female (13)**
Age 20 to 39	16		13	
Age 40 to 60	18		13	

[*]All subjects in acute pain were receiving analgesics every 4 to 6 hours.

Data were gathered during a 4-minute interaction by a trained nurse interviewer, a white female, while the interaction was transcribed by a second nurse recorder who was viewed by the patient as accompanying the nurse interviewer on routine rounds. The nurse interviewer was viewed as a helper in that she was regularly working with nursing students on the patient unit. Patients were able to spontaneously express information regarding the nature and intensity of their pain to a nurse who could provide relief. Four standard questions were used to initiate conversation related to the patients' comfort: "How are you or how are you feeling?" "Did you just have surgery?" "Are you comfortable?" "Can I help you in any way?" A detailed explicit pain assessment, with examples of descriptors, was specifically avoided. A reflective, nondirective technique was used throughout the 4-minute interaction. If the conversation ended before the 4 minutes had elapsed, the nurse performed routine assessment of dressings, drainage tubes, and so forth. At the end of the 4 minutes, patients were given a pain scale to determine whether the severity of pain affected their disclosure. Patients rated their pain on a five-point scale: 1, no pain; 2, slight pain; 3, moderate pain; 4, severe pain; and 5, unbearable pain. Analysis of the pain ratings comparing race, sex, and age indicated that the subjects did not differ significantly (Shuter and Miller, 1982).

Prior to data collection for this study, both the nurse interviewer and recorder were trained by the researchers. Role playing as well as their data collection on a pilot study of 10 patients interactions were critiqued.

Data were analyzed by use of content analysis of the process recordings of the interactions as well as use of analysis of variance to determine effects of sex, race, and age on pain disclosure. Two raters independently examined the process recordings of the nurse/patient interactions and rated words used by the patients as pain descriptors and pain intensifiers and further rated the words as maximally, moderately, or minimally descriptive. (See Table 2.) Interrater reliability was computed for pain descriptors as 0.89, for pain intensifiers as 0.88, and for pain disclosure statements as 0.91. Maximally descriptive words are those which provide highly specific information on the nature (pain descriptors) or intensity (pain intensifiers) of pain. Moderately descriptive words are those which provide moderately specific information about the nature (pain descriptors) or intensity (pain intensifiers) of pain. Minimally descriptive words are those which provide minimally specific information about the nature (pain descriptors) or intensity (pain intensifiers) of pain (Shuter and Miller, 1982).

RESULTS

Analysis of variance was used to determine whether sex, race, and age had any effect on (1) frequency of pain disclosure statements and (2) frequency of minimal, moderate, and maximum pain descriptors and pain intensifiers. In addition, variety or number of different types of descriptors and intensifiers were

TABLE 2   Selected pain descriptors and pain intensifiers

	Pain descriptors	Pain intensifiers
Minimal	Sore	Just mild
	Hurt	Slightly
	Ache	Not too bad
	Discomfort	A little
	Uncomfortable	Diminished
		Some
Moderate	Sharp	Not real, real severe
	Tender	Bearable
	Bloated	Worse, getting worse
	Cramping	Not good
	Spasm	More moderate
		Not very comfortable
Maximal	Burning	Severe
	Throbbing	A lot of
	Stabbing	Awful
	Exploding	Can't stand it
	Shooting	Really kills you
		Worst in the world
		So terrible
		So miserable
		Really bad
		So very painful

Reprinted with permission from Shuter, R., and Miller, J.: An exploratory study of pain expression styles among blacks and whites, Int. J. Intercultural Relations **6**:281-290, 1982. Copyright, Pergamon Press, Ltd.

examined. The least significant difference multiple comparison procedure was used to determine whether differences between individual means were significant at the 0.05 level.

Race, sex, and age did not interact on any measure. However, whites used significantly more maximum pain intensifiers than blacks did ($p < 0.05$, $f = 5.11$), and males used significantly more moderate pain intensifiers than females did, ($p < 0.01$, $f = 9.24$). Males also used a greater *variety* of pain intensifiers than did females ($p < 0.01$, $f = 9.24$), and whites used a greater *variety* of maximum pain intensifiers than did blacks ($p < 0.05$, $f = 5.48$). Whites used more pain disclosure statements than blacks did ($p < 0.05$, $f = 4.31$), and older patients (>40) used more pain disclosure statements than younger patients (<40) $p < 0.05$, $f = 4.58$) (Shuter and Miller, 1982). (See Tables 3, 4, and 5.)

DISCUSSION

It appears that both races provided nurses with minimal description of their pain. On the average, blacks and whites used less than one pain descriptor and

TABLE 3   **Race effects**

Variable	Black				White				f	p
	Number	Min.	Mod.	Max.	Number	Min.	Mod.	Max.		
Frequency of pain intensifiers	26 BM = 13 BF = 13	0.30	0.42	0.42	34 WM = 16 WF = 18	0.79	0.41	1.23	5.11	0.05
Variety of pain intensifiers	26 BM = 13 BF = 13	0.26	0.42	0.34	34 WM = 16 WF = 18	0.29	0.41	1.05	5.48	0.05
Frequency of pain descriptors	26 BM = 13 BF = 13	1.5	0.07	0.26	34 WM = 16 WF = 18	1.2	0.17	1.27	2.21	0.05
Variety of pain descriptors	26 BM = 13 BF = 13	0.84	0.03	0.11	34 WM = 16 WF = 18	0.76	0.14	0.17	1.04	0.05

CODE: BM = black males; BF = black females; WM = white males; WF = white females.

Reprinted with permission from Shuter, R., and Miller, J.: An exploratory study of pain expression styles among blacks and whites, Int. J. Intercultural Relations **6**:281-290, 1982. Copyright Pergamon Press, Ltd.

TABLE 4   **Sex effects**

Variable	Male				Female				f	p
	Number	Min.	Mod.	Max.	Number	Min.	Mod.	Max.		
Frequency of pain intensifiers	29	0.37	0.64	1.0	31	0.22	0.19	0.77	9.24	0.01
Variety of pain intensifiers	29	0.37	0.65	0.82	31	0.19	0.19	0.67	9.24	0.01
Frequency of pain descriptors	29	1.3	0.12	0.24	31	1.6	0.13	0.29	2.65	0.05
Variety of pain descriptors	29	0.79	0.10	0.13	31	0.80	0.09	0.16	1.84	0.05

Copyright Pergamon Press, Ltd.

TABLE 5   **Pain disclosure statements**

		Number	Mean	f	p
Race	Black White	26 34	4.4 6.3	4.31	0.05
Age	20-39 40-60	W = 16 25 B = 13 W = 18 38 B = 13	4.1 5.7	4.58	0.05

Copyright Pergamon Press, Ltd.

one pain intensifier during the 4-minute interactions; the variety of pain descriptors and intensifiers used by each race also averaged less than one.

This finding suggests that nurses have to be sensitive to the fact that patients in acute pain do not spontaneously disclose descriptive information about their pain states. Rather, patients in acute pain may expect nurses to be aware of the nature of their pain simply because they are in a setting which is supposed to be able to provide comfort. Nurses may need to anticipate providing pain relief measures without relying on patients' verbal reports to alert them to the nature of the patients' pain states. The importance of using a systematic pain assessment, observation of nonverbal cues, and physiologic changes to diagnose altered comfort states seems to be reinforced by this study. Nurses also need to avoid anticipating a familiar pain trajectory but to determine the nature of pain to each individual patient. Specific meaning of the pain event also needs to be investigated.

Patients' hesitancy to talk about their pain has been supported by Jacox (1979) and Jacox and Stewart (1973). Of the 102 patients interviewed with acute, progressive, or chronic pain, 70% of the patients did not like to discuss their pain or were ambivalent about doing so (Jacox, 1979). Patients' qualitative explanations had to do with hesitancy to burden others, overtly solicit sympathy, or be labeled a "complainer" (Jacox, 1979). Further investigation may be needed to determine whether hospitalized patients in acute postoperative pain are socialized by health care personnel to engage in the pain task of enduring pain more so than expressing pain. Fagerhaugh (1974) suggests that for some settings such as burn units, enduring pain, especially pain inflicted by treatments like tubbings and debridements, was valued more by the staff than pain expression. Nurses were more sympathetic to patients who were stoical "teeth gritters" than to patients who were overly expressive about their pain (Weiner, 1975).

Although blacks conveyed less information than whites (fewer number and variety of maximum pain intensifiers), the impact of the health care institution and black patients' trust of white health providers was not measured in this study but needs to be considered in future research. Whether or not differences in pain relief measures provided for patients whose verbal pain expression styles are elaborate and detailed compared to patients who suffer silently also needs to be studied.

Accurate diagnosis of pain is a complex inferential process and is dependent upon more than one source of data. The patients' spontaneous disclosure about the nature and intensity of pain may not be adequate for assessing pain states in all persons.

REFERENCES

Agnew, D.C., and Merskey, H.: Words of chronic pain, Pain **2:**73-81, 1976.
Baer, E., Davis, L., and Lieb, R.: Inferences of physical pain and psychological distress, in relation to verbal and nonverbal patient communication, Nurs. Res. **19:**388-392, 1970.

Bond, M.R., and Pilowsky, I.: Subjective assessment of pain and its relationship to the administration of analgesics in patients with advanced cancer, J. Psychosom. Res. **10:**203-208, 1966.

Carpenito, L.J.: Nursing diagnosis: application to clinical practice, Philadelphia, 1983, J.B. Lippincott Co.

Chapman, W.P., and Jones, C.M.: Variations in cutaneous and visceral pain sensitivity in normal subjects, J. Clin. Invest. **23:**81-91, 1944.

Dana, C.L.: The interpretation of pain and the dysaesthesias, JAMA **56:**787-791, 1911.

Fagerhaugh, S.: Pain expression and control on a burn care unit, Nurs. Outlook **22:**645-650, 1974.

Fagerhaugh, S., and Strauss, A.: Politics of pain management: staff-patient interactions, Menlo Park, Calif., 1977, Addison-Wesley Publishing Co.

Gordon, M.: Manual of nursing diagnosis, New York, 1982, McGraw-Hill Book Co.

Hilgard, E.: Pain as a puzzle for psychology and physiology, Am. Psychol. **24:**103-113, 1969.

Jacox, A.: Assessing pain, Am. J. Nurs. **79:**895-900, 1979.

Jacox, A., and Stewart, M.: Psychosocial contingencies of the pain experience, Iowa City, 1973, University of Iowa.

Kim, M.J., and Moritz, D., editors: Classification of nursing diagnoses—Proceedings of the Third and Fourth National Conferences, New York, 1982, McGraw Hill Book Co.

McCabe, G.: Cultural influences on patient behavior, Am. J. Nurs. **60:**1101-1104, 1960.

McCaffery, M.: Nursing management of the patient with pain, Philadelphia, 1979, J.B. Lippincott Co.

Meissner, J.: McGill-Melzack pain questionnaire, Nursing **80:**50-51, 1980.

Melzack, R., and Torgerson, W.S.: On the language of pain, Anesthesiology **34:**50-59, 1971.

Shuter, R., and Miller, J.F.: An exploratory study of pain expression styles among blacks and whites, Int. J. Intercultural Relations **6:**281-290, 1982.

Sternbach, R.A., and Tursky, B.: Ethnic differences among housewives in psychophysical and skin potential responses to electric shock, Psychophysiology **1:**241-246, 1965.

Strauss, A., Fagerhaugh, S., and Glaser, B.: Pain: an organizational-work-interactional perspective, Nurs. Outlook **22:**560-566, 1974.

Weisenberg, M., Kreindler, M., Schachat, R., and Werboff, J.: Pain: anxiety and attitudes in black, white and Puerto Rican patients. Psychosom. Med. **37:**123-135, 1975.

Wiener, C.: Pain assessment on an orthopedic ward, Nurs. Outlook **23:**508-516, 1975.

Winsberg, B., and Greenlick, M.: Pain response in Negro and White obstetrical patients, J. Health Soc. Behav. **8:**222-228, 1967.

Woodrow, K., Friedman, G., Siegelaub, A.B., and Collen, M.: Pain tolerance: difference according to age, sex, and race. In Weisenberg, M., editor: Pain: clinical and experimental perspectives, St. Louis, 1975, The C.V. Mosby Co.

Zborowski, M.: Cultural components in responses to pain, J. Soc. Issues **8:**16-30, 1952.

A description of self-concept as it is altered by the diagnosis of cancer

CAROL A. MORRIS, M.N., R.N.
NANCY R. LACKEY, Ph.D., R.N.

In 1973 the First National Conference on the Classification of Nursing Diagnoses was held in St. Louis. It was conceived as a starting point for a clear articulation of those health problems into a taxonomic system. Participants thought that such a system could be of value in nursing education, nursing research, and health record keeping. This taxonomy would contain words for describing states of the patient. Definitions of nursing diagnoses and a classification system would lead to greater consistency between investigations. Through compilation, evaluation, and validation of nursing diagnoses, a compendium of diagnoses could be developed which would add to the unique body of nursing knowledge.

Gordon and co-workers (1980) stated that prospective clinical studies using highly trained nursing diagnosticians were needed to provide a basis for standardization of diagnostic nomenclature. Diagnoses would provide a basis for developing a clinical science in nursing.

The goal of the National Group for Classification of Nursing Diagnoses was to standardize diagnostic labels so patients' problems and needs could be clearly communicated from one nurse to another and from one shift to another. These labels would then be tested by research and eventually lead to the establishment of specific outcome criteria and nursing interventions for each diagnosis. They requested that such work not be done in silence or in isolation but that collaboration would occur through conferences, publications, and correspondence (Dossey and Guzzetta, 1981).

PURPOSE

The purpose of this study was to validate the behavioral and emotional components, delineated from a review of the literature, of the psychological construct, self-concept, as it is altered through concept analysis. Utilizing a specified patient population, a study of these components was conducted. More specifically, the study was designed to answer the research question: What are the behavioral and emotional components of self-concept as altered by the diagnosis of cancer?

BACKGROUND

The review of the literature was divided into two major categories concerning self-concept: the nature of the phenomenon, and alteration by the diagnosis of cancer. The words of the authors cited formed the conceptual framework for this study.

Of all man's attributes, the self appears to be the most complex and most intangible. In reviewing psychologists' feelings about self-concept, Labenne and Greene (1969) defined self-concept as a psychological construct. They defined a construct as a concept of self-inferred behavior. Self-concept, as it was referred to in the professional literature, was a group of feelings and cognitive processes inferred from observed or manifest behavior. By way of a formal definition, they presented self-concept as the person's total appraisal of his appearance, background and origins, abilities and resources, and attitudes and feelings which culminated as a directing force in behavior.

The perceptual view as proposed by Combs and Snygg was discussed by Biehler (1974). They proposed "that man was in part controlled by and in part controller of his destiny." It viewed man as a growing, dynamic, creative being continuously in search of adequacy. Instead of an object at the mercy of environment, he was himself a purposive agent engaged in the never ending business of becoming.

Self-actualization was emphasized by Maslow (1962), who argued that an individual had within him a powerful desire to develop his potential to the fullest extent. He cited Freud's greatest discovery as being "the great cause of much psychological illness is the fear of knowledge of oneself, of one's emotions, impulses, memories, capacities, potentialities, of one's destiny." That kind of fear was termed defensive, in the sense that it was protection of one's self-esteem, of one's love and respect for the self. He found that man had a tendency to be afraid of any knowledge that could cause him to despise himself or make him feel inferior, weak, worthless, evil, or shameful. He would protect himself and his ideal image of himself by repression and similar defenses, which are essentially techniques by which he would avoid becoming conscious of unpleasant or dangerous truths.

Pediatric cancer survivors and the issues surrounding their marriages and the effect the diagnosis had on their adult adjustment were studied by Gogan and co-workers (1979). It was found that a life-threatening illness had an impact on the patient and those around him even many years after treatment. Negative effects ranged from serious psychological problems to milder difficulties, including occasional tension, emotional withdrawal, short temper, decreased appetite, insomnia, and anxiety about recurrence.

One-hundred-fourteen long-term survivors at the Sidney Farber Cancer Institute were investigated by O'Malley and associates (1979) in an attempt to measure the impact of cancer experience on their adjustment in later life. Fifty-nine percent of the sample of former patients were found to have at least mild psychiatric symptom formation, with 12% rated as markedly or severely impaired.

A descriptive study was designed by Johnson (1967) in which the role of communication before, during, and after cancer treatment was examined. In studying the sexual concerns of the cancer patient and his or her spouse, she found that, with the diagnosis of cancer, old values and concerns may disappear and new values and concerns may emerge. Individuals may feel differently about themselves and others; they may behave differently and communicate differently. The data obtained suggested that persons with cancer who had positive self-images did talk to their spouses about the cancer, its implications for their relationship, and the alterations required in their marriage. Persons with comparatively low self-image and much less self-esteem had been reluctant to talk about their illness with their spouse. Three persons indicated that they were having serious problems with the sexual aspects of their marital relationship, and they attributed those problems directly to the cancer.

Bard and Sutherland (1977) reported that for some women self-worth and acceptability as women have been predicated upon body attractiveness throughout their lives. Just the possibility of breast amputation could incite the feelings that life is no longer worth living. In some instances the patient's fearful projections of future rejection by people involved her most intimate relationships, such as those with her husband and children.

In discussing the psychological response to cancer Phipps and associates (1979) related that, once the diagnosis of cancer has been made, the patient and his family might be overwhelmed and immobilized. They might go through a period of denial during which there could be a delay in beginning therapy. Anxiety, depression, regressive behavior, and anger might be manifested.

Guilt was also cited by Phipps and co-workers (1979) as a frequent psychological response to the diagnosis of cancer. The cancer patient might feel that his disease was punishment for past actions of his life. He might also feel guilty if he had delayed seeking treatment. One of the most prevalent reactions described was a sense of isolation, of being cut off from those persons and things that were important to him. Perhaps the most profound isolation was psychological isolation, an inability to relate to and derive comfort from others, similar to the feeling of being alone in a crowd. They reported that some patients were overwhelmed with fantasies of death and dying. Most patients were more concerned with the process of dying, fearing pain, mutilation, and deterioration in both their physiologic and psychologic status, than with death itself.

A pilot study was conducted by Morris (1980) to investigate the self-concept as altered by the diagnosis of cancer. A structured-interview format was devised and descriptions of patients' emotions and behaviors after their diagnosis were collected. They were then categorized into feelings of depersonalization, altered identity, low self-esteem, altered body image, and role conflict.

Definition of Terms

To aid in comprehension and analysis, the following terms were defined. Common language was retained for terms not defined here.

Behavioral components. The identifiable action verbs delineated from the provisional criteria (Lackey, 1978)

Body-image. Sum of the conscious and unconscious attitudes the individual has toward his body; it includes present and past perceptions as well as feelings about size, function, appearance, and potential (Stuart and Sundeen, 1979).

Cancer. A collective term describing a large group of disease entities characterized by uncontrollable growth and spread of abnormal cells (Luckman and Sorensen, 1980)

Identity. Organizing principle of the personality system that accounts for the unity, continuity, uniqueness, and consistency of the personality; it is the awareness of the process of "being one-self" that is derived from self-observation and judgment and is the synthesis of all self-representation into an organized whole (Stuart and Sundeen, 1979)

Perception. Mental processes by which data—intellectual, sensory, and emotional—are organized meaningfully (Stuart and Sundeen, 1979)

Provisional criteria. Specific essential features or a group of characteristic features that can be utilized to identify or describe a concept (Wilson, 1971)

Self-actualization. The process of fulfilling one's potential

Self-concept. All of the notions, beliefs, and convictions that constitute an individual's knowledge of himself and influence his relationship with others (Stuart and Sundeen, 1979)

Self-esteem. The individual's personal judgment of his own worth obtained by analyzing how well his behavior conforms to his ideal (Stuart and Sundeen, 1979)

ASSUMPTIONS

In this study the following assumptions were made:

1. No two people have identical self-concepts (Stuart and Sundeen, 1979).

2. Because self-concept is the frame of reference through which the person interacts with the world, it is a powerful influence on human behavior (Stuart and Sundeen, 1979).

3. The diagnosis of cancer carries with it a connotation of prolonged, debilitating, painful death that evokes fear in most persons.

4. Uncertainty about the course of illness after diagnosis affects emotional reactions to malignant disease.

5. Persons who have cancer are frequently showered with compassion,

concern, and caring by family and friends, but their status as employees and productive members of society is jeopardized.

LIMITATION

This study was circumscribed by the fact that the data were collected through self-report and thus would only be as valid as patient recall and the amount of material the patient was willing to share.

METHOD
Subjects

Three groups were utilized in this study. The first group comprised three nurse experts in the field of oncology. Construct validity of both the checklist and the structured-interview format was determined by this panel. The second group, Study Group A, comprised 30 subjects who had been diagnosed as having cancer at least 3 months before. They completed the checklist twice for the purpose of obtaining reliability data on the checklist instrument. The third group, Study Group B, comprised 30 subjects over the age of 18 years who had been diagnosed as having cancer for the first time. They completed the interview and the checklist between 6 and 8 weeks after diagnosis. Subjects comprising Study Group B were interviewed in their homes between 6 and 8 weeks after diagnosis of cancer. Demographic data including age, sex, marital status, occupation, site of cancer, and days postdiagnosis when interviewed were obtained from each subject.

Instruments

Two instruments were used in this study: a structured-interview format to guide the interview and a checklist of the behavioral and emotional components completed by the subjects.

First, the investigator reviewed the literature. Then the structured-interview format was devised for use in a pilot study investigating self-concept altered by the diagnosis of cancer (Morris, 1980). The interview format was used with 10 subjects who had been diagnosed as having cancer. Following completion of the pilot study and analysis of the data, the structured-interview format was further refined. After a second review of the literature, a checklist of the behavioral and emotional components was compiled. The work of many theorists was used to compile the checklist. Since all of the behaviors and emotions extracted from the literature as the expected behaviors were all negatives, 20 of the items were changed to positive items and became the unexpected behaviors and emotions.

Construct validity of both the checklist and the structured-interview format was determined by a panel of nurses whose expertise was in the field of oncology. Reliability of the checklist was determined by administering the checklist to Study Group A on a test-retest basis at 48-hour intervals. Study Group A was comprised of 30 subjects who had been diagnosed as having cancer a minimum of 3 months prior to implementation of the study. Administrative feasibility of the structured-interview format was determined by the pilot study conducted. The structured-interview was conducted in the patients' home, and the checklist was administered after the interview was completed.

RESULTS

In order to obtain reliability data for the checklist instrument, the members of Study Group A completed identical copies of the instrument at 48-hour intervals. The data were analyzed by means of the Pearson *Product Moment Correlation Coefficient* calculated between the total scores of test one and test two.

The predominant form of data analysis used in this study was content analysis of the structured-interview responses. Percentages were used to analyze the checklist responses.

DISCUSSION OF THE FINDINGS

In this study, responses to the checklists raw scores were calculated for Study Group B. The raw scores were then converted to percentages. It was the belief of this investigator that percentages would be higher for the expected behaviors and emotions extracted from the literature than for the unexpected behaviors and emotions. Raw scores were tabulated and mean scores for each sample of expected and unexpected behaviors and emotions were calculated. A two-tailed t test was done to determine whether or not the responses to the expected behaviors and emotions were significantly higher than the responses to the unexpected behaviors and emotions. The unexpected items ranked significantly higher ($p = 0.001$) than the expected items. This investigator has to ask the question, does the diagnosis of cancer really alter the self-concept? Another question that naturally follows is Does the time span of 6 to 8 weeks since the patients were given the diagnosis of cancer give them time to move from altered self-concept soon after their diagnosis to adjustment and acceptance and wishing to get on with their lives by 6 to 8 weeks after diagnosis?

Based on this investigation, many questions remain unanswered and many new ones must be considered. One would question whether at 6 to 8 weeks after diagnosis of cancer some of the expected behaviors and emotions of the recently diagnosed cancer patient, as extracted from the literature, do really exist. Many patients report feeling hopeful, worthwhile, in control, calm, accepted, and loved. These findings are contrary to what is presented in the literature. Because of this conflict, it cannot be stated positively that the research question What are the behavioral and emotional component of self-concept as altered by the diagnosis? was answered. One can only speculate on possible causes for the results. Since no time frame is specified in the literature reviewed, it can be questioned if a different time frame might produce different results. Another area that poses question is the process of grief. Since this process appears to be very individualized, the stage in the grief process the patients were in when interviewed might also have produced varying results. Because of the incongruence between the checklist responses and the answers to the interview questions, it would seem a possibility that patients were not entirely honest about their behaviors and emotions, since in most instances a significant other was present for the interview. This situation may have had an influence on their answers. All of the patients were referred by physicians from their private practice. Through this method of selection the results may have been skewed by selecting patients who were coping well. Even though the data collected in this study did not show a difference in means scores on the unexpected items on the checklist with difference in age, one would have to question whether, if the sample was larger with a greater range in ages to include more younger clients, there might not be a greater difference. Rotter (1966) studied internal versus external locus of control. One would naturally question what effect maturity has on locus of control. The possibility that older subjects are more internally controlled as opposed to younger subjects, who are more externally controlled, would be an interesting area for exploration.

IMPLICATIONS FOR NURSING PRACTICE

This study has major implications for nursing. In reviewing the literature, it was found that self-concept, and altered self-concept in general, was frequently discussed and studied. The review of the literature revealed sparse information specifically concerning the self-concept as altered by the diagnosis of cancer. The results of this study will provide information to help fill that void and also provide a basis for further study in that specific area.

Hardy (1974) stated that knowledge of one's world is based on the use of concepts, hypotheses, and theories. She considered concepts to be the "bricks" of theory construction. Since nurses need to apply knowledge from theories in their practice, it is important that theories be composed of concepts that have been theoretically and operationally defined as well as empirically tested. The purpose of this study was to validate the behavioral and emotional components, delineated from a review of the literature, of the psychological construct self-concept as it is altered by the diagnosis of cancer.

Brill and Kilts (1980) stressed that nursing care that is organized around the individual's presenting behavior rather than isolated data is less fragmented and goal-oriented than task-oriented. Thus care is more comprehensive and individualized and recognizes the interrelationships within the total person. Through compilation, evaluation, and validation of nursing diagnoses, a compendium of diagnoses could be developed which would add to the unique body of nursing knowledge. Care would be improved and the profession would benefit by having a common language and a sharing of thought, since this compendium would be common to all.

Gordon and associates (1980) were in agreement when they stated that prospective clinical studies using highly trained nursing diagnosticians were needed to provide a basis for standardization of diagnostic nomenclature. They believed that such standardization would facilitate the incorporation of nursing diagnoses into educational programs and would improve communication in practice settings. Nursing diagnoses provide a focus for research on therapies for the various problems and provide a basis for developing a clinical science in nursing.

From the review of the literature, repeated citations were found stating that not only does the diagnosis of cancer alter the self-concept but the severity of the treatment regimens also results in altered self-concept, with specific behaviors and emotions occurring after the diagnosis. Those behaviors and emotions identified as being present after the diagnosis of cancer were extracted from the literature. Their perceived presence or absence was empirically tested on a specified population of patients. Inconclusive empirical data were received. Many of the behaviors and emotions identified in the literature were not identified by the subjects studied.

The information collected in this study is more specific than information collected to date. The results are detailed and provide valid and reliable information for inclusion in that specific expanded area of self-concept as altered by the diagnosis of cancer defined by the group collecting data for the classification system of nursing diagnosis.

From the review of the literature the patient diagnosed as having cancer was found to have many psychological needs that were not being met. The nursing profession must be cognizant of those needs and include measures in its plan of action for each individual patient to meet those needs. Nursing interventions must be planned specifically to help the patient meet those needs.

Since there is conflict between the literature reviewed and the data obtained from the study, this investigator must tell nurses to listen carefully to what patients are saying about their feelings. From the data obtained there appears to be a wide spread between the behaviors and emotions of each individual patient after the diagnosis of cancer. Nursing care of these patients will require a continual individualized approach. Specific implications must await the acquisition of less conflicting data.

RECOMMENDATIONS FOR FUTURE RESEARCH

Although research has been done in the area of psychological adaptation following the diagnosis of cancer, the emphasis has centered on the impact of the disease as it compares to other diseases and on methods found useful in assisting the patient to adjust. Based on the data obtained from this study and the preceding discussion, the following are recommended as areas for future research:

1. Changing the checklist to a semantic differential and conducting a longitudinal study 1 day after diagnosis and weekly for 3 months
2. Changing the checklist to a semantic differential and conducting a longitudinal study 1 day after diagnosis and weekly for 3 months along with the collection of data based on Rotter's locus of control
3. Conducting a descriptive study to determine if persons who personalize the term cancer cope more effectively than those who do not personalize the term cancer
4. Conducting a longitudinal study on a population of patients who have high risk for development of cancer to establish a base-line self-concept; then if diagnosed for cancer, how this self-concept changes
5. Replicating the study utilizing random selection of subjects, from a listing of all subjects entering an oncology clinic for inclusion in Group B
6. Conducting a study to determine what effect the type and length of therapy have on the self-concept
7. Conducting a study to determine the effect age has on locus of control
8. Conducting a study to determine if there is a correlation between coping strategies and the behaviors and emotions listed on the checklist
9. Doing a multiple regression analysis of the following factors: age, locus of control, coping strategies, and self-concept as altered by the diagnosis of cancer
10. Replicating the study and determining the position of the subjects in the grief process
11. Doing a comparative study between the *Tennessee Self-Concept Scale*, Rotter's *Locus of Control*, coping strategies, and a semantic differential of the checklist

REFERENCES

Bard, M., and Sutherland, A.M.: Adaptation to radical mastectomy. The psychological impact of cancer, pp. 55-71, Professional education publication, American Cancer Society, 1977.

Biehler, R.F.: Psychology applied to teaching, Boston, 1974, Houghton-Mifflin Co.

Brill, E.L., and Kilts, D.F.: Foundations for nursing, New York, 1980, Appleton-Century-Crofts.

Dossey, B., and Guzzetta, C.E.: Nursing diagnosis, Nursing '81, **6:**34-38, 1981.

Gogan, J.L., Koocher, G.P., Fine, W.E., Foster, D.J., and O'Malley, J.E.: Pediatric cancer survival and marriage: issues affecting adult adjustment, Am. J. Orthopsychiatry **19**(3):423-430, 1979.

Gordon, M., Sweeney, M.A., and McKeehan, K.: Nursing diagnosis: looking at its use in the clinical area, Am. J. Nurs. **4:**672-674, 1980.

Hardy, M.E.: Theories: components, development, evaluation, Nurs. Res. **23:**100-107, 1974.

Johnson, J.L.: A research brief: the sexual concerns of the cancer patient and his or her spouse, Counsel. Values **7:**186-188, 1967.

Labenne, W.D., and Greene, B.I.: Educational implications of the self-concept theory, Pacific Palisades, Calif., 1969, Goodyear Publishing Co., Inc.

Lackey, N.R.: Use of the computer in a concept analysis of emotional support. Unpublished doctoral dissertation, Texas, Woman's University, 1978.

Luckman, J., and Sorensen, K.: Medical surgical nursing: a psychophysiologic approach, Philadelphia, 1980, W.B. Saunders Co.

Maslow, A.H.: Toward a psychology of being, Princeton, N.J., 1962, D. Van Nostrand Co., Inc.

Morris, C.A.: Altered self-concept in cancer patients, validation of a nursing diagnosis. Unpublished manuscript, University of Kansas Medical Center, 1980.

O'Malley, J.E., Koocher, G., Foster, D., and Slavin, L.: Psychiatric sequelae of surviving childhood cancer, Am. J. Orthopsychiatry **49**(4):608-616, 1979.

Phipps, W.J., Long, B.C., and Woods, N.F.: Medical surgical nursing; concepts and clinical practice, St. Louis, 1979, The C.V. Mosby Co.

Rotter, J.B.: General experiences for internal versus external control of reinforcement, Psychol. Monogr. **80**:1-28, 1966.

Stuart, G., and Sundeen, S.: Principles and practice of psychiatric nursing, St. Louis, 1979, The C.V. Mosby Co.

Wilson, J.: Thinking with concepts, Cambridge, 1971, Cambridge University Press.

Poster presentations

Memory error: a new nursing diagnosis

LINDA S. BAAS, M.S.N., R.N., CCRN
GORDON A. ALLEN, Ph.D.

Currently, if a medication or treatment regimen is not followed correctly, a nursing diagnosis of noncompliance is made. Noncompliance is defined by Gordon (1982) as the failure to participate in carrying out the plan of care after indicating initial intention to comply. A second definition offered by Kim (1984) describes noncompliance as the person's informed decision not to follow a therapeutic regimen. Neither definition of noncompliance addresses the complex role of memory in following a prescribed plan of care. The purpose of this research is to establish memory error as a separate nursing diagnosis by documenting that two types of memory errors are possible when taking medications. Once a memory error is diagnosed, appropriate nursing interventions should be instituted.

MEMORY

Memory is the complex process that involves taking all of the experiences that we have and saving them for future use. Forgetting, or the inability to remember information, is a common and natural occurrence for all. It is important that nurses and other health professionals understand the normal process of memory and points in the process where errors can occur. After assessing the patient for the occurrence of memory errors, the health professional can develop strategies to effectively deal with these problems.

When a nurse is confronted with a patient who does not remember whether he or she has taken scheduled medications, it should not be assumed that the patient is recalcitrant. A thorough assessment of why the patient has not followed the schedule may reveal that it is the inability to remember that has caused the error. This assessment should include pathophysiologic factors such as neurologic, cardiovascular, pulmonary, hematologic, and endocrine parameters. Additionally, situational factors, such as complexity of therapeutic regimen, stressful or unpatterned life-style, or environmental distractions may interfere with memory.

Memory is currently viewed as comprising two major processes, short-term and long-term (Gleitman, 1981; Loftus, 1980).

Short-term memory is what a person is currently aware of, including events in the environment and recalled past memories. Its major characteristic is that it is volatile. Without active attention or rehearsal, information in short-term memory is lost within seconds.

Long-term memory is a relatively permanent information file of events, facts, and concepts. Its major characteristic is that the information must be organized in a manner so that it can be retrieved for use at a later time. It is common to know something but be unable to retrieve it at the appropriate time.

The movement of information from short-term to long-term memory is dependent upon practice, the organization of the information, the current level of environmental and emotional stress, and the physiological function of the individual (Loftus, 1980).

Memory error may be demonstrated in the area of patient education. A person may be able to answer questions about information just taught or read; however, after several minutes none of the information may be recalled. In this case the information was held in short-term memory but never transferred to long-term memory. Inability to transfer this information may be the result of environmental noise, interruptions, anxiety about health status, and physiologic factors such as a low hemoglobin, arterial oxygen, or blood sugar.

A second patient may use the hospital routines to organize the information that must be learned for self-care. The routine enhances the encoding process for long-term memory. However, when the patient returns home, this routine is broken, so that there are no cues to enable the patient to retrieve the information from long-term memory. Therefore the patient is not able to remember the self-care skills that were learned.

The most common type of information for which patients must be responsible is their own medication regimen. Remembering to take medications is more complex than most health professionals assume.

RESEARCH STUDY: MEMORY ERRORS WHEN TAKING MEDICATIONS
Purpose

Nursing and allied health professionals recognize that many patients do not adhere to their prescribed medication regimen.

When a patient does not remember to take his or her medication at the prescribed time, he or she commits a *schedule error,* an error that results in undermedication. Medication guides provide instructions on the action that should be taken when a patient realizes an error has been committed. The occurrence of schedule errors has been well documented (Haynes, 1979).

There is the potential for a second type of memory error, which has not been reported in the literature. An *event error* occurs when, after the prescribed time for taking the medication, the patient cannot recall whether or not the medication has been taken. Unlike the *schedule error,* the *event error* can lead to overmedication. Medication guides do not offer advice for this situation except to note that double dosing should be avoided for some drugs.

In one situation a patient may take the scheduled medication but later experience an *event error*. He can then choose to take the medication again, an action that will result in overmedication. In this same situation, if the patient chooses not to take the medication, the result will be correct dosage even though a memory error has been committed.

A second situation may occur in which the patient commits a *schedule error* and does not take the prescribed medication and later commits an *event error*. Taking a dose of medication after the second error will result in the correct medication, but choosing not to take the medication will result in undermedication.

Strategies for patients who experience schedule and event errors must be developed based on the severity of the results of either over- or undermedication. Additionally, the drug action, half-life, therapeutic serum levels, type, and frequency of error must be known since they determine the strategies for each prescribed medication.

The primary purpose of this research was to assess the frequency with which individuals on daily medications reported experiencing problems with both types of memory errors. Subjects were also asked what they did when they committed a memory error.

Method and design

The questionnaire contained two brief scenarios describing a situation in which a memory error was committed. Subjects answered questions related to the two scenarios. Scenarios were used to reduce the defensiveness of the respondents. Demographic information, including age, sex, medications prescribed, frequency of doses, length of time that the medication was prescribed, and sources of information about the drugs, was also obtained. The sample consisted of 224 men and women taking daily long-term medications. Respondents included 27 participants of a cardiac rehabilitation program, 45 members of self-help groups for diabetes, epilepsy, and parkinsonism, 113 college students, and 39 other subjects with a variety of medical problems.

Findings

The overall result was that subjects reported making both types of errors. Nearly everyone (94%) reported experiencing problems with remembering to take the medicine at the appropriate time *(schedule errors)*. Almost as many (83%) reported experiencing problems with remembering whether or not they had already taken their medicine *(event errors)*. The reported frequency of occurrence for both types of errors was about once a month, although *schedule errors* were made slightly more often than *event errors*. Only 15% of the respondents reported making more *event errors* than *schedule errors*. A limitation of the study was that subjects might make more schedule errors than reported but were unable to remember these occurrences.

The frequency with which *event errors* were made was not systematically related to any other variables—such as age, number of medications taken per day, number of times per day that medications were taken, or the length of time that the medication had been prescribed.

The frequency with which *schedule errors* were made was related to other variables. *Schedule error* frequency was related to age, with more errors being reported by younger people, i.e., the college-age group. (This finding is the opposite of what is generally believed to occur.) When only people over 21 years old were considered, this relationship disappeared although a relationship between the frequency of occurrence of *schedule errors* and the number of times per day a medication was taken did appear (r = 0.25).

If a patient cannot remember whether he or she has taken the medication, the next decision to be made is what to do. Should the patient take the medication and run the risk of overmedication? Or should the patient not take the medication and run the risk of undermedication? The correct choice depends upon the type of medication that the patient is taking and the severity of the consequences of over- or undermedication. Whether or not a medication error actually occurs depends upon the choice of the patient and whether the medication has been taken on schedule.

The respondents in our study, even within disease and/or medication groups, did not agree among themselves as to the appropriate strategy to follow after an *event error.* For example, among the people with Parkinson's disease, 50% thought the medicine should not be taken while 42% thought that it should be taken. The remaining 8% did not know what they would do. Among the people taking antibiotics, 25% thought the medication should not be taken, 40% thought it should be taken, and 34% thought it depended upon the circumstances.

This same lack of consensus was also apparent in responses to the question what should be done following a *schedule error.* Among the people taking antibiotics, 30% thought the medication should be taken, 56% thought it should not be taken, and 14% thought a partial dose should be taken. Similarly patients with Parkinson's disease indicated that 15% thought the medication should be taken, 51% thought it should not be taken, and 31% thought a partial dose should be taken. This is somewhat surprising, since many medications come with instructions on what to do following a *schedule error.*

By far, the most commonly reported (81%) memory aid was taking one's medicine at a specific event, such as at mealtime. People frequently reported that this did not work, as in the example "I always take my medicines with my breakfast orange juice but I never drink orange juice on weekends." Few subjects reported using an alarm clock (5%) or marking a calendar or diary (6%). Some had friends or relatives remind them (12%), although they did not mention how these people remembered to remind them.

Nearly half of the respondents (45%) had discussed their medications with their physicians. Few had discussed problems with nurses (10%), and fewer still with their pharmacist (4%). These statistics are interesting since nurses view themselves as providers of health education and responsible for teaching patients self-care skills. Pharmacists also view themselves as providers of information in addition to providers of the drugs.

The findings related to both types of error *(schedule* and *event)* demonstrate a need for more patient education regarding medications. This need is all the greater in light of the frequency with which memory errors are made. Patient education should include not only how and when to take the medications but also what strategy should be used for each type of error. Memory aids developed for a patient, to assist in remembering to take the medication, should consider the possible occurrence of both types of errors.

MEMORY ERROR: A NURSING DIAGNOSIS

Gordon (1982) defines nursing diagnosis as actual or potential health problems which nurses, by virtue of their education and experience, are capable and licensed to treat. In clinical practice, nursing diagnosis provides a common language for nurses to describe problems which are the basis for nursing actions. This research provides support for the identification of memory error as a nursing diagnosis since these common occurrences may result in actual or potential health problems. Memory error differs sufficiently from noncompliance, knowledge deficit, altered thought processes, and health maintenance impairment to be recognized as a separate nursing diagnosis (Kim, 1984).

A guideline for the use of memory error as a nursing diagnosis is found in Box 1, which presents the problem, etiology, and symptom format suggested by the North American Nursing Diagnosis Association (Kim, 1984). Although memory has a long research history, only recently has it been researched in everyday life. The entries in Box 1 are thought to be relevant to memory process, but it is difficult to find particular experiments that substantiate this belief. Further research to identify the sensitivity and specificity of the defining characteristics is needed.

For example, on theoretical grounds, one would expect a patient who leads a very stressful fast-paced life to commit many *schedule errors* because a simple habit would be difficult to establish in that life-style. On the other hand, a person who leads a routine or regimented life would be expected to commit few *schedule errors* but would commit many *event errors* since it would be easy to confuse today with yesterday. No research has yet been reported on life-style and particular memory errors even though it is needed.

BOX 1   **Memory error**

Definition: Inability to encode, maintain, or retrieve information
Etiological or contributing factors
   Pathophysiological
      Neurological
         CVA, tumor, edema
      Cardiovascular
         Low cardiac output
         Myocardial infarction, aortic stenosis, atherosclerosis
      Pulmonary
         Chronic obstructive pulmonary disease, pulmonary embolism
      Endocrine
         Diabetes, adrenal insufficiency
      Hematological
         Anemia
   Pharmacological
      Side effect
      CNS depressant
   Situational
      Interference
      Repetitive regimented life-style
      Unpatterned life-style
      Stressful life-style
      Traumatic event
   Encoding specificity
   Complexity of therapeutic regimen
   Excessive environmental distractions
Defining characteristics
   Verbalized difficulty in remembering to take medication
   Verbalized difficulty in recalling if medication was taken
   Subtherapeutic serum drug levels
   Toxic serum drug levels
   High pill count
   Low pill count

While this research examined the occurrence of memory error in the general population, the same diagnosis could be used in patients with neurological alteration resulting in memory deficit. These patients may require extensive retraining programs or cue systems to follow not only their therapeutic regimens but also their activities of daily living.

The nursing assessment should include questions related to the medication pattern, frequency of reported *schedule* and *event errors,* and actions taken when an error is realized. Other data that are helpful include serum drug levels and pill counts. Once the type and frequency of memory errors are determined, appropriate interventions can be planned. For example, a patient who reports frequent *schedule errors* might benefit from calendars, daily cues, or electronic pill reminders. Patients who report frequent *event errors* should avoid the use of daily event cues as reminders since the event of taking the medication on one day might not be distinguished from taking the medication on previous days and might result in more frequent errors. These individuals should be encouraged to maintain diaries or use compartmentalized pill containers.

One implication of the findings of this research is to make explicit the distinction between noncompliance and nonadherence. Even when a patient fully intends to comply with a prescribed regimen, there are variables such as memory errors which reduce the level of adherence. The appropriate nursing intervention for this patient is not to persuade or convince him or her to follow the schedule. Instead, it is to develop strategies to reduce memory errors.

REFERENCES

Gleitman, H.: Psychology, New York, 1981, W.W. Norton & Co., Inc.

Gordon, M.: Nursing diagnosis process and application, New York, 1982, McGraw-Hill Book Co.

Haynes, R., Taylor, D., and Sackett, D., editors: Compliance in health care, Baltimore, 1979, The Johns Hopkins University Press.

Kim, M., McFarland, G., and McLane, A., editors: Pocket guide to nursing diagnosis, St. Louis, 1984, The C.V. Mosby Co.

Loftus, E.: Memory, New York, 1980, Addison-Wesley Publishing Co.

Noncompliance as a nursing diagnosis: current use in clinical practice

KATHLEEN A. BREUNIG, M.N., R.N.
GENEE BRUKWITZKI, B.S.N., R.N.
JUDEEN SCHULTE, M.S., R.N.
LARAINE CRANE, M.S.N., R.N.
PAMELA M. SCHROEDER, M.S.N., R.N.
JANET LUTZE, B.S.N., R.N.

Noncompliance is being used as a nursing diagnosis in clinical practice; however, research to validate its use is lacking. This descriptive study was designed to explore the current use of the diagnosis, noncompliance, in nursing practice. The study was based on the assumptions that (1) the use of nursing diagnosis is essential to professional nursing practice and (2) the identification of nursing diagnosis influence on the care provided to the client.

During the Fifth National Nursing Diagnosis Conference it was determined that diagnoses could not be placed on the approved list without adequate research to support the diagnosis. In addition, diagnoses could not be removed from the approved list without adequate research to verify this position. When the noncompliance work group met to study this diagnosis at the Fifth National Conference, great concern was expressed regarding the effect of this diagnosis on the nursing care provided to clients. A list of questions was generated that required further study in order to determine the viability of noncompliance as a nursing diagnosis. One of our researchers was a member of this noncompliance work group. The information generated by this work group was subsequently disseminated to the members of the Southeastern Wisconsin Nursing Diagnosis Interest Group. Reservations regarding the use of noncompliance led to the formation of a research study group whose purpose was to develop a study which would describe the current use of noncompliance as a nursing diagnosis in clinical practice.

LITERATURE REVIEW

Several conceptual frameworks for noncompliance exist. Primarily they can be categorized into the areas of health beliefs, attitudes, motivation, and locus of control. The available literature generally shows research based on the medical model, lack of a clear definition for noncompliance, and inconsistency in defining characteristics. In addition, neither nursing theories nor the general nursing literature provides a consistent framework for noncompliance. Instead of offering specific definitions, the majority of references described a list of characteristics believed to be necessary to prove compliance or noncompliance to a particular health practice (Deyo, 1982; Jones and Russell, 1980; Spadaro, 1980). A generic definition of noncompliance stated "yielding to a wish, demand, or request; acquiescence. A disposition or tendency to yield to others" (Hoover, 1980).

Discrepancy also existed between the definitions provided by Gordon (1982) and those of the Third and Fourth National Conferences for the use of nursing diagnoses. The Proceedings (Kim and Moritz, 1982) identified noncompliance as a "person's informed decision not to adhere to a therapeutic recommendation." Gordon (1982) further expands this definition by referring to the client's expressed intention, "nonadherence to a therapeutic recommendation following informed decision and expressed intention to adhere or attain therapeutic goals."

Defining characteristics were offered only in relation to the medical disease entity being studied. For example, in diabetes care, Ketodiastix and blood sugar results were used as parameters for determining compliance or noncompliance. In contrast, Sackett and Haynes (1979) identified delay in seeking care, nonparticipation in health care, broken appointments, and the lack of following the prescribed regimen as indicators of noncompliance. The defining characteristics found in the Classification of Nursing Diagnoses from the Third and Fourth National Conferences (Kim and Moritz, 1982) provided a prototype for the general content areas found in the literature review. The most frequent defining characteristics found in the literature included self-report, pill counts, broken appointments, laboratory/clinical data, and failure to resolve the problem.

The compliance literature generally follows a medical model, regardless of the discipline addressing the issue. Only one article has addressed noncompliance as a nursing diagnosis and ultimately described reservations concerning its use. In that article Stanitis and Ryan (1982) cite the diagnosis as being value laden. They identify that nursing needs to consider the effect of the diagnosis on the client's and the nurse's behavior, the processes and factors nurses use to decide that a client is noncompliant, the specific behaviors in this label, and the relationship of compliant behavior to the client's involvement in developing treatment goals.

In summary, nursing literature on noncompliance as a nursing diagnosis is sparse. The general nursing literature on noncompliance does not provide a clear definition of defining characteristics to determine when compliance ceases and noncompliance becomes a problem. It generally reflects an underlying assumption that noncompliance is a problem. The nurse's role in treatment, preventing, and even creating the problem is not universally addressed.

Hence, the diagnosis remains vague. This discussion confirms the need for further study in order to address the abstractness of noncompliance, as well as its relationship to nursing.

METHOD

This was a study designed to describe how the nursing diagnosis of noncompliance is currently used in clinical practice. A five-item questionnaire was developed to address some of the issues identified by the noncompliance work group at the Fifth National Conference. A systematic sampling technique was used to select 100 subjects from the list of 400 participants at the Fifth National Nursing Conference. A questionnaire and stamped self-addressed return envelope were mailed to the selected sample. The researchers selected the Fifth National Nursing Diagnosis Conference participants as the sample because of their interest and familiarity with nursing diagnosis, and also with the assumption that this would increase the rate of return. The tool encompassed questions that dealt with the use of nursing diagnosis in clinical practice. Specifically it included the following questions:

1. Do you use nursing diagnosis in your nursing practice?
2. Do you use noncompliance as a nursing diagnosis?
3. If you do not use noncompliance as a nursing diagnosis:
   (a) Why don't you use noncompliance as a diagnosis?
   (b) Do you use an alternative nursing diagnosis?
   (c) Do you consider noncompliance an etiology?
   (d) Do you consider noncompliance a defining characteristic?
4. If you do use noncompliance as a nursing diagnosis, what are the characteristics necessary for arriving at this diagnosis?
5. Whether you currently use or do not use noncompliance as a nursing diagnosis, would you feel more comfortable with another term, and if so, what is it?

Demographic data were not solicited from the subjects. Response to the questionnaire indicated consent of the subjects to participate in the study.

RESULTS

Of the 100 questionnaires sent, 60 were returned. These responses were counted and subjected to content analysis.

The results indicated that 88% of the respondents used nursing diagnoses in their practice. Noncompliance as a nursing diagnosis was used by 52% of the respondents and was not used by 48%. The respondents who did not use noncompliance as a nursing diagnosis indicated responses which were coded into the categories of being a value-laden diagnostic label (42% of responses), not addressing the real problem (31% of responses), felt that the diagnosis

TABLE 1   **Frequency distribution of alternative nursing diagnoses used**

Nursing diagnosis	n
Altered coping	8
Knowledge deficit	8
Alteration in health management	5
Adherence/nonadherence	2
Participation/nonparticipation	2
Responses not labeled as diagnoses	4
Other	9
TOTAL	38

TABLE 2   **Frequency distribution of reported defining characteristics for noncompliance**

Defining characteristics	n
Nonadherence to therapeutic regimen	9
Failure to resolve problem	8
Nonadherence to medication regimen	6
Nonadherence after instruction	5
Gordon's characteristics	5
Verbalized not carrying out regimen	5
Attributions regarding behavior (unmotivated, uncooperative, etc.)	5
Observed noncompliance	3
Health care seeking behavior	3
Clinical data (serum/urine levels)	3
Verbalized lack of intent to comply	3
Previous verbal intent to comply	2
Impaired mental status	2
Value conflict with treatment	1
Perceived lack of problem/seriousness of problem	1
Denial of illness	1
Knowledge deficit	1
History of noncompliance	1
Inability to follow medical regimen	1
Behaviors dichotomous to mutually set goals	1
Proceedings from Third and Fourth Conference	1
Uncertain	1
TOTAL	68

TABLE 3   **Frequency distribution of preferred alternative terms**

Alternative term	n
Nonadherence	4
Knowledge deficit	4
Motivation deficit	2
Nonreliance on information	1
Nonrecognition of useful information	1
Refusal	1
Lack of adherence to medical regimen	1
Lack of adherence to nursing interventions	1
Alliance	1
Management, alteration or dysfunction in	1
Management of illness, alteration or dysfunction in	1
Management of health, alteration or dysfunction in	1
Self-care management deficit	1
Decreased incorporation of their therapeutic plan into life-style management	1
Ineffective individual coping	1
Denial	1
Limitation	1
Compromised health management	1
Ineffective self-control ability	1
TOTAL	26

denoted a lack of mutual decision making (18% of responses), and "other" (9% of responses). "Other" included issues regarding the legality of nursing diagnosis, lack of relevance to the subject's area of nursing, and that the label reflected a nonunderstanding professional.

If the subjects did not use noncompliance as a nursing diagnosis, they were asked if an alternative nursing diagnosis was used. Thirty percent of the respondents used an alternative diagnosis. The most frequent responses were altered coping, knowledge deficit, and alteration in health management (see Table 1).

Seventy-one percent of the sample indicated that noncompliance was not an etiology. Similarly, 50% indicated that they did not consider noncompliance a defining characteristic. There were 67 responses concerning the defining characteristics. They were categorized into 22 defining characteristics. The most frequently identified characteristics were nonadherence to the therapeutic regimen, nonadherence after instruction, the client verbalizes not carrying out the regimen, and Gordon's characteristics (see Table 2).

Both respondents who used noncompliance as a nursing diagnosis and those respondents who did not use noncompliance as a nursing diagnosis were asked if they would feel more comfortable with another term, and, if yes, to identify that term. Forty percent responded that they would feel more comfortable with an alternative term. Nineteen alternative terms were generated from the responses. The most frequent responses were nonadherence, knowledge deficit, and motivation deficit (see Table 3).

DISCUSSION

The study generated a high percentage of response for a mail survey. From this, we assume that noncompliance as a nursing diagnosis is an issue of great interest and controversy.

Currently we are dealing with a nursing diagnosis that is used by only 52% of the sample. In these responses there were numerous defining characteristics or groups of defining characteristics identified, which could imply that the diagnosis of noncompliance is abstract in nature, at the construct level. Also the variety of responses might reflect nursing's lack of a universal definition for this term. This is a reasonable assumption considering that the noncompliance literature also lacks a universal definition of this term.

The results indicate that there is no consensus for the use of noncompliance as a nursing diagnosis. Since the sample was divided on this issue, the viability of noncompliance as a nursing diagnosis should be questioned, since it may not describe a health problem that nurses diagnose and treat. If indeed noncompliance is to remain a viable diagnosis, nursing will require further research and education concerning this diagnostic label in order to build a universal language.

Since there are numerous frameworks or viewpoints from which to identify noncompliance, and since most frameworks are from outside the discipline of nursing, it is difficult to defend the use of this diagnosis in nursing practice. Nursing needs to consider if

- The compliance frameworks from other disciplines are applicable to nursing.
- Nursing has a unique framework from which noncompliance can be diagnosed and treated.
- Noncompliance is necessarily detrimental to the client.
- The diagnosis of noncompliance is self-serving to the profession and not the client, hence causing nurses to "diagnose by convenience."
- Noncompliance is either a viable problem that nurses treat or the outcome of a problem that was not identified and treated earlier.

In summary, we believe this study raises serious issues for our profession and indicates the need for further research.

FUTURE RESEARCH

1. Replication of this study using a larger sample
2. Replication using a sample from various practice areas
3. The definition of noncompliance
4. Ethical concerns about the use of noncompliance as a nursing diagnosis, specifically
   a. When and how is the diagnosis of noncompliance resolved?
   b. How does the diagnosis affect the quality of nursing care provided to the client?
   c. Does the diagnosis of noncompliance serve a purpose? If so, what is the purpose?
5. The extent and limitations of the use of this diagnosis
6. Legal issues concerning the use of noncompliance as a nursing diagnosis

CONCLUSION

The results of this study verify the lack of consensus among practitioners regarding the use and defining characteristics of noncompliance as a nursing diagnosis. This lack of consensus supports the need to continue questioning whether noncompliance should be included as an approved nursing diagnosis.

REFERENCES

Allen, A.F., and Perkins, N.: Patient factors in CAPD, J. Am. Assoc. Nephrol. Nurses **8**(5):19-23, 1981.

Aminoff, M.J., and Simon, R.P.: Status epilepticus: causes, clinical features, and consequences in 98 patients, Am. J. Med **69**(5):657-666, 1980.

Baldonado, A.A., and Phillips, K.M.: Is high quality health care a right or an obligation? Nephrol. Nurse **1**(5):23-26, 1979.

Basch, C.E., Gold, R.S., McDermott, R.J., and Richardsen, C.E.: Confounding variables in the measurement of cancer patient compliance, Cancer Nurs. **6**(4):285-293, 1983.

Beck, N.C., Shekim, W., Gilbert, F., and Fraps, C.: A cross validation of factors predictive of AMA discharge, Hosp. Commun. Psychiatry **34**(1):69-71, 1983.

Bollen, B.W., and Hart, L.K.: The relationship of health belief motivations, health locus of control and health valuing to dietary compliance of hemodialysis patients, J. Am. Assoc. Nephrol. Nurses **9**(5):41-47, 1982.

Bova, C.A.: Primary nursing: a greater opportunity for patient independence, Nurs. Admin. Q. **5**(4):56-59, 1981.

Buchanan, N., and others: Factors influencing drug compliance in ambulatory black urban patients, S. Afr. Med. J. **55**(10):368-373, 1979.

Carpenter, P.J., Morros, G.R., Del Gander, A., and Ritzler, B.: Who keeps the first outpatient appointment? Am. J. Psychiatry **138**(1):102-105, 1981.

Change, B.L.: Evaluation of health care professionals in facilitating self-care: review of the literature and a conceptual model, Adv. Nurs. Sci. **3**(1):43-58, 1980.

Daniels, L.M., and Kochar, M.S.: Monitoring and facilitating adherence to hypertension therapeutic regimens, Cardiovasc. Nurs. **16**(2):7-12, 1980.

Davidhezar, R.E.: Compliance by persons with schizophrenia: A research issue for the nurse, Issues Ment. Health Nur. **4**(3):233-255, 1982.

Deyo, R.: Compliance with therapeutic regimens in arthritis: issues, current status, and a future agenda, Semin. Arthritis Rheum. **12**(2):233-244, 1982.

Gever, L.N.: Nadolol: a new beta-blocker that may increase patient compliance, Nursing 80 **10**(10):57, 1980.

Gordis, L.M., Markowitz, M., and Lilienfeld, A.: Studies in the epidemiology and preventability of rheumatic fever. IV. A quantitative determination of compliance in children on oral penicillin prophylaxis, Pediatrics **43**(2):173-181, 1969.

Gordon, M.: Manual of nursing diagnosis, New York, 1982, McGraw-Hill Book Co.

Gordon, M.: Nursing diagnosis: process and application, New York, 1982, McGraw-Hill Book Co.

Guthrie, D.: Helping the diabetic manage his self-care, Nursing 80 **10**(2):57, 1980.

Hartman, J., Menefee, P., Shares, E., and Rogers, R.: Clients' reasons for dropping out of rehabilitation centers, Psychol. Rep. **51**:1307-1316, 1982.

Haynes, R.B., Sackett, D.L., and Taylor, D.W.: How to detect and manage low patient compliance in chronic illness, Geriatrics **35**(1):91-97, 1980.

Haynes, R.B., Taylor, W., and Sackett, D., editors: Compliance in health care, Baltimore, 1979, The John Hopkins University Press.

Hoover, J.: Compliance from a patient's perspective, Diabetes Educ. **6**(1):9-12, 1980.

Itano, J., and others: Compliance of cancer patients to therapy, West. J. Nurs. Res. **6**(1):5-20, 1983.

Jones, J., and Russell, W.: More noncompliance, Arch. Intern. Med. **140**(6):866-867, 1980.

Kellaway, G.S.M., and McCrae, E.: The effect of counseling on compliance—failure in patient drug therapy, N. Z. Med. J. **89**(631):161-165, 1979.

Kim, M.J., and Moritz, D.A., editors: Classification of nursing diagnoses—Proceedings of the Third and Fourth National Conferences, New York, 1982, McGraw-Hill Book Co.

Kirilloff, L.: Factors influencing the compliance of hemodialysis patients with their therapeutic regimen, J. Am. Assoc. Nephrol. Nurse Techn. **8**(4):15-20, 1981.

Korcok, M.: Balking at radiotherapy may signal underlying anxieties, J. Amer. Med. Assoc. **249**(4):454-455, 1983.

Kovacs, M., Rush, A.J., Beck, A., and Hollon, S.: Depressed outpatients treated with cognitive therapy or pharmacotherapy, Arch. Gen. Psychiatry **38**(1):33-39, 1981.

Lager, E., and Zweeling, I.: Time orientation and psychotherapy in the ghetto, Am. J. Psychiatry **137**(3):306-309, 1980.

Loustau, A., and Blair, B.: A key to compliance, Nursing 81 **11**(2):84-87, 1981.

Medina, J., and others: Comparative evaluation of two methods of natural family planning in Colombia. Am. J. Obstet. Gynecol. **138**(8):1142-1147, 1980.

Miller, D.J., and others: Predicting AWOL discharge at a community mental health center: a "split-half" validation, Am. J. Psychiatry **140**(4):479-482, 1983.

Oldridge, N., and others: Predictors of dropout from cardiac exercise rehabilitation, Am. J. Cardiol. **51**(1):70-74, 1983.

Paulen, A.: Patient compliance: Is that what we really want? Cancer Nurs. **4**(3):179, 1981.

Pippenger, C.E.: Rationale and clinical application of therapeutic drug monitoring, Pediat. Clin. North Am. **27**(4):891-925, 1980.

Richardson, B.: The real world of diabetic noncompliance, Nursing 82 **12**(1):68-73, 1982.

Robinson, K.D., and Little, G.L.: One-day dropouts from correctional drug treatment, Psychol. Rep. **51**(2):409-410, 1982.

Scobie, I.N., Rafferty, A.B., Franks, P.C., and Sonksen, P.H.: Why patients were lost from follow-up at an urban diabetic clinic, Br. Med. J. **286**(6360):189-190, 1983.

Shillinger, F.: Locus of control: implications for clinical nursing practice, Image **15**(2):58-63, 1983.

Simons, R.D.: Medication "contracts" bring pain relief, RN **43**(4):123, 1980.

Sklar, C.: You and the law, Can. Nurse **76**(1):15-18, 1980.

Spadaro, D.C.: Factors involved with patient compliance, Pediatr. Nurs. **4**(1):27-29, 1980.

Stanitis, M.A., and Ryan, J.: Noncompliance—an unacceptable diagnosis? Am. J. Nurs. **82**(6):941-942, 1982.

Steckel, S.B.: Patient contracting, New York, 1982, Appleton-Century Crofts.

Steinglass, P., Grantham, C.E., and Hertzman, M.: Predicting which patients will be discharged against medical advice: a pilot study, Am J. Psychiatry **137**(11):1375-1389, 1980.

Stewart, R.B., Springer, P.K., and Adams, J.E.: Drug-related admissions to an inpatient psychiatric unit, Am. J. Psychiatry **137**(9):1093, 1980.

Tirrell, B.E., and Hart, L.K.: The relationship of health beliefs and knowledge to exercise compliance in patients after coronary bypass, Heart Lung **9**(3):487-493, 1980.

Villeneuve, M.E.: The patient compliance puzzle, Nurs. Manage. **13**(5):54-56, 1982.

Witt, R.: Medication compliance among discharged psychiatric patients, Issues Ment. Health Nurs. **3**(4):305-317, 1981.

Youngren, D.E.: Improving patient compliance with a self-medication teaching program, Nursing 81 **11**(3):60-61, 1981.

Nursing diagnosis as a descriptor for nursing care provided under DRGs

LYNNE CHEATWOOD, B.S.N., R.N.
PATRICIA A. MARTIN, M.S., R.N.

PROBLEM

The skyrocketing cost of health care has caused the American public to demand a halt to this trend. The Federal Government has increasingly passed legislation designed to reduce the government spending for health care. The Tax Equity and Fiscal Responsibility Act of 1982 (TEFRA) changed the focus of hospital payment from reimbursement for monies spent to a prospectively predetermined payment based on a patient's diagnosis related group (DRG). In addition to TEFRA, the Reagan administration proposes another package of budget cuts called "health incentive reforms" reported in *The Washington Report of Medicine and Health/Perspectives*, on February 7, 1983.

Nursing must be accountable to identify its portion of health care costs. This identification is necessary to provide the safe, high-quality nursing care needed by consumers. An extensive study about the cost of nursing care utilizing a method called Relative Intensity Measures (RIM's) was developed in New Jersey (Grimaldi and Micheletti, 1982). A debate about the limitations of this model was published in *Nursing Management* (Caterinicchio, 1983); however, Curtin (1983a) points out that, without viable alternatives, the limitations may well be ignored and this model implemented. Curtin wrote an article (1983b) outlining a method of determining costs of nursing services per DRG. She lists the problems with her method as being "inaccurate assignment of DRG, inaccurate nursing assessments of patient needs, and allowance for the difference, if any, between the care needed and the care received by the patient." Riley and Schaefers (1983) reported their study of costing nursing services at St. Paul–Ramsey Medical Center, St. Paul, Minnesota. Their research demonstrated that nursing intensity varied among DRGs and suggested that nursing staffing can be analyzed and should be planned for on this basis.

Research needs to be continued to develop an acceptable, usable method for costing nursing services and to analyze the actual cost to the hospital for a given patient's care. According to Curtin (1983a) "any item that constitutes

Thanks are expressed for the research assistance provided by Patricia A. Hatton, R.N., and Marietta Baer, hospital volunteer.

as large a share of any hospital's budget as does the nursing department budget simply must be justified."

PURPOSE

The primary purpose in conducting this study was to develop a usable methodology for correlating nursing diagnosis and nursing personnel hours based on an acuity system with medical DRGs. The intent of the study included identifying the nursing diagnoses associated with various DRGs as a descriptor for needed nursing care, the nursing personnel hours based on an acuity system, as a descriptor of the time, and therefore dollars, associated with providing this care and the relationship of age and length of stay (LOS) to the range of nursing resources utilized within a DRG category.

In addition to the development of a methodology, this study provides an analysis of the DRG specific profile variables of nursing diagnoses, acuity pattern, acuity totals, age, and length of stay (LOS). The study is ongoing as the data collected to date is insufficient to identify needed nursing care that can be calculated as a specific portion of DRG reimbursement. Within the setting for this study, acuity and nursing diagnosis are readily available for analysis to enlarge the knowledge base for decision making concerning nursing productivity.

DESIGN

An ex post facto descriptive correlational design was developed to describe subjects throughout their acute hospital stay. In this field study, the medical record and the acuity system were reviewed to obtain the data after routine recording by the staff. Acuity data was routinely entered in the computer on the nursing unit every 8 hours. The independent variables were the patient's age and the DRG assignment. The dependent variables were nursing diagnoses, patient acuity, and LOS.

DESCRIPTION OF SUBJECTS AND SAMPLE SIZE

The population consisted of all patients whose hospital bills would be paid by Medicare and who were admitted to four similar general medical/surgical units over a 2-week period. The hospital setting was a 772 bed urban nonprofit regional referral center located in the East North Central region for DRG reimbursement. The total number of patients studied was 55, with an age range from 35-94 years old. There were two patients under 65, 37 from age 65 to 79, and 16 from age 80 to 94.

DATA COLLECTION

Researchers identified Medicare admissions daily by going to each of the four units and reading the unit admission book. The patients' admission face sheet was used to affirm Medicare status, age, and admission diagnosis (potential DRG). The patient's nursing care plan was checked for nursing diagnoses. Each patient's records were checked daily throughout their hospital stay for new nursing diagnoses. LOS was determined when the patient was discharged, expired, or transferred to a DRG-exempt unit such as psychiatry or rehabilitation. After discharge, medical records personnel assigned a DRG for each patient using Health Systems International's DRG grouper.

Patient acuity was printed from the computer on a daily basis and compiled by a volunteer at the end of the patient's hospitalization. (The computer system at present does not calculate total nursing care time per patient for more than an 8-hour time span.)

DATA ANALYSIS

The subjects were grouped by medical record assigned DRG after discharge. There were a total of 55 patients in 32 different DRG categories. DRG 127, heart failure and shock, had 10 patients; DRG 014, specific cerebrovascular disorders except transient ischemic attack (TIA), had 5 patients. There were three DRGs with 3 patients each: 088, chronic obstructive pulmonary disease; 142, syncope-collapse age less than 70 without complications and comorbidity; and 294, diabetes age 36 and older. All others had just one or two patients in each category. For each DRG, all nursing diagnoses were listed and reviewed for similarities within the DRG.

Using the computerized acuity system, direct care hours for RN, LPN, and TA (trained attendant) were totaled and then averaged. The average cost was determined using a mean salary times the hours. The average cost of nursing care per DRG is not reported in this paper, as this would vary from hospital to hospital based on salaries. However, average hours can be translated into dollars by each institution. Age and LOS range and mean were also calculated per DRG. The categories reported are the five with three or more patients per DRG.

In addition, the mean of the total required nursing care hours of patients 65 to 79 was compared with required nursing care hours of patients 80 to 95.

MAJOR FINDINGS

The methodology used was satisfactory for gathering appropriate data, but the actual number of subjects per DRG was insufficient to reach conclusions and the cost of data collection was high ($17.50 per subject, including the time and services of two RNs and the medical records DRG coordinator). The volunteer's time was free and therefore not included in the cost. The cost could be reduced by using unit based clerical workers for part of the data collection and by using a computerized acuity system that keeps retrospective totals of hours of required nursing care.

Only the five DRG categories with three or more patients are reported in

TABLE 1   **Characteristics of patients in five DRG categories**

	DRG				
	127 **(n = 10)**	**014** **(n = 5)**	**088** **(n = 3)**	**142** **(n = 3)**	**294** **(n = 3)**
Age range (yr)	70-94	76-93	71-82	46-68	73-84
Mean (yr)	81	83	75	60	78
LOS range (days)	3-18	11-17	5-12	3-11	5-13
Mean (days)	8	14	9	6	9
RN range (hours)	15-80	43-96	22-56	14-62	25-57
Mean (hours)	40	67	39	30	41
LPN range (hours)	0-5	1-14	1-6	0	0-2
Mean (hours)	2	7	4	0	1
TA range (hours)	0-20	2-34	0-25	1-4	3-17
Mean (hours)	8	20	10	2	11
Total range (hours)	17-91	51-144	27-88	15-66	27-71
Mean (hours)	49	94	53	32	52
Nursing range (hours/day)	4-11	4-9	5-6	5-6	5-7
Mean (hours/day)	7	7	6	6	6

TABLE 2   **Nursing resources consumed**

	n	$\bar{\chi}$
Young-old (65 to 79 yr)	37	47.458
Old-old (80 to 95 yr)	16	68.394

this paper. Table 1 gives the findings on age, LOS, required RN hours, required LPN hours, required TA hours, total required nursing hours, and average nursing hours per day.

A comparison of nursing resources consumed by subjects 65 to 79 years old (young-old) and those resources consumed by subjects 80 to 95 (old-old) is shown in Table 2.

There was also an attempt to associate nursing diagnoses with DRGs though results in this endeavor were very limited. There were two patients out of ten with DRG 127, heart failure and shock, who had nursing diagnoses of impaired physical mobility. In DRG 014, specific cerebrovascular disorders except TIA, there were two patients with nursing diagnoses of potential for injury and potential for trauma and two patients with impairment of skin integrity: actual.

Other than these examples, there were no commonalities in nursing diagnoses per DRG.

SIGNIFICANCE

A prospective payment system has forced nursing to develop methodologies for collecting baseline data on nursing care costs per DRG. Only when we know what we currently use in nursing resources per DRG can we identify ways to reduce that cost. The percentage of a hospital budget allocated for nursing care is reported to be anywhere from 14% to 21% (Walker, 1983), to 30% to 60% (Davis, 1983). Until we know what we currently use in nursing resources per DRG, we will find it very difficult to determine where and how we can reduce the cost for these resources.

Continued research on the cost of nursing care related to individual nursing diagnosis is also needed. Nursing diagnoses should be an integral part of the patient's acuity system with the nursing interventions required having a time factor calculated in acuity just as a bed bath or Foley catheter has a weighted standard time calculated in acuity.

Age is currently a factor in the DRG decision tree, with patients over 70 being allocated a larger amount of money than those under 70 for the same medical diagnosis. However, it is the finding of these researchers that the young-old (65 to 79) require less resources than the old-old (80 and above) (see Table 2). This preliminary finding needs additional research.

According to Davis (1983) there is 30 million dollars in the Health Care Financing Administration (HCFA) budget to be used for research and development related to Medicare reimbursement and coverage issues. Nursing needs to tap this available resource and study the issue of nursing costs for hospitalized patients.

REFERENCES

Caterinicchio, R.P.: A debate: RIM's and the cost of nursing care, Nurs. Manage. **14**(5):36-41, 1983.

Curtin, L.: A debate: RIM's and the cost of nursing care (editorial), Nurs. Manage. **14**(5):36, 1983a.

Curtin, L.: Determining costs of nursing services per DRG, Nurs. Manage. **14**(4):16-19, 1983b.

Davis, C.K.: The federal role in changing health care financing, Nurs. Econ. **1**:98-104, 1983.

Grimaldi, P.L., and Micheletti, J.A.: DRG reimbursement: RIM's and the cost of nursing care, Nurs. Manage. **13**:12-22, 1982.

Riley, W., and Schaefers, V.: Costing nursing services, Nurs. Manage. **14**(12):40-43, 1983.

Walker, D.: The cost of nursing care in hospitals, J. Nurs. Admin. **13**(3):13-18, 1983.

The Washington report on medicine and health/perspectives, Washington, D.C., 1983, McGraw-Hill Book Co.

Nursing diagnoses in a nurse-managed wellness resource center

RICHARD J. FEHRING, D.N.Sc., R.N.
MARILYN FRENN, M.S.N., R.N.

In recent years the health care system in the United States has undergone considerable criticism for its approach in delivering health care. Much of the criticism is based upon the narrow focus of the health care system, the astronomical cost of delivering that care, and the diminishing returns in terms of life expectancy and overall disease patterns. There is now a realization that there is a need for a greater emphasis on disease prevention, health promotion, and the modification of life-styles that contribute to the major degenerative diseases prevalent in our modern society. The importance of greater access to health care, self-responsibility, and the need for different models and approaches to health are also being promoted in health care circles.

As of late, the nursing profession has become more involved with the accessibility and delivery of health care. Nurse-managed health clinics are now being developed throughout the United States (Mezey and Chiamulera, 1980; Ossler and associates, 1982; Reisch and associates, 1980). These clinics allow nurses to have direct access to clients and allow nurses to focus their care on health promotion and disease prevention in a more independent manner. Many of these nurse-managed clinics are based on nursing models of health; they promote self responsibility, utilize nursing diagnoses, rely heavily on health education, and allow clients to have direct access to the services of a professional nurse.

In order to bring together some of the recent changes of emphasis in health care delivery (especially the focus on health promotion and self responsibility) and to utilize nursing diagnoses and a nursing model of health in an independent setting, an academic-based nurse-managed wellness clinic was developed by the Marquette University College of Nursing (MUCN) faculty. The purpose of this paper is to describe the MUCN nurse-managed Wellness Resource Center (WRC). Included within this description will be a presentation of the type of care the nurses provide, the types and patterns of nursing diagnoses being made, and the ongoing diagnostic revision process being utilized. One of the most frequent nursing diagnoses made in the WRC, Health maintenance: blood pressure, will be elaborated on.

DESCRIPTION OF THE WRC

There were two major purposes for developing an academic-based nurse-managed wellness resource center. The first purpose was to enable the maintenance and promotion of health within the Marquette University community. The second purpose was to provide a setting for students and faculty of the MUCN to practice, teach, and research well-health care. The WRC was established not to replace primary medical care but rather to expand and augment the existing system. The WRC also allows faculty and students to explore different types of health care delivery other than those provided in the traditional medical care system.

Before the WRC was developed, the plan was to originally develop a nurse-managed clinic at the existing College of Nursing. However, because the College of Nursing was being moved into new facilities on the University campus, the development of a University-based center was not immediately possible. Because of the move a church-based outreach site was developed before the centralized campus clinic. Future plans envision having a centralized campus-based wellness resource center at the College of Nursing, with accessible outreach sites in the surrounding community. These outreach sites will be at places that are accessible and convenient to a given population. Of particular interest are sites that have low-income and indigent populations, such as low-income housing projects and inner city churches. Whether the outreach sites will be at a church or other type of facility, the intent is to include a spiritual (holistic) approach to the delivery of health care.

In order to develop the first outreach WRC at the church, two faculty members from the MUCN negotiated with the pastors and key members of the church about the feasibility of starting a WRC. One of the faculty members is a member of the church and knew there was interest at the church for starting such a project. A proposal was written and presented to the church's Council of Ministries (COM). The COM agreed upon the project and appointed an implementation committee. This eventually developed into a formal committee composed of a nurse-liaison director from the MUCN, a codirector from the COM, a pastoral representative from the church, a physician liaison from the church, a treasurer, a secretary, and a lay church representative, all from the church. A coordinator of nursing staff from MUCN and the chairperson from the MUCN WRC committee completed the church committee. Besides developing a committee structure, this committee also was involved with securing rooms at the church for a physical site, developing brochures, setting hours of operation, and conducting a needs assessment of the health needs of the church members. The needs assessment gave the committee ideas for hours, services, and resources.

Meanwhile, the MUCN-WRC committee (made up of faculty, students, volunteer community nurses) and a University pastoral representative developed the conceptual basis for the health and nursing services. They developed forms, recruited volunteer professional nurses from the MUCN faculty and local community, obtained equipment and supplies, and facilitated legal negotiations between the Dean of the College, the University officials, and representatives from the church. Several of the faculty were also involved in writing for grant money from various federal and private organizations. One of the private organizations that granted money was the Wisconsin United Methodist Foundation. Because the center was to be a resource for health promotion, health promotion materials for self-health such as books, cassette tapes, home practice biofeedback monitors, and calorie counters were sought through the grant.

Since the College of Nursing's conceptual focus is based on a model of self-care, self-care was chosen as the conceptual basis for the WRC and was operationalized through the modification of Gordon's twelve functional health patterns. A self-health assessment guide was developed based on these twelve functional patterns, with the twelfth pattern modified to help assess spiritual well-being. Besides a self-health guide, a physical assessment form, a functional pattern assessment guide for the nurse, a nursing diagnosis problem page, a short assessment form, and progress notes were developed. The functional self-health assessment form and the functional assessment guide enabled the nursing staff to assess clients and to make nursing diagnoses. The types of diagnoses made at the WRC will be elaborated in another section of this paper. The committee also developed the proposed services for the center, which included health screening and assessment, health consultation, nutritional assessment and maintenance, stress management, community and medical referral, and spiritual health services. Spiritual health services were operationalized by inclusion of self-spiritual assessment guides, referral to pastoral services, inclusion of a spiritual focus in nursing interventions (for example, use of meditative prayer in helping clients with stress management), and developing the staff's spiritual lives through discussion, prayer, and literature.

In order to initiate the start of the WRC and to publicize its existence, an open house and ribbon cutting ceremony were conducted. The open house included booths on various topics of health that were manned and developed by the MUCN nursing faculty, aerobic jump rope demonstrations, and blood pressure and hearing screenings. The ribbon initiating opening of the WRC was cut by the senior pastor from the church and the Dean from the College of Nursing. Since the open house, the clinic has been functioning for three fourths of a year. Accomplishments since that time will now be presented.

Since opening in October 1982, there have been over 400 client visits at the WRC. Most of these visits have been for blood pressure monitoring. Some clients have consulted the professional staff for more in-depth problems such as uncontrolled anxiety, alterations in nutritional status, coping with family stress, and body image concerns.

In view of our mission to provide a place for faculty and students to develop independent nursing practice, considerable attention has been devoted to quality assurance. All of the client records were audited over the summer to determine what clients' chief concerns were, what nursing diagnoses were made, what strategies were used in helping the person promote their own wellness, and what outcomes were achieved. These data were viewed along with results of the self-health assessment. A secondary purpose of the audit was to arrive at information which would be the basis for the creative development of protocols for the common nursing diagnoses being utilized in the WRC. These protocols would be used by current clinic nurses to enhance quality of care as well as a tool for education of new nurses who would be oriented to providing care in this setting.

Box 1 is a summary of the nursing diagnoses seen in our client population. As shown, the most frequent diagnoses were those related to people's concern and maintenance of their blood pressure. This is probably so because people readily recognize taking blood pressure as a "function of nursing" and feel comfortable approaching the nurse for that service. There are also a great number of people who have problems related to blood pressure. However, we have found that once the client makes the initial contact with the nurse there are many other underlying health problems. The diagnosis related to blood pressure as listed in the box (Health maintenance: blood pressure) is not a label found on the current list of diagnoses sanctioned by the National Group for Classification of Nursing Diagnoses (the North American Nursing Diagnosis Association). The blood pressure label was developed in order to meet responses that were not covered by the current list but were being diagnosed and treated at the WRC.

The list of diagnoses from the 6-month audit probably will change (in regard to variety and frequency) as the clients become more familiar with the types

---

BOX 1   **Nursing diagnoses identified in the nurse-managed Wellness Center***

Health maintenance: blood pressure
Alteration in nutrition: greater than body requirements
Anxiety: moderate
Stress related to unemployment
Ineffective stress management
Maladaptive stress response (mild) related to family problems
Anxiety related to pain
Altered comfort related to cold and stress
Anxiety (mild) related to performing on the piano
Sleep pattern disturbance related to impaired coping with husband's illness
Lack of knowledge related to self-breast examination, pulse measurement, and low-sodium diet.

---

*In order of frequency.

BOX 2   **Protocol for the diagnosis (based on 62 client records) Health maintenance: blood pressure (B/P)**

Definition: Diagnosis referring to clients who know they have high blood pressure (hypertension) and seek help to adhere to their self-management
Indicators
    Need for help regarding low-salt diet
    Expressed interest in losing weight
    Need for periodic blood pressure checks
    Advice on how to stop smoking
    Need for nutritional information
    Knowledge deficit of risk factors for heart disease
    Need for periodic heart rate check
    Need for education regarding medications, diet, physical activity, stress management
    Need for physical activity advice
    Need for stress management
Etiology
    Lack of thorough teaching by health provider
    Need for reinforcement of blood pressure maintenance
    Unavailability of teaching B/P information
    Impaired self-care responsibility
Plan of care
    B/P check and advice on frequency of checks
    Client to bring record of B/P checks to give to MD on next visit
    Client education
        Diet regimen: Weight loss, low-salt, balanced
        Medication regimen: What the medication is, its effect on body, when to take it, how to adhere to schedule for taking it
        Risk factor information: For example, smoking
        Stress management
        Physical exercise
        Self-responsibility: Need to take responsibility for care
    Stress management
        Why important (relate to B/P)
        Relaxation technique, Benson's (give written paper)
        Home practice relaxation tapes
        Self-evaluation of effectiveness
        Stress symptom check list (optional)
        Recent life changes (discuss)
        Diet, exercise, sleep, importance of
        Evaluation of spiritual outlook
    Physical exercise
        Explore with client best type of aerobic exercise
        Teach client how to take heart rate
    Adherence techniques for diet, medications, and other areas of B/P maintenance
    Use of simple contingency contracting

Continued.

BOX 2	**Protocol for the diagnosis (based on 62 client records) Health maintenance: blood pressure (B/P)—cont'd**

Evaluation
    Blood pressure, pulse, weight loss
    Review knowledge of medications, diet, stress management, exercise
    Individual indicators
        Number of cigarettes
        Miles walked per day
        Calorie count
        Number of times doing relaxation technique
        Number of times doing exercise

of service the nurses can offer and as the nurses' diagnostic capacities develop. In the future repeat audits of total nursing diagnoses will be conducted. When completed, it will be interesting to compare the list in Box 1 with new lists and with lists from other settings (scuh as acute hospital settings). For example, Leslie (1981) completed a frequency list of nursing diagnoses in a long-term care setting. Impaired mobility was the most frequent diagnosis and pain was ranked ninth. On the other hand, Gordon and associates (1980) completed a frequency list of discharge diagnoses from an acute care setting. The most frequent diagnoses were grouped under the Role/relationship pattern.

Since completing this audit, two of the faculty have developed an initial protocol for clients with the nursing diagnosis of *Health maintenance: blood pressure*. A copy of this protocol is found in Box 2.

CONCLUSION

Besides developing individual evaluation schemes for specific nursing diagnoses into protocols, future plans include completing audits of specific diagnoses and designing simple evaluation tools and criteria in order to evaluate effectiveness of on-going treatment of large numbers of clients. There is also a plan to continue to develop and refine specific nursing diagnoses in terms of definitions, signs and symptoms (indicators), etiology, treatment, and evaluation, as illustrated with the diagnosis of *Health maintenance concerns: blood pressure*. Evaluation of referrals in terms of numbers, appropriateness, and preventing acute medical problems is also of concern.

Although the above diagnostic and evaluation process could and is being accomplished in hospital settings, the uniqueness of the nurse-managed WRC allows for greater freedom and clarity of independent nursing. As such, the WRC serves as an ideal vehicle to examine the nursing profession and to develop and evaluate the practice of nursing. Furthermore, the WRC offers an alternative model for health care that can and does augment the existing health care system. Developing and evaluating the effectiveness of treating nursing diagnoses, demonstrating cost effectiveness, and demonstrating a need through fee for services are some of the major tasks confronting nurse-managed centers in the future.

REFERENCES

Gordon, M., Sweeney, M.A., and McKeehan, K.: Nursing diagnosis: looking at its use in the clinical area, Am. J. Nurs. **10:**672-674, 1980.
Leslie, F.M.: Nursing diagnosis: use in long-term care, Am. J. Nurs. **11:**1012-1014, 1981.
Mezey, M., and Chiamulera, D.N.: Implementation of a campus nursing and health information center in the baccalaureate curriculum. I, J. Nurs. Educ. **19:**7-10, 1980.
Ossler, C.C., Goodwin, M.E., Mariani, M., and Gilliss, C.L.: Establishment of a nurse clinic for faculty and student clinical practice, Nurs. Outlook **30:**402-405, 1982.
Reisch, S., Felder, E., and Strauder, C.: Nursing centers can promote health for individuals, families, and communities, Nurs. Admin. Q. **4:**1-8, 1980.

Nursing diagnosis case study: community system as client

DOROTHEA FOX JAKOB, M.A., R.N.

Few, if any, studies exist of nursing diagnosis being used in relation to the nursing of community systems. This paper describes the identification and treatment of a community-wide "health maintenance alteration," i.e., an "inability to identify, manage, and/or seek out help to maintain health," in this case, regarding oral health. This category label was a specification of a new nursing diagnosis accepted for clinical testing at the Fifth National Conference for Classification of Nursing Diagnoses, 1982.

CLINICAL EVIDENCE

The author identified and addressed the prevalence of this health problem while functioning as a public health nurse (PHN), assigned 4 half-days per week to an elementary school with approximately 700 children, ages 4 to 13, during the two school years 1982 to 1984. As a result of affixing colored "flag" tags to school health records during the August 1982 record review, one could easily see that the visiting Department of Public Health dental hygienist had identified 38% of the students as having untreated cavities and 21% with neglected hygiene or periodontal disease. After the May 1982 teaching survey was completed, written notification of the defects was given to the students for their family's information; the notice also included information and a consent for parental signature for tax-paid dental treatment at the closest children's dental clinic (located just across a busy street).

As a new staff member with the Department of Public Health and the school, the author proceeded to gather much information about the school population and families, the school staff systems, and Department of Public Health resources. Only summary information will be presented.

The school itself is geographically located within a culturally diverse inner-city neighborhood; approximately 70% of the students learned Portuguese as a mother tongue, and the majority of families work long hard hours in blue-collar jobs without many fringe benefits other than provincially organized medical and hospital insurance. Various strengths were also identified among the student and family clients; most pivotal for this endeavor was the presence

The author gratefully acknowledges the support and assistance of Carolyn Cruickshank, R.N., M.Ed., Personal Health Services Supervisor (Nursing), City of Toronto, Department of Public Health, Western Health Area, Parkdale Area Office, in the refinement of the poster presentation and discussion paper.

of supportive and influential bonds among multitudes of sibling and cousin networks and neighborhood peers. By October 1982, few of the many students needing dental care had received any despite the proximity of a no-cost dental resource. Many students said "I'm going to the dentist next week . . . next week . . . next week" or "Yeah, Miss, O.K. I'll bring the card back to you." Some parents seemed to think "the baby teeth will fall out anyway." Health care workers who had dealt with the problem for several years felt "most of the parents don't care . . . the kids don't care."

TARGET SYSTEMS AND RESOURCES

Among school leadership and staff a climate of concern and response resulted when this health problem and its prevalence were factually described. The principal encouraged and facilitated the involvement of staff: two key bilingual secretaries, two translator/counselors, a teacher's aide, and all the classroom teachers. Elder students gave invaluable assistance and leadership.

The City of Toronto, Department of Public Health, was in a period of flux after the full implementation of a decentralization/reorganization process in July 1982. The guiding document, *Public Health in the 1980s,* was in the process of becoming a reality. All school students had access to a wide variety of Department of Public Health resources, but in this case/example certain resources were critical: part-time public health nurse, school survey/teaching hygiene team, dental staff of the two closest (part-time) school dental clinics, and the hygiene staff of the closest children's dental prophylaxis (full-time) clinic.

PHN'S OPERATIONAL FRAMEWORK AND ASSUMPTIONS

The following beliefs and assumptions were inherent in the nursing approach:
- Open systems (Hanchett, 1979, Stewart, 1982) and unitary human models (Kim and Moritz, 1982) were used.
- Careful identification of contributing factors to the existence and intensity of the problem would provide direction and leverage for much nursing intervention (see Fig. 1).
- Children and parents value good health, including oral health.
- Good oral health is not the no. 1 priority for many families.
- The lack of a dental clinic in the target school is arbitrary.
- Special efforts would be needed to begin a momentum for responding to this poorly known "epidemic."
- Multidisciplinary stimulation and collaboration would be needed to interrupt this many-faceted health problem.
- Many staff would expend extra efforts.
- Modeling, body-image valuing, peer support, and genuine concern would be healthy stimuli for responsive health maintenance behavior.

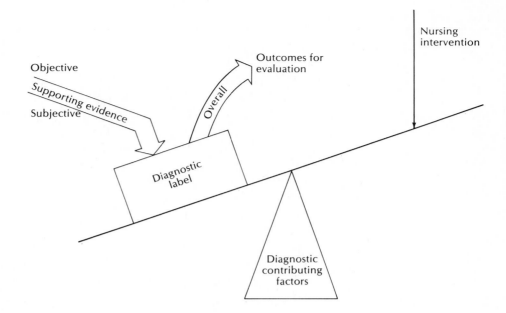

FIGURE 1

OVERALL OUTCOMES

Without reservation, the discrete clinical outcomes displayed in Table 1 confirmed successful efforts. All of the key school and Department of Public Health employees extended themselves personally and professionally. Student participation was clearly crucial in turning the attitudinal tides.

SUMMARY OF CLINICAL METHODOLOGY

As indicated, the nursing interventions geared to decrease the "community-wide health maintenance alteration regarding oral health practices" emerged from a careful identification of four key contributing factors and the PHN's stated assumptions. A summary of the clinical methodology is presented in Table 2.

DISCUSSION

Utilizing nursing diagnosis on a community scope raised several questions for the author. Where are the clinical nurse specialists who practice as community health nurses?

In this brief discussion I propose to link: (1) our current opportunities to develop nursing diagnosis nomenclature with (2) an increasing challenge in the literature for community health nurses to focus on client populations. I also will suggest that the underdeveloped clinical specialist role in *community health nursing* (as opposed to parent/child, geriatric, or mental health nursing) likely presents a formidable barrier to significantly addressing either of these.

TABLE 1   Overall outcomes

Time frame (mo)	Desired	Actual
10	50% lower in students with cavities	45% lower
	50% lower in students with neglected oral hygiene/periodontal disease	68%
	Escalating education program and "hype" about oral health	A "rock dental play" culminated year's efforts
		More than 220 students registered at oral prophylaxis clinic
15	Maintain statistical progress	Above figures essentially maintained
		15% lower in cavity formation
18	Significant student attitudinal change about oral health maintenance	Three to four students per week request referral to DPH dental services

The purpose of this paper is to stimulate discussion among community health nursing colleagues.

NURSING DIAGNOSIS OPPORTUNITY

Over the last 15 years the generation and classification of nursing diagnoses have led to a scientific revolution/evolution for the nursing profession (Kritek, 1978; Warren, 1983). At this stage the concepts of nursing diagnosis are still in flux; no hardening of the definitions or category labels has yet taken place. In April 1982 the Fifth National Nursing Diagnosis Conference in St. Louis presented a new broader-based organization: the North American Nursing Diagnosis Association. At that Conference, Shoemaker presented a definition of nursing diagnosis, derived from her doctoral investigation, which may become a useful alternative to those offered by the Conference group, Gordon (1982b), Mundinger and Jauron (1975), or others:

. . . a clinical judgment about an individual, family, or community derived through a deliberate, systematic process of data collection and analysis. It provides the basis for prescriptions for definitive therapy for which the nurse is accountable. It is expressed concisely and includes the etiology of the condition when known.

Currently 50 nursing diagnosis category terms have been "accepted for clinical testing" by the five Nursing Diagnosis Conference groups and none are cast in stone. In addition, 15 other diagnostic terms were recognized as "to be developed" because insufficient time was available to adequately address them. Other diagnostic terms have emerged from specific authors or projects and could be seen as useful to help bridge many obvious gaps in the span of category labels (Campbell, 1978; Gordon, 1982a; Jones and Jakob, 1982; Simmons, 1980).

TABLE 2   Summary of clinical methodology for community-wide health maintenance alteration regarding oral health practices

Related to (contributing factors)	Intervention objectives	Nursing interventions	Desired specific outcomes
A. Knowledge deficit (student and family) about Basic dental treatment and reasonable self-care behavior Importance of baby teeth vis-à-vis permanent teeth Tax-supported Department of Public Health (DPH) services and how to use them Secondary to misconceptions, lack of exposure, and nonuse of information Secondary to language and educational and life-style barriers between many parents and DPH staff	A. Students and parents will be focus of educational effort Families will be able to understand dental information sent home All consenting families will obtain appointments All students will receive new toothbrush during Dental Week	A. Seek principal's support Engage prioritized students in teaching and encouragement Facilitate multidisciplinary teaching efforts Invite parental consent for DPH dental care Request translation of information Facilitate appointments when necessary Request donation of toothbrushes	A. Prioritized students will begin treatment Interested students will register for prophylaxis care DPH survey hygienist will maximize teaching at school Knowledgeable older students will become resources Material sent home will be straightforward and bilingual Treatment resources will be more successfully accessed Teaching hygienst and dental clinic will distribute toothbrushes
B. Unavailability of adults to accompany students to dental resources	B. Young or fearful students will be accompanied Peer support for older stu-	B. Role model importance of adult escort Facilitate peer accompani-	B. Someone else will eventually coordinate escort arrangements

Secondary to economic and energy priorities of many struggling immigrant families regarding work absenteeism or costly dental care	dents to come to hygiene clinic	ment during appointment making	Students/families will increasingly request dental referrals
C. Knowledge deficits and uncoordinated efforts by many school and DPH personnel about scope and severity of problem	C. Knowledge about scope and contributing factors and system's bugs will form basis for multidisciplinary collaboration	C. Share all information with principal. Explore possibility of increasing available dental services. Reinforce smooth effective working relationships and be advocate for students. Share marks of progress with key personnel	C. Teachers will be urged to include a dental unit. Expanded dental treatment hours. School teaching program will be student participatory: a "rock" dental play. Multidisciplinary communication will increase. Proponents of dental clinic cutbacks will receive expressions of concern
D. Avoidance tactics by students fearful of uncomfortable dental treatment	D. Fearful children will receive treatment with minimal emotional trauma	D. Offer more support and teaching to fearful students. Arrange most feasible escort. Distribute coloring stencils depicting dentists giving treatment	D. Fear and discomfort will be acknowledged frankly and will not sabotage treatment. Positive inoculation regarding dental treatment through age-oriented media

COMMUNITY SYSTEM AS CLIENT

During 1982-1983 several community health nursing authors reiterated the challenge for clinicians to focus on population groups, as well as individual and family clients.

Fry explored a fundamental "moral tension" between "two conflicting ethics" of nursing and aggregate-oriented public health; she maintained that accountability in community health nursing must become refocused toward the population as a whole, and she concluded that grappling with the moral requirements of these ethical principles could determine the future direction and influence of the discipline.

With stinging insight Drehar identified conservative ("thinking small") tendencies of public health nursing theory and practice that interface with transcending a clinical focus with individual families. Rather than attempting to reorganize a chaotic and confusing health care system, she sees educators and clinicians emphasizing the role of patient advocate or counsellor to help the client negotiate or adjust to the system.

Hamilton (1983) observes that "much of the work concerning nursing diagnosis seems to be more applicable to the care of individuals than to the nursing of entire communities." She points out that several authors convey assumptions about the applicability of the diagnostic process and possibly the nomenclature to the nursing care of client groups, systems, aggregates, populations, or communities; to date this has not been tested or analyzed in an actual practice context, although Lunny (1982) and Gordon (1982b) have promoted the notion.

CLINICAL NURSE SPECIALIST ROLE IN COMMUNITY HEALTH NURSING

Gordon (1982b) identifies the clinical nurse specialist (CNS) as probably the most sophisticated practitioner who has a responsibility for studying new or unlabeled diagnoses and consulting about differential nursing diagnoses. (Clinical) "specialty practice is at the growing edge of the profession" (American Nurses' Association, 1980). All other nursing practice areas make use of the CNS for direct care of complex client situations, role modeling, role clarification, colleagial consultation and collaboration, and advancement of the professional as well as the specialty field.

Where are those nurses with graduate education in community health nursing who are directly involved in practice as opposed to education or administration and supervision? As Chavigny and Kroske (1983) observed in their timely, thought-provoking article, ". . . clinical specialization as a public health nurse is viewed as a strange hybrid . . ." where is community health nursing's counterpart to the practicing CNS's in gerontology, parent/child health, pediatrics, mental health, etc.? Where are those who function as practitioners with a strong population focus?

My own observation is that the CNS role has been minimally explored in community or public health nursing by either organizations or by the literature. Williams (1977) identified "(a) the paucity of service settings in which the individualistic clinical approach of nursing . . . and the basic public health strategy of dealing with aggregates are effectively merged and practiced." I would like to suggest that the absence of a clinical ladder (apart from seniority) in community or public health nursing is an important issue worthy of consideration.

Chavigny and Kroske (1983) believe that "role confusion is probably the most salient factor in the problems of public health nursing today." Anderson's (1983) study results from 305 members of the public health nursing section of the American Public Health Association in regard to their community-focused functions seem to confirm this. Fifty functions were identified by the author from basic texts of public health nursing and were viewed as important by the practitioner, educator, and administrator participants. Overall, the participants viewed the administrators as having the major responsibilities for carrying out the functions, but the administrators "differed significantly in perceptions as to who was responsible for performance for various functions."

I believe that now is the time to further explore the role of the CNS at the district level in community health nursing as we grapple with specialty-specific nursing diagnosis development, multidisciplinary service frameworks, and shrinking resources.

Unless community nurses can differentiate their area of practice and expertise from the area of those adapting an expanded community orientation within their fields, it is possible that community health nursing could be integrated out of existence (Archer and Fleshman, 1974).

REFERENCES

American Nurses' Association: Nursing: a social policy statement, Kansas City, Mo., 1980, The Association.

Anderson, E.T.: Community focus in public health nursing: whose responsibility? Nurs. Outlook **31**:44-48, 1983.

Archer, S.E., and Fleshman, R.: Community health nursing: a typology of practice, Nurs. Outlook **23**:358-364, 1974.

Campbell, C.: Nursing diagnosis and intervention in nursing practice, New York, 1978, John Wiley & Sons, Inc.

Chavigny, K., and Kroske, M.: Public health nursing in crisis, Nurs. Outlook **31**(6):312-316, 1983.

Drehar, M.C.: The conflict of conservatism in Public Health Education, Nurs. Outlook **30**:504-509, 1982.

Fry, S.: Dilemma in Community Health Ethics, Nurs. Outlook **31**:176-179, 1983.

Gordon, M.: Manual of nursing diagnosis, New York, 1982a, McGraw-Hill Book Co.

Gordon, M.: Nursing diagnosis: process and application. New York, 1982b, McGraw-Hill Book Co.

Hamilton, P.: Community nursing diagnosis, Adv. Nurs. Sci. **5**(3):21-32, 1983.

Hanchett, E.: Community health assessment: a conceptual tool kit, New York, 1979, John Wiley & Sons, Inc.

Jakob, D., and Jones, P.: Nursing diagnosis; differentiating fear and anxiety, Nurs. Papers **13**(4):20-29, 1981.

Jones, P., and Fox Jakob, D.: Definition of nursing diagnosis, Toronto, 1982, University of Toronto, Faculty of Nursing.

Kim, M.J., and Moritz, D.A., editors: Classification of nursing diagnoses—Proceedings of the Third and Fourth National Conferences, New York, 1982, McGraw-Hill Book Co.

Kritek, P.: Generation and classification of nursing diagnosis; toward a theory of nursing, Image **10**(2):33-40, 1978.

Lunny, M.: Framework to analyze a taxonomy of nursing diagnoses. In Kim, M.J., McFarland, G., and McLane, A., editors: Classification of nursing diagnoses—Proceedings of the Fifth National Conference, St. Louis, 1984, The C. V. Mosby Co.

Mundinger, M., and Jauron, D.: Developing a nursing diagnosis, Nurs. Outlook **23**(2):95-98, 1975.

Shoemaker, J.: Essential features of nursing diagnosis. In Kim, M.J., McFarland, G., and McLane, A., editors: Classification of nursing diagnoses—Proceedings of the Fifth National Conference, St. Louis, 1984, The C. V. Mosby Co.

Simmons, D.: Classification scheme for client problems in community health nursing, Hyattsville, Md., 1980, Department of Health and Human Services, Pub. no. HRA 80-16.

Stewart, M.: Community health assessment; a systematic approach, Nurs. Papers **14**(1):30-46, 1982.

Warren, J.: Accountability and nursing diagnosis, J. Nurs. Admin. **13**(10):34-37, 1983.

Williams, C.: Community health nursing; what is it? Nurs. Outlook **25**(4):250-254, 1977.

The applicability of nursing diagnoses[*]

PHYLLIS E. JONES, M.Sc., R.N.

At previous National Conferences on the Classification of Nursing Diagnoses in 1978, 1980, and 1982, work at the University of Toronto was reported on the development of nursing diagnosis terminology (Jones 1982a to 1982c; Jones and Jakob, 1984). Those papers reported partial early findings of a project which proceeded in three phases between 1976 and 1982, supported throughout by funds awarded by the National Health Research and Development Program.[*] The purpose which guided this project was to discover, document, and define the terms that nurses use to describe the patient situations for which they provide care. The results of all three phases have been reported in full elsewhere (Jones and Jakob, 1982). The purpose of this paper is to share with this audience as sequel to the previous Conferences a summary of the completed work, to comment on the results in terms of their applicability to the practice of nursing, and to raise further questions.

BACKGROUND

As a framework for this three-phased investigation, nursing was viewed as aiming to enhance the coping behavior of individuals, families, and groups as they respond to health-related situations. Nursing aims to assist clients in achieving health, as mirrored in healthful behavior, and in this context coping was viewed as a function, or strategy, of adapting to a situation. The process by which nursing achieves this aim includes four phases: (1) assessing, (2) planning (3) implementing, and (4) evaluating the outcome (Fig. 1).

This investigation focused on the assessment phase during which the nurse, in interaction with the client, gathers information about the client and the client's responses and interprets the information to derive an understanding of the level of wellness, the response, and level of coping. Data collection leads to making a nursing diagnosis, which was defined as a statement of a person's response to a situation or illness which is actually or potentially unhealthful and which nursing intervention can help to change in the direction of health. The statement of the nursing diagnosis has two components: the response and the related contributing factors.

[*]NHRDP project nos. 606-1399-46, 6606-1610-46, 6606-1830-46, and 6606-1567-50A.

The contribution of Dorothea Fox Jakob, Research Assistant, and of the nurses who participated in this project over a period of 8 years is gratefully acknowledged.

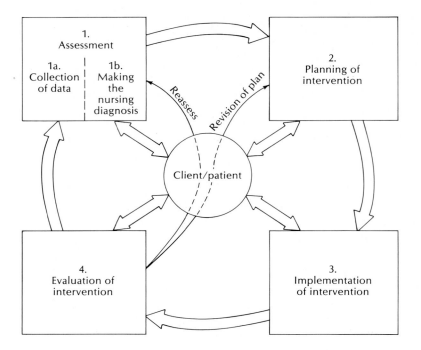

FIGURE 1

Among the assumptions underlying this study were that participating nurses use a form of problem solving in their practice which leads to a nursing diagnosis or label and that this diagnostic label is derived from the identification of those aspects of the client and his environment that are threatening his integrity. Thus it was reasoned that if clinicians judged the categories of nursing diagnoses to be useful in the process of caring for clients, there is likelihood that the identified terminology reflects the real world of nursing from which it was drawn.

PROCEDURES

The procedures of this project were outlined to the 1980 Conference (Jones, 1982b) and will be only summarized here. An initial pilot phase provided for the field test of a list of nursing diagnoses which had been developed during preceding months and enabled the refinement of procedures for data-gathering and analysis, including the revision of the original draft list of nursing diagnoses.

Using these refined procedures and revised list of nursing diagnoses, Phase 2 followed a similar strategy; that is, clinical nurse specialists and nurse clinicians were provided with the revised list, instructions, and definitions and were asked to (1) select from the list those terms which described the client responses identified during 10 nurse-client encounters, (2) provide data to support their selection, (3) comment on the usefulness, clarity, and completeness of the list, and (4) suggest new terms for the list. All completed returns were reviewed and coded separately by two nurse-reviewers associated with the project in order to appraise the congruence between the reported nursing diagnoses and the supporting data. Criteria for acceptance of a nursing diagnosis were

- A human response, i.e., cognitive-affective, behavioral, and/or biophysiological
- A state which was actually or potentially unhealthful
- Supporting data which could be obtained and analyzed by the nurse in the light of nursing knowledge
- Supporting data which would show two or more related facts

Analyses of these data were used in drafting a revised list of diagnostic categories which was subjected to review by a conference of the nurse-participants. The resulting *list of Nursing Diagnoses, 1980,* contained 64 nursing diagnostic terms ordered alphabetically according to major concepts, accompanied by definitions to which nurse-participants had major input.

Following similar procedures, the resulting *List of Nursing Diagnoses, 1980,* was then tested in a third phase as to its usefulness, clarity, and completeness through use in the practice of a non-random sample of registered nurses in a wide range of clinical settings. Analysis of the submitted nursing diagnoses and related data led to the revision of the 1980 *list,* which was similarly subjected to review and revision through discussion with nurses who had participated in at least two phases of this investigation.

It is to be noted here that in each of the last two phases of the project, when reports of related category identification began to be available, the work of systematic revision of the *List of Nursing Diagnoses* and the development of associated definitions included comparison with other relevant works, that is, the Second National Conference on the Classification of Nursing Diagnoses (Campbell, 1978; Gebbie, 1976), and the National Group for Classification of Nursing Diagnoses (Kim and Moritz, 1982). The procedures of these three phases are summarized in Fig. 2.

SELECTED RESULTS AND DISCUSSION

From the large volume of data resulting from this project the major outcome is the *List of Nursing Diagnoses and Their Definitions, 1982.* Attention is focused here on the *List* and its applicability.

List of nursing diagnoses and their definitions, 1982

The *List of Nursing Diagnoses and Their Definitions, 1982,* emerges from the incremental nature of the data derived from the three phases of this 8-year

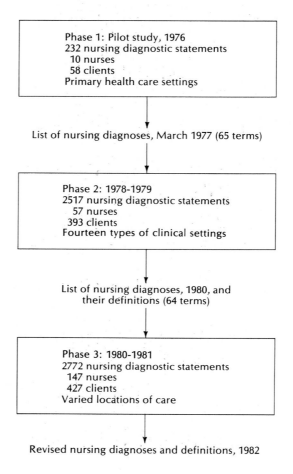

Phase 1: Pilot study, 1976
232 nursing diagnostic statements
10 nurses
58 clients
Primary health care settings

List of nursing diagnoses, March 1977 (65 terms)

Phase 2: 1978-1979
2517 nursing diagnostic statements
57 nurses
393 clients
Fourteen types of clinical settings

List of nursing diagnoses, 1980, and
their definitions (64 terms)

Phase 3: 1980-1981
2772 nursing diagnostic statements
147 nurses
427 clients
Varied locations of care

Revised nursing diagnoses and definitions, 1982

FIGURE 2

project. It reflects the clinical judgment of 214 nurses in caring for 878 clients/ patients in a wide range of settings in which nursing is practiced. These data are summarized in Table 1.

Of the 214 nurses, 123 (57.5%) had university nursing preparation (baccalaureate or higher) and 91 (42.5%) had diploma nursing preparation. About 80% of participating nurses had completed their most recent nursing education in 1970 or later. Clients were from all age groups, and their primary medical diagnoses were in all classifications of the *International Classification of Diseases* (World Health Organization, 1977).

These nurses and clients have influenced, indeed generated, the development and revision of the diagnostic terms and their definitions. Derived from the study's framework, the *List* should be viewed as being comprised of descriptions of human responses to health-related situations which are actually

TABLE 1   **Data from three Phases "the definition of nursing diagnoses"**

	Phases			Total
	1	2	3	
Nurse participants	10	57	147	214
Client encounters	58	393	427	878
Reported nursing diagnoses	232	2517	2772	5521
Mean acceptance rate of diagnoses	67%	66%	76%	*
List reported complete for client encounters	*	3%	66%	*
Terms reported clear for client encounters	*	9%	71%	*
List reported useful for client encounters	*	41%	81%	*

*Not available.

or potentially unhealthful; through actions which assist persons with coping, nursing can help to change these unhealthful situations in the direction of health. Attention is drawn to the importance of the modifiers, potential (at risk), actual, or possible, in describing patient/client responses of concern in promoting and maintaining health. It is also noted that the terms may be used in combination with descriptors of intensity (such as mild, moderate, severe) or of duration (such as acute, recovering, chronic).

The *List of Nursing Diagnoses and Their Definitions, 1982*, contains 71 terms which summarize and label the judgments made by nurses about client-related data gathered during the assessment activities in the nursing process. Terms are ordered alphabetically in two major groups: (1) individual client and (2) other than individual client. We recognize that alphabetical listing in such gross categories makes for some difficulty for use in clinical practice. However, at the time of the development of this List it seemed counterproductive to adopt an organizing scheme which might differ substantially from current work such as that of the nurse theorists in conjunction with the National Conference Group for Classification of Nursing Diagnoses (Roy, 1982). The subsequent publication of Gordon's *Manual* (1982b) offers other typology of functional health patterns.

As noted earlier, the development of the *List* included reference to concurrent reports of category identification. For example, in the report which emerged from the Second National Conference on the Classification of Nursing Diagnoses, Gebbie (1976) reported 35 diagnoses accepted by the USA Conference and 13 yet to be considered; all appeared on the list which resulted from Phase 2 (Jones and Jakob, 1980). Similarly, in the final third phase, other sources such as Campbell (1978) and Kim and Moritz (1982) were considered in the drafting of the emerging list of nursing diagnoses. Of the 42 categories accepted for clinical testing by the National Group for Classification of Nursing Diagnoses (Kim and Moritz, 1982), 24 appeared on the Toronto list of 71 terms. Since the publication of Gordon's *Nursing Diagnosis: Process and Application* (1982) and its accompanying *Manual of Nursing Diagnosis*, a similar comparison reveals that, of the 77 diagnostic categories listed by Gordon, 38 appear on the Toronto list.

Applicability

The question of applicability in nursing practice of the developing terms was addressed by two measures: first, the level of respondent-reviewer agreement for the reported nursing diagnoses (acceptance rate) achieved in each phase (as shown in Table 1) which in Phase 3 reached 76%; and second, the responses regarding usefulness, completeness, and clarity of the terms. Since, as already noted, the comments regarding completeness and clarity of the terms influenced the final version of the list, comment at this point focuses on the question of the usefulness of the categories in the *List of Nursing Diagnoses, 1982*.

As noted earlier, responding nurses were asked, Are the diagnostic statements useful? It is interesting to note (as shown in Table 1) the marked increase in positive responses in the final phase of the project: the terms were judged to be useful for 82% of clients in Phase 3, compared with 41% in Phase 2. The available data cannot tell us whether this increase in usefulness is a result of improved terminology and definitions or of increased familiarity and competence among nurses with the diagnostic process. After all, data for Phase 2 were gathered in 1978 and for Phase 3 in 1980-1981, a period during which the rate of publication regarding nursing diagnoses was increasing markedly. Phase 3 findings shed additional light on this variable since nurses in this phase were asked to judge the usefulness of the *List* in each of the four steps of the nursing process. Usefulness was reportedly much higher in assessing (by 81% of the respondents) than in planning (63%, implementing (53%), or evaluating (49%). Whether or not this is a function of the study design or of how nurses view the nursing process is not at all clear. It could be, for example, that as others have observed (Allen, 1981) to date there has been a greater emphasis on assessment and planning than on implementation and evaluation. When nursing develops greater understanding of strategies for intervention and their outcome, practitioners may be able to see more clearly the relevance of nursing diagnoses to implementation and evaluation.

IMPLICATIONS

The level of respondent-reviewer agreement (76%) regarding the selection of diagnostic category and the judged usefulness in patient care (in 81% of client encounters) provided indication of the clinical applicability of the identified nursing diagnoses. These findings regarding applicability, together with the level of comparability of the list with other categorizations, noted above, led to the recommendation that the *List of Nursing Diagnoses and Their Definitions, 1982,* should be used by nurses in clinical practice. At the same time other recommendations in the *Final Report* (Jones and Jakob, 1982) included some caution in its use:

Continued use of the *List of Nursing Diagnoses, 1982* and its component terms should include testing in clinical settings and with a wide range of client populations. Such testing could include a variety of approaches and should contribute to refinement of listed terms and their definitions, to validation of terms, to deletion of terms, etc.

Newly identified terms should be added to the *List* as they become available.

The results of such testing should be communicated through publication and through the ongoing work of the North American Nursing Diagnosis Association.

Clearly the findings of this investigation suggest that those listed nursing diagnoses with the lowest acceptance rate require further investigation, as do those which have not appeared on other lists resulting from classification activities such as that of the National Group for Classification of Nursing Diagnoses (Kim and Moritz, 1982) and Gordon (1982ab). Some diagnostic terms fell into both categories, that is, had a low acceptance rate and do not appear in other lists of nursing diagnoses (for example, *Significant other's impaired coping; Grieving difficult; Fluid volume deficit; Role adaptation disturbance; Parenting maladaptive; Sexual pattern impaired),* and these should have early study.

Finally, it should be emphasized that this study was undertaken to discover and document the terms which nurses use in describing the patient situations for which they are caring, that is, the label. It did not address the very important area of how nurses make these judgments, that is, the process. Nevertheless, the responses and their analyses constantly suggested questions regarding the cognitive processes, the required knowledge base, clinical inference, etc. These questions led to our recommendation that research should continue on the diagnostic process used by nurses and its impact on the care of clients.

REFERENCES

Allen, M.: Nursing in new settings. In Allen, M., Frasure-Smith, N., and Gottlieb, L., editors: Models of nursing practice in a changing health care system, Montreal, 1980, School of Nursing, McGill-University.

Campbell, C.: Nursing diagnosis and intervention in nursing practice, New York, 1978, John Wiley & Sons, Inc.

Gebbie, K.: Summary of the Second National Conference on Classification of Nursing Diagnoses, St. Louis, 1976, The C.V. Mosby Co.

Gordon, M.: Nursing diagnosis: process and application, New York, 1982a, McGraw-Hill Book Co.

Gordon, M.: Manual of nursing diagnosis, New York, 1982b, McGraw-Hill Book Co.

Jones, P.E.: Developing terminology: a University of Toronto experience. In Kim, M.J., and Moritz, D.A., editors: Classification of nursing diagnoses—Proceedings of the Third and Fourth National Conferences, New York, 1982a, McGraw-Hill Book Co.

Jones, P.E.: The revision of nursing diagnosis terms. In Kim, M.J., and Moritz, D.A., editors: Classification of nursing diagnoses—Proceedings of the Third and Fourth National Conferences, New York, 1982b, McGraw-Hill Book Co.

Jones, P.E.: Developing nursing diagnoses: Three phases. In Zilm, G., Hilton, A., and Richmond, M., editors: Nursing research—a base for practice, service and education, Vancouver, 1982c, University of British Columbia School of Nursing.

Jones, P.E., and Jakob, D.F.: The definition of nursing diagnoses: Phase 3 and Final Report, Toronto, 1982, University of Toronto Faculty of Nursing.

Jones, P.E., and Jakob, D.F.: Anxiety revisited—from a practice perspective. In Kim, M.J., McFarland, G., and McLane, A., editors: Classification of nursing diagnoses—Proceedings of the Fifth National Conference, St. Louis, 1984, The C.V. Mosby Co.

Kim, M.J., and Moritz, D.A., editors: Classification of nursing diagnoses—Proceedings of the Third and Fourth National Conferences, New York, 1982, McGraw-Hill Book Co.

Roy, C.: Historial perspective of the theoretical framework for the classification of nursing diagnoses. In Kim, M.J., and Moritz, D.A., editors: Classification of nursing diagnoses—Proceedings of the Third and Fourth National Conferences, New York, 1982, McGraw-Hill Book Co.

World Health Organization: International classification of diseases, Geneva, 1977, The Organization.

Relationship among nursing diagnoses and between medical and nursing diagnoses

PATRICIA A. MARTIN, M.S., R.N.
KAREN A. YORK, M.S.N., R.N.

The use of nursing diagnosis (ND) has a long history at Miami Valley Hospital (MVH), a 772-bed private not-for-profit teaching hospital and member of Voluntary Hospitals of America. In 1976, the use of ND was formally introduced to the staff during inservice associated with the move to primary nursing. Since then ND has been a fundamental part of most staff development activities. Individual ND served as monthly themes, providing a framework around which to organize educational offerings. In contrast, the Quality Assurance (QA) Committee had been limited to developing standards of nursing care based primarily on medical diagnosis because medical records could be retrieved only by medical diagnoses, a severe limitation for nursing.

In 1982, at the Fifth National Conference on Classification of Nursing Diagnoses, Martin and York reported a study completed at MVH which showed the incidence of ND and identified the ten most prevalent ND from a hospital-wide concurrent study. This report seemed to serve as a catalyst for a surge of interest in ND. Tanner and Hughes (1984) state that this "momentum results from perceptions that nursing diagnosis can contribute significantly to the practice of nursing by defining and organizing knowledge as a basis of practice and by providing a method of communicating this knowledge in a systematic way." Medical Records Department personnel agreed to abstract up to four coded ND from each patient's care plan, similar to the abstracting done for medical diagnoses, starting in March 1983. At about the same time, the QA Committee began converting to a ND framework for standards development and subsequent audit. These two developments made it possible for the first time to analyze records of all discharged patients for incidence of ND. This information was expected to be useful to administrators, educators, and clinical practitioners in efforts to systematically advance the quality of nursing (Kiley and co-workers, 1983).

The Division of Nursing's philosophy of primary nursing identifies the nurse caring for the patient as the nursing "expert"; therefore, the nurses decide on the wording of ND for their patients and assign appropriate code numbers.

Thanks are expressed for the data collection assistance provided by Norma Keefer, R.N., M.S. and Barbara Kellerstrass, R.N., M.S., and for the assistance with data management provided by Ann Block during her temporary service as research assistant.

425

Nursing diagnosis is seen as pivotal to decision making in the nursing process, and lies within the scope of the care giver's responsibility (Bruce and Snyder, 1982; Putzier and Padrick, 1984). The nurses use a suggested list of ND but are aware that this list is not "complete" (Kim and Moritz, 1982). They have been encouraged to use the list when appropriate, but also told that they, as primary nurses, retain responsibility for naming the nursing problems. The reference books used extensively by the nurses are Gordon's (1982) *Manual of Nursing Diagnosis* and the Kim and Moritz (1982) *Conference Proceedings.*

The design was an ex post facto descriptive study of the use of ND. The information about ND and their relationship to other nursing and medical diagnoses was available only as raw data. An adequate analysis and reporting system remained undeveloped, in part because of lack of access to a computer. A manual method was developed to identify the incidence of occurrence of ND and which medical diagnoses were associated with the most frequently occurring ND. This method took 8 to 16 hours per month for data extraction from the monthly Medical Records report and did not permit complete analysis of the data.

The ND were all given a two-digit code. The numbers were assigned as follows: 01 to 10 were assigned to the ten most prevalent ND, as identified by Martin and York in 1982. An alphabetized list of ND accepted for clinical testing by the North American Nursing Diagnosis Association (NANDA) at the 1982 Conference was assigned numbers 11 to 53 (Kim and Moritz, 1982). Records with no ND were coded as 00. Medical records abstractors always record the numbers in numerical sequence (e.g., 01 before 05). Records having more than 4 ND have the first 3 ND identified and the last two spaces are designated "NN." The code numbers are assigned by the nurses caring for the patient. ND which are not the same or similar in concept to any listed ND are all numbered 99. For example, *Alteration in bowel elimination: constipation* and *Constipation* are both coded 13 since they refer to the same concept; *Uncompensated immature temperature regulation* is coded 99 by the nurses who use this in their care of newborns, since this concept is not represented by any ND accepted by NANDA.

Any records arriving in Medical Records with ND having no code are also assigned 99. Any care plan with some ND coded and some not are abstracted by the code numbers identified plus 99 for those not coded. All records have at least one two-digit number, 00 to 99, with 01 to 53 representing coded ND.

Diagnostic skills are new to many practicing nurses (Mallick, 1983); therefore, inservices were held for the nursing staff when the coding system was initiated and periodically since then. Two major recurring themes to these inservices were critical for implementation: (1) nursing diagnosis was defined (Gordon, 1979) and (2) it was differentiated from medical diagnosis (Carnevali, 1984). Pocket cards with the code numbers and ND were distributed to all nurses (see Box 1). Medical Records identified areas where ND were seldom

BOX 1   **Miami Valley Hospital Division of Nursing**

January 1983 list of nursing diagnoses and code numbers

01 Ineffective airway clearance
02 Ineffective breathing patterns
03 Alteration in comfort: pain
04 Potential for injury: potential for trauma
05 Knowledge deficit
06 Impaired physical mobility
07 Alterations in nutrition: <body requirements
08 Alterations in parenting: actual or potential
09 Impairment of skin integrity: actual
10 Impairment of skin integrity: potential
11 Activity intolerance
12 Anxiety
13 Alteration in bowel elimination: constipation
14 Alteration in bowel elimination: diarrhea
15 Alteration in bowel elimination: incontinence
16 Alteration in cardiac output: decreased
17 Impaired verbal communication
18 Ineffective individual coping
19 Ineffective family coping: compromised
20 Ineffective family coping: disabling
21 Family coping: potential for growth
22 Diversional activity deficit
23 Alteration in family process
24 Fear
25 Alteration in fluid volume: excess
26 Actual fluid volume deficit
27 Potential fluid volume deficit
28 Impaired gas exchange
29 Anticipatory grieving
30 Dysfunctional grieving
31 Health maintenance alteration
32 Impaired home maintenance management
33 Noncompliance
34 Alterations in nutrition: >body requirements
35 Alterations in nutrition: potential for >body requirements
36 Alteration in oral mucous membrane
37 Powerlessness
38 Rape-trauma syndrome
39 Self-care deficit
41 Disturbance in self-concept: body image
42 Disturbance in self-concept: self-esteem
43 Disturbance in self-concept: role performance
44 Disturbance in self-concept: personal identity
45 Sensory-perceptual alterations
46 Sexual dysfunction

Continued.

BOX 1 **Miami Valley Hospital Division of Nursing—cont'd**

47 Sleep pattern disturbance
48 Social isolation
49 Spiritual distress (distress of the human spirit)
50 Alteration in thought processes
51 Alteration in tissue: perfusion
52 Alteration in patterns of urinary elimination
53 Potential for violence (self-directed or directed at others)

coded and this information was used to increase motivation on those nursing units. The reports from division-wide audits also provided motivation through competition, as well as identifying targets for intensive staff development.

The Medical Records personnel abstract the code numbers onto an abstract form (see Fig. 1), which is processed into a monthly report. *Special case request E* is the report, including ND, and is available on microfiche (see Box 2). The report is prepared from the abstracts by a shared computer service for health

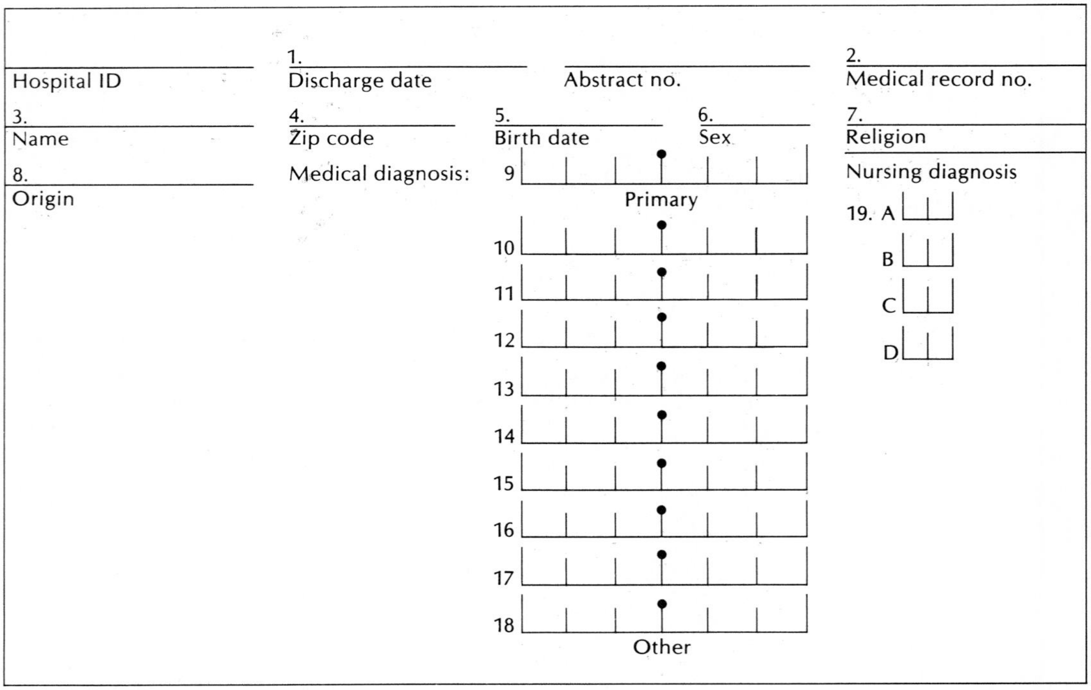
Hospital ID
1. Discharge date
Abstract no.
2. Medical record no.
3. Name
4. Zip code
5. Birth date
6. Sex
7. Religion
8. Origin
Medical diagnosis: 9
Primary
10
11
12
13
14
15
16
17
18
Other
Nursing diagnosis
19. A
B
C
D

FIGURE 1

BOX 2   **Sample report—Special case request E***

Primary medical diagnosis	Other medical diagnoses			Nursing diagnoses		
V25.2	625.9	626.9	465.9	01	03	
			V25.2			
650.	V25.2		V22.2	01	03	
732.0	250.00		732.0	01	03	04
530.0	428.0	496	052.9	01	03	06
	710.0	574.20	530.0	NN		

*Illustrates only 7 columns of the 24 columns on the real form.

care data processing and therefore has a non-negotiable format for abstracting. The information on these reports for March-December 1983 was manually tabulated. This represented 20,309 records. Of these 18% had no ND, 24% had uncoded ND, and 58% (or 11,818 records) represented the sample available to data analysis (Fig. 2, Table 1).

Due to the large volume of care plans and the manual method used, only simple frequency counts were attempted. For each ND the associated primary medical diagnosis was recorded. From this listing, the most prevalent ND were identified. The most prevalent medical diagnoses associated with any one ND were also identified from this list. The ND associated with the four most prevalent ND were then tabulated. No attempt has been made to determine how findings are affected by the overall incidence of either the medical diagnoses or ND (see Table 2 for list of most common medical diagnoses).

There were 12 ND which accounted for more than half of all the coded ND (Table 3). Minor monthly variations in rank order can be seen in Table 4. *Alteration in comfort: pain* (Pain) was always the most frequently coded ND and accounted for 13% of all coded ND in the 10-month period. *Knowledge deficit* (Knowledge) was the second most frequently occurring ND and accounted for 9% of all coded ND. *Anxiety* was the third most prevalent ND, accounting for 6% of coded ND. *Potential for injury* (Injury) was the fourth most prevalent ND, accounting for 5% of all coded ND. *Impairment in skin integrity* (Skin) accounted for 5% of coded ND when actual and potential were totaled together. *Health maintenance alteration* ranked sixth (accounting for 4% of all coded ND). This ND was unique in that before October, it was never ranked higher than seventh. In October printed ND stickers were introduced in the maternity area, and the frequency of use of *Health maintenance* went from ninth in September, to fourth in October and November, to finally third in December. *Self-care deficit* ended seventh in rank and accounted for 4% of all coded ND. The next four each accounted for 3% of all coded ND. They

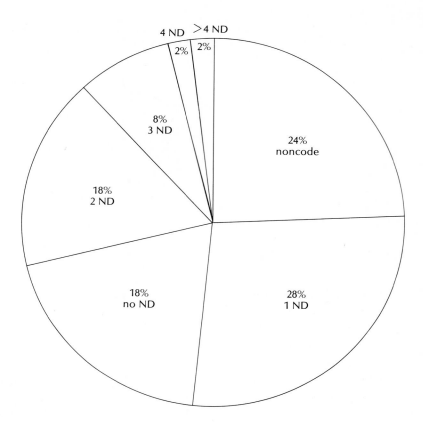

FIGURE 2

TABLE 1   Frequency of nursing diagnoses (NDs)

	Mar	Apr	May	June	July	Aug	Sept	Oct	Nov	Dec	Total	% of all Records Reviewed
Records n =	680	1680	2412	2411	2473	2394	1617	2230	2163	2236	20,296	
No ND f =	160	268	349	434	399	419	292	343	427	528	3619	18
No code f =	200	650	759	607	446	435	341	446	490	495	4869	24
One ND f =	139	317	562	672	804	696	472	687	690	723	5762	28
Two ND f =	103	239	450	398	483	525	331	482	372	349	3732	18
Three ND f =	43	144	184	195	221	222	142	189	125	111	1576	8
Four ND f =	24	19	37	37	39	52	16	41	35	19	319	2
>Four ND f =	11	43	71	68	74	45	23	42	24	21	422	2
Coded care plans n =	320	762	1304	1370	1628	1540	984	1441	1246	1223	11,818	58
Total care plans n =	520	1412	2063	1977	2074	1975	1325	1887	1736	1708	16,677	82

TABLE 2   **Twenty most common final medical diagnoses (excluding newborn) at Miami Valley Hospital (January to June 1983)**

	Percentage of all discharges
Fetal distress, affecting management of mother, delivered	1.7
Chronic ischemic heart disease, unspecified	1.4
Delivery in a completely normal case (best estimate of normal newborn)	1.3
Congestive heart failure	1.3
Uterine scar from previous surgery, with delivery	1.3
Senile cataract, unspecified	1.3
Acute alcohol intoxication, unspecified	1.2
Forcep delivery, not otherwise stated	1.2
Cholelithiasis with cholecystectomy	1.0
Displacement of lumbar intervertebral disc without myelopathy	1.0
Maintenance chemotherapy	.9
Unspecified cataract	.8
Delivery with cord entangled, not elsewhere classified	.8
Chronic airway obstruction, not elsewhere classified	.7
Unilateral inguinal hernia	.7
Pneumonia, organism unspecified	.7
Depressive psychosis, unspecified	.7
Coronary atherosclerosis	.6
Benign neoplasm of leiomyoma of uterus, unspecified	.6
Acute, but ill-defined, cerebrovascular disease	.6

were, in order (eighth to eleventh)—*Alterations in nutrition: less than body requirements* (Nutrition), *Impaired physical mobility* (Mobility), *Ineffective breathing patterns,* and *Ineffective individual coping.* The twelfth ranked ND is *Alteration in bowel elimination: constipation* (Constipation), which accounted for 2% of all coded ND. These 12 together accounted for 60% of all coded ND. The top four accounted for approximately one third of the sample.

These top four ND had some interesting medical diagnoses associated with them (see Table 5). There were two main associated primary medical diagnoses accounting for 7% of the 3035 care plans where pain was identified as a ND. *Spinal disc displacement* (4%) and *Back pain* (3%) were the primary medical diagnoses for these patients. These findings suggest target populations needing pain assessment. There were three associated primary medical diagnoses having an incidence over 2% each for the ND *Knowledge deficit: fetal distress and death* (8%), *alcohol intoxication* (6%), and *coronary artery disease* (3%). The care plans with these three medical diagnoses totaled 326, or 17% of all

TABLE 3   Frequency of most prevalent and percent of all coded nursing diagnoses (ND)

	Mar	Apr	May	June	July	Aug	Sept	Oct	Nov	Dec	ND total	Percent of all coded (22,515)
1. Pain	83	209	438	345	380	383	282	359	276	280	3035	13
2. Knowledge deficit	47	89	212	218	248	271	112	264	259	209	1929	9
3. Anxiety	37	91	148	170	188	196	134	189	135	99	1387	6
4. Potential injury	42	98	131	167	148	161	91	130	99	90	1157	5
5. Skin												
Actual	17	41	70	81	106	100	47	63	54	67	646	3
Potential	16	27	54	80	79	66	40	63	53	33	511	2
Total	33	68	124	161	185	166	87	126	107	100	1157	5
6. Altered health maintenance	9	56	93	79	113	99	70	141	126	177	963	4
7. Self care	27	58	80	101	108	106	77	100	78	72	807	4
8. Nutrition: less than	18	56	106	118	111	94	71	56	71	63	764	3
9. Mobility	24	47	73	96	95	100	56	76	65	52	684	3
10. Breathing patterns	14	47	67	88	76	71	66	68	28	57	582	3
11. Individual coping	10	35	87	68	72	69	50	62	58	54	565	3
12. Constipation	25	54	79	58	65	82	43	62	37	41	546	2
Monthly total	369	908	1638	1669	1789	1798	1139	1633	1339	1294	13,576	60
All coded	687	1507	2527	2842	2823	2957	1873	2680	2369	2250	22,515	—
Monthly total ÷ All coded	54%	60%	65%	59%	63%	61%	61%	61%	56%	58%	60%	—

TABLE 4   **Rank order for frequency of nursing diagnoses**

	Mar	Apr	May	June	July	Aug	Sept	Oct	Nov	Dec	Average
1. Pain	1	1	1	1	1	1	1	1	1	1	1
2. Knowledge	2	4	2	2	2	2	3	2	2	2	2
3. Anxiety	4	3	3	3	3	3	2	3	3	4	3
4. Injury	3	2	4	4	6	6	4	5	8	7	4
5/6. Skin Actual Potential	5/6	5/6	5/6	5/6	4/5	4/5	5/6	6/7	5/6	5/6	5/6
7. Health maintenance	15	8/9	8	11	7	9	9	4	4	3	7
8. Self care	7	7	10	8	9	7	7	8	9	8	8
9. Nutrition	9	8/9	7	7	8	10	8	15	10	9	9
10. Mobility	9	11/12	12	9	10	8	11	9	11	13	10
11. Breathing pattern	12/13	11/12	13	10	12	15	10	10	16	11	11
12. Coping (I) (individual)	14	13	9	13	13	14	12	12/13	12	12	13
13. Constipation	8	10	11	14	14	12	14	12/13	14	14	12
14. Airway clearance	17	15	14	15	15	13	13	14	13	15	14

A: Pain
B: Knowledge deficit
C: Anxiety
D: Potential for injury
E: Impaired skin integrity
F: Health maintenance alteration
G: Self-care deficit
H: Alteration in nutrition: less than body requirements
I: Impaired mobility
J: Ineffective breathing patterns
K: Ineffective individual coping
L: Constipation

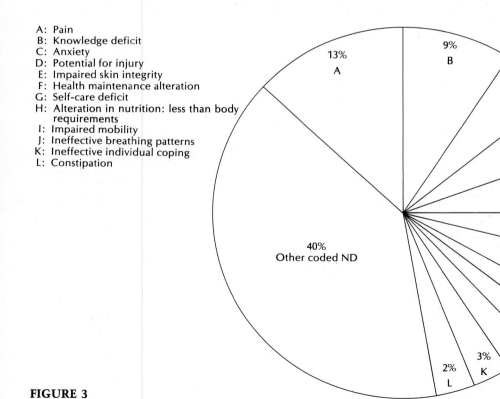

FIGURE 3

TABLE 5   Most prevalent nursing diagnoses (NDs) and associated medical diagnoses (MDs)

ND	Mar	Apr	May	June	July
03 Pain (TOTAL)*	MD (f) % 722 (3) 4 724 (6) 7 (83)	MD (f) % 722 (12) 6 724 (12) 6 (209)	MD (f) % 722 (20) 5 724 (14) 3 (438)	MD (f) % 722 (11) 3 724 (7) 2 (345)	MD (f) % 722 (17) 4 724 (15) 4 (380)
05 Knowledge (TOTAL)	303 (5) 11 656 (3) 6 414 (5) 11 (47)	303 (9) 10 656 (6) 7 414 (8) 9 (89)	303 (18) 8 656 (14) 7 414 (7) 3 (212)	303 (19) 9 656 (7) 3 414 (7) 3 (218)	303 (14) 6 656 (13) 5 414 (5) 2 (248)
12 Anxiety (TOTAL)	414 (3) 8 366 (2) 5 (37)	414 (2) 2 366 (2) 2 (91)	414 (4) 3 366 (0) 0 (148)	414 (3) 2 366 (0) 0 (170)	414 (3) 2 366 (2) 1 (188)
04 Injury (TOTAL)	366 (7) 17 V30 (0) 0 (42)	366 (5) 5 V30 (0) 0 (98)	366 (21) 5 V30 (44) 11 (411)	366 (24) 14 V30 (0) 0 (167)	366 (31) 21 V30 (0) 0 (148)
31 Health mainte-nance (TOTAL)	V30 (8) 39 (9)	V30 (42) 75 (56)	V30 (80) 86 (93)	V30 (66) 84 (79)	V30 (96) 85 (113)

*Monthly total of nursing diagnoses in this code

Key to MD code numbers

722 = *Spinal disc displacement*   414 = *Coronary artery disease*
724 = *Back pain*   414 = *Chronic ischemic heart disease*
303 = *Acute alcohol intoxication*   366 = *Cataract*
656 = *Fetal distress and death*   V30 = *Healthy newborn*

TABLE 6   Most common nursing diagnoses (NDs) and associated nursing diagnoses (ANDs)

	Mar	Apr	May	June	July
03 Pain (TOTAL)	AND (f) % 05 (11) 13 12 (5) 6 (83)	AND (f) % 05 (11) 5 12 (16) 8 (209)	AND (f) % 05 (39) 9 12 (30) 7 (438)	AND (f) % 05 (24) 7 12 (31) 9 (345)	AND (f) % 05 (43) 11 12 (38) 10 (380)
05 Knowledge deficit (TOTAL)	03 (11) 23 08 (0) 0 18 (2) 4 12 (2) 4 (47)	03 (11) 12 08 (1) 1 18 (9) 10 12 (5) 6 (89)	03 (39) 18 08 (4) 2 18 (20) 9 12 (11) 5 (212)	03 (24) 11 08 (2) 1 18 (18) 8 12 (9) 4 (218)	03 (43) 17 08 (9) 4 18 (9) 4 12 (20) 8 (248)
12 Anxiety (TOTAL)	03 (5) 14 05 (2) 5 (37)	03 (16) 18 05 (5) 5 (91)	03 (30) 20 05 (11) 7 (148)	03 (31) 18 05 (9) 5 (170)	03 (38) 20 05 (20) 11 (188)
04 Potential for injury (TOTAL)	05 (2) 5 39 (9) 21 (42)	05 (5) 5 39 (12) 12 (98)	05 (10) 8 39 (21) 16 (131)	05 (11) 7 39 (33) 20 (167)	05 (12) 8 39 (29) 20 (148)

Key to AND code numbers

03, 04, 05, and 12 = Same as for ND   18 = *Ineffective individual coping*
08 = *Alterations in parenting*   39 = *Self-care deficit*

Aug	Sept	Oct	Nov	Dec	Total
MD (f) %	MD (f) %	MD (f) %	MD (f) %	MD (f) %	MD (f) %
722 (15) 4	722 (15) 5	722 (7) 2	722 (9) 3	722 (12) 4	722 (121) 4
724 (13) 3	724 (5) 2	724 (13) 4	724 (6) 2	724 (8) 3	724 (99) 3
(383)	(282)	(359)	(276)	(280)	(3035)
303 (15) 6	303 (7) 6	303 (10) 4	303 (10) 4	303 (6) 3	303 (113) 6
656 (25) 9	656 (13) 12	656 (27) 10	656 (25) 10	656 (18) 9	656 (151) 8
414 (12) 4	414 (6) 5	414 (6) 2	414 (5) 2	414 (1) ½	414 (62) 3
(271)	(112)	(264)	(259)	(209)	(1929)
414 (8) 4	414 (8) 6	414 (8) 5	414 (3) 2	414 (3) 2	414 (45) 3
366 (3) 2	366 (5) 4	366 (4) 3	366 (6) 4	366 (0) 0	366 (24) 2
(196)	(134)	(189)	(135)	(99)	(1387)
366 (27) 17	366 (14) 15	366 (23) 18	366 (7) 7	366 (12) 13	366 (171) 12
V30 (0) 0	V30 (0) 0	V30 (1) 1	V30 (1) 1	V30 (2) 2	V30 (48) 3
(161)	(91)	(130)	(99)	(90)	(1437)
V30 (67) 69	V30 (40) 57	V30 (98) 70	V30 (95) 75	V30 (110) 62	V30 (702) 73
(99)	(70)	(141)	(126)	(177)	(963)

Aug	Sept	Oct	Nov	Dec	Total
AND (f) %	AND (f) %	AND (f) %	AND (f) %	AND (f) %	AND (f) %
05 (22) 6	05 (17) 6	05 (33) 9	05 (27) 10	05 (21) 8	05 (248) 8
12 (35) 9	12 (27) 10	12 (32) 9	12 (13) 5	12 (16) 6	12 (243) 8
(383)	(282)	(359)	(276)	(280)	(3035)
03 (22) 8	03 (17) 15	03 (33) 12	03 (27) 10	03 (21) 10	03 (248) 13
08 (54) 20	08 (10) 9	08 (39) 15	08 (75) 29	08 (42) 20	08 (236) 12
18 (15) 6	18 (16) 14	18 (9) 3	18 (15) 6	18 (15) 7	18 (128) 7
12 (16) 6	12 (14) 13	12 (21) 8	12 (7) 3	12 (6) 3	12 (111) 6
(271)	(112)	(264)	(259)	(209)	(1929)
03 (35) 18	03 (27) 20	03 (32) 17	03 (13) 10	03 (16) 16	03 (243) 18
05 (16) 8	05 (14) 10	05 (21) 11	05 (7) 5	05 (6) 6	05 (111) 8
(196)	(134)	(189)	(135)	(99)	(1387)
05 (11) 7	05 (6) 6	05 (8) 6	05 (11) 11	05 (6) 7	05 (82) 7
39 (24) 15	39 (19) 21	39 (17) 13	39 (14) 14	39 (16) 18	39 (194) 17
(161)	(91)	(130)	(99)	(90)	(1157)

those where "Knowledge deficit" was an identified ND. There were two identifiable primary medical diagnoses associated with anxiety, *Chronic ischemic
heart disease* (on 3% of the care plans) and *Cataracts* (on 2% of the 1387 care
plans), where anxiety was an identified ND. Cataracts also accounted for 12%
of the care plans where injury was an identified ND. Normal newborn (3%)
was the only other identifiable primary medical diagnosis associated with
injury.

These top four ND, where the top medical diagnoses never are associated
with more than 12% of the total, illustrate the wide range of medical diagnoses
associated with any one ND. Compare this to the ND "health maintenance"
where 73% of the medical records had a primary medical diagnosis of "normal
newborn." From this comparison it is easy to see the influence of the printed
ND stickers available in the Maternity areas.

The associated nursing diagnoses (ANDs) also form some interesting patterns (see Table 6). The two most prevalent ANDs for the ND of *Pain* were
Knowledge deficit and *Anxiety*, which were each associated with pain on
approximately 8% of 3035 care plans. For the ND of *Knowledge deficit* besides
Pain (13%), the ANDs were *Alterations in parenting* (on 12%) and *Ineffective
individual coping* (on 7%). Besides the AND of *Pain* on 17% of the 1387 care
plans where *Anxiety* was a ND, the only two frequently appearing ANDs were
Constipation (on 3% of the care plans) and *Alterations in patterns of urinary
elimination* (on 2%). On the 1157 care plans where *Potential for injury was
identified as a ND, the ANDs were Self-care deficit* (on 17%) and *Knowledge
deficit* (on 7%). An overall pattern of association was noted between pain,
knowledge deficit, and anxiety.

These findings offer some concrete descriptions of the nursing care provided
by the nurses at one large acute care hospital. This information can be used
by nursing administrators in their strategic planning. The Quality Assurance
Committee can use the prevalence to prioritize nursing standards for development or further work. Standards based on ND provide a big step toward
outcome measures for efficiency of nursing care. Staff development activities
such as inservice and orientation can consider these findings when setting
priorities for content. Decisions about resource allocation of staff and support
services can be based in part on these descriptors of the nursing care provided
from March to December 1983. Knowledge of the associated medical diagnoses
can assist with targeted admission assessments to improve the efficiency of
nursing care. Computer assistance seems likely in 1984 so that more sophisticated analysis will be possible for assessing relationships among ND, and
between ND and medical diagnoses.

REFERENCES

Bruce, J.A., and Snyder, M.E.: The right and responsibility to diagnose, Amer. J. Nurs. **82:**645-646, 1982.

Carnevali, D.L.: Nursing diagnosis: An evolutionary view, Top. Clin. Nurs. **5:**10-20, 1984.

Gordon, M.: The concept of nursing diagnosis, Nurs. Clin. North Am. **14:**483-485, 1979.

Gordon, M.: Manual of nursing diagnosis, New York, 1982, McGraw-Hill Book Co.

Kiley, M., and others: Computerized nursing information systems, Nurs. Manage. **14**(7):26-29, 1983.

Kim, M.J., and Moritz, D.A., editors: Classification of nursing diagnoses—Proceedings of the Third and Fourth National Conferences, New York, 1982, McGraw-Hill Book Co.

Mallick, M.J.: Nursing diagnosis and the novice student, Nurs. Health Care **4:**455-459, 1983.

Martin, P., and York, K.: Incidence of nursing diagnosis. In Kim, M.J., McFarland, G.K., and McLane, A., editors: Classification of nursing diagnoses—Proceedings of the Fifth National Conference, St. Louis, 1984, The C.V. Mosby Co.

Putzier, D., and Padrick, K.P.: Nursing diagnosis: a component of nursing process and decision making, Top. Clin. Nurs. **5:**21-29, 1984.

Tanner, C.A., and Hughes, A.M.G.: Nursing diagnosis: Issues in clinical practice research, Top. Clin. Nurs. **5:**30-38, 1984.

Anticipatory/dysfunctional grieving and inappropriate aggression: a descriptive study[*]

GERTRUDE K. McFARLAND, D.N.Sc., R.N.[*]
CHARLOTTE NASCHINSKI, M.S., R.N.[*]

Anticipatory grieving and *Dysfunctional grieving* are nursing diagnoses accepted at the Fourth National Conference on the Classification of Nursing Diagnoses (Kim and Moritz, 1982) as well as by the Fifth National Conference (Kim and associates, 1984ab). Defining characteristics, as well as etiology, have likewise been identified for these two diagnoses by the National Conference Group. In fact, work on these diagnoses goes back to the First National Conference, held in 1973, when a total of seven nursing diagnoses focusing on various aspects of grieving were identified. At the Fourth Conference it was suggested that developmental work continue for both *Anticipatory grieving* and *Dysfunctional grieving* (Kim and Moritz, 1982).

Potential for violence was accepted at the Fourth and Fifth Conferences (Kim and Moritz, 1982; Kim and associates, 1984ab). At the Fifth Conference, a number of diagnoses to be developed were identified in this general behavioral area—*Aggressive coping mode, Aggressive responsive state, Rational anger state,* and *Self-harm* (Kim and associates, 1984ab). The authors propose *inappropriate aggression* as a nursing diagnosis in this area of focus. Obviously, continuing developmental work is still needed in this area.

Over the past 4 years extensive literature research has been conducted, clinical observations were made, and input was sought from numerous psychiatric nurses in the areas of grieving, aggression, and communication. This data base, along with input from NANDA's work, was utilized in developing the nursing diagnostic labels—*Anticipatory grieving, Dysfunctional grieving, Impaired communication,* and *Inappropriate aggression*—along with etiologies, defining characteristics, and goals and nursing interventions (McFarland and Naschinski, 1986; McFarland and Wasli, 1982, 1984, 1986, and one in press).

A descriptive study was conducted in order to determine professional judgments regarding the relevancy of the etiological factors and defining charac-

[*]The opinions expressed herein are those of Dr. Gertrude K. McFarland and Ms. Charlotte Naschinski, R.N., M.S., and do not necessarily reflect those of the Division of Nursing, Health Resources and Services, Adminstration, Department of Health and Human Services, or those of Saint Elizabeth's Hospital, National Institute of Mental Health, USDHHS, respectively.

teristics of these four diagnoses. This report will focus on describing that portion of the study and results focusing on three of the four diagnostic labels— anticipatory/dysfunctional grieving and inappropriate aggression.

STATEMENT OF PURPOSE

The purposes of the descriptive study were to (1) validate and/or identify etiological factors and defining characteristics for the nursing diagnostic labels *Anticipatory grieving* and *Dysfunctional grieving* and (2) validate and/or identify etiological factors and defining characteristics for the diagnostic label *Inappropriate aggression.*

METHODOLOGY

The convenience study sample consisted of 25 nurses with a master's or doctoral degree in nursing plus a minimum of 2 years' clinical experience in psychiatric nursing. The subjects were currently employed at the same large, federal, mental hospital and were involved in providing a wide range of treatment modalities and services to a variety of psychiatric clients.

The data base which has been generated was utilized to develop a survey tool. On this tool were listed the etiological factors and defining characteristics for each nursing diagnosis. The subjects were asked to validate the etiologies and defining characteristics by documenting their opinion in checking either the "yes" or "no" column. Blanks were available for the participants to specify any other possible etiological factors and defining characteristics.

In addition, a client observation tool was developed for the diagnosis of inappropriate aggression on which were listed the defining characteristics of this diagnosis. Five subjects were asked to observe one client experiencing inappropriate aggression, for a total of five tours of duty. At the end of each tour of duty, the subject checked off those defining characteristics observed in the clients during the indicated time span. Client observational tools were not developed for the diagnoses of *Anticipatory grieving* or *Dysfunctional grieving,* due to the paucity of clients at the participating agency experiencing these diagnoses.

RESULTS AND DISCUSSION

The data generated from the survey tool and the client observation tools were tabulated and reported as both raw numbers and as percentages of respondents validating the identified etiological factors and defining characteristics of each nursing diagnosis.

The findings of the RN Survey on anticipatory grieving, dysfunctional grieving, and inappropriate aggression are documented in Tables 1 to 6. The number of responding RNs agreeing that the specified etiological factors and defining characteristics are valid for the respective diagnoses are documented in column

TABLE 1   **Etiology of anticipatory grieving**

Factors (see p. 441 for symbols)	RN Survey (n = 25)	
	n	%
○ Perceived potential loss of significant person	24	96
+ Perceived potential loss of significant animal	24	96
* Perceived potential loss of prized material possession(s)	24	96
+ Perceived potential loss of body part(s) or function(s)	24	96
○ Perceived potential loss of physiopsychosocial well-being	24	96
+ Perceived potential loss of social role	24	96
+ Perceived potential developmental or role transitional loss(es)	22	88
+ Perceived impending death of self	24	96

From McFarland, G., and Wasli, E.: In Thompson, J., and others, editors: Clinical nursing, St. Louis, 1986, The C.V. Mosby Co.

TABLE 2   **Defining characteristics of anticipatory grieving**

Factors (see p. 441 for symbols)	RN survey (n = 25)	
	n	%
* Normal grieving initiated upon anticipation of a significant loss	24	96
○ Denial of potential loss	20	80
+ Shock	20	80
+ Disbelief	21	84
+ Avoiding focusing on loss	21	84
+ Physiological symptoms	22	88
+ Decreased muscular power	18	72
+ Feeling of emptiness in stomach	23	92
* Tightness in throat	23	92
* Choking sensation	20	80
+ Shortness of breath	20	80
+ Sighing	21	84
+ Perspiration	18	72
+ Flushed face	18	72
* Exhaustion	19	76
○ Changes in eating habits, e.g., decreased appetite	22	88
+ Internal preoccupation	21	84
* Disinterest or difficulty in carrying out activities of daily living	21	84

TABLE 2 **Defining characteristics of anticipatory grieving—cont'd**

Factors (see p. 441 for symbols)	RN survey (n = 25)	
	n	%
○ Anger	24	96
+ Hostility or irritability toward others	23	92
○ Guilt	22	88
+ Self-accusation of negligence	21	84
+ Weeping	22	88
+ Feelings of loss and loneliness	23	92
+ Emotional distance from others	22	88
+ Sense of unreality	21	84
○ Alterations in sleep patterns	23	92
* Social isolation and inhibition	21	84
○ Altered communication patterns	21	84
* Speech pressure	16	64
* Reduced communication	19	76
○ Alterations in activity level	21	84
* Psychomotor retardation	19	76
* Restlessness with inability to engage in organized activities	20	80
+ Withdrawal	21	84
+ Decreased acceleration of grieving, increased defense mechanisms as death or loss approaches	21	84
+ Hope regarding action(s) to prevent actual loss	22	88
+ Realization or resolution of impending death or loss	21	84

From McFarland, G., and Wasli, E.: In Thompson, J., and others, editors: Clinical nursing, St. Louis, 1986, The C.V. Mosby Co.

1, followed by a calculation of the percentage of respondents validating this in column 2.

The findings from the observation tool are recorded in column 3 for the diagnosis *Inappropriate aggression.*

Tables containing etiological factors and defining characteristics for all diagnoses except inappropriate aggression are coded utilizing three symbols:

○ Identifies an etiological factor or defining characteristic accepted at the Fifth National Conference (Kim and associates, 1984ab)

* Identifies a modification of an etiological factor or defining characteristic accepted at the Fifth National Conference

+ Identifies a new etiological factor or defining characteristic

TABLE 3   **Etiology of dysfunctional grieving**

Factors (see p. 441 for symbols)	RN survey (n = 25)	
	n	%
* Perceived/actual loss of significant person	21	84
+ Perceived/actual loss of significant animal	21	84
* Perceived/actual loss of prized material possession(s)	21	84
* Perceived/actual loss of body part(s) or function(s)	21	84
* Perceived/actual loss of physiopsychosocial well-being	21	84
* Perceived/actual loss of social role(s)	22	88
+ Perceived/actual developmental or role transition loss(es)	19	76
+ Multiple previous or concurrent losses	24	96
* Previous unresolved or interlocking grief reactions	25	100
+ Lack of adequate social supports	23	92
+ Difficulty/inability in expressing feelings freely	21	84
+ Unresolved guilt related to deceased person	25	100
* Sudden, untimely, unexpected death or loss	22	88
+ Prolonged or stressful anticipated loss	23	92
+ Unrevealed secrets or unfinished business with the deceased person	23	92
+ Loss sustained when confronted with important tasks or need to emotionally sustain others	19	76
+ Previous pattern of delayed or dysfunctional grief reactions	24	96
+ Secondary gain from others to maintain grieving	24	96
+ Powerful, but silent, contracts with deceased	24	96
+ Overidentification with deceased	25	100
+ Dysfunctional grieving process of parents	22	88
+ Unconscious family maneuvers to alleviate guilt or control fate	20	80

From McFarland, G., and Wasli, E.: In Thompson, J., and others, editors: Clinical nursing, St. Louis, 1986, The C.V. Mosby Co..

For the diagnostic label *Anticipatory grieving* all eight of the identified etiological factors were supported by 80% or more of the respondents. For *Dysfunctional grieving* 80% or more of the respondents checked "yes" for all but two of the 22 etiological factors. For *Inappropriate aggression*, all but one of the 18 etiologies were supported by 80% or more of the respondents. The following etiologies were suggested by individual project participants:

Anticipatory grieving
Recent history of unexpected loss
Perceived failure to reach personal, interpersonal, or career goals

Inappropriate aggression
Threat to vital interests (e.g., property, self, or family)
Threat to need for consistency

TABLE 4   **Defining characteristics of dysfunctional grieving**

Factors (see p. 441 for symbols)	RN survey (n = 25)	
	n	%
+ Arrested/excessive time in any step of normal grieving	25	100
+ Excessive distorted, exaggerated, and/or delayed emotional reaction	25	100
* Prolonged/excessive denial of loss	25	100
* Extreme difficulty in concentration and/or pursuit of tasks	22	88
* Prolonged developmental regression	23	92
* Maladaptive behavior interfering with life functioning	24	96
* Continuous reliving of past experiences	24	96
* Excessive idealization of lost person	24	96
+ Severely impaired self-esteem	23	92
+ Excessive self-blame or self reproach	25	100
* Protracted withdrawal	24	96
+ Protracted symptoms similar to those of dead person	21	84
* Protracted hyperactivity or irritability	24	96
+ Stereotyped, repetitious behaviors	20	80
+ Being overwhelmed by protracted grief	24	96
+ Severe feelings of loss of identity	23	92
+ Loss of interest in and planning for future	21	84
+ Resurrection-of-the-dead syndrome	21	84
+ Unabated searching behavior or yearning for lost object	25	100
+ Feeling or behaving as if loss occurred yesterday	23	92
+ Inability to remove material possessions of deceased	21	84
+ Psychosomatic conditions	20	80
* Social withdrawal/isolation	21	84
+ Engaging in self-detrimental activities	21	84
+ Unusual dependency	19	76
* Expansive overactivity without sense of loss	23	92
+ Prolonged depression, agitated depression	25	100
+ Irrational despair, severe hopelessness	24	96
+ Suicidal thoughts/fantasies	23	92
* Extremely labile affect	23	92
* Extreme anger/hostility	21	84
+ Furious, persistent hostility toward specific persons	21	84
* Prolonged guilt	24	96
+ Protracted apathy	20	80

From McFarland, G., and Wasli, E.: In Thompson, J., and others, editors: Clinical nursing, St. Louis, 1986, The C.V. Mosby Co.   *Continued*

TABLE 4   Defining characteristics of dysfunctional grieving—cont'd

Factors (see p. 441 for symbols)	RN survey (n = 25)	
	n	%
+ Inappropriate affect	18	72
+ Excessive ambivalence along with inability to deal with it	24	96
+ Prolonged panic attacks	22	88
+ Intense separation anxiety	23	92
+ Schizophrenic-like features	18	72
+ Refusal to follow prescribed treatment regimen especially by clients experiencing chronic mental illness	19	76

TABLE 5   Etiology of inappropriate aggression (+)

	RN survey (n = 25)	
	n	%
Frustration	23	92
Loss of dignity	24	96
Feelings (e.g., anxiety, fear, guilt, anger)	24	96
Need to test reality	17	68
Physical impairment (e.g., minimal brain dysfunction)	22	88
Threat to satisfaction of need for love and belonging	25	100
Repressed resentment, hate, or hostility	25	100
Grief (anger phase)	23	92
Threat to satisfaction of basic physiological needs	23	92
Threat to satisfaction of need for security	23	92
Perceptual or cognitive distortion	25	100
Social milieu (e.g., rejection from significant others, subculture expression of aggression)	23	92
Helplessness	24	96
Thwarting of goals (e.g., career progression)	23	92
Thwarting of needs for power, control, authority, attention	25	100
Ward milieu (e.g., staff conflict, overcrowding)	25	100
Threat to self-esteem	24	96
Substance abuse disorder(s)	25	100

From McFarland, G., and Wasli, E.: In Brunner, L., and Suddarth, D., editors: The Lippincott manual of nursing practice, Philadelphia, 1982, J.B. Lippincott Co.; McFarland, G., and Walsi, E.: Nursing diagnosis and process in psychiatric mental health nursing, Philadelphia, J.B. Lippincott Co. (In press.)

TABLE 6   **Defining characteristics of inappropriate aggression** (+)

	RN survey (n = 25)		Client observations
	n	%	n = 5
Scape-goating	21	84	1
Acting-out	24	96	2
Overuse of mental mechanisms	16	64	1
Gossiping	18	72	0
Round-about derogation	21	84	0
Derogatory jokes	21	84	1
Slamming doors	23	92	0
Temper tantrums	25	100	1
Negativism	19	76	2
Resentment	20	80	1
Irritability	20	80	2
Postponements	17	68	0
Verbal hostility	21	84	3
Physical assault/injury of others	25	100	1
Violence	25	100	1
Cursing	22	88	2
Screaming/shouting	23	92	1
Damaging inanimate objects	21	84	1
Physical assault/injury of animals	25	100	0
Inappropriate forceful goal directed verbal or physical action	22	88	0
Inappropriate defensive verbalizations	19	76	2
Inappropriate physical defensive actions	20	80	0
Destructive offensive actions	23	92	1
Intimidation	23	92	2
Self-inflicted physical harm	25	100	1
Passive aggressive behavior	21	84	2

From McFarland, G., and Wasli, E.: In Brunner, L., and Suddarth, D., editors: The Lippincott manual of nursing practice, Philadelphia, 1982, J.B. Lippincott Co.; McFarland, G., and Wasli, E.: Nursing diagnosis and process in psychiatric mental health nursing, Philadelphia, J.B. Lippincott Co. (In press.)

For the diagnostic label *Anticipatory grieving* all but seven of the 38 defining characteristics were supported by 80% or more of the respondents. For *Dysfunctional grieving* 80% or more of the respondents checked "yes" for all but four of the 40 defining characteristics. Additional defining characteristics for this diagnosis suggested by individual project participants included suicide attempt, weeping, difficulty in acknowledging loss, and distortion of facts regarding the cause of death. For inappropriate aggression, all but five of the 26 defining characteristics were supported by 80% or more of the respondents.

For the client observation on *Inappropriate aggression* 19 of the 26 defining characteristics were observed at least once in the five clients being observed by the five psychiatric nurses.

An obvious limitation of this study is the sample size, particularly in regard to the number of clients observed for the presence of defining characteristics of the diagnostic label of inappropriate aggression. Since the sample of psychiatric nurse experts was a convenience population employed at the same institution, generalization of findings is limited to this and similar populations.

RECOMMENDATIONS

Continued validation for the proposed etiologies and defining characteristics for all three nursing diagnostic labels—*Anticipatory grieving, Dysfunctional grieving,* and *Inappropriate aggression*—is needed. Through replication studies, it will be possible to begin to eliminate those etiologies or defining characteristics that are not supported by clinical judgment and observation of clients by the majority of nurse experts. The studies should be replicated in a variety of clinical settings representing differing client populations and geographic locations.

The proposed nursing interventions for each of the four nursing diagnoses are found in other publications (McFarland and Naschinski, 1986; McFarland and Wasli, 1986 and one in press). The present study did not attempt to test these intervention strategies. It is suggested that research in this arena be conducted.

As previously noted, the initial data base, which included nurse expert input, led the authors to propose the diagnostic label *Inappropriate aggression.* The 25 psychiatric nurse experts participating in the descriptive study did not comment negatively on the use of this diagnostic label and could readily observe the "phenomenon" in the clients observed. It is thus recommended that further consideration be given to this proposed diagnostic label.

REFERENCES

Kim, M.J., McFarland, G., and McLane, A., editors: Classification of nursing diagnoses: Proceedings of the fifth national conference, St. Louis, 1984a, The C.V. Mosby Co.

Kim, M.J., McFarland, G., and McLane, A.: Pocket guide to nursing diagnoses, St. Louis, 1984b, The C.V. Mosby Co.

Kim, M.J., and Moritz, D.A., editors: Classification of nursing diagnoses: Proceedings of the third and fourth national conferences, New York, 1982, McGraw-Hill Book Co.

McFarland, G., and Naschinski, C.: Communication pattern. In Thompson, J., and others, editors: Clinical nursing, St. Louis, 1986, The C.V. Mosby Co.

McFarland, G., and Wasli, E.: Psychiatric nursing. Part II in Brunner, L., and Suddarth, D.: The Lippincott manual of nursing practice, ed. 3, Philadelphia, 1982, J.B. Lippincott Co.

McFarland, G., and Wasli, E.: Potential dysfunctional grieving, dysfunctional grieving. In Kim, M.J., McFarland, G., and McLane, A., editors: Pocket guide to nursing diagnoses, St. Louis, 1984, The C.V. Mosby Co.

McFarland, G., and Wasli, E.: Stress-coping tolerance pattern. In Thompson, J., and others, editors: Clinical nursing, St. Louis, 1986, The C.V. Mosby Co.

McFarland, G., and Wasli, E.: Nursing diagnosis and process in psychiatric mental health nursing, Philadelphia, J.B. Lippincott Co. (In press.)

Empirical validation of defining characteristics of constipation: a study of bowel elimination practices of healthy adults

AUDREY M. McLANE, Ph.D., R.N.
RUTH E. McSHANE, M.S., R.N.

This is an initial report of a larger study of bowel elimination practices of healthy individuals. The purposes of the study were to refine and validate the defining characteristics of the nursing diagnosis of constipation, to identify etiologies for the diagnosis, and to describe bowel elimination health practices for three groups: older adults, middle-aged adults, and adolescents.

The discussion in this paper is limited to the analysis and interpretation of the data collected to provide empirical support for the list of defining characteristics and to identify the etiologies of constipation from the perspective of the client. Earlier efforts to establish validity from the perspective of practicing nurses (using the nurse validation model) were abandoned because practicing nurses limited their assessments to the presenting signs and symptoms rather than the patient's pattern of bowel elimination. A detailed discussion of the preliminary work is reported elsewhere (McShane and McLane, In press).

CONCEPTUAL FRAMEWORK

The conceptual framework for the study included Gordon's (1982) typology of 11 functional health patterns (elimination patterns) and the conceptual categories of diagnostic indicators for the nursing diagnosis of constipation (McLane and associates, 1984). The bowel elimination pattern (referring to excretory function) is one of 11 functional health patterns developed by Gordon to provide a framework for assessment, diagnosis, and treatment of phenomena of concern to nursing.

The importance of pattern recognition as the major cognitive task within the diagnostic process is well established in the nursing diagnosis literature (McLane and Fehring, 1984). Two conceptual schemas for nursing diagnoses incorporate patterns of elimination: Gordon (1982) explicitly included elimination pattern as one of 11 functional health patterns; and the nurse theorists (Kim and Moritz 1982) implicitly included elimination within the pattern of material exchange, one of the patterns of unitary man. According to Gordon, patterns (sequences of historical and current behavior across time) are constructed from the client's descriptions and the nurse's observations. Furthermore, she emphasized the interaction and interdependence of functional patterns with specific reference to etiological concerns, "Explanations of one pattern may lie in other pattern areas" (Gordon 1982), and "the search for causal explanations, (is) usually outside the problem category" (Gordon 1982). It is this notion of the interaction and interdependence of patterns, confirmed by an earlier study (McLane and associates, 1984) that guided the conceptualization of this study.

Although the multicausal nature of phenomena is well accepted in the scientific community, single factor research continues to be prevalent. During the seventies, bowel elimination research in health-related literature reflected a concern for inadequate fiber as the cause of constipation. The status of fiber research was reviewed by Godding (1980), who recommended more attention to quantification of constipation. The need for more accurate and reliable measures of a phenomenon (in this instance, constipation) cannot be disputed. However, the search for better explanations of the complex nature of a phenomenon or a functional health pattern and the interaction and interdependence of functional health patterns, must take precedence in nursing research. Both the conceptual framework and the instrument used in this study reflect the researchers' commitment to the preceding perspective.

The conceptual categories of diagnostic indicators, developed from a qualitative study of healthy older adults who had experienced constipation (McLane and associates, 1984), provided structure for the variables included in this study of bowel elimination health practices.

Bowel elimination, alteration in: constipation—conceptual categories of diagnostic indicators

I. Signs and symptoms
   A. Description of constipated stool
      1. Character qualities, for example, color or consistency
      2. Amount
      3. Frequency (lapse of time between bowel movements, BMs)
   B. Feelings and sensations: physical feelings and sensations associated with constipation, for example, stomachache and bloating
II. Etiology: contributing factors, for example, diet, fluids, inadequate exercise, medication, and change in routine
III. Attending behaviors: consistent use of measures for the expressed purpose of alleviating or preventing constipation
   A. Treatment: measures taken to relieve constipation
   B. Prevention: measures taken to avoid an occurrence of constipation (action oriented)
IV. Health behaviors: use of measures to influence normal elimination, for example, diet, fluid, and exercise

---

Continued.

Bowel elimination, alteration in: constipation—conceptual categories of diagnostic indicators—cont'd

  V. Patterning: behaviors related to production of bowel movement, including toilet routine
- A. Expected frequency: perception of normal frequency
- B. Timing
    1. Actual frequency of bowel movement(s)
    2. Time of day of bowel movement(s)
- C. Stimulus behaviors
    1. Actions taken to stimulate a bowel movement, short-term within the hour, for example, drink hot water
    2. Actions as part of daily routine that result in a bowel movement, for example, breakfast
- D. Response to reflexes: behaviors in response to the urge to defecate

---

The conceptual categories of diagnostic indicators are congruent with the functional health patterns and, like the patterns, reflect the interaction and interdependence of phenomena.

METHODOLOGY
Design

This was a descriptive study of bowel elimination practices of healthy adults. A researcher-designed questionnaire was used to conduct a survey of three groups of healthy individuals (adolescent, middle aged, older adults).

Sample

The sample was composed of 300 individuals: 100 older adults who participated in an exercise program at senior citizen centers in the Midwest; 100 middle-aged adults working in a variety of occupational settings (industrial, educational, and a health care agency); and 100 adolescents enrolled in a high school health class. The older adults ranged in age from 57 to 79 ($\bar{x}$ 66.9), with 92% in the 57 to 75 age category. Seventy-nine percent were women. The middle-aged respondents ranged in age from 20 to 63 ($\bar{x}$ 35.8), with 74% in the 20 to 45 age group. Seventy-seven percent of this group were women. The adolescents ranged in age from 14 to 20 ($\bar{x}$ 14.9), with 83% in the 14 to 15 age category. Seventy percent were females. The older adults were primarily retired (61%). All the middle-aged adults, except one, were employed in a variety of settings. All adolescents were students who attended a coeducational high school in the Midwest and completed the survey as part of a required health class.

Instrument

The instrument used for this study was Health Practices Tool; *Elimination: Client Perspective*, the second of two instruments developed to validate the defining characteristics of the nursing diagnosis *Bowel elimination, alteration in: constipation.*

The initial instrument was designed to gather data from practicing nurses who recorded their practice each time they diagnosed and treated a patient with constipation. The second was designed to obtain data from clients about their bowel elimination practices. Content validity was established through a systematic review of the literature (conceptual, empirical, anecdotal) and use of a panel of experts. Initial construct validity was established as part of a qualitative study of older adults who reported experiencing constipation (McLane and associates, 1984; McShane and associates, In press).

FINDINGS
Signs and symptoms

The respondents identified 22 defining characteristics for the nursing diagnosis of *Constipation*. Nine of the 22 had been identified at the Fourth National Conference on Classification of Nursing Diagnoses (Kim and Moritz, 1982). An analysis of the historical development of consensual and empirical validation of the diagnostic indicators (Table 1) demonstrates the progress made at six conferences (McLane and McShane, In press).

There was a difference in frequency of bowel elimination among the three groups of respondents, with more middle-aged (working) adults and adolescents reporting longer periods of time between bowel movements than the older adults (Table 2). The older adults, however, were members of an exercise class at senior citizen centers, which could have accounted for the difference.

TABLE 1   **Historical development of consensual and empirical validation—diagnostic indicators: Constipation**

1973 1st National Conference	1975 2nd National Conference	1978 3rd National Conference	1980 4th National Conference	1982 5th National Conference	1984 6th Conference
	Abdominal mass	Abdominal mass	Abdominal mass Abdominal pain	↓ Bowel sounds Abdominal mass Abdominal pain ↑ Abdominal pressure	Abdominal distention Δ Abdominal growling Abdominal mass Abdominal pain ↑ Abdominal pressure Δ Abdominal size

Continued

TABLE 1   Historical development of consensual and empirical validation—diagnostic indicators: Constipation—cont'd

1973 1st National Conference	1975 2nd National Conference	1978 3rd National Conference	1980 4th National Conference	1982 5th National Conference	1984 6th Conference
	Appetite impairment	Appetite impairment	Appetite impairment	↓ Appetite	↓ Appetite
					Blood with stool
	Hard, formed stool	Hard, formed stool	Hard, formed stool	Hard, formed stool	Dry hard stool
Infrequent stools	Frequency <3 times per week	Frequency < 3 times per week	Frequency <usual patterns	Frequency <usual patterns	Δ Flatus Δ Frequency
	Headache	Headache	Headache	Headache Nausea	Headache Indigestion Mass in rectum Oozing liquid stool
	Rectal fullness Rectal pressure	Rectal fullness Rectal pressure	Rectal fullness Rectal pressure	Rectal fullness Rectal pressure	Rectal fullness Rectal pain with BM Rectal pressure
	Straining at stool	Straining at stool	Straining at stool	Less than usual amount of stool Straining at stool	Small volume of stool Straining at stool
					Swollen rectal veins
Difficult evacuation of feces					Unable to pass stool

From McLane, A.M., and McShane, R.E.: In Mosby's advanced nursing reference, St. Louis, The C.V. Mosby Co., In press.

TABLE 2   Signs/symptoms: frequency

	Old	Adol.	Mid.
>3/day	3	1	1
2-3/day	25	21	19
1/day	62	47	52
1 every other day	6	20	17
1 every 3 or more days	0	7	5

χ^2 $p \le .05$

Etiology

Ten etiological factors were reported by the respondents (Box 1). The most common factors given for an instance of constipation were being worried/upset and feeling down. Factors related to meals (missed mealtime, missed meals, and usual foods not available) received the second highest frequency rating. Sweating was the next most frequent factor given, with 36 adolescents, 23 middle-aged adults, and 12 older adults reporting constipation produced by sweating. Medications (antacids and codeine), increase in body temperature, and vomiting were also suggested by respondents as contributing to a change in their pattern of bowel elimination.

BOX 1   **Etiology: reason for missed bowel movement**

Worried/upset	Sweating
Feeling down	Antacid use
Change in meal times	Codeine use
Missed meals	Increased body temperature
Usual foods not available	Vomiting

Attending behaviors: treatment

There was no difference among the three groups in their use of oral laxatives to treat an instance of constipation. However, use of suppositories and enemas was reported more often by older adults than the other two groups (middle-aged adults and adolescents).

Health behaviors: diet

The use of cereal, fruits, and cooked vegetables was reported as a health practice by the respondents. There was a difference ($p \leq 0.01$) in the number of times the individuals in each group ate the following foods each week: prunes, cereal, cooked vegetables, fresh fruit, and cooked fruit. Older adults reported eating prunes, cooked vegetables, fresh fruit, and cooked fruit more often than the other two groups, while adolescents reported eating cereal more often than the other two groups. There was no difference in the amount of fluids consumed among the three groups.

Health behaviors: exercise

There was a difference ($p \leq 0.01$) among the groups in the time spent (hours/week) engaged in strenuous activity. In addition, the types of strenuous activities varied. Adolescents reported running, jogging, team sports, swimming, and hiking; middle-aged adults reported swimming, walking, hiking, running, and jogging; and older adults reported exercise, walking, hiking, golfing, and bowling. The individual respondent applied the label of strenuous activity. It is interesting to note that the activities reported by the adolescents required a higher expenditure of energy. However, the exercise sessions attended by the older adults were described by the data collectors as fast paced and vigorous.

Patterning: stimulus behavior

Participants reported whether they responded to the defecation reflex:

	Old	Adol.	Mid.
Most always	91	50	98
Seldom	3	6	2
Never	1	6	—
Did not know	1	37	—

Older and middle-aged adults were more aware of the pattern of their response to the defecation reflex. Thirty-seven percent of the adolescents did not know whether they responded to the urge to defecate.

DISCUSSION AND RECOMMENDATIONS

Data provided initial validation for nine defining characteristics of *Elimination, alteration in: constipation* (Fourth National Conference). Thirteen additional signs and symptoms were identified. In addition, changed or missed meals, stress, and depression were perceived as major factors contributing to constipation. Significant differences among the groups were found for attending behaviors; health behaviors related to diet and exercise; and frequency of bowel elimination.

Recommendations include further refinement and validation of signs, symptoms, and contributing factors of alterations in bowel elimination: constipation. Furthermore, it is recommended that Sixth Conference (NANDA) participants consider adding the etiologies of constipation identified in this study to the approved list for clinical testing and use.

REFERENCES

Godding, E.W.: Physiological yardsticks for bowel function and the rehabilitation of the constipated bowel, Pharmacology **20:**88-103, 1980.

Gordon, M.: Nursing diagnosis: Process and application, New York, 1982, McGraw-Hill Book Co.

Kim, M.J., McFarland, G.K., and McLane, A.M., editors: Classification of nursing diagnoses—Proceedings of the Fifth National Conference, St. Louis, 1984, The C.V. Mosby Co.

Kim, M.J., and Moritz, D.A., editors: Classification of nursing diagnoses—Proceedings of the Third and Fourth National Conferences, New York, 1982, McGraw-Hill Book Co.

McLane, A.M., and McShane, R.E.: Elimination pattern. In Mosby's Clinical nursing reference, St. Louis, The C.V. Mosby Co., In press.

McShane, R.E., and McLane, A.M.: Constipation: consensual and empirical validation, Nurs. Clin. North Am., In press.

McLane, A.M., McShane, R.E., and Sliefert, M.: Constipation: conceptual categories of diagnostic indicators. In Kim, M.J., McFarland, G.K., McLane, A.M., editors: Classification of nursing diagnoses—Proceedings of the Fifth National Conference, St. Louis, 1984, The C.V. Mosby Co.

Nursing diagnoses in nursing practice

AUDREY M. McLANE, Ph.D., R.N.
JANE LANCOUR, M.S.N., R.N.
PAMELA GOTCH, M.S.N., R.N.

Interest in studying the use of nursing diagnoses in nursing practice grew out of an earlier study of the implementation of nursing diagnoses in nursing education (McLane, 1982). The extent to which nursing diagnoses are used in nursing practice has been reported for single agencies (Martin and York, 1984; Miaskowski and associates, 1984; Silver and associates, 1984; Sweeney and Gordon, 1983), but no data are available which reflect the extent to which nursing diagnoses are used within a geographic area.

The single agency studies were done by researchers who were interested in identification of the most commonly used nursing diagnoses, the extent to which practicing nurses used the National Conference Group's list of nursing diagnoses, and evaluation of the quality of the diagnoses. The methods used to evaluate the quality of the diagnoses were described more fully in some studies than in others. Martin and York (1984) used a panel of ten experts to evaluate each diagnostic label using a series of five questions. Miaskowski and associates (1984) focused their evaluation on the relationship of the supporting signs and symptoms to the diagnostic label but did not describe how evaluators reached agreement on the congruence of a diagnostic label with daily recordings of patient observations. Sweeney and Gordon (1983) used functional health patterns, a modification of Gordon's initial functional framework, to categorize diagnostic labels used by registered nurses in the referral of obstetrical-gynecological patients. Silver and co-workers (1984) used a panel of national experts to refine a classification system to evaluate diagnostic labels. The classification system consisted of sixteen categories which served as a model for developing a language analysis system for this study.

PURPOSE

The purposes of this study were to refine an instrument, a questionnaire, designed to obtain data about the use of nursing diagnoses in clinical practice and to use this instrument to study the use of nursing diagnoses in clinical practice.

CONCEPTUAL FRAMEWORK

The typology of 11 functional health patterns developed by Gordon (1982) was used as a framework for this study. The typology grew out of efforts to develop

456

a unified assessment structure that could be used with any model of nursing. According to Gordon, patterns are sequences of historical and current behavior across time which are constructed by a nurse from data obtained from a client and the nurses's observations. In this study, the typology served as a framework for organizing each diagnostic label into one of the 11 categories of functional health patterns (Gordon, 1982):

Health perception–health management pattern
Nutritional-metabolic pattern
Elimination pattern
Activity-exercise pattern
Cognitive-perceptual pattern
Sleep-rest pattern
Self-perception–self-concept pattern
Role-relationship pattern
Sexuality-reproductive pattern
Coping-stress-tolerance pattern
Value-belief pattern

The framework is appropriate for the study of nursing diagnoses in a variety of settings and geographic areas since it incorporates both traditional and contemporary areas of nursing practice and is useful with many models of nursing.

METHODOLOGY
Design

This was a descriptive study of registered nurses' use of diagnostic labels in nursing practice. A researcher-designed questionnaire was used to survey registered nurses practicing in a variety of health care settings and geographic locations.

Sample

A convenience sample of 228 registered nurses practicing in a variety of health care settings in rural and metropolitan areas in Eastern Wisconsin participated in this study. Years in active practice ranged from less than 1 year experience as a registered nurse to 40 years. The distribution was as follows: 0 to 4 years, 50; 5 to 10 years, 58; 11 to 20 years, 61; 21 to 40 years, 51. Eight participants did not specify the number of years in active practice. Nurses who graduated from diploma schools of nursing were most represented in the study (107) while those with a bachelor's degree in nursing ranked second (64). Those with a master's degree or above numbered twenty-two (22) while nineteen (19) held an associate degree. Sixteen (16) participants had a bachelor's degree outside of nursing. Employing agencies were primarily acute care settings (184). Other settings included education (11), long-term care (8), community/home health (7), and mental health (8). Ten respondents did not specify the setting in which they practiced. Of the 228 registered nurses, 146 indicated that nursing diagnoses had been integrated into clinical practice in their setting; 54 said they were in the planning stages; and 28 reported no integration and no plans to do so.

Instrument and procedure

The instrument used in this study, The Nursing Diagnoses in Nursing Practice Questionnaire (Box 1), was a modification of one used to collect data about the use of nursing diagnosis in nursing education (McLane, 1982). The questionnaire was refined in a pilot study using a random sample of registered nurses employed in acute health care agencies. It was designed to gather information about the use of nursing diagnosis in nursing practice, the most commonly used nursing diagnoses in the respondent's practice, and problem areas. The refined instrument was completed on a voluntary basis by registered nurses who attended continuing nursing education courses at a university or health care agency in Eastern Wisconsin.

Data analysis

The diagnostic labels were initially classified by one of the researchers into one of Gordon's 11 functional health patterns. The diagnostic labels within the categories were then analyzed individually by the researchers and classified into 17 categories, adapted from Silver and associates (1984) and the unpublished work of Miller with the developmentally disabled. Classifications by individual researchers were compared and disagreements discussed until a consensus was reached (Table 1).

BOX 1   **Nursing diagnoses in nursing practice**

1. What resources did you use to develop your knowledge of nursing diagnosis? (Check all that apply.)
   a. _____ Nursing school content
   b. _____ Graduate school content
   c. _____ Inservice programs
   d. _____ Continuing education courses
   e. _____ Publications
   f. _____ Peer interactions
   g. _____ Other (Please specify) _____
2. Do you think you are sufficiently prepared to utilize nursing diagnoses in your practice?
   a. _____ Yes   b. _____ No
3. If the above answer is "no," which of the following learning opportunities would you utilize to improve your skill?

BOX 1   **Nursing diagnoses in nursing practice—cont'd**

    a. _____ Baccalaureate education
    b. _____ Graduate education
    c. _____ Inservice programs
    d. _____ Continuing education courses
    e. _____ Publications
    f. _____ Other (Please specify) _____

4. Has nursing diagnosis been integrated into clinical practice in your agency?

    a. _____ Yes   b. _____ No   c. _____ Planning for integration

5. If the above answer is "yes," how is nursing diagnosis being integrated into clinical practice?

    a. _____ Nursing history/data base
    b. _____ Problem list
    c. _____ Patient care plan
    d. _____ Discharge planning
    e. _____ Interagency referrals
    f. _____ Progress notes/nurses' notes
    g. _____ Care planning conferences
    h. _____ Change of shift report
    i. _____ Nursing audit
    j. _____ Standard nursing care plans
    k. _____ Nursing research
    l. _____ Basis for inservice programs
    m. _____ Other (Please specify) _____

6. List three nursing diagnoses that are most common to your practice.

    a. _____
    b. _____
    c. _____

7. Do you utilize a "list" of labels when identifying a nursing diagnosis?

    a. _____ Yes   b. _____ No

8. If the above answer is "yes," which of the following is utilized?

    a. _____ Gordon's functional patterns
    b. _____ Fourth and Fifth National Conference listing
    c. _____ Agency list
    d. _____ Other (Please specify) _____

9. What do you see as "problematic" in the utilization of nursing diagnoses? (Check all that apply.)

    a. _____ Inadequate knowledge of the concept of nursing diagnosis and its utilization
    b. _____ Absence of a classification system for diagnostic labels
    c. _____ Absence of standardization of diagnostic labels
    d. _____ Absence of a practical system within which nursing diagnoses can be documented

Continued.

BOX 1   Nursing diagnoses in nursing practice—cont'd

 e. _____ Insufficient organizational support
 f. _____ Time consuming
 g. _____ Other (Please specify) _____

Demographic data

Years in active nursing practice _____
Highest level of education _____

Type of agency in which you are practicing:

_____ Community _____ Nursing home

_____ Long-term care _____ Acute care hospital

_____ Home health _____ Other (Please specify)

_____ Hospice   _____

What is the size of your agency (beds)?

_____ 50 or less _____ 201 to 300

_____ 51 to 100 _____ 301 to 500

_____ 101 to 200 _____ Greater than 500

TABLE 1   Nursing diagnoses in nursing practice

Category	Definition	Interpretation
1. NANDA Diagnostic Category	Diagnostic category of the Third, Fourth, or Fifth National Conferences on Classification of Nursing Diagnoses	
2. Variation of NANDA Diagnostic Category	Diagnostic category which refers to a pattern of human response similar to a NANDA category	Nursing diagnosis
3. Human Response Pattern	Human response identified by researchers as representing diagnostic category	
4. Somatic dysfunction	Term or phrase which describes potential or actual generalized physiological deviation	
5. Client Need	Term or phrase which describes a client/family deficiency	Precursors to identification of diagnostic category
6. Nursing problem	Term or phrase which describes a nurse's difficulty in coping with client/family care	
7. Assessment	Term or phrase which refers to information obtained through ongoing monitoring or data collection processes	

TABLE 1   **Nursing diagnoses in nursing practice—cont'd**

Category	Definition	Interpretation
8. Intervention	Term or phrase which describes an action taken to help meet a client/family goal	Nursing process components
9. Goal	Term or phrase which describes an intended expectation of client/family health status at certain point in time	
10. Sign or symptom	Term or phrase which describes subjective or objective indicator of client/family health status	
11. Risk factor	Term or phrase which describes fact, circumstance, or pattern of behavior which tends to put client/family at higher than normal probability of incurring alteration in health	Data base components
12. Side effects/complications	Term or phrase which describes actual or potential undesirable result of a therapeutic intervention	
13. Equipment	Term or phrase which describes apparatus used in care of client/family	
14. Diagnostic test	Term or phrase which describes examination or procedure performed for purpose of gathering information	
15. Medical Diagnosis or surgical procedure	Term or phrase which appears in *International Classification of Diseases* specifically adapted for use in North American hospitals (H-ICDA)	Miscellaneous
16. Multiple title	Phrase which refers to two or more patterns of human responses	
17. Nebulous	Term or phrase that is unintelligible/indefinite	

Adapted from the work of Silver, McShane, Nowak, Halfmann, and Hunt as presented at the Fifth National Conference on Classification of Nursing Diagnoses and work done by J. Miller, Central Wisconsin Center for the Developmentally Disabled, Madison, Wisconsin.

Findings

The nurses reported using 372 diagnostic labels in their practice. Three-hundred-four labels fit within a functional health pattern (Table 2). It is interesting to note that the greatest number of responses was in the cognitive-perceptual functional health pattern while no responses were identified for sleep-rest, sexuality-reproductive, and value-belief health patterns. Most of the responses in the cognitive-perceptual functional health pattern centered about altered comfort states.

TABLE 2   **Functional health patterns—language analysis**

	Responses (n = 304)	NANDA category	NANDA variation	Human response
Health Perception–Health Management	7	5	0	2
Nutritional-Metabolic	59	10	43	6
Elimination	30	0	30	0
Activity-Exercise	51	14	36	1
Cognitive-Perceptual	106	13	92	1
Self-Perception–Self-Concept	31	23	7	1
Role Relationship	6	2	3	1
Coping–Stress Tolerance	14	2	12	0
Sleep-Rest	0	0	0	0
Sexuality-Reproductive	0	0	0	0
Value-Belief	0	0	0	0

Other (n = 68): precursors, nursing process components, data base components, and miscellaneous subcategories.

The 304 nursing diagnoses fell into three broad categories: NANDA diagnostic categories (62), a variation of NANDA (181), and human response patterns (12), diagnoses that were not a NANDA diagnostic category or a NANDA variation. The latter were *Depression, Loneliness, Potential for infection, Restlessness, Alterations in body temperature, Adaptive grief, Localized edema,* and *Comfort alterations: nausea and vomiting.*

Further language analysis was done with those responses (68) that did not fit into the three categories. The 68 responses were categorized as follows: precursors, nursing process components, data base components, and miscellaneous. For this study, somatic dysfunction, client need, and nursing function were considered to be precursors. Nursing process components included assessment factors, interventions, and goal statements. Sign/symptoms, risk factors, side effects/complications were placed into the data base components. The miscellaneous category included equipment, diagnostic test, medical diagnosis or surgical procedure, multiple titles, and nebulous words. Problematic aspects related to the use of nursing diagnosis were identified by the registered nurses. Approximately one-half of the respondents (163) reported inadequate knowledge in the use of nursing diagnosis. Other problem areas included: absence of a classification system (93), time constraints/time consuming (91), absence of a practical documentation system (90), absence of standardized diagnostic labels (88), insufficient organizational support (72), and 22 miscellaneous problems.

DISCUSSION OF FINDINGS

More than 90% of the diagnostic labels reported by the nurses could be categorized into a functional health pattern despite the fact that 163 of the 228 respondents identified inadequate knowledge as a problem in the use of nursing diagnoses. Diagnostic labels in the NANDA variation category outnumbered those in the NANDA category in seven of the eight functional health patterns represented in the responses. The self-perception–concept pattern was the only one within which NANDA labels outnumbered NANDA variations (Table 2).

The absence of diagnostic labels within some functional health patterns in this study had some similarities with other studies. For example, Gordon (1983) found no diagnoses within value-belief and sleep-rest patterns. Silver and co-workers (1984) also reported an absence of diagnoses in one of the same patterns, sleep-rest. In this study there were no diagnoses within value-belief, sleep-rest, and sexuality-reproductive. In the latter category only two diagnoses were listed by Gordon (1983).

There was an improvement in the language selected by nurses to label the nursing diagnoses they were using when compared with those classified by Silver and associates. The areas of greatest improvement were less frequent use of somatic dysfunctions, sign/symptoms, risk factors, medical diagnoses, and multiple titles to label patient problems.

CONCLUSIONS AND RECOMMENDATIONS

The study provides some insight into the use of nursing diagnosis in the Eastern region of Wisconsin. Nurses are moving away from a medical to a nursing perspective when viewing patient problems, as evidenced by the 304 diagnoses (>80%) which were classified within eight functional health patterns. However, the findings of this study support the need for nursing diagnosis educational programs as explicitly identified by 163 of the nurses. The absence of diagnoses in three of the functional health patterns and the 68 labels which were not nursing diagnoses provide evidence of the need for more educational opportunities for registered nurses.

REFERENCES

Gordon, M.: Nursing diagnosis; process and application, New York, 1982, McGraw-Hill Book Co.

Kim, M.J., and Moritz, D.A., editors: Classification of nursing diagnoses—Proceedings of the Third and Fourth National Conferences, New York, 1982, McGraw-Hill Book Co.

Martin, P.A., and York, K.A.: Incidence of nursing diagnoses. In Kim, M.J., McFarland, G.K., and McLane, A.M., editors: Classification of nursing diagnoses—Proceedings of the Fifth National Conference, St. Louis, 1984, The C.V. Mosby Co.

McLane, A.M.: Nursing diagnosis in baccalaureate and graduate education. In Kim, M.J., and Moritz, D.A., editors: Classification of nursing diagnoses—Proceedings of the Third and Fourth National Conferences, New York, 1982, McGraw-Hill Book Co.

Miaskowski, C., Spangenberg, S., and Garofallou, G.: An evaluation study of the implementation of nursing diagnosis. In Kim, M.J., McFarland, G.K., and McLane, A.M., editors: Classification of nursing diagnoses—Proceedings of the Fifth National Conference, St. Louis, 1984, The C.V. Mosby Co.

Miller, J.: Unpublished data, Central Wisconsin Center for the Developmentally Disabled, Madison.

Sliver, S.M., and others: The identification of clinically recorded nursing diagnoses and indicators. In Kim, M.J., McFarland, G.K., and McLane, A.M., editors: Classification of nursing diagnoses—Proceedings of the Fifth National Conference, St. Louis, 1984, The C.V. Mosby Co.

Sweeney, M.A., and Gordon, M.: Nursing diagnosis; implementation and incidence in an obstetrical-gynecological population. In Chaska, N.L., editor: The nursing profession; a time to speak, New York, 1983, McGraw-Hill Book Co.

A study of nursing diagnoses in an oncologic patient population

CHRISTINE A. MIASKOWSKI, M.S., R.N.
GRAMATICE GAROFALLOU, M.S., R.N.

As part of a larger project of identifying the characteristics of an oncologic patient population in a tertiary care facility without a designated oncology unit, consideration was given to identifying the nursing diagnoses written for this specific group of patients. This study would provide preliminary data on the kinds of diagnoses practitioners were writing for this population. Comparisons would be made to the medical diagnoses and medical problem lists. The goal was to determine the physical and psychosocial needs of these patients and begin to develop standards of nursing care to meet those needs.

PURPOSE

The purpose of this evaluation study was to identify nursing diagnoses written for an oncology patient population in a tertiary care facility without a specifically designated oncology unit.

METHODOLOGY

The Departments of Nursing and Quality Assurance jointly conducted the studies. A concurrent 3-month review was performed. Data were obtained on the age of the population, sex distribution, average length of stay, admitting medical diagnosis, discharge diagnosis, types of admission, reason for admission, medical problems, treatment modalities utilized, types and numbers of medical referrals, supportive services required, documentation of teaching, and the number and types of nursing diagnoses. A brief summary of the findings will be presented in this paper.

SAMPLE SIZE AND CHARACTERISTICS

The total number of patients identified during the 3-month period totaled three hundred and forty eight (n = 348). The average of the total patient population was 59.4 years. The sex distribution was one hundred and thirty seven males (39.4%) and two hundred and eleven females (60.6%). The length of stay ranged from 1 day for nineteen patients (5.5%) to 124 days for one patient (0.3%). The average length of stay was 12.8 days.

The 10 most common admitting medical diagnoses are listed in Table 1. These diagnoses accounted for 66.8% of the patient population. In comparing

TABLE 1   Ten most common admitting medical diagnoses

	n	%
Lung cancer	43	12.4
Breast cancer	38	10.9
Bladder cancer	35	10.1
Ovarian cancer	34	9.8
Colon cancer	24	6.9
Prostate cancer	16	4.6
Cervical cancer	15	4.3
Lymphoma	9	2.6
Rectal cancer	9	2.6
Gastric cancer	9	2.6

TABLE 2   Ten most common medical problems

	n	%
Anemia	40	6.7
Hypertension	37	6.2
Diabetes	34	5.7
Atherosclerotic heart disease/myocardial infarction	22	3.7
Fever	16	2.7
Pain	16	2.7
GI bleeding	16	2.7
Anorexia/nutritional problems	15	2.5
Arrhythmias	14	2.4
Pleural effusion	13	2.2

the data on admitting medical diagnoses with national statistics, it should be noted that lung cancer is the leading cause of death in males and breast cancer is the leading cause of death in females.

Eighty-eight percent of the patients were admitted for a diagnostic workup, initial treatment, or follow-up workup and/or treatment of their malignancies. Only 12% of the patients were admitted for palliative or supportive care.

An analysis was done of the medical problems listed for each patient. The average number of medical problems for this population was two. The minimum number of problems listed was zero, and the maximum number of problems identified was ten. The 10 most common medical problems are listed in Table 2. It can be seen from the list that many of these patients had other medical problems (i.e., hypertension, diabetes, atherosclerotic heart disease) in addition to their oncologic diagnoses and their associated sequelae (i.e., pain, fever, anemia, etc.).

TABLE 3   Frequency distribution of nursing diagnoses

No. of diagnoses	No. of patients	%
0	16	5.7
1	61	21.6
2	80	28.4
3	59	20.9
4	40	14.2
5	17	6.0
6	8	2.8
7	1	0.4
TOTAL	282	100.0

TABLE 4   Actual nursing diagnoses

	Frequency	%
Alteration in comfort/pain	97	17.4
Anxiety	69	12.3
Alteration in respiratory integrity	51	9.1
Alteration in gastrointestinal integrity	50	8.9
Alteration in genitourinary integrity	43	7.7
Alteration in skin integrity	26	4.7
Alteration in nutritional status	23	4.1
Lack of knowledge	22	3.9
Preoperative teaching	20	3.6
Alteration in metabolism	20	3.6

NURSING DIAGNOSIS DATA

An analysis was performed on the number and types of nursing diagnoses written for this population. It should be noted that sixty-six patients were eliminated from this portion of the study because they were admitted for short stays. Patients who were admitted for between 24 and 48 hours did not require a nursing care plan with the formulation of nursing diagnoses. Therefore a total of two hundred and eighty-two (n = 282) patient charts were evaluated for nursing diagnoses.

The average number of nursing diagnoses was 2.5. A frequency distribution is given in Table 3. The minimum number of diagnoses was zero and the maximum number was seven.

The nursing diagnoses were divided into two groups: actual, totaling 560 (78.9%), and potential, totaling 149 (21.1%). There were a total of 42 different diagnoses in the latter category. The 10 most common actual nursing diagnoses are listed in Table 4. There were a total of 27 different potential diagnoses identified. The 10 most common diagnoses in this category are listed in Table

TABLE 5   **Potential nursing diagnoses**

	Frequency	%
Potential for alteration in respiratory integrity	28	18.9
Potential for infection	25	16.8
Potential for alteration in skin integrity	15	10.1
Potential for alteration in fluid and electrolytes	10	6.7
Potential for cardiac complications	8	5.4
Potential for alteration in genitourinary integrity	8	5.4
Potential for alteration in hemodynamics	6	4.0
Potential for alteration in gastrointestinal integrity	5	3.4
Potential for bleeding	5	3.4
Potential for chemotherapy side effects	4	2.7

5. In general, the nursing diagnoses were written as broad categories. In some cases, the "related to" added clarity and specificity. These data were not analyzed as part of this evaluation study.

It is of interest when comparing the medical problem list with the nursing diagnoses identified to note that pain was identified as a medical problem in 16 cases and as a nursing problem in 97 cases. There seems to be very little correlation between the medical problems identified and the nursing problems identified, with the exception perhaps of nutrition in the patient population. This finding may warrant further investigation.

SUMMARY

This study was an attempt to provide preliminary data on the nursing diagnoses written on an oncologic patient population in an acute care inpatient setting. Further work needs to be done on analyzing descriptions which led to these diagnoses, the accurateness and completeness of these diagnoses to each patient, and the appropriateness of the interventions to each of these problems.

A nursing diagnosis–oriented charting system in obstetrics

CHRISTINE A. MIASKOWSKI, M.S., R.N.
GRAMATICE GAROFALLOU, M.S., R.N.
NANCY HNAT, B.S.N., R.N.

The *clinical* implementation, utilization, and evaluation of nursing diagnoses are vital to the concept's growth and development. Our institution began utilizing a nursing diagnosis oriented documentation system in the fall of 1980. At the time of implementation, the authors envisioned that specialty areas would make adaptations in the generic system.

The obstetrical service was one of the first specialty units to modify the generalized approach. The focus of this article is to describe (1) the issues explored in the development of a postpartum nursing diagnosis oriented documentation system, (2) the actual tools used in the documentation and their integration into the multidisciplinary record, and (3) the process of evaluating the system.

DEVELOPMENTAL ISSUES

The priority question in developing this system was: "Could a nursing diagnosis oriented charting system be implemented on an obstetrical service that delivers over 300 infants per month?" The goal was to develop a system that would establish standards of nursing care for the postpartum patient and her family. The system needed to be both comprehensive and flexible. A major concern voiced by nursing personnel was the time factor involved in writing an acceptable plan of care when the turnover of these patients was so rapid and the volume was so large. Nursing time spent in direct patient care activities and patient and family teaching was the priority. The documentation system had to be useful, workable, and not time consuming.

Another major concern was whether our method of charting in obstetrics would allow the nurse to formulate individualized plans of care, particularly for our high-risk mothers. If the system was too rigid or complicated, there would be poor compliance.

There were two additional objectives to be achieved.

The *first* was to establish a coordinated system of assessment, nursing-directed patient care, patient education, and discharge planning. The assessment process would begin in the labor and delivery suite. The data obtained would be structured in a way that would facilitate the formulation of individualized nursing diagnosis. The established nursing diagnoses, goals, and interventions for the obstetrical service would serve as the foundation for nursing directed patient care. Incorporated into the nursing interventions and evaluation criteria would be utilization of the postpartum teaching guide and principles of discharge planning.

The *second* objective was to develop a standard of nursing care for the postpartum patient that would serve as a teaching tool for the orientation of new employees in the obstetrical unit. This nursing diagnosis oriented and goal directed care plan would serve as a blueprint for the orientee. It would help the practitioner to prioritize the patient's nursing problems, establish realistic and measurable goals, and integrate nursing care with teaching activities. In addition, the care plan would provide a systematic method of evaluation of the patient's progress toward goal achievement and specific standards of documentation.

Each of these issues was given careful consideration during the development of the postpartum nursing diagnosis–oriented documentation system. An evaluation of the system after its implementation would determine whether the objectives had been accomplished.

DOCUMENTATION SYSTEM

The system that was instituted consisted of a nursing diagnosis–oriented assessment tool and a formalized postpartum nursing care plan. The development of the system began with a review of the literature on nursing diagnoses being utilized on obstetrics. There was very little documentation on the subject.

Working with the accepted list of nursing diagnoses published by the Third National Conference (Kim and Moritz, 1982), the American Nurses' Association *Standards of Maternal Child Health Nursing Practice* (ANA, 1983), and the *Obstetrical, Gynecologic, and Neonatal Nursing Functions and Standards* published the Nurses' Association of the American College of Obstetricians and Gynecologists (1974), the actual assessment tool and nursing care plan was completed.

The assessment process began in the labor and delivery area and was completed in the postpartum area. Emphasis was placed on health maintenance habits such as diet, exercise, and smoking and various aspects of women's health, including the practice of breast self-examination. Data were also obtained on attitudes and reactions to the labor and delivery experience and present expectations and concerns. The nurse assessed the need for discharge planning by ascertaining whether the family was prepared for the infant, who would help at home after discharge, and who was caring for other children at home.

The postpartum nursing diagnosis oriented care plan consisted of ten nursing diagnoses (see Box 1). It was utilized for both normal, spontaneous deliveries

BOX 1   **Postpartum nursing diagnoses**

1. Return to nonpregnant state related to termination of pregnancy
2. Alteration in comfort related to perineal healing process and uterine involution
3. Alteration in breast integrity related to bottle- or breastfeeding
4. Alteration in elimination related to diuresis after delivery and perineal discomfort
5. Alteration in body image related to postpartum state
6. Potential for postpartum blues related to emotional and hormonal changes
7. Alteration in life-style related to birth of an infant
8. Alteration in parent-child relationship related to birth of a sibling
9. Alteration in sexual integrity related to return to nonpregnant state
10. Potential for postoperative complications related to cesarean section

and cesarean sections. Specific patient-centered goals, nursing interventions, and evaluation criteria were delineated (see Table 1). This care plan established the standards of nursing practice for each postpartum patient. The plan was individualized in a variety of ways. Additional interventions were added to each specific nursing diagnosis based on ongoing assessment of the patient and her family. Patient progress was documented on the progress notes and on the formalized postpartum teaching guide. This method of documentation provided a clear, concise summary of the patient's care, patient education, and discharge planning.

TABLE 1   **Postpartum nursing care plan**

Nursing diagnosis	Goal	Nursing interventions	Evaluation
1. Return to non-pregnant state related to termination of pregnancy	Demonstrate understanding of involutionary process within 24 hours Experience normal involutionary process by discharge	1. Involutionary process check q24h 2. Provide instruction on normal involutionary process 3. Encourage participation in physical examination 4. Encourage attendance at formal classes	Monitor progressive descent of fundus q24h and document on graphic sheet Evaluate knowledge of involution process and document on teaching guide prior to discharge
2. Alteration in comfort related to perineal healing process and uterine involution	Decrease in perineal and uterine discomfort within 24 hours after delivery	1. Offer pain meds q3-4h 2. Instruct in pericare 3. Use sitzbaths and tucks prn 4. Instruct in proper sitting position 5. Encourage ambulation	Monitor for decrease in subjective complaints and objective signs of discomfort (minimal discoloration and swelling of perineum, increased ambulation) and document on graphic sheet q24h

Continued

TABLE 1   Postpartum nursing care plan—cont'd

Nursing diagnosis	Goal	Nursing interventions	Evaluation
3. Alteration in breast integrity related to bottle or breast feeding	Demonstrate proper care of breast dependent on type of feeding prior to discharge	1. Perform breast exam per routine 2. Teach breast self-exam 3. Follow teaching guide for breast feeding techniques and care 4. Follow teaching guide for breast care when bottle feeding.	Observe condition of breast, including nipples, per routine and document on graphic sheet Evaluate understanding of breast care and document on teaching guide prior to discharge
4. Alteration in elimination related to diuresis after delivery and perineal discomfort	Adequate urinary output and normal bowel function prior to discharge	1. Bladder check per routine 2. Follow postpartum orders for bladder distention 3. High bulk diet 4. Fluid intake—2000 cc/day 5. Give laxative per routine 6. Fleet enema per routine	Monitor urinary output ×2 and document on progress notes Monitor for return of normal bowel function and document on progress notes prior to discharge
5. Alteration in body image related to postpartum state	Verbalize knowledge of nutritional needs and postpartum exercises prior to discharge	1. Follow postpartum teaching guide entitled *Nutrition and Exercise*	Observe return demonstration of exercises and document on teaching guide
6. Potential for postpartum blues related to emotional and hormonal changes	Verbalize potential for postpartum blues as a normal process and recognize methods of coping prior to discharge	1. Follow postpartum teaching guide entitled *Emotionality of the PostPartum Period*	Observe following behaviors and document emotional status on progress notes ×1 prior to discharge: a. Absence of crying, social withdrawal, poor eating or sleeping b. Participation in self-care and infant care activities
7. Alteration in life-style related to birth of infant	Initiation of bonding process by time of discharge	1. Orient parents to family-centered care 2. Assist with infant care 3. Provide support and encouragement to parent-infant interaction	Observe for appropriate bonding response and document on progress notes ×1 prior to discharge
8. Alteration in parent-child relationship related to birth of sibling	Able to cope with the occurrence of sibling rivalry prior to discharge	1. Follow postpartum teaching guide entitled *Sibling Rivalry*	Verbally demonstrate knowledge of sibling rivalry and can state methods of coping prior to discharge and document on teaching guide
9. Alteration in sexual integri-	Understand postpartum sexuality and contracep-	1. Follow postpartum teaching guide entitled	Demonstrate knowledge of sexuality and contra-

TABLE 1   Postpartum nursing care plan—cont'd

Nursing diagnosis	Goal	Nursing interventions	Evaluation
ty related to return to non-pregnant state	tive methods prior to discharge	*Sexuality and Contraception*	ception and document on teaching guide
10. Potential for postoperative complications related to cesarean section	Free of postoperative complications for length of stay	1. Vital signs q4h till stable, then each shift 2. Turn and position q4h prior to ambulation 3. Ambulate 24 hr postoperatively 4. Cough and deep breathe q4h 5. Antiembolic stockings for varicosities prn 6. Abdominal exam each shift 7. Intake and output each shift 8. Incisional check each shift	Evaluate for signs and symptoms of postoperative complications and document progress on progress notes q24h

EVALUATION

The entire documentation system was evaluated 6 months after its implementation. The audit criteria included (1) the compliance with completing the obstetrical and postpartum admission assessments and the nursing care plan, according to the established guidelines, (2) whether the flow sheets and progress notes showed documentation of the nursing interventions and evaluation criteria specified in the postpartum care plan, and (3) whether there were additional nursing diagnoses written reflecting individualization of the plan of care.

The results of the evaluation studied showed between 80 and 100% compliance with completing the forms and documenting based on the established criteria. In 98% of the cases, when an additional nursing diagnosis was warranted, it was documented in the nursing care plan.

Anecdotal reports from the staff regarding this method of documentation were extremely positive. The system was clear, concise, and time-sparing. It also served as an excellent orientation tool for new personnel.

SUMMARY

A formalized nursing diagnosis oriented charting system was successfully implemented in a tertiary care, high-risk obstetrical service. Several objectives were achieved through this system, including: (1) the establishment of nursing standards of care for the postpartum patient, (2) a coordinated documentation system, (3) individualization of the nursing plan of care, and (4) the formulation of an orientation tool.

The actual nursing diagnoses defined for the postpartum patient need to be tested clinically and the defining characteristics elucidated. This paper was presented to encourage further exploration and refinement.

REFERENCES

American Nurses' Association: Standards of maternal child health nursing practice, Kansas City, Mo., 1983, The Association.

Kim, M.J., and Moritz, D.A., editors: Classification of nursing diagnoses—Proceedings of the Third and Fourth National Conferences, New York, 1982, McGraw-Hill Book Co.

Nurses' Association of the American College of Obstetricians and Gynecologists: Obstetrical, gynecologic, and neonatal nursing functions and standards, Chicago, 1974, The Association.

Staff nurses' identification of nursing diagnoses from a simulated patient situation*

JUDITH L. MYERS, M.S.N., R.N.
ANNE G. PERRY, M.S.N., R.N.
RAMONA WESSLER, Ph.D., R.N.
ANN BECKER, M.S.N., R.N.
MARION RESLER, M.S.N., R.N.
MARTHA SPIES, M.S.N., R.N., CCRN
NORMA METHENY, Ph.D., R.N.

In 1972 nursing diagnosis was first included in nurse practice acts (Mahoney, 1977), and in 1973 nursing diagnosis was incorporated into the American Nurses' Association Standards of Practice (ANA, 1973). Since that time, interest in nursing diagnosis has increased, as evidenced by the National Conferences on the Classification of Nursing Diagnoses. There has been a significant increase in the number of books and articles about nursing diagnosis. Numerous regional special interest groups have been formed to support the work on nursing diagnosis in the last ten years. In addition, nurses are conducting more research to validate nursing diagnosis labels.

Currently, nursing practitioners make limited use of nursing diagnosis in developing care plans. There is inconsistent use of terms to identify nursing diagnoses, and sometimes the terminology is unique to an agency. Goals, symptoms, and interventions are frequently used as diagnostic labels (Mundinger and Jauron, 1975; Silverthorn, 1979). However, research has been done to validate specific nursing diagnoses (Beck, 1977; Draye and Pesznecker, 1979; LeSage and associates, 1979). In addition, other researchers have studied the criteria that nurses use to make inferences about patient behaviors and to select a course of nursing action (Grobe, 1971; Keller, 1967). There is lack of agreement among nurses about the relationship between nursing education, nursing experience, and the ability to make nursing diagnoses (Aspinall, 1976; Beck, 1977; Zuehls, 1979).

Aspinall (1979) found that nurses lacked the theoretical knowledge enabling them to evaluate data and focus on problems responsible for specific client behaviors. Matthews (1979) noted that nurses were poor diagnosticians and lacked the critical thinking skills necessary to discriminate the abstract con-

*Supported in part by the Beaumont Fund, Saint Louis University Graduate School, and in part by the Research Fund, Saint Louis University School of Nursing.

cepts associated with nursing diagnoses. The study concluded that nurses could learn these cognitive skills and improve their diagnostic abilities.

When nurses tend to see and record rather than analyze and synthesize, there is perpetual fragmentation of nursing care. The formulation of a nursing diagnosis is a cognitive process. Utilization of this process forces the nurse to expand skills, depth of knowledge, and sensitivity to patient behaviors. Such an expansion of nursing competencies optimizes the selection of nursing actions.

For the purposes of this study, a nursing diagnosis was defined as a judgment or conclusion that occurs as a result of a nursing assessment. It describes an actual or potential health problem which nurses are able and licensed to treat. This definition is consistent with the definition proposed by the North American Nursing Diagnosis Association (NANDA).

OBJECTIVES AND HYPOTHESES

The specific objectives of this study were to (1) determine the ability of coronary care staff nurses to formulate nursing diagnoses, (2) determine the extent to which the nursing diagnoses made by the coronary care staff nurses are comparable to those formulated by the Conferences for the Classification of Nursing Diagnoses, and (3) compare formulations of nursing diagnoses by relevant subgroups of coronary care staff nurses, taking into account such variables as basic nursing education; years of nursing experience; and preparation in the use of nursing diagnoses.

The study investigated the following hypotheses.

1. Nurses with a bachelor of science in nursing (BSN) would spontaneously generate nursing diagnostic labels and would identify their occurrence from a checklist more frequently than would diploma (DI) or associate degree (AD) nurses.
2. Nurses with 3 or more years of general nursing experience would spontaneously generate and identify from a checklist a greater number of correct nursing diagnostic labels regardless of the basic level of nursing preparation.
3. Nurses with 3 or more years of experience in the coronary care unit would spontaneously generate and identify from a checklist a greater number of correct nursing diagnostic labels.
4. Nurses with preparation in nursing diagnosis would spontaneously generate and identify more diagnostic labels from a checklist than those nurses without this preparation.

METHOD

A convenience sample of 54 registered nurses from eight metropolitan hospitals who have direct patient care in coronary care units was obtained for the study.

TABLE 1   **Characteristics of subjects' preparedness**

Education	Occurrence	
	Absolute	Relative
Degree		
Associate	12	22.2
Baccalaureate	22	40.7
Diploma	20	37.7
Years of nursing experience		
Less than 3	9	16.7
3 or more	45	83.3
Years of cardiovascular experience		
Less than 3	30	55.6
3 or more	24	44.4
Nursing diagnosis preparation		
None	31	57.4
Some	23	42.6

The characteristics of the subjects in regard to nursing education preparation, years of experience in nursing, years of experience in a coronary care unit, and preparation in nursing diagnosis are summarized in Table 1.

INSTRUMENTATION

The instrumentation involved the use of (1) a 10-minute videotape simulating client behaviors that depicted nursing diagnoses commonly seen in a patient with an acute myocardial infarction, (2) a written instrument to be completed in conjunction with the viewing of the videotape, asking subjects to spontaneously generate nursing diagnoses and to identify nursing diagnoses from a checklist of established nursing diagnoses and (3) a demographic data form.

The videotape was prepared for the purpose of this study. The validity of using videotape as an effective means of evaluating individuals' clinical competencies and observation skills has been established (Hubbard, 1971). The videotape simulation ensured that all the subjects were exposed to the same patient situation when asked to identify nursing diagnoses. Nursing diagnoses commonly identified in the patient with an acute myocardial infarction were utilized in preparing the videotape script (Rossi and Haines, 1979). These seven nursing diagnoses represent both the physiological and psychosocial dimensions of nursing practice. Content validity of the script was determined by five nurse educators prior to the videotape production. The videotape was prepared by persons with media production education and experience. Volunteers, known to the researchers, served as performers in the videotape simulation. The completed videotape was viewed by a panel of five cardiovascular nurse clinicians to validate the inclusion of client behaviors that should produce the agreed upon nursing diagnoses.

After viewing the videotape, subjects were asked to complete the instrument. The written instrument was designed to obtain data regarding staff nurses' identification of the nursing diagnoses portrayed in the videotape. The instrument asked the subjects first to spontaneously generate nursing diagnostic labels and second to select from the checklist diagnostic labels depicted by the videotape simulation. While over forty nursing diagnoses have been established by the national conferences, only fifteen were selected by Matthews (1979), who noted that as the number of diagnoses increased, the ability to identify correct diagnoses decreased because of cognitive strain.

PROCEDURE

After the necessary approvals were obtained, the directors of nursing of eight metropolitan hospitals were contacted, explaining the need for subjects and requesting written permission to contact potential subjects within the institution. The hospitals chosen for the study all contained a coronary care unit.

BOX 1   **Subject tool—nursing diagnosis checklist**

Please check those nursing diagnoses identified on the videotape.

_____ Alteration in comfort level*

_____ Alteration in cardiac output/activity tolerance*

_____ Altered sleep patterns*

_____ Coping, ineffective family

_____ Diversional activity deficit

_____ Grieving

_____ Knowledge deficit*

_____ Maladaptive coping*

_____ Mobility, impairment

_____ Noncompliance*

_____ Nutritional alterations

_____ Role disturbance

_____ Self-concept (body image), alteration of*

_____ Sexuality, altered patterns of

_____ Thought processes, impaired

---

*Diagnoses portrayed on videotape.

They represented large and small, teaching and non-teaching facilities. Potential subjects were asked to meet with the investigators for an explanation of the expectations and rights of subjects participating in the study. All volunteers were accepted as subjects. A time was designated for the data collection, avoiding all times when the staff nurses had responsibility for patient care or when the nurses might be unusually fatigued, to eliminate risk to subjects.

After subjects provided informed consent, demographic data were collected. Subjects were given written directions that included (1) the definition of a nursing diagnosis, (2) comparison of nursing and medical diagnoses, and (3) examples of nursing and medical diagnoses. The written directions instructed the subjects to record spontaneously generated nursing diagnoses and to select from a checklist (Box 1) nursing diagnoses portrayed on the videotape. The data collector did not give any verbal directions or answer questions about nursing diagnosis. The data collectors had been instructed by the investigators to answer questions only to clarify the procedure for data collection.

RESULTS AND DISCUSSION
Data analysis

Statistical methods utilized to analyze the data in relation to the hypotheses included content analysis, a percentage of agreement corrected for chance, a chi-square test of homogeneity for correlated proportions, and chi-square tests of homogeneity for independent samples.

Content analysis was used to classify the spontaneously generated nursing diagnoses obtained in this study. The responses included medical diagnoses, disease symptoms, nursing goals, and interventions. Very few subjects were able to generate diagnostic labels that agreed with the proposed labels from NANDA. Since 57.4% of the subjects reported no preparation in nursing diagnosis, this may account for their inability to generate diagnoses that reflect the work done at the conferences. It is of interest to note that 72.2% of the subjects reported that they currently use nursing diagnosis in some form in their practice setting. Only 50% of the subjects reported some level of confidence in their ability to use nursing diagnosis.

The diagnostic categories were then compared to the established labels to determine the percentage of agreement and its standard error per established label. The spontaneously generated nursing diagnoses were also compared with the diagnoses obtained on the recognition task. A percentage of agreement corrected for chance and a chi-square test of homogeneity for correlated proportions (Fleiss, 1973) was used to determine the correspondence between nursing diagnoses generated spontaneously and those identified on the checklist. Finally, chi-square tests of homogeneity for independent samples were used to measure the influence of the various demographic variables on the nurses' identification of each of the established nursing diagnoses.

Analysis of the data showed no statistical significance in the ability of nurses to spontaneously generate nursing diagnoses, or correctly identify nursing diagnoses from a checklist based on type of basic nursing education, years of experience, and preparation in nursing diagnosis (Tables 2 to 7).

A further analysis of individual nursing diagnoses revealed that there was a significant difference between the level of education and the incidence of checking the nursing diagnosis *Noncompliance* at the 0.005 level. According to the data, nurses with a diploma education were better able to identify this diagnosis than were nurses with a BSN or an Associate degree (Table 8). It is difficult to interpret this particular result, considering that all the other data for the various variables and the other individual diagnoses were not significant. The sample size is small, so conclusions about the importance of the finding are limited. The geographic area in which the data was collected has a large number of diploma nursing programs, thus accounting for 37.7% of the subjects.

TABLE 2   **Relationship between level of basic education and ability to spontaneously generate nursing diagnoses**

Group	Mean	f-Statistic (df = 2/51)
AD (n = 12)	−3.83	0.572*
BSN (n = 22)	−3.00	
Diploma (n = 20)	−3.14	

*Not significant at the 0.05 level.

TABLE 3   **Relationship between level of basic education and performance on checklist**

Group	Mean	f-Statistic (df = 2/51)
AD (n = 12)	10.08	2.83*
BSN (n = 22)	9.27	
Diploma (n = 20)	10.50	

*Not significant at the 0.05 level.

TABLE 4   **Relationship between number of years of experience as nurse and ability to spontaneously generate nursing diagnoses**

Group	Sample size	Mean	SD	t-Statistic (df = 52)
Less than 3 years	9	−3.44	1.94	−0.83*
Three years or more	45	−3.0	2.62	

*Not significant at the 0.05 level.

TABLE 5   **Relationship between number of years of experience as nurse and score on checklist**

Group	Sample size	Mean	SD	t-Statistic (df = 52)
Less than 3 years	9	9.22	1.92	− 1.29*
Three years or more	45	10.04	1.70	

*Not significant at the 0.05 level.

TABLE 6   **Relationship between level of preparation in nursing diagnoses and ability to spontaneously generate those diagnoses**

Group	Sample size	Mean	SD	t-Statistic (df = 52)
None	31	− 3.32	2.63	− 0.59*
Some	23	− 2.91	2.37	

*Not significant at the 0.05 level.

TABLE 7   **Relationship between level of preparation in nursing diagnoses and score on checklist**

Group	Sample size	Mean	SD	t-Statistic (df = 52)
None	31	10.12	1.80	1.08*
Some	23	9.30	1.67	

*Not significant at the 0.05 level.

TABLE 8   **Relationship between level of education and the incidence of checking the nursing diagnosis *Noncompliance***

	Item checked		
	No	Yes	
AD	12 (100.0)*	0 (0.0)	12 (100%)
BSN	19 (86.4)	3 (13.6)	22 (100%)
Diploma	11 (55.0)	9 (45.0)	20 (100%)

Chi-square = 10.37; df = 2
*Significant at the 0.005 level.

As regional and national groups continue to develop a taxonomy to classify nursing diagnoses, it will be important to identify those variables that influence a nurse's diagnostic skill. The results of this study support the need to have a common language for nursing diagnoses. Having a prepared list of approved diagnoses to draw from may be more time-efficient than asking a nurse to generate diagnoses from assessment data.

REFERENCES

Abdellah, F.G.: Method of identifying covert aspects of nursing problems, Nurs. Res. **57:**4-23, 1957.

American Nurses' Association: Standards of nursing practice, Kansas City, Mo., 1973, The Association.

Aspinall, M.J.: Nusring diagnosis—the weak link, Nurs. Outlook **24:**433-437, 1976.

Aspinall, M.J.: Use of a decision tree to improve accuracy of diagnosis, Nurs. Res. **28:**182-185, 1979.

Beck, R.: A study of the relevance of nursing diagnosis labels to maternity nursing. Unpublished master's thesis, University of Wisconsin–Milwaukee, 1977.

Draye, M.A., and Pesznecker, B.L.: Diagnostic scope and certainty: an analysis of FNP practice, Nurs. Pract. **4**(1):42-43, 1979.

Fenn, J., and Fassel, B.: Research in critical care education: Production of videotapes for in-hospital use, Heart Lung **8:**313-318, 1979.

Fleiss, J.L.: Statistical methods for rates and proportions, New York, 1973, John Wiley & Sons, Inc.

Fox, D.J.: Fundamentals of nursing research, ed. 3, New York, 1976, Appleton-Century-Crofts.

Gebbie, K., and Lavin, M.A.: Classifying nursing diagnoses, Missouri Nurse **42:**10-14, 1973.

Gebbie, K., and Lavin, M.A., editors: Classification of nursing diagnoses, St. Louis, 1975, The C.V. Mosby Co.

Gordon, M.: Nursing diagnosis and the diagnostic process, Amer. J. Nurs. **76:**1298-1300, 1976.

Gordon, M., and Sweeney, M.A.: Methodological problems and issues in identifying and standardizing nursing diagnoses, Adv. Nurs. Sci. **2**(1):1-15, 1979.

Grobe, B.A.: A study of criteria used to determine priorities of patient care. Unpublished master's thesis, Saint Louis University, 1971.

Hubbard, J.P.: An objective evaluation of clinical competence, N. Engl. J. Med. **272:**1321-1328, 1965.

Hubbard, J.P.: Measuring medical education, Philadelphia, 1971, Lea & Febiger.

Keller, M.J.: A study of clinical inferences in nursing. Unpublished master's thesis, St. Louis University, 1967.

Kritek, P.: The generation and classification of nursing diagnoses: toward a theory of nursing, Image **10:**33-40, 1978.

LeSage, J., Beck, C., and Johnson, M.: Nursing diagnosis of drug incompatibility: a conceptual process, Adv. Nurs. Sci. **1**(1):63-77, 1979.

Mahoney, E.A.: Some implications for nursing diagnosis of pain, Nurs. Clin. North Am. **12:**613-619, 1977.

Matthews, C.A., and Gaul, A.L.: Nursing diagnosis from the perspective of concept attainment and critical thinking, Adv. Nurs. Sci. **2**(1):16-26, 1979.

Mundinger, M.A., and Jauron, G.D.: Developing a nursing diagnosis, Nurs. Outlook **23:**94-98, 1975.

Nuftulin, D.: A comparison of videotaped and live patient interview examinations and written examinations in psychiatry, Amer. J. Psychiatry **134:**1093-1096, 1977.

Rossi, L.P., and Haines, V.M.: Nursing diagnosis related to acute myocardial infarction, Cardiovasc. Nurs. **15:**11-15, 1979.

Silverthorn, A.: Nursing care plans: a vital tool, Canad. Nurse **75:**36-69, 1979.

Stein, R.F., Steele, L., Fuller, M., and Langhoff, H.F.: A multimedia independent approach, Nurs. Res. **21:**436-447, 1972.

Tardiff, K.: Evaluation of a videotape technique for measuring clinical psychiatric skills of medical students, J. Med. Educ. **53:**438-441, 1978.

Weber, S.: Nursing diagnosis in private practice, Nurs. Clin. North Am. **14:**433-439, 1979.

Zuehls, K.S.C.: Nursing diagnosis and clinical cues, Nurs. Diagn. **6**(1):2, 1979.

A study to determine the defining characteristics of the nursing diagnosis of knowledge deficit

BARBARA E. POKORNY, M.S.N., R.N.C.

ABSTRACT

Nursing diagnoses are concise statements of the actual or potential health problems that nurses treat. A taxonomy of diagnoses and their defining characteristics has been inductively generated through the work of the North American Nursing Diagnosis Association (NANDA). The defining characteristics must be clinically researched to establish their use as empiric indicators of the diagnosis. The diagnosis of knowledge deficit was selected for study because no previous efforts to investigate it were found.

A descriptive study was designed to answer the following questions: (1) What defining characteristics are present when the diagnosis of knowledge deficit is made? (2) With what frequency does each occur? (3) Do any of the defining characteristics constitute a critical defining characteristic?

A random sample of 120 discharged patient charts on which the diagnosis of knowledge deficit had been made was selected from the inpatient population of a federal hospital. Data were collected via retrospective chart review, using a tool designed for the study.

One or more defining characteristics were present in 51 of the 120 cases examined (42.5%). Seven of the eight defining characteristics proposed by NANDA were documented at least once. No instances were found of demonstration of inappropriate or exaggerated behavior. No critical defining characteristics were found, though the data suggest that an important indicator of the diagnosis is the patient's verbal statement of a need for information or clarification.

Nursing diagnoses are concise statements of the actual or potential health problems that nurses treat. Over the last 12 years the National Group for the Classification of Nursing Diagnoses and its successor, the North American Nursing Diagnosis Association (NANDA), have developed a taxonomy of diagnostic labels and a set of proposed defining characteristics for each (Kim and Moritz, 1982).

The diagnoses have been inductively generated on the basis of the clinical experience of the nurses involved, and each must be supported on the basis of clinical research (Gordon, 1982b). Gordon and Sweeney (1979) recognized the dual needs for research studies to establish the clinical validity of each nursing diagnosis and for studies that supported the clinical occurrence of the proposed defining characteristics.

Three models of research were described by Gordon and Sweeney (1979) to meet those needs. One, the nurse validation model, was recommended as particularly suited to determining the defining characteristics of a nursing diagnosis. It called for the tabulation of the defining characteristics found each time a given diagnosis was made and a determination of the actual frequency of each (Gordon and Sweeney, 1979). No instances of the use of this method were found in the literature.

The nursing diagnosis of knowledge deficit is a statement by the nurse that the patient lacks the information needed to be an informed participant in his health care. The usual intervention for knowledge deficit has been patient education. However, it is unclear from the literature exactly what clinical findings the nurse relies on to indicate the need for patient education. These findings would constitute the defining characteristics of knowledge deficit. No research studies were found that attempted to establish the defining characteristics.

The purpose of this descriptive study was to identify the defining characteristics documented by nurses to support the nursing diagnosis of knowledge deficit. The study was directed at answering the following questions: (1) What defining characteristics are present when the diagnosis of knowledge deficit is made? (2) With what frequency does each occur? (3) Do any of the defining characteristics constitute a critical defining characteristic?

The study was conducted on a random sample of 120 charts of adult patients discharged from a federal research hospital in the Eastern United States for whom the nursing diagnosis of knowledge deficit had been made. Data were collected from each chart using a tool designed specifically for this study (Pokorny, 1984). The defining characteristics proposed by NANDA (Kim and Moritz, 1982) and Gordon (1982a) were noted as present or absent, and space was provided in which to note any additional defining characteristics that were documented by the nurse. Content validity was established through review by a panel of nurse researchers (Pokorny, 1984). Descriptive statistics were used to answer the research questions, and the chi-square statistic was calculated at the $p = 0.05$ level of significance to measure association between variables.

FINDINGS

One or more defining characteristics were present in 51 of the 120 cases examined (42.5%). A verbalized statement of inadequate knowledge was the defining characteristic found most often. It was present in 25.8% of all cases examined and in 60.8% of those cases in which any defining characteristics were present (Table 1).

Other frequently found defining characteristics included verbalized inad-

TABLE 1   **Distribution of defining characteristics of knowledge deficit**

	n	Percent of total*	Percent of subgroup†
Verbalized inadequate recall of information	13	10.8	25.5
Verbalized inadequate understanding of information	16	13.3	32.0
Verbalized statement of inadequate knowledge	31	25.8	60.8
Evidence of information misinterpretation	4	3.3	7.8
Evidence of inaccurate follow-through of instructions	12	10.0	23.5
Inadequate performance of a test	1	0.8	1.9
Inadequate demonstration of a skill	9	7.5	17.6
Demonstration of inappropriate or exaggerated behavior	0		
TOTAL	86		

*n = 120.
†Subgroup is cases where any defining characteristics are documented (n = 51).

equate understanding of information (13.3%), verbalized inadequate recall of information (10.8%), and evidence of inaccurate follow-through of instructions (10.0%). One or more of the three defining characteristics that depend on a verbal statement by the patient were present in 49.9% of the total sample and in 86.2% of the cases in which any defining characteristics were documented.

No instances were found in which a demonstration of inappropriate or exaggerated behavior was used as a defining characteristic of knowledge deficit. The other seven defining characteristics proposed by NANDA were documented at least once in the sample. No critical defining characteristics were identified, nor were any defining characteristics found other than those proposed by NANDA.

The absence of any documented defining characteristics was found to be associated with two subgroups of patients. Those with one of four medical diagnoses collectively termed *invasive diagnostic procedures* (cardiac catheterization, bronchoscopy, liver biopsy, and skin biopsy) were significantly less likely to have any defining characteristics documented on the chart, $\chi^2(1, n = 120) = 4.63$, p = 0.03. An association approaching significance was found between the nursing diagnosis of lack of knowledge of the role of normal volunteer, one of 12 subtypes of knowledge deficit at the institution, and the absence of any documented defining characteristics, $\chi^2(1, n = 120) = 3.37$, p = 0.06.

DISCUSSION

"The purpose of an information system is to provide the data that are needed to make decisions. An information system for nursing practice should include, therefore, the facts that nurses need to know to make nursing diagnoses" (Grier, 1981). The system can be programmed to require that each diagnosis be substantiated by documentation of the cluster of signs and symptoms that led the nurse to apply a particular diagnostic label (Spotts, 1982).

The medical information system used at the institution does not require that the nurse substantiate a given nursing diagnosis by documenting any defining characteristics. The nursing diagnosis can be made without any documentation of the rationale for its selection or on the basis of an assessment indicating that a learning need exists. Though various assessment, observation, and implementation panels are included in the system, none lists the NANDA-proposed defining characteristics of the nursing diagnosis of knowledge deficit. With few exceptions, the data documenting defining characteristics must be entered by the nurse in a narrative form.

The design of the system may be responsible for the absence of any defining characteristics in 57.5% (69) of the records reviewed. In those cases either no documentation of the rationale behind the diagnosis was found, or the only explanation was stated in terms of the existence of a learning need. The latter statement is itself diagnostic in nature and sheds no light on the data points that led the nurse to identify the presence of a learning need.

Two categories of patients illustrate the difficulty. Patients who were admitted as normal volunteers, i.e., healthy individuals used as control subjects or as sources of normative data in medical research protocols, were given the nursing diagnosis of lack of knowledge of the role of the normal volunteer in every instance examined. However, those patients were less likely (p = 0.06) to have had any defining characteristics of the diagnosis documented on their charts. In the absence of any data to the contrary, it may be that nursing personnel considered all such patients to lack the knowledge needed for transition into unfamiliar role expectations and applied the diagnosis of knowledge deficit without documenting the data to support it.

Those patients who underwent invasive diagnostic procedures were similar. They were significantly more likely (p = 0.03) to have no defining characteristics documented on the chart. Again it is possible that nurses judge all patients about to undergo a cardiac catheterization or other invasive procedure to lack the knowledge needed to participate in the procedure and the recovery from it. If the diagnosis and the accompanying intervention of patient education are automatically applied in such cases, it may explain the lack of documented defining characteristics. This is consistent with studies reported in the literature in which education was provided without evidence of an assessment supporting its need (Dumas and Leonard, 1963; Healy, 1968; King and Tarsitano, 1982; Lindeman and Van Aernam, 1971; Maiman and associates, 1979; Mezzanote, 1970).

In examining the cases in which one or more defining characteristics were documented, a pattern similar to that found by Nicoletti, Reitz, and Gordon (1982) emerges. While no critical defining characteristics were found, a cluster of three characteristics occurred such that one or more appeared in 86.5% of the cases. This subgroup consisted of the three defining characteristics concerned with the patient's verbal statements: verbalized inadequate recall of information, verbalized inadequate understanding of information, and verbalized statement of inadequate knowledge. It may be that the critical indicator is the patient's self-report of a knowledge deficit, or it may be that the patient's self-reported need for knowledge is so obvious that it demands recognition by the nurse while more subtle indicators are more easily overlooked in the assessment process.

Limited support was found for three of the four remaining defining characteristics proposed by NANDA: evidence of inaccurate follow-through of instructions, evidence of information misinterpretation, and inadequate demonstration of a skill. Some examples found were demonstration of an incorrect self-injection technique and the failure to adhere to a self-medication regime while on a brief pass. These are similar to the possiblities suggested by Speers and Turk (1982).

The only defining characteristic not found in the sample was that of demonstration of inappropriate or exaggerated behavior. Though the charts reviewed did indicate that some patients manifested hostile or agitated behavior, nothing in the narrative linked the behavior to a state of inadequate knowledge. In several instances the behavior was noted as a defining characteristic of another nursing diagnosis, usually ineffective individual coping. The failure to establish any clinical substantiation for this indicator is congruent with the facts that no support was found for it in the literature and that it was given a marginally acceptable rating by the panel of raters who validated the tool.

Syred (1981) has suggested that nurses accept the nursing process (Yura and Walsh, 1983) intellectually but do not consistently operationalize it, particularly the assessment phase. The present study can neither support nor refute the suggestion, but it indicates that if nurses do consistently assess patients' needs, they do not consistently document the findings from the assessment. It further suggests that some categories of patients are given the nursing diagnosis of knowledge deficit routinely without documentation to support its accuracy. The failure to record baseline data handicaps the quality assurance process. If there is no documentation of the signs and symptoms of a diagnosis, one is unable to verify that a specific intervention (in this case, patient teaching) was effective in eliminating the signs and symptoms of knowledge deficit (Gordon, 1982b; Spotts, 1982).

CONCLUSIONS

On the basis of the findings of the study, limited clinical support is provided for the following defining characteristics of the nursing diagnosis of knowledge deficit: verbalized inadequate recall of information, verbalized inadequate understanding of information, verbalized statement of inadequate knowledge, and evidence of inaccurate follow-through of instructions. Evidence of information misinterpretation, inadequate performance of a test, and inadequate demonstration of a skill were found, but with insufficient frequency to establish their usefulness as defining characteristics of knowledge deficit.

The study findings provide no support for the use of demonstration of inappropriate or exaggerated behavior as a defining characteristic of knowledge deficit.

The study findings do not support the presence of a critical defining characteristic for the nursing diagnosis of knowledge deficit. The findings do, however, suggest that an important indicator of the diagnosis is the patient's verbal statement of a need for information or clarification.

RECOMMENDATIONS

On the basis of the foregoing it is recommended that
1. The study be replicated in a nonresearch hospital with a more representative patient population
2. A population of nonhospitalized patients be used
3. The study takes place in a setting where the nursing documentation system demands that one or more defining characteristics will be noted whenever a nursing diagnosis is made
4. A study be designed to look specifically at the use of the defining characteristic of demonstration of inappropriate or exaggerated behavior
5. The nursing diagnosis *Knowledge deficit* be investigated using a design based on Gordon and Sweeney's (1979) clinical model
6. The methodology used in this study be applied in the investigation of other nursing diagnoses

REFERENCES

Dumas, R.G., and Leonard, R.C.: The effect of nursing on the incidence of postoperative vomiting, Nurs. Res. **12:**12-15, 1963.

Gordon, M.: Manual of nursing diagnosis, New York, 1982a, McGraw-Hill Book Co.

Gordon, M.: Nursing diagnosis: process and application, New York, 1982b, McGraw-Hill Book Co.

Gordon, M., and Sweeney, M.A.: Methodological problems and issues in identifying and standardizing nursing diangoses, Adv. Nurs. Sci. **2:**1-15, 1979.

Grier, M.R.: The need for data in making nursing decisions. In Werley, H.H., Grier, M.R., editors: Nursing information systems, New York 1981, Springer Publishing Co., Inc.

Healy, K.M.: Does preoperative instruction make a difference? Am. J. Nurs. **68:**62-67, 1968.

Kim, M.J., and Moritz, D.A., editors: Classification of nursing diagnoses—Proceedings of the Third and Fourth National Conferences, New York, 1982, McGraw-Hill Book Co.

King, I., and Tarsitano, B.: The effect of structured and unstructured pre-operative teaching: a replication, Nurs. Res. **31**:324-329, 1982.

Lindeman, C.A., and Van Aernam, B.: Nursing intervention with the presurgical patient—the effects of structured and unstructured preoperative teaching, Nurs. Res. **20**:319-332, 1971.

Maiman, L.A., Green, L.W., Gibson, G., and MacKenzie, E.J.: Education for self-treatment by adult asthmatics, JAMA **241**(18):1919-1922, 1979.

Mezzanote, E.J.: Group instruction in preparation for surgery, Am. J. Nurs. **70**:89-91, 1970.

Nicoletti, A.M., Reitz, S.M., and Gordon, M.: A descriptive study of the parenting diagnosis. In Kim, M.J., and Moritz, D.A., editors: Classification of nursing diagnoses—Proceedings of the Third and Fourth National Conferences, New York, 1982, McGraw-Hill Book Co.

Pokorny, B.E.: A study to determine the defining characteristics of the nursing diagnosis of knowledge deficit. Unpublished master's thesis, Washington, D.C., The Catholic University of America, 1984.

Speers, M.A., and Turk, D.C.: Diabetes self-care: knowledge, beliefs, motivation, and action, Patient Counsel. Health Educ. **3**:144-149, 1982.

Spotts, S.J.: Nursing information systems. In Kim, M.J., and Moritz, D.A., editors: Classification of nursing diagnoses—Proceedings of the Third and Fourth National Conferences, New York, 1982, McGraw-Hill Book Co.

Syred, M.E.J.: The abdication of the role of health education by hospital nurses, J. Adv. Nurs. **6**:27-33, 1981.

Yura, M., and Walsh, M.B.: The nursing process: assessing, planning, implementing, evaluating, ed. 4, New York, 1983, Appleton-Century-Crofts.

The nursing diagnosis of noncompliance: a pilot study

POLLY RYAN, M.S.N., R.N.
SUZANNE M. FALCO, Ph.D., R.N.

Noncompliance has been accepted as a nursing diagnosis by the North American Nursing Diagnosis Conference Group. As a nursing diagnosis, it is in its early developmental phase. The use of the diagnosis of noncompliance by practitioners indicates that the phenomenon is recognized in the clinical situation and strategies are employed to handle the problem. A question arises: To what are these practitioners responding when they diagnosis a patient as noncompliant? The purpose of this pilot study, then, was to determine (1) the presence of selected etiologies and defining characteristics in individual patients, (2) the comprehensiveness of the generated list for all clinical findings, and (3) the nurse's perceptions of the importance of these etiologies and defining characteristics to making the diagnosis of noncompliance.

METHOD

A descriptive survey approach was used for this study. The descriptive approach allowed for the exploration of the topic without the need for hypotheses. The survey strategy provided an efficient mechanism for collecting a large amount of data from the subjects. This approach, however, did not allow for randomization, control, and manipulation of variables.

SAMPLE

A convenience sample of 22 registered nurses was obtained through contacts with colleagues and professional groups. All of the subjects were requested to complete the survey if they actively worked with patients whom they identified as noncompliant. Of the 22 nurses who responded, 10 had their master's degree, 7 had a baccalaureate, and 5 had diplomas. Their experience in nursing ranged from 7 months to 35 years.

INSTRUMENT

As a result of a thorough review of the literature and an extensive clinical practice with noncompliant patients, a list of those items which characterized the beliefs and behaviors of noncompliant individuals was generated (Ryan, in press). This list was utilized to develop an instrument consistent with the general format of the North American Nursing Diagnosis Association. The instrument listed the etiologies and their defining characteristics for the diagnosis of noncompliance.

Once developed, the list contained eleven etiologies which clustered into four categories: (1) cognition—the client's ability to obtain or process information; (2) perception—the client's beliefs, feelings, and values; (3) social support—factors related to significant other, job, church, community, or material resources; and (4) the health care system—its persons, processes, facilities, or resources. Within these clusters, etiologies and defining characteristics were identified and organized.

The identified etiologies and defining characteristics were organized into the survey instrument such that the defining characteristics followed their etiology. For each item on the instrument, there was an 8-point Likert scale whose values ranged from 1, least important, to 8, most important. Sample items included

( )　Inadequate motivation 　　　　　　　　　　　1 2 3 4 5 6 7 8

( )　a. Does not perceive illness or risk to be 　　　1 2 3 4 5 6 7 8
　　　　serious

( )　b. Does not feel susceptible to risks or 　　　　1 2 3 4 5 6 7 8
　　　　effects of illness

The instrument's directions required the subjects to check the items which applied to a chosen patient and then circle the number that best reflected the importance of the chosen item in making the diagnosis of noncompliance for that patient. Each item was scored based on the number circled.

The developed instrument, consisting of 66 items, was reviewed by three masters' prepared clinical nurse specialists who work with patients identified as noncompliant. As a result of this review, minor changes were made to clarify the directions. Demographic information on the subjects was collected for the purposes of describing the sample. The instrument made no attempt to identify patient demographics as these have been shown to be unrelated to noncompliance.

DATA COLLECTION PROCEDURES

Over a 3-month period, registered nurses were asked to participate in the study. All who indicated a willingness to participate were provided with a packet which contained the general description and purpose of the study, instructions for completion of the instrument, a copy of the instrument, and a self-addressed stamped envelope. Because the purpose of the survey was to collect data specific to a patient and not to the nurse's perception of noncompliance in general, the respondent had to be working with an individual who was identified as noncompliant. Completed surveys were returned to the investigator by mail.

Participation in the study was voluntary and return of the completed instrument constituted consent to participate. Anonymity was ensured as those who returned the survey could not be identified. The subjects were provided with the name, address, and phone number of the investigator, and participants were encouraged to contact the investigator if there were questions or problems. The investigator was contacted by several individuals to relate that they did not use the diagnosis of noncompliance because they felt it to be too judgmental.

RESULTS

A total of 28 surveys were returned by the twenty-two subjects. Fourteen of the surveys indicated that the respondent established the diagnosis of noncompliance weekly; eight monthly; four several times a year; and two did not respond to the item.

In evaluating the etiologies and defining characteristics, descriptive statistics were used. The results indicated that all of the items on the instrument were chosen at least once and one of the items was chosen 24 times. The average number of items chosen was 21, with a range of 7 to 60. The most frequently chosen items were personal statement of noncompliance (24), direct observation (22), does not perceive the illness or risk to be serious (21), does not want information (21), and verbal denial (17). The five least frequently chosen items were unavailability of medical follow-up (1), the system fails to provide information (1), inadequate material or equipment (3), lack of transportation (3), and disturbance in memory (3).

Items chosen at least 50% of the time were subjected to further scrutiny. Six defining characteristics had percentages ranging between 50 and 75. Four of these were components of the health belief model and two were related to denial. Two characteristics—personal statement and direct observation—had percentages of 75, while only one—does not perceive risk as serious—had greater than 75. None of the etiologies met this 50% criterion.

The importance of the chosen items was then evaluated. Every item on the instrument was rated over 4 in importance. Fifty of the 66 items had average ratings between 6.0 and 7.5. Three items had the highest average rating of 7.7: behavioral denial, system inadequacy, and inaccurate feedback. The least important items were transportation (4.3), failure to provide referral (4.5), and failure to provide supervision (4.9).

Seven items were found to rank high both in terms of importance and frequency: behavioral denial, verbal denial, direct observation, personal statement, does not feel susceptible, does not feel vulnerable, and does not believe in the efficacy of therapy. The Spearman Brown rank order correlation procedure was used to determine if a relationship existed between an item's frequency of choice and its relative importance. The results indicated that frequency did not correlate with importance.

To evaluate the comprehensiveness of the instrument's items, subjects were encouraged to add other items they considered when making the diagnosis of noncompliance. A number of items were added by the respondents. These additional items included cultural barriers, nontherapeutic relationship with health care provider, failure of significant other to value the health care regimen, outdated patient's knowledge, and drastic change in the patient's lifestyle.

An effort was made to determine if there were relationships between the demographic characteristics of the subject and the items selected. The demographic characteristics of educational preparation, experience, and frequency of diagnosis use were found to have significant relationships with selected items on the instrument.

Education correlated significantly with only one item. Subjects with master's degrees selected direct observation with greater frequency (Kendall's tau $B = 0.378$, $p < 0.024$). Using the Pearson's product moment correlation procedure, greater years of experience were correlated with greater importance for the items: failure to keep appointments ($r = 0.779$, $p < 0.034$); belief in therapy but inability to change behavior ($r = 0.732$, $p < 0.031$), and unable to identify specific plan to change behavior ($r = 0.852$, $p < 0.007$). Greater years of experience was also correlated with lesser importance for the items: does not feel vulnerable in terms of risk ($r = -0.507$, $p < 0.022$); does not perceive illness or risk to be serious ($r = -0.431$, $p < 0.029$); and does not feel susceptible to the risk or effects of the illness ($r = -0.688$, $p < 0.001$).

Greater frequency of use of the nursing diagnosis noncompliance was correlated with greater importance for the item anger ($r = 0.771$, $p < 0.005$). Greater frequency was also correlated with lesser importance for the following items: low priority in value system ($r = -0.766$, $p < 0.013$); and alteration in affective state ($r = -0.794$, $p < 0.002$).

DISCUSSION

The instrument was so constructed that each etiology was followed by specific defining characteristics. One of the purposes of the study was to determine if the items on the list of etiologies and defining characteristics were present in individual patients. The results indicated that all of the items were so identified. The subjects, however, did not view the etiologies and defining characteristics as a unit. In many cases, characteristics were chosen independently of the etiology. Such selections could mean that the units were incorrectly constructed. It is quite possible that the etiologies and defining characteristics are, in reality, independent entities, or that additional factors need to be identified before cohesive units can be developed. It is also possible that the subjects' responses were on a different level of abstraction than that used in the instrument construction.

The general defining characteristics of noncompliance as identified in the proceedings of the Fourth National Conference and from the health belief model were selected with a high degree of frequency. The fact that these items were selected frequently may reflect the perceived strength of their relationship to noncompliance or may indicate the subjects' prior acquaintance with these two works. Interestingly, nurses with more experience identified those items associated with the health belief model to be of significantly less importance than that of other items on the instrument. Thus, although these items were chosen frequently, the weighting of importance varied, raising questions about the nature of noncompliance.

It is interesting to note that the majority of subjects who selected items taken from the health belief model also identified denial to be present in the noncompliant patient. Are patients denying their illness if they do not identify the illness or risk to be serious, identify themselves to be susceptible or vulnerable, or believe in the efficacy of the therapy? Is denial the cause of the patient's noncompliance or is it a related phenomenon? Clearly, there is the need for further investigation of the relationship between denial and noncompliance.

Etiologies related to social support and the health care system were chosen less frequently than other items. Since the subject's responses were based upon the patient population, the patient was still involved with the health care system and therefore, the subject may not have been in a position to select health care related items. Depending on the nature of the selected patient population, social system items may also not have been relevant. Since the characteristics of the patients were not determined, it is impossible to determine the impact of these factors.

The second purpose of the study was to determine the comprehensiveness of the list. As previously noted, several additions were made to defining characteristics. These additions were identified as defining characteristics and were not associated with any one etiology. No additions were made to the etiologies. None of the subjects made any comments regarding the appropriateness of the defining characteristics to the etiologies. One potential subject who declined to complete the instrument because the term noncompliance was "value laden," identified the phenomena in clinical practice as a specific behavioral diagnosis, such as "failure to quit smoking related to . . . ."

The last purpose was to determine the nurse's perception of the importance of the items to making the diagnosis of noncompliance. All the items were felt to be important as the diagnosis of noncompliance was made. This addition of items coupled with the choosing of all possibilities reflects the failure of the instrument to provide for discrimination among the items. This failure to discriminate is particularly evident in the measurement of importance. All items were felt to be at least moderately important. Adjusting the instrument to request priorities might provide for increased discrimination.

IMPLICATIONS

As this study indicates, validation of the nursing diagnosis of noncompliance is a difficult and complex task. The problems associated with identifying etiologies, defining characteristics, and models are only part of the larger whole. Should the items be considered as units? What are the prevalent patterns? Is a specified level of education or amount of experience necessary for the accurate diagnosis of noncompliance? Is there priority structure to the etiologies and defining characteristics? Decidedly not an inclusive list, these are but a few of the questions raised by this study that clearly demonstrate a need for more work in this area.

REFERENCE

Ryan, P.: The nursing diagnosis of noncompliance. In Thompson, J., and others, editors: Clinical nursing, St. Louis, 1986, The C.V. Mosby Co.

Clinical validation of respiratory nursing diagnosis: a model

KAREN A. YORK, M.S.N., R.N.
PATRICIA A. MARTIN, M.S., R.N.

The project of classification of nursing diagnoses was started by the Task Force in 1973 and has been carried on since that time. The process began as a part of a conference format, where nurses attending the conference utilized an inductive approach to develop diagnostic categories, based on their recollections of clinical experiences (Gordon, 1982).

As part of this work, not only have diagnostic categories been developed, but also suggested etiologies and defining characteristics (DCs). Clinical studies are needed to validate these empirical classifications, etiologies, and defining characteristics (Kim, 1982).

The number of studies of clinical validation available in the literature is limited. Of that number, only a few attempt to validate DCs (Castles, 1982; Kim and associates, 1982). Validation of the DC as an appropriate basis for making a nusring diagnosis is crucial to the evolution of the nursing care planning process (Tanner and Hughes, 1984).

Three of the nursing diagnoses so identified relate directly to respiratory dysfunctions: (1) *Ineffective breathing patterns* (IBPs), (2) *Ineffective airway clearance* (IAC), and (3) *Impaired gas exchange* (Gordon, 1982; Kim and Moritz, 1982). Definitions, etiologies, and defining characteristics of these three respiratory nursing diagnoses (RNDs) have been identified empirically but are somewhat unclear, with much overlap (Carpenito, 1983; Kim and Moritz, 1982).

This study attempted to use the clinical validation process to organize and clarify the etiologies and DCs for these RNDs. The study design was based upon a model developed by the researchers to guide the clinical validation process of RND. However, this model could be a useful basis for validation of other diagnostic categories. The validation process is envisioned as a continuous evolutionary process based on input from the NANDA membership and the researchers' professional experience. The process moves forward by gathering input from staff nurses, evaluating research results, and producing validated nursing diagnosis information to return to NANDA.

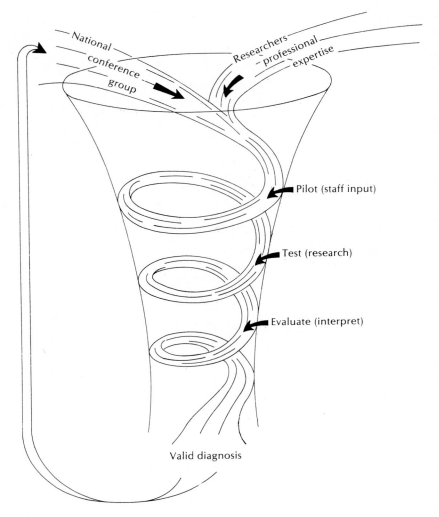

FIGURE 1

PURPOSE

This study sought to validate the RNDs and to identify the critical DC associated with each. The study was based on five hypotheses identified by the researchers:

1. Nurses who work regularly with respiratory patients will identify the appropriateness of defining characteristics and etiologies as established by NANDA.
2. The questionnaire will prove to be reliable in a test-retest situation.
3. There are critical DCs associated with and differentiating each RND.

4. The DC most frequently associated with *Ineffective airway clearance* will reflect presence of increased respiratory secretions.
5. The DC most frequently associated with *Ineffective breathing patterns* will reflect abnormal respiratory mechanics.

This clinical validation will provide NANDA with findings on which to base revisions and clarification of the classification system of RND.

DESIGN

The design was divided into two phases.

Phase I consisted of a simple evaluation questionnaire administered to nurses (RNs) expert in the care of people with respiratory dysfunctions in the acute care setting. The questionnaire asked the RNs to rate the appropriateness or inappropriateness of etiologies and DCs for the three RNDs. The etiologies and DCs considered were those accepted for testing at or before the Fifth National Conference for Classification of Nursing Diagnoses (1982).

The questionnaire was first piloted by five RNs to identify problems with clarity of directions. A test-retest design was used to test the reliability of the tool. Ten RNs answered the questionnaire on two occasions, 2 weeks apart (See Box 1).

BOX 1   **Revised questionnaire**

The researchers feel that you, the primary nurses of 5E, are the true clinical nurse experts in respiratory nursing care. Please check the appropriate column for each defining characteristic below. You may check more than one column if you feel the defining characteristic applies to both nursing diagnoses.

	Ineffective airway clearance	*Ineffective breathing patterns*	Neither
Respiratory mechanics Dyspnea/shortness of breath			
Respiratory distress			
Abnormal respiratory depth			
Labored respirations			
Accessory muscle use			

Continued.

BOX 1   Revised questionnaire—cont'd

	Ineffective airway clearance	Ineffective breathing patterns	Neither
Prolonged expiration			
Increased A-P diameter			
Tachypnea (rr >20)			
Bradypnea (rr <10)			
Apnea			
Nasal flaring			
3-Point position			
Orthopnea			
Oxygenation Abnormal P_{O_2} (<80 − >100)			
Abnormal P_{CO_2} (>45 − <35)			
Cyanosis			
Pale			
Breath sounds and cough Cough			
Sputum			
Difficulty expectorating			
Rales/crackles			
Rhonchi/wheezes			
Tracheal suctioning			
Decreased breath sounds			
Tubular breath sounds			
Gurgling breath sounds			
Mental status Confusion			

BOX 1   **Revised questionnaire—cont'd**

	Ineffective airway clear- ance	Ineffective breath- ing pat- terns	Neither
Somnolence			
Restlessness			
Irritability			
(above are chronic)			
Other			

Phase II was designed to identify the clinical presence or absence of DCs in those patients with a RND. The researcher reviewed care plans on the acute respiratory care unit (RCU) at Miami Valley Hospital, a 772-bed nonprofit regional referral center. Care plans which contained an RND made by an RN regularly assigned to the RCU made up the sample. The clinical rcecord was reviewed by the researcher (K.Y.) to identify the presence or absence of DCs supporting that RND. The RN who made the RND was then interviewed to identify all DCs present at the time the diagnosis was made. This was done to capture data lost through the documentation process. The interview took place within 7 days of the date of the identification of the diagnosis. Care plans which contained more than one RND were excluded from the sample (see Box 2).

The data collection tools for Phase II were piloted and revised before the beginning of this study. Definitions of the DC were clarified by the researchers (see Box 3).

The RNs voluntarily responded to the interview format. Again the RNs were assured that their responses were anonymous and that only grouped data would be reported. These RNs whose schedules prevented the researchers from interviewing them within the allotted time were excluded from this study. Diagnoses made by RNs who worked weekends or nights only were excluded. Records of chart review information only were kept when the RN was un- available for interview. Data from records where no interview was possible

BOX 2   **Clinical validation of RND**

_____ (RN) made the nursing diagnosis
_____ 0100 *Ineffective airway clearance*
_____ 0200 *Ineffective breathing patterns*
_____ 2800 *Impaired gas exchange*

On _____ (patient)   On _____ (date)
Etiology:
R/T _____

Medical record review date _____

RN interview date _____

	Medical record	RN interview	Total
Respiratory mechanics Dyspnea/shortness of breath			
Respiratory distress			
Abnormal respiratory depth			
Labored respirations			
Accessory muscle use			
Prolonged expiration			
Increased A-P diameter			
Tachypnea (rr >20)			
Bradypnea (rr <10)			
Apnea			
Nasal flaring			
3-Point position			
Orthopnea			
Oxygenation Abnormal Po_2 (<80 − >100)			
Abnormal Pco_2 (>45 − <35)			
Cyanosis			
Pale			

BOX 2   **Clinical validation of RND—cont'd**

	Medical record	RN interview	Total
Breath sounds and cough Cough			
Sputum			
Difficulty expectorating			
Rales/crackles			
Rhonchi/wheezes			
Tracheal suctioning			
Decreased breath sounds			
Tubular breath sounds			
Gurgling breath sounds			
Mental status Confusion			
Somnolence			
Restlessness			
Irritability			
(above are chronic)			
Other			

have been excluded from this report because there was a variance in data from RNDs where record review and interview were completed versus those where only record review was completed.

The evaluation tool was completed on 11 samples, of each of two of the RNDs IAC and IBP. There were insufficient samples of *Impaired gas exchange* to complete the study.

BOX 3   **Definitions of terms**

The following definitions indicate parameters and terms that will be accepted, whether found in the medical record or reported by the nurse.

- Dyspnea/Shortness of breath—verbatim, includes dyspnea on exertion, DOE, PND (paroxysmal nocturnal dyspnea), SOB. (In clinical use in this institution these 2 terms are used interchangeably.)
- Labored respirations, —write in verbatim
- Difficulty breathing, —write in verbatim
- Respiratory distress, —write in verbatim
- Cough—verbatim
- Sputum—also with mucus, productive (cough)
- Tachypnea—respiratory rate >20; highest rate recorded on graphic sheet
- Cyanosis—skin coloring to include dusky, gray, bluish
- Abnormal breath sounds—verbatim or decreased or diminished breath sounds but not
     Rales*—verbatim
     Crackles*—verbatim
     Wheezes*—verbatim
     Rhonchi*—verbatim
- Changes in rate or depth of respiration
  Rate—change of greater than 4 breaths per minute in 1 hour (in same state of consciousness)
  Depth—shallow, deep
- Abnormal blood gases
  pH <7.35
  pH >7.45
  Pco_2 <35
  Pco_2 >45
  HCO_3 <20
  HCO_3 >28
  Po_2 <80
  Po_2 >100
- Difficulty expectorating sputum—verbatim or noted separately
- Nasal flaring—verbatim
- Pursed lip breathing (PLB)—verbatim
- Prolonged expiratory phase
  Prolonged expiration (exhalation)
  Slow expiration (exhalation)
  I:E ratio ↑, >1:2
- Increased A-P diameter—barrel chest
- Use of accessory muscles—verbatim or
  use of neck muscles
  use of abdominal muscles
  use of intercostal muscles

---

*Accepted as terminology when used but not considered (defined as) abnormal breath sounds.

BOX 3   **Definitions of terms—cont'd**

- Fremitus—vocal fremitus increased or decreased
- Assumption of 3 point (shoulders elevated by pressing on elbows or hands)
- Hypercapnia—$P_{CO_2} > 45$
- Hypoxia—$P_{O_2} < 80$
- Confusion—verbatim, not oriented
- Somnolence—sleepy, difficult to arouse
- Restlessness—verbatim
- Irritability—verbatim
- Inability to move secretions—verbatim

SUBJECTS/SAMPLE

RNs who are regularly assigned to the 34-bed RCU were recruited to participate in the study. These RNs comprise a stable population, and all have worked with patients with respiratory problems on this RCU for at least 1 year. The researchers considered these RNs to be clinical nurse experts in respiratory care.

Phase I: The first questionnaire was distributed to all RNs attending a regularly scheduled staff meeting. All ten of these RNs voluntarily completed the questionnaire. The instructions for the questionnaire included the statement that it was being administered to these RNs because they were considered to be clinical nurse experts in this field, and that their input was considered essential.

Phase II: Patients' records were identified for inclusion in the study by review of the nursing care plans and selection of all who had an RND made by an RN regularly assigned to the RCU. The RND and etiology were recorded verbatim, in addition to the name of the RN who wrote the care plan, and the patient's medical diagnosis. The patient's name was recorded only to facilitate communication with the RN and was removed after the patient left the hospital. The patient record was reviewed for documentation of DCs associated with an RND. Nurse interviews were then sought to complete the data collection and to furnish any DC which had been present but was not recorded in the patient record. Eleven samples of IAC and IBP each were completed.

RESULTS

Verbal comments indicated that these RNs felt that the etiologies and DCs had been identified by experts and that therefore they must be appropriate. The tabulation of the questionnaires bears this out.

BOX 4   **Questionnaire results**

	Survey I	Survey II
I. *Ineffective breathing patterns* (IBP) R/T decreased lung expansion	70%	100%
Defining characteristics		
Fremitus	70%	70%
Cough	70%	50%
Assumption of 3-point position	90%	70%
Pursed lip breathing/prolonged expiratory phase	60%	60%
Increased A-P diameter	30%	80%
II. *Impaired gas exchange*		
R/T alveolar-capillary membrane alterations	70%	70%
R/T altered oxygen carrying capacity of blood	80%	70%
All defining characteristics considered appropriate by 80% or more of clinical nurse experts		
III. *Ineffective airway clearance* (IAC) All etiologies and defining characteristics considered appropriate by 80% or more of nurses		

Phase I: The test-retest results (Box 4) indicated that it was a reliable tool but the small sample size requires further testing. Only two DCs were consistently considered appropriate by less than 70% of the RNs. These two were cough and prolonged expiratory phase when used as definers of IBP. Comments indicated that cough is a DC of IAC and would not contribute to a diagnosis of IBP. Prolonged expiratory phase was felt to be a treatment modality and not a symptom to be used in arriving at a diagnosis.

Phase II: IAC: Two DCs were present in 100% of the sample: cough and sputum. Four additional DCs were present in 91%: dyspnea/SOB, tachypnea, abnormal or decreased breath sounds, and rhonchi/wheezes.   IBP: One DC was present in 100% of the sample: dyspnea/SOB. One additional DC was present in 91%: abnormal blood gases.

SIGNIFICANCE

Despite reinforcement of the expertise of the RNs sampled, they were unwilling to challenge the opinions of the printed lists of DCs and etiologies.

Phase I: The findings were not highly significant. A replication of this portion of the study might elicit less inferiority feelings if it was not based wholly on the NANDA approved list. The researchers plan a revised approach using the format of the data collection tool used in Phase II. This format would

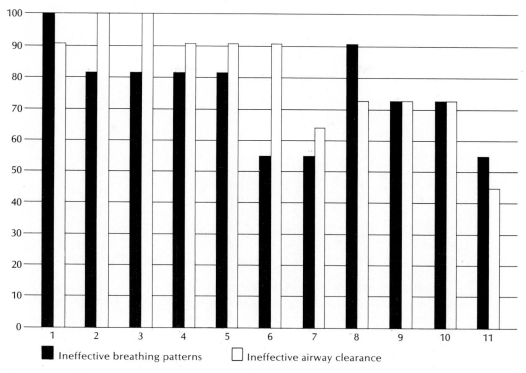

Ineffective breathing patterns   Ineffective airway clearance

FIGURE 2

feature a listing of all DCs and ask the RN to indicate which are appropriate to each individual RND (see Box 1).

Despite these results, when the questionnaire was first presented for the RNs to complete as clinical nurse experts, their comments included several versions of "It's about time somebody asked us!" The RNs' recognition of the importance of their input is reflected by the 100% return of not one but two questionnaires.

Phase II: There was a difference in the rank order of the DCs for two of the three RNDs in this study. Due to the sample size these findings were not considered conclusive, and further study is necessary. The findings of the rank ordering of the DCs were generally supportive of hypotheses 4 and 5. Cough, sputum production, and abnormal breath sounds were most commonly found in patients with IAC. The DCs most associated with IBP included dyspnea/SOB and accessory muscle use.

The study developed, piloted, and tested a model for clinical validation of RNDs which can serve as a basis for further study. The design was intended to be a workable method for use by researchers who must conduct research in addition to other job responsibilities. This design can be incorporated readily

BOX 5   **Characteristics associated with diagnoses***

Ineffective breathing patterns
    1. Dyspnea/SOB
    8. Abnormal ABG
  11. Accessory muscle use
Ineffective airway clearance
    2. Cough
    3. Sputum
    4. Wheezing
    5. Tachypnea
    6. Abnormal or decreased breath sounds
    7. Rales/crackles

*Characteristics were found in both diagnoses but most frequent association as identified.

into clinical practice duties which require chart review of respiratory patients and interaction with their nurses. A design featuring direct patient assessment might increase the validity of the findings, but also increase the time commitment necessary for the researcher, and possibly increase inconvenience of the patients involved. These researchers also feel strongly that it is essential to have the involvement of the nurses who work most closely with the patients. This involvement guarantees more clinical validity and usefulness of the resulting data. This method also increases their feeling of ownership for the end product and should increase application of findings, a long-standing criticism of research.

One disadvantage of the design was the dependence on nursing diagnoses and care plans written by a specific group of RNs. Patients on the RCU had frequently been admitted through the Emergency Room and/or transferred from other units in the hospital. The RNDs had often been written by RNs in those areas, so that those records could not be included in the study, even though the problem continued to exist and require nursing intervention. A modification of the design to utilize verbal identification of the RND by a clinical nurse expert could eliminate this disadvantage.

This study presents a simple and workable model for clinical validation of DCs for RNDs which can also be applied to other nursing diagnostic categories. Hopefully, the simplicity will encourage more sites for validation projects to greatly enlarge the data base.

REFERENCES

Carpenito, L.: Nursing diagnosis application to clinical practice, Philadelphia, 1983, J.B. Lippincott Co.

Castles, M.: Interrater agreement in the use of nursing diagnosis. In Kim, M.J., and Moritz, D.A., editors: Classification of nursing diagnoses—Proceedings of the Third and Fourth National Conferences, New York, 1982, McGraw-Hill Book Co.

Gordon, M.: Manual of nursing diagnosis, New York, 1982, McGraw-Hill Book Co.

Kim, M.J., and others: Clinical use of nursing diagnosis in cardiovascular nursing. In Kim, M.J., and Moritz, D.A., editors: Classification of nursing diagnoses—Proceedings of the Third and Fourth National Conferences, New York, 1982, McGraw-Hill Book Co.

Kim, M.J., and Moritz, D.A., editors: Classification of nursing diagnoses—Proceedings of the Third and Fourth National Conferences, New York, 1982, McGraw-Hill Book Co.

Tanner, C., and Hughes, A.M.G.: Nursing diagnosis: issues in clinical practice research, Top. Clin. Nurs. **5:**30-38, 1984.

Validation of nursing diagnoses on urinary elimination

ANNE MARIE VOITH, B.S.N., R.N.
DEBORAH ANN SMITH, B.S.N., R.N.

With the increasing importance placed on nursing diagnoses to develop and define our body of knowledge and improve patient care, research aimed at validation of nursing diagnoses must be pursued. The purpose of this research was to establish content validity of the nursing diagnosis of Urinary Retention.

The method used was adapted from work by Fehring. A questionnaire was distributed to 200 registered nurses from seven units at a 400-bed teaching hospital in Milwaukee. Part One of the questionnaire asked the participants to rank from 1 to 5 on a Likert-type scale the degree of association of signs and symptoms and etiologic factors to the diagnosis *Urinary retention.* Urinary retention was defined as high urethral pressure inhibiting voiding until high abdominal pressure causes urine to be involuntarily lost, or high urethral pressure inhibiting complete emptying of the bladder. In Part Two, subjects were asked to identify a nursing diagnosis for another clinical problem. The list of signs and symptoms, etiological factors, and definitions was developed for Columbia Hospital as part of a nursing care information system.

Fifty-three questionnaires (27%) were returned.

In Part One, frequencies, means, and standard deviations were calculated to determine what signs and symptoms and etiologic factors were associated with the defined diagnosis, contributing to diagnostic content validity. Etiologic factors and signs and symptoms were accepted if the mean rank was 3.0 or greater. Items were termed critical if the value was greater than 4.0.

Seventy-four percent of the signs and symptoms listed on the questionnaire were seen as indicators of urinary retention. Of those, 36% were termed critical indicators. These were: distention; small, frequent voidings; no urine output; sensation of bladder fullness; and dribbling. Sixty-three percent of the etiologic factors listed were confirmed as contributing to urinary retention. Ranking of etiologic factors may have been influenced by how frequently a particular factor was seen by the clinical expert based on specific patient populations with which the individual nurse worked.

In Part Two, participants were asked to suggest a label for the problem defined: urine is involuntarily expelled by bladder contraction as inhibitory controls fail or urine is not held by the bladder at all. Seventy-nine percent gave the diagnosis Urinary Incontinence.

   This study was valuable in suggesting commonality of terms describing alterations in urinary elimination. It may be implied from the results that urinary retention communicates a similar clinical picture to most nurses participating.

The effect of progressive relaxation in the anticipation phase of the pain experience on the actual postoperative pain sensation with increased activity

ELLEN G. WILSON M.S.N., R.N.

ABSTRACT

The purpose of this study was to explore the effect of progressive relaxation on postoperative comfort levels during a subject's first attempt at getting out of bed. The study was conducted on a general surgery ward, on an orthopedic ward, and in the surgical intensive care unit of an 1800-bed general medical, surgical, and psychiatric hospital. The subjects were thirty-eight male patients who did not have a psychiatric history but who required postoperative care. Nineteen patients received preoperative teaching and training in progressive relaxation, while the remainder of the patients were the control group and received preoperative teaching followed by a question and answer period. Comparisons of blood pressure, heart rate, and respiratory rate prior to surgery and after the first attempt to get out of bed were reported. Reports of surgical pain and body distress were measured using Johnson's *Pain and Distress Scale.* Reports of pain intensity were measured using Stewart's *Pain-Color Scale.*

Four categories of narcotic intake were established for the study. Patients' scores were placed for analysis in one of the categories. Patients in Category A received narcotic injections within 3 hours of getting up. Those in Category B received narcotic injections greater than 3 hours of getting up. Category C patients received oral narcotics within 4 hours of getting up, and those in Category D received oral narcotics greater than 4 hours of getting up. Study results after a multivariate analysis of variance indicated decreased distress in patients taught progressive relaxation and receiving injectable narcotics within 3 hours of getting out of bed.

Approved nursing diagnoses accepted for clinical testing

This section contains the nursing diagnoses, to the extent they have been developed with definitions, etiologies, and defining characteristics, which have been accepted by the North American Nursing Diagnosis Association for clinical testing. The list includes those diagnoses accepted at the Fourth and Fifth National Conferences. There has been no attempt to capture the refining process that these diagnoses have undergone since their inception. The reader is referred to the Proceedings of the Third and Fourth Conferences (Kim and Moritz, 1982) and the Proceedings of the Fifth Conference (Kim and associates, 1984) for further exploration. An asterisk (*) next to a defining characteristic in all the diagnoses indicates a critical defining characteristic (must be present for the diagnosis to be made).

NURSING DIAGNOSES ACCEPTED AT THE FOURTH NATIONAL CONFERENCE (1982)

Airway clearance, ineffective
Bowel elimination, alteration in: constipation
Bowel elimination, alteration in: diarrhea
Bowel elimination, alteration in: incontinence
Breathing pattern, ineffective
Cardiac output, alteration in: decreased
Comfort, alteration in: pain
Communication, impaired verbal
Coping, ineffective individual
Coping, ineffective family: compromised
Coping, ineffective family: disabling
Coping, family: potential for growth
Diversional activity, deficit
Fear
Fluid volume deficit, actual†
Fluid volume deficit, potential
Gas exchange, impaired
Grieving, anticipatory
Grieving, dysfunctional
Home maintenance management, impaired
Injury, potential for; poisoning, potential for; suffocation, potential for; trauma, potential for
Knowledge deficit (specify)
Mobility, impaired physical
Noncompliance (specify)
Nutrition, alteration in: less than body requirements
Nutrition, alteration in: more than body requirements
Nutrition, alteration in: potential for more than body requirements
Parenting, alteration in: actual
Parenting, alteration in: potential

†Two sets of defining characteristics with two etiologies for the same nursing diagnosis.

Rape-trauma syndrome: rape trauma, compound reaction, silent reaction

Self-care deficit (specify level): feeding, bathing/hygiene, dressing/grooming, toileting

Self-concept, disturbance in: body image, self-esteem, role performance, personal identity

Sensory-perceptual alteration: visual, auditory, kinesthetic, gustatory, tactile, olfactory

Sexual dysfunction

Skin integrity, impairment of: actual

Skin integrity, impairment of: potential

Sleep pattern disturbance

Spiritual distress (distress of the human spirit)

Thought processes, alteration in

Tissue perfusion, alteration in: cerebral, cardiopulmonary, renal, gastrointestinal, peripheral

Urinary elimination, alteration in patterns

Violence, potential for

LIST OF NURSING DIAGNOSES ACCEPTED AT THE FIFTH NATIONAL CONFERENCE (1984)

Activity intolerance

Activity intolerance, potential

Anxiety

Family processes, alteration in

Fluid volume, alteration in: excess

Health maintenance alteration

Oral mucous membrane, alteration in

Powerlessness

Social isolation

The nursing diagnoses

ACTIVITY INTOLERANCE

Etiology

Bedrest/immobility

Generalized weakness

Sedentary life-style

Imbalance between oxygen supply/demand

Defining characteristics

* Verbal report of fatigue or weakness

Abnormal heart rate or blood pressure response to activity

Exertional discomfort or dyspnea

Electrocardiographic changes reflecting arrhythmias or ischemia

ACTIVITY INTOLERANCE, POTENTIAL

Etiology

To be developed

Defining characteristics

History of previous intolerance

Deconditioned status

Presence of circulatory/respiratory problems
Inexperience with the activity

AIRWAY CLEARANCE, INEFFECTIVE

Etiology

Decreased energy/fatigue
Tracheobronchial
Infection
Obstruction
Secretion
Perceptual/cognitive impairment
Trauma

Defining characteristics

Abnormal breath sounds (rales [crackles], rhonchi [wheezes])
Changes in rate or depth of respiration
Tachypnea
Cough, effective/ineffective, with or without sputum
Cyanosis
Dyspnea

ANXIETY

Definition

A vague uneasy feeling whose source is often nonspecific or unknown to the individual

Etiology

Unconscious conflict about essential values/goals of life
Threat to self-concept
Threat of death
Threat to or change in health status
Threat to or change in socioeconomic status
Threat to or change in role functioning
Threat to or change in environment
Threat to or change in interaction patterns
Situational/maturational crises
Interpersonal transmission/contagion
Unmet needs

Defining characteristics

I. Subjective
Increased tension
Apprehension
Painful and persistent increased helplessness
Uncertainty
Fearful
Scared
Regretful
Overexcited
Rattled
Distressed
Jittery

Feelings of inadequacy
Shakiness
Fear of unspecific consequences
Expressed concerns re change in life events
Worried
Anxious
II. Objective
*Sympathetic stimulation—cardiovascular excitation, superficial vasoconstriction, pupil dilation
Restlessness
Insomnia
Glancing about
Poor eye contact
Trembling/hand tremors
Extraneous movement (foot shuffling, hand/arm movements)
Facial tension
Voice quivering
Focus "self"
Increased wariness
Increased perspiration

BOWEL ELIMINATION, ALTERATION IN: CONSTIPATION

Etiology

To be developed

Defining characteristics

Decreased activity level
Frequency less than usual pattern
Hard formed stools
Palpable mass
Reported feeling of pressure in rectum
Reported feeling of rectal fullness
Straining at stool

Other possible defining characteristics

Abdominal pain
Appetite impairment
Back pain
Headache
Interference with daily living
Use of laxatives

BOWEL ELIMINATION, ALTERATION IN; DIARRHEA

Etiology

To be developed

Defining characteristics

Abdominal pain
Cramping
Increased frequency

Increased frequency of bowel sounds
Loose liquid stools
Urgency

Other possible defining characteristics
Change in color

BOWEL ELIMINATION, ALTERATION IN: INCONTINENCE

Etiology
To be developed

Defining characteristic
Involuntary passage of stool

BREATHING PATTERN, INEFFECTIVE

Etiology
Neuromuscular impairment
Pain
Musculoskeletal impairment
Perception/cognitive impairment
Anxiety
Decreased energy/fatigue

Defining characteristics
Dyspnea
Shortness of breath
Tachypnea
Fremitus
Abnormal arterial blood gas
Cyanosis
Cough
Nasal flaring
Respiratory depth changes
Assumption of 3-point position
Pursed-lip breathing/prolonged expiratory phase
Increased anteroposterior diameter
Use of accessory muscles
Altered chest excursion

CARDIAC OUTPUT, ALTERATION IN: DECREASED

Etiology
To be developed

Defining characteristics
Variations in blood pressure readings
Arrhythmias
Fatigue
Jugular vein distention
Color changes, skin and mucous membranes
Oliguria

Decreased peripheral pulses
Cold clammy skin
Rales
Dyspnea
Orthopnea
Restlessness

Other possible defining characteristics

Change in mental status
Shortness of breath
Syncope
Vertigo
Edema
Cough
Frothy sputum
Gallop rhythm
Weakness

COMFORT, ALTERATION IN: PAIN

Etiology

Injuring agents
Biological
Chemical
Physical
Psychological

Defining characteristics

Subjective
Communication (verbal or coded) of pain descriptors
Objective
Guarding behavior, protective
Self-focusing
Narrowed focus (altered time perception, withdrawal from social contact, impaired thought process)
Distraction behavior (moaning, crying, pacing, seeking out other people and/or activities, restlessness)
Facial mask of pain (eyes lack luster, "beaten look," fixed or scattered movement, grimace)
Alteration in muscle tone (may span from listless to rigid)
Autonomic responses not seen in chronic stable pain (diaphoresis, blood pressure and pulse rate change, pupillary dilatation, increased or decreased respiratory rate)

COMMMUNICATION, IMPAIRED VERBAL

Etiology

Decrease in circulation to brain
Physical barrier, brain tumor, tracheostomy, intubation
Anatomical deficit, cleft palate
Psychological barriers, psychosis, lack of stimuli
Cultural difference
Developmental or age-related

Defining characteristics

* *Unable to speak dominant language
* *Speaks or verbalizes with difficulty
* *Does not or cannot speak
* Stuttering
* Slurring
* Difficulty forming words or sentences
* Difficulty expressing thought verbally
* Inappropriate verbalization
* Dyspnea
* Disorientation

COPING, INEFFECTIVE INDIVIDUAL

Definition

Impairment of adaptive behaviors and problem-solving abililties of a person in meeting life's demands and roles

Etiology

Situational crises
Maturational crises
Personal vulnerability

Defining characteristics

* *Verbalization of inability to cope or inability to ask for help
* Inability to meet role expectations
* Inability to meet basic needs
* *Inability to problem-solve
* Alteration in societal participation
* Destructive behavior toward self or others
* Inappropriate use of defense mechanisms
* Change in usual communication patterns
* Verbal manipulation
* High illness rate
* High rate of accidents

COPING, INEFFECTIVE FAMILY: COMPROMISED

Definition

Insufficient, ineffective, or compromised support, comfort, assistance, or encouragement usually by a supportive primary person (family member or close friend); client may need it to manage or master adaptive tasks related to his or her health challenge

Etiology

Inadequate or incorrect information or understanding by a primary person
Temporary preoccupation by a significant person who is trying to manage emotional conflicts and personal suffering and is unable to perceive or act effectively in regard to client's needs
Temporary family disorganization and role changes
Other situational or developmental crises or situations the significant person may be facing
Little support provided by client, in turn, for primary person
Prolonged disease or disability progression that exhausts supportive capacity of significant people

Defining characteristics

Subjective

Client expresses or confirms a concern or complaint about significant other's response to his or her health problem

Significant person describes preoccupation with personal reactions (e.g., fear, anticipatory grief, guilt, anxiety, to client's illness or disability or to other situational or developmental crises)

Significant person describes or confirms inadequate understanding or knowledge base which interferes with effective assistive or supportive behaviors

Objective

Significant person attempts assistive or supportive behaviors, with less than satisfactory results

Significant person withdraws or enters into limited or temporary personal communication with the client at time of need

Significant person displays protective behavior disproportionate (too little or too much) to the client's abilities or need for autonomy

COPING, INEFFECTIVE FAMILY: DISABLING

Definition

Behavior of a significant person (family member or other primary person) that disables his or her own capacities and the client's capacities to effectively address tasks essential to either person's adaptation to the health challenge

Etiology

Significant person with chronically unexpressed feelings of guilt, anxiety, hostility, despair, etc.

Dissonant discrepancy of coping styles for dealing with adaptive tasks by the significant person and client or among significant people

Highly ambivalent family relationships

Arbitrary handling of family's resistance to treatment, which tends to solidify defensiveness as it fails to deal adequately with underlying anxiety

Defining characteristics

Neglectful care of the client in regard to basic human needs and/or illness treatment

Distortion of reality regarding the client's health problem, including extreme denial about its existence or severity

Intolerance

Rejection

Abandonment

Desertion

Carrying on usual routines, disregarding client's needs

Psychosomaticism

Taking on illness signs of client

Decisions and actions by family which are detrimental to economic or social well-being

Agitation, depression, aggression, hostility

Impaired restructuring of a meaningful life for self, impaired individualization, prolonged overconcern for client

Neglectful relationships with other family members

Client's development of helpless, inactive dependence

COPING, FAMILY: POTENTIAL FOR GROWTH

Definition

Effective managing of adaptive tasks by family member involved with the client's health challenge, who now is exhibiting desire and readiness for enhanced health and growth in regard to self and in relation to the client

Etiology

Needs sufficiently gratified and adaptive tasks effectively addressed to enable goals of self-actualization to surface

Defining characteristics

Family member attempting to describe growth impact of crisis on his or her own values, priorities, goals, or relationships

Family member moving in direction of health-promoting and enriching life-style which supports and monitors maturational processes, audits and negotiates treatment programs, and generally chooses experiences which optimize wellness

Individual expressing interest in making contact on a one-to-one basis or on a mutual-aid group basis with another person who has experienced a similar situation

DIVERSIONAL ACTIVITY, DEFICIT

Etiology

Environmental lack of diversional activity, as in

Long-term hospitalization

Frequent lengthy treatments

Defining characteristics

Patient's statements regarding

Boredom

Wish there were something to do, to read, etc.

Usual hobbies cannot be undertaken in hospital

FAMILY PROCESSES, ALTERATION IN

Etiology

Situational transition and/or crises

Developmental transition and/or crisis

Defining characteristics

Family system unable to meet physical needs of its members

Family system unable to meet emotional needs of its members

Family system unable to meet spiritual needs of its members

Parents do not demonstrate respect for each other's views on child-rearing practices

Inability to express/accept wide range of feelings

Inability to express/accept feelings of members

Family unable to meet security needs of its members

Inability of the family members to relate to each other for mutual growth and maturation

Family uninvolved in community activities

Inability to accept/receive help appropriately

Rigidity in function and roles

Family not demonstrating respect for individuality and autonomy of its members

Family unable to adapt to change/deal with traumatic experience constructively

Family failing to accomplish current/past developmental task
Unhealthy family decision-making process
Failure to send and receive clear messages
Inappropriate boundary maintenance
Inappropriate/poorly communicated family rules, rituals, symbols
Unexamined family myths
Inappropriate level and direction of energy

FEAR

Definition

Feeling of dread related to an identifiable source which the person validates

Etiology

To be developed

Defining characteristics

Ability to identify object of fear

FLUID VOLUME, ALTERATION IN: EXCESS

Etiology

Compromised regulatory mechanism
Excess fluid intake
Excess sodium intake

Defining characteristics

Edema
Effusion
Anasarca
Weight gain
Shortness of breath, orthopnea
Intake greater than output
S_3 heart sound
Pulmonary congestion: chest x-ray
Abnormal breath sounds: crackles (rales)
Change in respiratory pattern
Change in mental status
Decreased hemoglobin and hematocrit
Blood pressure changes
Central venous pressure changes
Pulmonary artery pressure changes
Jugular vein distention
Positive hepatojugular reflex
Oliguria
Specific gravity changes
Azotemia
Altered electrolytes
Restlessness and anxiety

FLUID VOLUME DEFICIT, ACTUAL (1)

Etiology

Failure of regulatory mechanisms

Defining characteristics
>
> Dilute urine
> Increased urine output
> Sudden weight loss

Other possible defining characteristics
>
> Possible weight gain
> Hypotension
> Decreased venous filling
> Increased pulse rate
> Decreased skin turgor
> Decreased pulse volume/pressure
> Increased body temperature
> Dry skin
> Dry mucous membranes
> Hemoconcentration
> Weakness
> Edema
> Thirst

FLUID VOLUME DEFICIT, ACTUAL (2)

Etiology
>
> Active loss

Defining characteristics
>
> Decreased urine output
> Concentrated urine
> Output greater than intake
> Sudden weight loss
> Decreased venous filling
> Hemoconcentration
> Increased serum sodium

Other possible defining characteristics
>
> Hypotension
> Thirst
> Increased pulse rate
> Decreased skin turgor
> Decreased pulse volume/pressure
> Change in mental state
> Increased body temperature
> Dry skin
> Dry mucous membranes
> Weakness

FLUID VOLUME DEFICIT, POTENTIAL

Etiology
>
> Extremes of age
> Extremes of weight
> Excessive losses through normal routes, e.g., diarrhea
> Loss of fluid through abnormal routes, e.g., indwelling tubes

Deviations affecting access to or intake or absorption of fluids, e.g., physical immobility
Factors influencing fluid needs, e.g., hypermetabolic state
Knowledge deficiency related to fluid volume
Medications, e.g., diuretics

Defining characteristics

Increased output
Urinary frequency
Thirst
Altered intake

GAS EXCHANGE, IMPAIRED

Etiology

Ventilation perfusion imbalance

Defining characteristics

Confusion
Somnolence
Restlessness
Irritability
Inability to move secretions
Hypercapnea
Hypoxia

GRIEVING, ANTICIPATORY

Etiology

To be developed

Defining characteristics

Potential loss of significant object
Expression of distress at potential loss
Denial of potential loss
Guilt
Anger
Sorrow
Choked feelings
Changes in eating habits
Alterations in sleep patterns
Alterations in activity level
Altered libido
Altered communication patterns

GRIEVING, DYSFUNCTIONAL

Etiology

Actual or perceived object loss (*object loss* is used in the broadest sense); objects may include people, possessions, a job, status, home, ideals, parts and processes of the body

Defining characteristics

Verbal expression of distress at loss
Denial of loss

Expression of guilt
Expression of unresolved issues
Anger
Sadness
Crying
Difficulty in expressing loss
Alterations in
  Eating habits
  Sleep patterns
  Dream patterns
  Activity level
  Libido
Idealization of lost object
Reliving of past experiences
Interference with life functioning
Developmental regression
Labile effect
Alterations in concentration and/or pursuits of tasks

HEALTH MAINTENANCE ALTERATION

Definition

Inability to identify, manage, and/or seek out help to maintain health

Etiology

Lack of, or significant alteration in, communication skills (written, verbal and/or gestural)
Lack of ability to make deliberate and thoughtful judgments; perceptual/cognitive impairment (complete/partial lack of gross and/or fine motor skills)
Ineffective individual coping dysfunctional grieving
Unachieved developmental tasks
Ineffective family coping: disabling spiritual distress
Lack of material resources

Defining characteristics

Demonstrated lack of knowledge regarding basic health practices
Demonstrated lack of adaptive behaviors to internal/external environmental changes
Reported or observed inability to take responsibility for meeting basic health practices in any or all functional pattern areas
History of lack of health seeking behavior
Expressed interest in improving health behaviors
Reported or observed lack of equipment, financial and/or other resources
Reported or observed impairment of personal support systems

HOME MAINTENANCE MANAGEMENT, IMPAIRED

Definition

Inability to independently maintain a safe growth-promoting immediate environment

Etiology

Individual/family member disease or injury
Insufficient family organization or planning
Insufficient finances

Unfamiliarity with neighborhood resources
Impaired cognitive or emotional functioning
Lack of knowledge
Lack of role modeling
Inadequate support systems

Defining characteristics

Subjective

*Household members express difficulty in maintaining their home in a comfortable fashion

*Household requests assistance with home maintenance

*Household members describe outstanding debts or financial crises

Objective

Disorderly surroundings

*Unwashed or unavailable cooking equipment, clothes, or linen

*Accumulation of dirt, food wastes, or hygienic wastes

Offensive odors

Inappropriate household temperature

*Overtaxed family members, e.g., exhausted, anxious

Lack of necessary equipment or aids

Presence of vermin or rodents

*Repeated hygienic disorders, infestations, or infections

INJURY: POTENTIAL FOR

Etiology

Interactive conditions between individual and environment which impose a risk to the defensive and adaptive resources of the individual

Internal factors, host

Biological
Chemical
Physiological
Psychological perception
Developmental

External environment

Biological
Chemical
Physiological
Psychological
People/Provider

Defining characteristics

Internal

Biochemical

Regulatory function

Sensory dysfunction
Integrative dysfunction
Effector dysfunction

Tissue hypoxia
Malnutrition
Immune-autoimmune
Abnormal blood profile

Leukocytosis/leukopenia
Altered clotting factors
Thrombocytopenia
Sickle cell
Thalassemia
Decreased hemoglobin
Physical
  Broken skin
  Altered mobility
Developmental
  Age
    Physiological
    Psychosocial
Psychological
  Affective
  Orientation
External
  Biological
    Immunization level of community
    Microorganism
  Chemical
    Pollutants
    Poisons
    Drugs
      Pharmaceutical agents
      Alcohol
      Caffeine
      Nicotine
      Preservatives
      Cosmetics and dyes
      Nutrients (vitamins, food types)
  Physical
    Design, structure, and arrangement of community, building, and/or equipment
    Mode of transport/transportation
    Nosocomial agents
  People/provider
    Nosocomial agent
    Staffing patterns
    Cognitive, affective, and psychomotor factors

A. POISONING: POTENTIAL FOR

Definition

Accentuated risk of accidental exposure to or ingestion of drugs or dangerous products in doses sufficient to cause poisoning

Defining characteristics

Internal (individual)
  Reduced vision
  Verbalization of occupational setting without adequate safeguards
  Lack of safety or drug education

Lack of proper precaution
Cognitive or emotional difficulties
Insufficient finances
External (environmental)
Large supplies of drugs in house
Medicines stored in unlocked cabinets accessible to children or confused persons
Dangerous products placed or stored within the reach of children or confused persons
Availability of illicit drugs potentially contaminated by poisonous additives
Flaking, peeling paint or plaster in presence of young children
Chemical contamination of food and water
Unprotected contact with heavy metals or chemicals
Paint, lacquer, etc., in poorly ventilated areas or without effective protection
Presence of poisonous vegetation
Presence of atmospheric pollutants

B. SUFFOCATION: POTENTIAL FOR

Definition
Accentuated risk of accidental suffocation (inadequate air available for inhalation)

Defining characteristics
Internal (individual)
Reduced olfactory sensation
Reduced motor abilities
Lack of safety education
Lack of safety precautions
Cognitive or emotional difficulties
Disease or injury process
External (environmental)
Pillow placed in an infant's crib
Propped bottle placed in an infant's crib
Vehicle warming in closed garage
Children playing with plastic bags or inserting small objects into their mouths or noses
Discarded or unused refrigerators or freezers without removed doors
Children left unattended in bathtubs or pools
Household gas leaks
Smoking in bed
Use of fuel-burning heaters not vented to outside
Low-strung clothesline
Pacifier hung around infant's head
Person who eats large mouthfuls of food

C. TRAUMA: POTENTIAL FOR

Definition
Accentuated risk of accidental tissue injury, e.g., wound, burn, fracture

Defining characteristics
Internal (individual)
Weakness

Poor vision
Balancing difficulties
Reduced temperature and/or tactile sensation
Reduced large or small muscle coordination
Reduced hand-eye coordination
Lack of safety education
Lack of safety precautions
Insufficient finances to purchase safety equipment or effect repairs
Cognitive or emotional difficulties
History of previous trauma
External (environmental)
 Slippery floors, e.g., wet or highly waxed
 Snow or ice collected on stairs, walkways
 Unanchored rugs
 Bathtub without hand grip or antislip equipment
 Use of unsteady ladders or chairs
 Entering unlighted rooms
 Unsturdy or absent stair rails
 Unanchored electric wires
 Litter or liquid spills on floors or stairways
 High beds
 Children playing without gates at the top of the stairs
 Obstructed passageways
 Unsafe window protection in homes with young children
 Inappropriate call-for-aid mechanisms for bed-resting client
 Pot handles facing toward front of stove
 Bathing in very hot water, e.g., unsupervised bathing of young children
 Potential igniting gas leaks
 Delayed lighting of gas burner or oven
 Experimenting with chemicals or gasoline
 Unscreened fires or heaters
 Wearing plastic apron or flowing clothes around open flame
 Children playing with matches, candles, cigarettes
 Inadequately stored combustible or corrosives, e.g., matches, oily rags, lye
 Highly flammable children's toys or clothing
 Overloaded fuse boxes
 Contact with rapidly moving machinery, industrial belts, or pulleys
 Sliding on coarse bed linen or struggling within bed restraints
 Faulty electrical plugs, frayed wires, or defective appliances
 Contact with acids or alkalis
 Playing with fireworks or gunpowder
 Contact with intense cold
 Overexposure to sun, sun lamps, radiotherapy
 Use of cracked dishware or glasses
 Knives stored uncovered
 Guns or ammunition stored unlocked
 Large icicles hanging from roof
 Exposure to dangerous machinery
 Children playing with sharp-edged toys

High-crime neighborhood and vulnerable client
Driving a mechanically unsafe vehicle
Driving after partaking of alcoholic beverages or drugs
Driving at excessive speeds
Driving without necessary visual aids
Children riding in the front seat in car
Smoking in bed or near oxygen
Overloaded electrical outlets
Grease waste collected on stoves
Use of thin or worn potholders or mitts
Unrestrained babies riding in car
Nonuse or misuse of necessary headgear for motorized cyclists or young children carried on adult bicycles
Unsafe road or road-crossing conditions
Play or work near vehicle pathways, e.g., driveways, laneways, railroad tracks
Nonuse or misuse of seat restraints

KNOWLEDGE DEFICIT (SPECIFY)

Etiology

Lack of exposure
Lack of recall
Information misinterpretation
Cognitive limitation
Lack of interest in learning
Unfamiliarity with information resources

Defining characteristics

Verbalization of the problem
Inaccurate follow-through of instruction
Inaccurate performance of test
Inappropriate or exaggerated behaviors, e.g., hysterical, hostile, agitated, apathetic

MOBILITY, IMPAIRED PHYSICAL

Etiology

Intolerance to activity/decreased strength and endurance
Pain/discomfort
Perceptual/cognitive impairment
Neuromuscular impairment
Musculoskeletal impairment
Depression/severe anxiety

Defining characteristics

Inability to purposefully move within the physical environment, including bed mobility, transfer, and ambulation
Reluctance to attempt movement
Limited range of motion
Decreased muscle strength, control, and/or mass
Imposed restrictions of movement, including mechanical, medical protocol
Impaired coordination

Suggested code for functional level classification†
- 0 Completely independent
- 1 Requires use of equipment or device
- 2 Requires help from another person, for assistance, supervison or teaching
- 3 Requires help from another person and equipment or device
- 4 Dependent, does not participate in activity

NONCOMPLIANCE (SPECIFY)

Definition

A person's informed decision not to adhere to a therapeutic recommendation

Etiology

Patient value system
  Health beliefs
  Cultural influences
  Spiritual values
Client-provider relationships

Defining characteristics

*Behavior indicative of failure to adhere (by direct observation or by statements of patient or significant others)
Objective tests (physiological measures, detection of markers)
Evidence of development of complications
Evidence of exacerbation of symptoms
Failure to keep appointments
Failure to progress

NUTRITION, ALTERATIONS IN: LESS THAN BODY REQUIREMENTS

Etiology

Inability to ingest or digest food or absorb nutrients due to biological, psychological, or economic factors

Defining characteristics

Loss of weight with adequate food intake
Body weight 20% or more under ideal
Reported inadequate food intake less than RDA††
Weakness of muscles required for swallowing or mastication
Reported or evidence of lack of food
Aversion to eating
Reported altered taste sensation
Satiety immediately after ingesting food
Abdominal pain with or without pathology
Sore, inflammed buccal cavity
Capillary fragility

---

†Adapted from Jones, E., and others: Patient classification for long-term care: user's manual, HEW Publication no. HRA-74-3107, November 1974.
††Recommended daily allowance.

Abdominal cramping
Diarrhea and/or steatorrhea
Hyperactive bowel sounds
Lack of interest in food
Perceived inability to ingest food
Pale conjunctival and mucous membranes
Poor muscle tone
Excessive loss of hair
Lack of information, misinformation
Misconceptions

NUTRITION, ALTERATIONS IN: MORE THAN BODY REQUIREMENTS

Etiology

Excessive intake in relation to metabolic need

Defining characteristics

Weight 10% over ideal for height and frame
*Weight 20% over ideal for height and frame
*Triceps skin fold greater than 15 mm in men, 25 mm in women
Sedentary activity level
Reported or observed dysfunctional eating patterns
   Pairing food with other activities
   Concentrating food intake at end of day
   Eating in response to external cues such as time of day, social situation
   Eating in response to internal cues other than hunger, e.g., anxiety

NUTRITION, ALTERATIONS IN: POTENTIAL FOR MORE THAN BODY REQUIREMENTS

Etiology

Hereditary predisposition
Excessive intake during late gestational life, early infancy, and adolescence
Frequent closely spaced pregnancies
Dysfunctional psychological conditioning in relation to food
Membership in lower socioeconomic group

Defining characteristics

*Reported or observed obesity in one or both parents
*Rapid transition across growth percentiles in infants or children
Reported use of solid food as major food source before 5 months of age
Observed use of food as reward or comfort measure
Reported or observed higher baseline weight at beginning of each pregnancy
Dysfunctional eating patterns
   Pairing food with other activities
   Concentrating food intake at end of day
   Eating in response to external cues such as time of day, social situation
   Eating in response to internal cues other than hunger such as anxiety

ORAL MUCOUS MEMBRANE, ALTERATIONS IN

Etiology

Pathological conditions—oral cavity (radiation to head and/or neck)
Dehydration
Trauma
Chemical, e.g., acidic foods, drugs, noxious agents, alcohol
Mechanical, e.g., ill-fitting dentures, braces, tubes (endotracheal/nasogastric), surgery in oral cavity
NPO for more than 24 hours
Ineffective oral hygiene
Mouth breathing
Malnutrition
Infection
Lack of or decreased salivation
Medication

Defining characteristics

Oral pain/discomfort
Coated tongue
Xerostomia (dry mouth)
Stomatitis
Oral lesions or ulcers
Lack of or decreased salivation
Leukoplakia
Edema
Hyperemia
Oral plaque
Desquamation
Vesicles
Hemorrhagic gingivitis
Carious teeth
Halitosis

PARENTING, ALTERATIONS IN: ACTUAL OR POTENTIAL

Definition

Ability of a nurturing figure(s) to create an environment which promotes the optimum growth and development of another human being (It is important to state as a preface to this diagnosis that adjustment to parenting in general is a normal maturational process that elicits nursing behaviors of prevention of potential problems and health promotion.)

Etiology

Lack of available role model
Ineffective role model
Physical and psychosocial abuse of nurturing figure
Lack of support between/from significant other(s)
Unmet social/emotional maturation needs of parenting figures
Interruption in bonding process, i.e., maternal, paternal, other

Unrealistic expectation for self, infant, partner
Perceive threat to own survival, physical and emotional
Mental and/or physical illness
Presence of stress: financial, legal, recent crisis, cultural move
Lack of knowledge
Limited cognitive functioning
Lack of role identity
Lack or inappropriate response of child to relationship
Multiple pregnancies

Defining characteristics

For actual and potential
Lack of parental attachment behaviors
Inappropriate visual, tactile, auditory stimulation
Negative identification of infant/child's characteristics
Negative attachment of meanings to infant/child's characteristics
Constant verbalization of disappointment in gender or physical characteristics of the infant/child
Verbalization of resentment towards the infant/child
Verbalization of role inadequacy
*Inattentive to infant/child needs
Verbal disgust at body functions of infant/child
Noncompliance with health appointments for self and/or infant/child
*Inappropriate caretaking behaviors (toilet training, sleep/rest, feeding)
Inappropriate or inconsistent discipline practices
Frequent accidents
Frequent illness
Growth and development lag in the child
*History of child abuse or abandonment by primary caretaker
Verbalizes desire to have child call him/herself by first name versus traditional cultural tendencies
Child receives care from multiple caretakers without consideration for the needs of the infant/child
Compulsively seeking role approval from others
For actual
Abandonment
Runaway
Verbalization, cannot control child
Incidence of physical and psychological trauma

POWERLESSNESS

Definition

Perception that one's own action will not significantly affect an outcome; a perceived lack of control over a current situation or immediate happening

Etiology

Health care environment
Interpersonal interaction
Illness-related regimen
Life-style of helplessness

Defining characteristics

Severe

Verbal expressions of having no control or influence over situation

Verbal expressions of having no control of influence over outcome

Verbal expressions of having no control over self-care

Depression over physical deterioration which occurs despite patient compliance with regimens

Apathy

Moderate

Nonparticipation in care or decision making when opportunities are provided

Expressions of dissatisfaction and frustration over inability to perform previous tasks and/or activities

Does not monitor progress

Expression of doubt regarding role performance

Reluctance to express true feelings, fearing alienation from care givers

Passivity

Inability to seek information regarding care

Dependence on others that may result in irritability resentment, anger, and guilt

Does not defend self-care practices when challenged

Low

Expressions of uncertainty about fluctuating energy levels passivity

RAPE-TRAUMA SYNDROME

Definition

Forced violent sexual penetration against the victim's will and consent (The trauma syndrome that develops from this attack or attempted attack includes an acute phase of disorganization of the victim's life-style and a long-term process of reorganization of life-style.) This syndrome includes the following three subcomponents: A, B, C.

A. RAPE TRAUMA

Defining characteristics

Acute phase

Emotional reactions

Anger

Embarrassment

Fear of physical violence and death

Humiliation

Revenge

Self-blame

Multiple physical symptoms

Gastrointestinal irritability

Genitourinary discomfort

Muscle tension

Sleep pattern disturbance

Long-term phase

Changes in life-style (changes in residence; dealing with repetitive nightmares and phobias; seeking family support; seeking social network support)

B. COMPOUND REACTION

Defining characteristics

All defining characteristics listed under rape trauma

Reactivated symptoms of such previous conditions, i.e., physical illness, psychiatric illness

Reliance on alcohol and/or drugs

C. SILENT REACTION

Defining characteristics

Abrupt changes in relationships with men

Increase in nightmares

Increased anxiety during interview, i.e., blocking of associations, long periods of silence, minor stuttering, physical distress

Pronounced changes in sexual behavior

No verbalization of the occurrence of rape

Sudden onset of phobic reactions

SELF-CARE DEFICIT: FEEDING, BATHING/HYGIENE, DRESSING/GROOMING, TOILETING

Etiology

Intolerance to activity, decreased strength and endurance

Pain, discomfort

Perceptual or cognitive impairment

Neuromuscular impairment

Musculoskeletal impairment

Depression, severe anxiety

A. SELF-FEEDING DEFICIT (LEVEL 0 TO 4)†

Defining characteristics

Inability to bring food from a receptacle to the mouth

B. SELF-BATHING/HYGIENE DEFICIT (LEVEL 0 TO 4)†

Defining characteristics

*Inability to wash body or body parts

Inability to obtain or get to water source

Inability to regulate temperature or flow

C. SELF-DRESSING/GROOMING DEFICITS (LEVEL 0 TO 4)†

Defining characteristics

*Impaired ability to put on or take off necessary items of clothing

Impaired ability to obtain or replace articles of clothing

---

†For definition of code, see **Mobility, impaired physical.**

Impaired ability to fasten clothing
Inability to maintain appearance at a satisfactory level

D. SELF-TOILETING DEFICIT (LEVEL 0 TO 4)†

Etiology (broad categories)

Impaired transfer ability
Impaired mobility status
Intolerance to activity, decreased strength and endurance
Pain, discomfort
Perceptual or cognitive impairment
Neuromuscular impairment
Musculoskeletal impairment
Depression, severe anxiety

Defining characteristics

*Unable to get to toilet or commode
*Unable to sit on or rise from toilet or commode
*Unable to manipulate clothing for toileting
*Unable to carry out proper toilet hygiene
Unable to flush toilet or empty commode

SELF-CONCEPTS, DISTURBANCE IN: BODY IMAGE, SELF-ESTEEM, ROLE PERFORMANCE, PERSONAL IDENTITY

Definition

Disruption in the way one perceives one's body image, self-esteem, role performance, and/or personal identity (These four subcomponents, in turn, have their own etiologies and defining characteristics [Fig. 1].)

A. BODY IMAGE, DISTURBANCE IN

Etiology

Biophysical
Cognitive perceptual
Psychosocial
Cultural or spiritual

Defining characteristics

A or B must be present to justify the diagnosis of body image, alteration in:
*A. Verbal response to actual or perceived change in structure and/or function
*B. Nonverbal response to actual or perceived change in structure and/or function
The following clinical manifestations may be used to validate the presence of A or B:
Objective
Missing body part
Actual change in structure and/or function

---

†For definition of code, see **Mobility, impaired physical.**

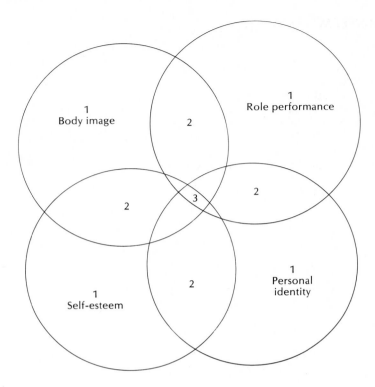

FIGURE 1

 Not looking at body part
 Not touching body part
 Hiding or overexposing body part (intentional or unintentional)
 Trauma to nonfunctioning part
 Change in social involvement
 Change in ability to estimate spatial relationship of body to environment
Subjective
 Verbalization of
  Change in life-style
  Fear of rejection or of reaction by others
  Focus on past strength, function, or appearance
  Negative feelings about body
  Feelings of helplessness, hopelessness, or powerlessness
 Preoccupation with change or loss
 Emphasis on remaining strengths, heightened achievement
 Extension of body boundary to incorporate environmental objects
 Personalization of part or loss by name
 Depersonalization of part or loss by impersonal pronouns
 Refusal to verify actual change

B. SELF-ESTEEM, DISTURBANCE IN

Etiology

To be developed

Defining characteristics

Inability to accept positive reinforcement
Lack of follow-through
Nonparticipation in therapy
Not taking responsibility for self-care (self-neglect)
Lack of eye contact
Self-destructive behavior

C. ROLE PERFORMANCE, DISTURBANCE IN

Etiology

To be developed

Defining characteristics

Change in self-perception of role
Denial of role
Change in others' perception of role
Conflict in roles
Change in physical capacity to resume role
Lack of knowledge of role
Change in usual patterns of responsibility

D. PERSONAL IDENTITY, DISTURBANCE IN

Definition

Inability to distinguish between self and nonself

Etiology

To be developed

Defining characteristics

To be developed

SENSORY-PERCEPTUAL ALTERATIONS: VISUAL, AUDITORY, KINESTHETIC, GUSTATORY, TACTILE, OLFACTORY

Etiology

Altered environmental stimuli, excessive or insufficient
Altered sensory reception, transmission and/or integration
Chemical alterations, endogenous (electrolyte), exogenous (drugs, etc.)
Psychological stress

Defining characteristics

Disoriented in time, in place, or with persons
Altered abstraction
Altered conceptualization
Change in problem-solving abilities
Reported or measured change in sensory acuity

Change in behavior pattern
Anxiety
Apathy
Change in usual response to stimuli
Indication of body-image alteration
Restlessness
Irritability
Altered communication patterns

Other possible defining characteristics

Complaints of fatigue
Alteration in posture
Change in muscular tension
Inappropriate responses
Hallucinations

SEXUAL DYSFUNCTION

Etiology

Biopsychosocial alteration of sexuality
Ineffectual or absent role models
Physical abuse
Psychosocial abuse, e.g., harmful relationships
Vulnerability
Values conflict
Lack of privacy
Lack of significant other
Altered body structure or function: pregnancy, recent childbirth, drugs, surgery, anomalies, disease process, trauma, radiation
Misinformation or lack of knowledge

Defining characteristics

Verbalization of problem
Alterations in achieving perceived sex role
Actual or perceived limitation imposed by disease and/or therapy
Conflicts involving values
Alteration in achieving sexual satisfaction
Inability to achieve desired satisfaction
Seeking confirmation of desirability
Alteration in relationship with significant other
Change of interest in self and others

SKIN INTEGRITY, IMPAIRMENT OF: ACTUAL

Etiology

External (environmental)
Hyper- or hypothermia
Chemical substance
Mechanical factors
Shearing forces
Pressure

        Restraint
Radiation
Physical immobilization
Humidity
Internal (somatic)
  Medication
  Altered nutritional state: obesity, emaciation
  Altered metabolic state
  Altered circulation
  Altered sensation
  Altered pigmentation
  Skeletal prominence
  Developmental factors
  Immunological deficit
  Alterations in turgor (change in elasticity)

Defining characteristics
  Disruption of skin surface
  Destruction of skin layers
  Invasion of body structures

SKIN INTEGRITY, IMPAIRMENT OF: POTENTIAL

Etiology
  Not applicable

Defining characteristics
  External (environmental)
    Hypo- or hyperthermia
    Chemical substance
    Mechanical factors:
      Shearing forces
      Pressure
      Restraint
    Radiation
    Physical immobilization
    Excretions/secretions
    Humidity
  Internal (somatic)
    Medication
    Alterations in nutritional state (obesity, emaciation)
    Altered metabolic state
    Altered circulation
    Altered sensation
    Altered pigmentation
    Skeletal prominence
    Developmental factors
    Alterations in skin turgor (change in elasticity)
    Psychogenic
    Immunologic

SLEEP PATTERN DISTURBANCE

Definition

Disruption of sleep time; causes discomfort or interferes with desired life-style

Etiology

Sensory alterations
  Internal
    Illness
    Psychological stress
  External
    Environmental changes
    Social cues

Defining characteristics

* Verbal complaints of difficulty falling asleep
* Awakening earlier or later than desired
* Interrupted sleep
* Verbal complaints of not feeling well-rested
  Changes in behavior and performance
    Increasing irritability
    Restlessness
    Disorientation
    Lethargy
    Listlessness
  Physical signs
    Mild fleeting nystagmus
    Slight hand tremor
    Ptosis of eyelid
    Expressionless face
    Dark circles under eyes
  Thick speech with mispronunciation and incorrect words
    Frequent yawning
    Changes in posture

SOCIAL ISOLATION

Definition

Aloneness experienced by the individual and perceived as imposed by others and as a negative or threatened state

Etiology

Factors contributing to the absence of satisfying personal relationships, such as:
  Delay in accomplishing developmental tasks
  Immature interests
  Alterations in physical appearance
  Alterations in mental status
  Unaccepted social behavior
  Unaccepted social values
  Altered state of wellness

Inadequate personal resources
Inability to engage in satisfying personal relationships

Defining characteristics
Objective
Absence of supportive significant other(s): family, friends, group
Sad dull affect
Inappropriate or immature interests/activities for developmental age/stage
Uncommunicative, withdrawn, no eye contact
Preoccupation with own thoughts, repetitive, meaningless actions
Projects hostility in voice, behavior
Seeks to be alone, or exists in a subculture
Evidence of physical/mental handicap or altered state of wellness
Shows behavior unaccepted by dominant cultural group
Subjective
Expresses feelings of aloneness imposed by others
Expresses feelings of rejection
Experiences feelings of difference from others
Inadequacy in or absence of significant purpose in life
Inability to meet expectations of others
Insecurity in public
Expresses values acceptable to the subculture but unacceptable to the dominant
cultural group
Expresses interests inappropriate to the developmental age/stage

SPIRITUAL DISTRESS (DISTRESS OF THE HUMAN SPIRIT)

Definition
Disruption in the life principle which pervades a person's entire being and which
integrates and transcends one's biological and psychosocial nature

Etiology
Separation from religious/cultural ties
Challenged belief and value system, e.g., due to moral/ethical implications of therapy,
due to intense suffering

Defining characteristics
*Expresses concern with meaning of life/death and/or belief systems
Anger toward God
Questions meaning of suffering
Verbalizes inner conflict about beliefs
Verbalizes concern about relationship with deity
Questions meaning of own existence
Unable to participate in usual religious practices
Seeks spiritual assistance
Questions moral/ethical implications of therapeutic regimen
Gallows humor
Displacement of anger toward religious representatives
Description of nightmares/sleep disturbances
Alteration in behavior/mood evidenced by anger, crying, withdrawal, preoccupation,
anxiety, hostility, apathy, etc.

THOUGHT PROCESSES, ALTERATION IN

Etiology
>To be determined

Defining characteristics
>Inaccurate interpretation of environment
>Cognitive dissonance
>Distractibility
>Memory deficit/problems
>Egocentricity
>Hyper- or hypovigilance

Other possible defining characteristics
>Inappropriate nonreality-based thinking

TISSUE PERFUSION, ALTERATION IN: CEREBRAL, CARDIOPULMONARY, RENAL, GASTROINTESTINAL, PERIPHERAL

Etiology
>Interruption of flow, arterial
>Interruption of flow, venous
>Exchange problems
>Hypovolemia
>Hypervolemia

Defining characteristics with estimated sensitivities and specificities

	Chances that characteristic will be present in given diagnosis	Chances that characteristic will not be explained by any other diagnosis
Skin temperature: cold extremities	High	Low
Skin color		
Dependent, blue or purple	Moderate	Low
*Pale on elevation, color does not return on lowering of leg	High	High
*Diminished arterial pulsations	High	High
Skin quality: shining	High	Low
Lack of lanugo	High	Moderate
Round scars covered with atrophied skin		
Gangrene	Low	High
Slow-growing, dry, thick brittle nails	High	Moderate
Claudication	Moderate	High
Blood pressure changes in extremities		
Bruits	Moderate	Moderate
Slow healing of lesions	High	Low

URINARY ELIMINATION, ALTERATION IN PATTERNS

Etiology

Multiple causality, including
Anatomical obstruction
Sensory motor impairment
Urinary tract infection

Defining characteristics

Dysuria
Frequency
Hesitancy
Incontinence
Nocturia
Retention
Urgency

VIOLENCE, POTENTIAL FOR (SELF-DIRECTED OR DIRECTED AT OTHERS)

Etiology

Antisocial character
Battered women
Catatonic excitement
Child abuse
Manic excitement
Organic brain syndrome
Panic states
Rage reactions
Suicidal behavior
Temporal lobe epilepsy
Toxic reactions to medication

Defining characteristics

Body language: clenched fists, tense facial expressions, rigid posture, tautness indicating effort to control
Hostile threatening verbalizations: boasting to or prior abuse of others
Increased motor activity: pacing, excitement, irritability, agitation
Overt and aggressive acts: goal-directed destruction of objects in environment
Possession of destructive means: gun, knife, weapon
Rage
Self-destructive behavior, active aggressive suicidal acts
Suspicion of others, paranoid ideation, delusions, hallucinations
Substance abuse/withdrawal

Other defining characteristics†

Increasing anxiety levels
Fear of self or others
Inability to verbalize feelings
Repetition of verbalizations: continued complaints, requests, and demands

---

†From unpublished dissertation by P. Clunn.

Anger
Provocative behavior: argumentative, dissatisfied, overreactive, hypersensitive
Vulnerable self-esteem
Depression (specifically, active, aggressive, suicidal acts)

References

Kim, M.J., and Moritz, D.A., editors: Classification of nursing diagnoses—Proceedings of the Third and Fourth National Conferences, New York, 1982, McGraw-Hill Book Co.

Kim, M.J., McFarland, G., and McLane, A., editors: Classification of nursing diagnoses—Proceedings of the Fifth National Conference, St. Louis, 1984, The C.V. Mosby Co.

Kim, M.J., McFarland, G. and McLane, A., editors: Pocket guide to nursing diagnoses, St. Louis, 1984, The C.V. Mosby Co.

Section V **Segment 1:**

Business meeting

MARJORY GORDON, Ph.D., R.N., FAAN

The first meeting of the North American Nursing Diagnosis Association is called to order. Our first order of business is the roll call. The by-laws specify that a quorum requires 20% of membership. The total membership is 701. We require 141 for a quorum. There are 260 members present. We have a quorum for this meeting.

On behalf of the Board of Directors, I wish to extend a warm welcome to you at the first business meeting of the North American Nursing Diagnosis Association. There will be no acceptance of minutes; this is our first meeting. As you know from your membership and conference packets, by-laws were accepted in April, 1982, and the organization was formally structured. Your packet includes an agenda and reports. There are no resolutions from the Board at this time. The Board has had two meetings; one was in August, 1983, in Boston, Massachusetts. The second was April 3, 1984, in St. Louis. The Board is planning two more meetings at this convention. The rules for business this morning will be that the chair will entertain any motions from the floor under new business or under the reports; each committee will be allotted 5 minutes and will entertain any questions or discussion within that time period.

As President, the focus for my term of office is to promote the classification of nursing diagnoses and to establish collaborative relationships with the American Nurses Association related to practice issues around nursing diagnosis—for example, implementation of nursing diagnosis, computerization, quality assurance, reimbursement, and other issues of practice. These come directly out of the by-laws, which state that the purpose of the Association is to develop, refine, and promote a taxonomy of nursing diagnostic terminology of general use to the profession. The functions of the Association, as you are aware, are to conduct conferences, publish documents, facilitate research, and serve as an information resource in order to promote a taxonomy of nursing diagnoses. The liaison with the American Nurses' Association has been established through the Steering Committee on Classification of Nursing Practice Phenomena. Nursing practice phenomena are currently defined by the Steering Committee as phenomena relevant to nursing practice, not just nursing diagnoses. Some people have commented that phenomena of concern in nursing practice would possibly be nursing diagnoses, interventions, outcomes, roles and functions of nurses, and classification of nurses. The emphasis thus far in the Steering Committee is on nursing diagnosis and looking at that as

547

perhaps an organizing framework for looking at the other phenomena of concern. NANDA will have a program at the American Nurses Association convention in 1984, and the Board has begun to consider whether or not it would be possible to get a NANDA program on the ICN. At the last International Council of Nurses convention, we were unable to do that. In a sense, there are rules for that association and although we had six countries supporting it, we did not get on the program. We are starting early this time and hope that the program will be possible. I think it is very important to start thinking about participation of other countries, outside of North America. Currently to our knowledge, diagnoses are being translated in Colombia and Japan. There is interest in a French translation by a person in Canada. People who have traveled to other countries have suggested that there is a great deal of interest in countries like New Zealand and Australia. If we look to the future, the need does exist for an international classification of nursing diagnoses. Perhaps we need to decide if we can support other countries in validating nursing diagnoses. They themselves might contact us. These issues are under consideration by the Board.

Although no survey exists, it is my impression that the interest in nursing diagnosis in North America appears to have increased considerably in the last few years. Structurally the Association continues to maintain a clearinghouse for nursing diagnoses and a newsletter. We have appointed an Executive Director for the NANDA office at St. Louis University School of Nursing. Karen Murphy, whom you all know, has assumed this responsibility. I believe our future needs should include consideration of methods to facilitate information exchange to a greater degree than we do at the present. This is needed in the areas of classification of nursing diagnoses as well as implementation of nursing diagnoses. Perhaps we need to look at better methods of doing this.

I believe a second future effort is the promotion of research on nursing diagnoses. You will hear the plans and progress in this area during the Research Committee report.

The third area of current concern is the development of a master plan. The by-laws require that we have an Ad Hoc Master Planning Committee which would translate our purposes and functions into operational programs. This may be a 2-year, 5-year, or 10-year plan.

As you can see in the committee reports, the new Association has been organized according to the by-laws and has begun the planning for implementation of the Association's purposes and functions. Anyone interested in participating in any of the committees please use your yellow card to indicate your name, address, and the particular committee in which you would like to participate.

Let us consider the business before the membership. I would now like to call for committee reports. (Appendix A.)

PROGRAM COMMITTEE: Audrey McLane

On page 1 you will find the committee report. There is one addition. I have two new members of the committee: Laura Rossi and Mary Ann Kelly. That will make up our five members of the committee. We will probably be meeting tomorrow. There has not been time to do anything other than plan the national conference. Are there any questions?

At this point the Board has not made any decision about the time and place for the 1986 Conference, that is, whether it will be in St. Louis or somewhere else. We may need a large convention center because of the size of the group.

I move that we accept the report from the Program Committee.

We have a second. Accepted by majority vote.

PUBLICATION COMMITTEE: Kristine Gebbie

You have the report of the Publications Committee in front of you. The Committee is charged to provide the Board with direction on any official publications of the organization. At present there are two major publications: the newsletter and the proceedings. As you can see from the document, one of the major issues has been the clarification of policy regarding placement of the work of the Association in the public domain. The statement will be useful to you if you have had any questions about the public domain status of nursing diagnoses.

The newsletter editor, Mary Woods, is a member of our Committee. The newsletter will become a major item of planning and discussion in the coming year in regard to format and content. We have not spent much time on it to date. We are concerned about (1) growing from the base of the previously published proceedings, while maintaining the high quality of editorial work and useful information, and (2) finding a speedier process for turnaround so that materials are available a little more quickly. The latter is a difficult process, but we are working on it. We are considering regular publications, other than proceedings. We will be working on methodology for identifying needed publications, perhaps with other committees, and then taking the necessary steps to get them out. We would be happy to answer any questions. We do have one vacancy on this committee. If you have a particular interest in publication, make sure you indicate that on your cards.

Questions

Joanne McCloskey, the University of Iowa: I appreciate your efforts to have a speedier process for publishing the proceedings. But from my quick reading of number three, it sounds as if you're looking for a technical editor of this next volume rather than a nurse with professional skills. Is that a correct reading of number three?

Kristine Gebbie: No, although we did not specify it there. Our advertisement for the editor has only been through nursing channels, in our own newsletter, and schools of nursing. The applicants we have to date are nurses, several of whom have previous experience with nursing diagnosis. We discussed with the Board of Directors the concern that we not select an editor who would have no content information, because there is a need to understand the material as well as understand basic English.

Carol Hayes Christiansen, Gainesville, Florida: I was noticing you said we would need permission to cite. I was wondering if you were going to make any stipulation as to how much could be cited without written permission; like the *AJN* says, you can do 50 words, or something like that.

Kristine Gebbie: Most publishers have standard rules. We would expect those to be followed in the usual kind of format.

Harriet Werley, University of Wisconsin, Milwaukee: Since one of your concerns has been the delay in the availability of the published volumes, I think it would be well for your committee to consider how you might have some established format that authors should follow and see that your format is followed in detail and that your membership recognizes that the delay is frequently not something that you blame on publishers but that goes back to the authors not having done a good enough job with their papers, or not having done a good enough job with their referencing and what not. Therefore, the editors have to get back to them, and back to them, and back to them, and all that delays it. So, I do think you need a professional editor, and you need some guidelines for your authors in their strict adherence to good scholarly preparation of their paper so that it won't be held up.

Kristine Gebbie: I think the existing editors will just give you a gold medal, Harriet, for saying that. In conjunction with the Program Committee, we will be looking at stricter guidelines for incoming manuscripts. Was there another question? If not, I move the adoption of the Publication Committee report.

We have a second. Accepted by majority vote.

MEMBERSHIP COMMITTEE: Ann Becker

The committee has not met, as such, except by mail. We will be meeting tomorrow. Our major focus is to make nurses throughout the United States and Canada more aware of us and increase our membership. We are also trying to determine the information that we need to have on our membership applications so that we will have various types of available information and be able to retrieve this from a computer. We are in the process, as you see in number three, of looking at the possibility of including the newsletter as part of the membership fee. That will be discussed at the Board meeting this week. I do want to tell you one thing. As of last week, we had 710 members. We also have, again as of last week, 1,038 newsletter subscriptions. The reason for the discrepancy between the two is that we have people and institutions who are receiving the newsletter who are not members of the Association.

Questions

Juanita Theile, Wisconsin: I recently returned from Australia and in Adelaide, Australia, I spoke before a group of over 100 nurses who are keenly interested in nursing diagnosis and are very actively using it. I wonder if there is any provision by this organization, to think of other countries and their possible membership. Australian nurses were very keen to receive information and get in contact with nurses in America.

Ann Becker: Yes, indeed, this came up at the Board meeting and we are discussing that. The Public Relations Committee will also be considering this. I am aware that we have received letters recently from Queensland, Australia, as well as many other countries.

Nancy Creason, Illinois: I think you're the appropriate person to talk to about this. My concern is establishing a better form of rather quick networking, and it would seem to me if you're going to collect data about the members, one should make an effort to get some idea of their interest area and their expertise area of nursing diagnosis so that could be communicated to everybody with the membership list once a year, or something. This is not just to collect data, but to help us network with other people.

Ann Becker: We are looking into this, and one of the things we're checking with the Board is how much information will be disseminated and when it will be disseminated.

Harriet Werley, University of Wisconsin-Milwaukee: My comment ties in with membership, but it also ties in with something that Marjory said earlier. If you are interested in having a program at the ICN, you are already too late for the call for abstracts. That was the 15th of February. So I would suggest that you get busy and see if, organization to organization, you can get a program in there. That would have a great bearing on your membership.

Ann Becker: Are there any other questions or comments? If not, I move to accept the Membership Committee report.

We have a second. Accepted by majority vote.

PUBLIC RELATIONS COMMITTEE: Derry Ann Moritz

There are a couple of things I want to point out as our major targets or goals. As a Public Relations Committee, we want to get into the public media. (My goal in life is *The New York Times* or something like that.) This is obviously just the beginning. The Public Relations Committee has met by phone once and yesterday over lunch. We identified a number of goals. We're going to try to get press releases in numerous professional journals. We want to determine our articulation, as a committee, with the Publications Committee, the Membership Committee, and the Program Committee. All of these committees interdigitate and we need to work together. This was the first year for all of us. I think that the Public Relations Committee obviously can do much more to publicize a convention like this, to publicize membership, and to work in various fronts. I would appreciate any input. We have essentially a full membership for our committee, but I would like any ideas or volunteers from different parts of the country. Membership of the Committee consists of Oregon, two people from Connecticut, and one person from British Columbia. We do not have Mexico, Australia, or various other parts of the world represented even as ad hoc advisory people. I would really appreciate help.

Comments

Participant: I have relatives in England and Australia who are very interested in our organization. So I volunteer.

Derry Ann Moritz: Are there any questions or recommendations? If not, I move acceptance of the report.

We have a second. Accepted by majority vote.

Marjory Gordon: I can add one more thing that happened at noontime yesterday. A regional radio station interviewed Ann Becker and me regarding what nursing diagnosis is and, of course, the DRG issue.

NOMINATIONS COMMITTEE: Joyce Shoemaker

The report is contained in your packet, and I have only a couple things that I want to add to it. I neglected to tell you who the membership is, and I think you should know that: Patricia Clunn from Florida, Nancy Lengel from Pennsylvania, and Winnifred Mills from British Columbia. We have an election coming up next year, and so the Nominating Committee will be working in the next few months, attempting to establish a slate. I invite you, if you are interested in running for office, to let either myself or Winnifred Mills know during the course of this meeting. And, in fact, Winni, would you stand up so that people can recognize you, because I think it is important that you get to us if you have some interest. As it indicates in my report, the office of president, the office of secretary, three board members, and one member of the nominating committee will be elected to serve beginning July 1985. Are there any questions?

Questions

Rona Levin, New York: I just wondered if you could mention some of the process in terms of how you decide upon the nominees, what criteria you use, etc.

Joyce Shoemaker: That's a very good question. The Nominating Committee has not yet met. One of the goals of the Committee is to determine a process. Obviously, if we're inundated with nominees for a particular office, we need to have some type of process. I believe that there is implicit in our charge the notion of having some geographic distribution as well as distribution of the membership in terms of functional interest. However, at this point in time, we do not have a process established to share with you. Are there any other questions? I move acceptance of the report of the Nominating Committee.

We have a second. Accepted by majority vote.

RESEARCH COMMITTEE: Gertrude McFarland

The Research Committee report is contained in the business report in front of you. We met in an extensive work session last evening and we have made some additional suggestions and some additional goals that I wish to share with you. Of course, these will be submitted to the Board for review. The goals that were revised were the 2a and 2b, and they now read as follows: (2a) Supporting or co-sponsoring research conferences by other professional nursing organizations such as ANA, MNRS, SCRB, MARNA, National Nursing Research Conference of Canada, etc. (2b) was revised as follows: Developing a research session in NANDA's newsletter and editing/publishing research articles. We were somewhat of a group of dreamers last evening; we made an additional goal that we will be submitting to the Board for consideration. That is, 2d, which reads: Providing seed money for conducting nursing diagnosis research, requesting and reviewing proposals, and developing pilot projects. In addition to revising the goals, we looked at the development of the committee structure. We are proposing a subcommittee structure co-chaired by the official committee membership. If this is approved by the Board, we certainly will be calling upon those of you interested in working with the Research Committee to serve on the subcommittees. So anyone interested in serving on a research subcommittee may so indicate on the yellow cards. We did have an excellent turnout yesterday at the research special interest group: over seventy people. A lot of discussion took place. At that meeting, also, we had an excellent response of people indicating their interest in serving on the Research Committee. We made several recommendations, and I will not go into these in detail. We keep submitting to the officers for their consideration such things as the newsletter, how we perceive perhaps a name change to reflect a more scholarly and research-type publication from the organization. We also considered making some suggestions to the Membership Committee to include an area on the application form to begin to collect some data on past research that has been done by potential members of the organization and also current research endeavors. We can begin to collect data that will serve to develop a data base that we can share and disseminate among the membership. We developed an action plan and set a timetable for the submission of progress reports. Are there any questions?

Questions

Juanita Theile, Wisconsin: I'm wondering if the Research Committee's focus is perhaps broader than what your goals state. Maybe it's my misunderstanding of what your purpose really is, but will not the research be aimed at nursing phenomena, as was identified earlier this morning? We're looking at not only nursing diagnosis but related interventions (evaluation, in other words), the totality of nursing process that nursing diagnosis fits into rather than specifically stating nursing diagnosis. Or is that understood in these goals?

Gertrude McFarland: At this point in time in our committee discussion and in meetings of the Board, the words "nursing diagnosis research" have seemed to be floating around. Perhaps that is an issue we need to take a closer look at. Any other questions? I move that the report be accepted.

We have a second. Accepted by majority vote.

TAXONOMY AND DIAGNOSIS REVIEW COMMITTEES: Phyllis Kritek

The first report is the Taxonomy Committee report and, as indicated, the bylaws require that this committee develop and regularly review a taxonomic system for diagnoses and promote this both within and without the organization. The committee has not yet deliberated, nor made any determination on that. I think that we will need to spend some time doing what is listed there under 2a, reviewing all possible options before any action is taken. The rest of the activities of the committee will flow from that. I think probably the most critical issue in this report is that we would like to consider at the Seventh Conference a review of a NANDA Taxonomic System. That is, at the next conference, a general assembly would debate such an issue. It might just be helpful to say that we hope that in the next 2 years (the taxonomy group that met yesterday discussed this to some degree), between this and the next scheduled conference, that the discipline and particular members of NANDA will give some attention to the whole question of taxonomic structure and their desires, and that that would be reflected in nursing's public literature so we have some opportunity to deliberate prior to any formal action.

Questions

Rosemary Hogan, Kent State University: I would just see this as one of the highest priorities (and I realize all of the problems in developing a taxonomic structure), but an alphabetized list clinically is very difficult to use. What I see happening is that people are developing their own organizing structure to make that alphabetized list clinically useful and developing assessment tools to use. I think maybe that's the way we have to go, but I see it like the Tower of Babel—everybody out there saying something different—and given all the problems, it would be ideal if we could get some kind of agreement on a taxonomic structure.

Phyllis Kritek: Needless to say, I concur with your viewpoint. That was nice of you to say it so it sounded like a movement. We felt, since the membership at large (the general assembly and the membership) did not have an opportunity to deliberate to any degree on the work of the Fifth Conference Group and the taxonomic structure proposed, that it seems somewhat premature and that we really need some internal discussion and exploration. I guess I want people to feel pretty good about it when it happens. It is in the bylaws that one shall be developed and regularly reviewed. That is a bylaw requirement of this Committee and will be pursued accordingly. Thank you for your observation. I would just make one other point. If anyone has any other visions, suggestions, insights, hopes, dreams, etc., please do share them. I would be most receptive to them (including "I used your tree and it's crazy!"). I move we accept the report of the Taxonomy Committee.

We have a second. The report is accepted by majority vote.

I want to take a little more time with the Diagnosis Review Committee report because I think it's the one that's a major transition. This I chair by reason of office, vice-presidency, and I think it's the most overt change in the Conference for those of you who have been to several prior conferences. I want to go through this process because several people have approached me with questions. This committee also has to create a large number of mechanisms and appropriate forms to accompany them. The bylaws require that this Committee review proposed diagnoses and recommend acceptance, modification, rejection; that they appoint review task forces; that they designate the format for submission; and that they prepare proposed diagnoses, as are recommended, for membership voting. In addition, the bylaws call under the general assembly statement, which is Article 8.2, that the general assembly reviews and comments on proposed diagnoses. Prior to any vote of the membership, the general assembly would have a review and comment session. That would seem to indicate that our cycle for review, acceptance, approval, etc., would be tied to meetings of the general assembly. I would hope that there would be a very expeditious membership vote immediately after general assembly review and comment. This Committee's charge, from my perception at least, is to create a review process, set guidelines, mechanisms, rules of the game, expectations, standards, and make them functional, implement them, and create a cyclic pattern. That cyclic pattern is theoretically endless. We do have some assumptions listed that were discussed with the Board. I think they're important to know about, in part because if you're waiting breathlessly to change some diagnoses right now, that you really think are appalling, we are giving changes second priority. First, there is a need to create a new mechanism. We have about 25 diagnoses that have been submitted. These include everything from twelve-page documents and theses to a word. We have to set up some guidelines for what can be submitted under what conditions. It's a problem if we encourage people to send diagnoses in and then send them back and say we're very sorry, but they are not in the format. We are going to have to say that unless you can give at least these basic components, no review group can address it. In addition, because the membership will want to know how things are going with each step, we will be using the NANDA newsletter to keep the membership informed, to the degree it attempts to stay informed through the newsletter. The established rules of public domain will persist. None of this is formalized yet. You will get news of each piece of this as we proceed. We are hoping to find a mechanism so that those who submit diagnoses know their submission is going to be in the review cycle for a while. If you consent, we'll put your name and the area you're looking at in the newsletter so that people can begin to communicate with you even though your diagnosis is in the cycle. The activities of the committee have been listed in some detail (what has to be done yet). Finally, it is our hope that the general assembly review and comment will occur for the first time at the Seventh Conference. This should be feasible to achieve. Do you have any questions?

Questions

Joanne McCloskey, University of Iowa: It was my understanding that we had guidelines for submission of a new diagnosis, namely those published in Marge Gordon's book. Are you saying that those guidelines are going to be revised, that new guidelines are going to be set up, or that we're still using those?

Phyllis Kritek: I think we're going to review them, not necessarily revise them. I'm not saying either of those things or any of those things, I guess. But we were not

NANDA when those were used and, indeed, they were not acted on by any formal body to any degree. They tended to be a program planning mechanism at that point. We need to determine as a committee, and I think even as a Board probably, if these make sense or not. In addition, if we formally act on them and make them part of NANDA's procedures, I think it then gives some message to those who wish to send in diagnoses that it is not simply the caprice of some individual. While I'm concerned because part of me wants very much to encourage the submission of these phenomena and realize a person's hard work on it, we simply are going to have to have some degree of structuring, I think.

Helena Lee, Wisconsin: I think we've heard from the chairpersons of the various committees about the interrelationship in the NANDA structure of the various committees. Particularly the Diagnosis Review Committee and the Taxonomic Committee seem to be so interrelated that I'm wondering how the criteria for the diagnosis can be established prior to the taxonomic system, which would be the overall framework within which we would accept diagnoses that would be reflective of nursing phenomena. Have you given consideration to that?

Phyllis Kritek: Personally I have; in all honesty, I can't speak for anybody else. The committees have not formally met, so I can't really answer from their perspective. I'm chairing Diagnosis Review because of the by-laws. I was interested in taxonomy so I'll be able at least to talk to myself about these two things. I do think they're interactive rather than a cause-effect kind of patterning. I'm not anxious about that, though I do hope that the interaction is real. It seems to me that if we have survived for eleven years with the alphabet, this is no time to be faint-hearted. I'm very conscious of people in both the organization and nursing at large being more invested in generation of labels than they are in creation of taxonomies, on the whole. It seems imperative that we become responsive to that activity and the discipline. To some degree I hope that the taxonomy can grapple with that input. That's my own view, only. Are there any other questions? I move acceptance of this report.

We have a second. The report is accepted by majority vote. The vice-president will take over the chair while the president gives the report as per the bylaws on the Master Plan Ad-Hoc Committee.

MASTER PLAN AD HOC COMMITTEE: Marjory Gordon

As was referred to in my previous comments, the Master Plan Ad-Hoc Committee has not met. The reasoning behind that was that the master plan arises out of our committees and the committees reflect our functions and purposes. Out of their goals comes our first master planning. As chair of that committee, I would be very interested in the membership's input, and I have thought of a way to do that. Members of the Association who are presently here, please take a piece of paper; there will be a box outside the meeting rooms today. Place in that box one issue or plan, in whatever specificity that you think should be high priority focus. The reasoning behind that is that if we get one from everyone, they might be able to be tabulated tonight and influence the decisions of the Board in terms of master planning. Also, in terms of participating on that committee, that is open. Thank you. I move we accept the report of the Master Plan Committee.

We have a second. Accepted by majority vote.

FINANCIAL REPORT: Kristine Gebbie, Treasurer

Some of you know in my other life that I deal with budgets that could never be placed on one piece of paper and follow formats and guidelines that go on till next Tuesday. We have only operated a few months with a formal budget and do not have a good method of reporting to you either income or expenses as compared with budget so that you can really track where the organization is going.

As is evident, however, from the financial report that you have, we are quite solvent, particularly as compared to previous days. Some of you remember when we didn't even have a dime for a postage stamp. The conference was clearly intended to help with that solvency. It's one of the few mechanisms we have right now of generating reserve funds that can help support the activities. We have not, to date, had, for example, any budget for committees, and that's one of the reasons you've seen slow progress, because they've had no support for the work that they might have done. In developing the budget for the next fiscal year, we'll be able to more accurately project both income and expenses. I think we will be able to budget for committee work and by the time you get a financial report for the following fiscal period, all members will be able to track our projections and our actual expenditures in a better way. At that time I will be able to talk about longer range fiscal planning. With all of those caveats and explanations, I would be happy to answer any questions about the budget and expenditures to date or about the plans.

Questions

Participant: I would just like to know if any of these rather large funds are invested in any way in order to be adding to particularly a source of research funding?

Kristine Gebbie: At the present time (again, this relates to the historic development of this orgnaization) all of our funds are at St. Louis University, which has been providing all of our business support since this whole process began. One of the issues is how to separate those funds and really get them under the management of the Association so that they can be appropriately invested. That is our intent with as short a turnaround time as possible. I can assure you, I hate to see them going uninvested, but at this point until we are a formal organization and until we clear the relationship with St. Louis University, this is not possible. We . . . were getting so much free from them that it was a little difficult to say "And besides that, we want to take our money out of your bank account and invest it somewhere else." We didn't want to lose more than we could gain. Other questions? I move acceptance of the treasurer's report.

We have a second. The financial report of the organization is accepted.

The Chair will entertain discussion in regard to new business.

Lynda Carpenito, Delaware: We were discussing in our Mid-Atlantic Regional meeting last night the possibility and the question of having a regional meeting group come under NANDA. Are there any regional groups that presently come under NANDA as an umbrella? No? Has that been discussed at all with the Board?

Marjory Gordon, President: I'll refer that to Audrey McLane, Program Committee. Yes, there has been discussion. She will cite the regional groups; a meeting was held today.

Audrey McLane, Program Committee Chairperson: With the work on taxonomy and diagnosis review being such a high priority, the Board has not had time nor the money to invest in supporting regional groups. And at this conference, that's a step we're trying to take. We're having a breakfast meeting tomorrow morning and asking one representative from each established group to meet with us and to raise some of the questions and issues about how the regional groups are organized. Currently, as far as I know, there's no mechanism for them to be organized under NANDA. In Wisconsin, we're organized under the Wisconsin Nurses Association. Some states have them as free standing organizations. There are multiple ways of doing this, but that's the purpose of the meeting. So, if you didn't hear my invitation before, any established group registered with Karen, come to the meeting. (We're not interested at that breakfast in having people who just want to establish a group.) If you want to establish a group, go to one of the group meetings. At future conferences, we'll probably have some more to report to you.

Lynda Carpenito. Delaware: Just one comment. I don't think, necessarily, we have to say that it has to be a financial relationship. In other words, in our particular group, we're not looking for financial aid from NANDA. We are searching for a group perhaps. We are presently under MARNA, which is a group that umbrellas the whole area, and we're looking at other alternatives.

Marjory Gordon, President: I do think we should spend the time tomorrow and work on some of those issues. Maybe we could make a report to the assembly about the wishes of the regional groups before this meeting ends on Friday.

The Board has also considered the articulation between the Membership Committee, the Program Committee, and the Public Relations Committee. We appreciate the interaction among these committees in terms of helping regions and states to get organized, obtain resource people, and start networking. That also influences membership as well as activities and public relations. Depending on the objectives that are set up by regional and state groups, the activities may very well impact on the other committee activities as listed on your program, such as Diagnosis Review. There is no formal regional structure, as Audrey has said, but this is an important item for Board consideration. Perhaps Dorothea Jakob from Canada is going to comment on regions. We have to get some way of looking at North America by regions.

Dorothea Jakob, Toronto: Yes, I was going to speak to share the information with the group that there are no regional associations that I'm aware of in Canada. But I bring greeting from a very small group in Toronto that began meeting in September, a group of eight individuals. We have informally gathered under the title of the Toronto Nursing Diagnosis Interest Group. We're presenting a clinical session at the Registered Nurses Association Meeting of Ontario (RNAO) in May, and we're hoping to incite the small group–grass roots meeting of people with, perhaps, a 2- or 3-year down-the-line goal of developing regional group. We would enjoy the support of people.

Marjory Gordon, President: New business, discussion?

Participant: This isn't really new business. I just want to say that I'm impressed with what I've heard go on here today in the business meeting (the work of the committees and the work of the Board) and I want to commend you for the hard work that's gone on in a very short period of time. I'm really impressed with you.

Marjory Gordon, President: I reflect that compliment to the people that you elected. It's been extremely enjoyable and I think, as you are saying, productive, in terms of the work they've done in such a short time. If there is no new business, I will ask for a motion for adjournment. So moved. This first meeting of the North American Nursing Diagnosis Association is adjourned. Remember, jot down those high-priority master plan suggestions for the box that is outside. Thank you very much. Have a very good day.

Committee reports

Report of the Program Committee

MEMBERSHIP

The Planning Committee for the Sixth Conference is a subcommittee of the Program Committee.

A. McLane, Chairperson
A. Becker, Co-Chairperson
R. Fehring
M. J. Kim

With the exception of R. Fehring, all are members of the Program Committee.

ISSUES CONSIDERED

The Committee met in Milwaukee to plan the Sixth Conference and in Chicago to make the final selection of research/scholarly papers.

One-hundred-four abstracts were submitted. Members of NANDA with research preparation participated in a blind review of the abstracts. The Planning Committee, with the assistance of K. Murphy, summarized the reviews and made the final selection of papers and posters to be presented.

An awards ceremony was scheduled for the opening session of the Sixth Conference to recognize nurse leaders who had made significant contributions to the work of NANDA. It is recommended that a more formal process be established by the Board of Directors to nominate and select future award recipients.

The Planning Committee, with the assistance of the President, submitted a program to the ANA for the Convention in New Orleans in June. The program was approved and will be presented on Tuesday, June 26, 1984, from 1:00 PM to 2:45 PM. The title of the program is "Nursing Diagnoses: Current and Future Challenges." NANDA is the official sponsor of the program. Presenters and titles of their presentations are as follows:

Decisions and directions
Speaker: Audrey McLane, Ph.D., R.N.
Implementation of nursing diagnoses: choosing goals and strategies
Speaker: Jane Lancour, M.S.N., R.N.
"Nursing is. . . " The human response dilemma: toward interpretation of the social policy statement
Speaker: Marjory Gordon, Ph.D., R.N.

The Planning Committee for the Seventh Conference will be appointed following the April meeting in St. Louis so that work can begin immediately. The two vacancies on the Program Committee will be filled after the location of the next conference is announced by the Board of Directors.

Report of the Publications Committee

MEMBERSHIP

Kristine Gebbie, Chairperson
Mary Hurley
Joyce Shoemaker
Mary Woods

ISSUES CONSIDERED TO DATE

1. Public domain

Because it is in the Association's interest to have nursing diagnoses (including the diagnostic and etiological labels, defining characteristics and definitions) and taxonomies of diagnosis (including category labels and definitions) widely used by the profession, it is the policy of the Association to consider these terms in the public domain, and therefore available for duplication and distribution by nurses. The Association expects that the usual scholarly standards for source citation will be followed.

Materials other than diagnoses and taxonomy appearing in proceedings or publications of the Association (including invited papers, transcripts or summaries of discussions, or replications of audiovisual presentations) are copyrighted. While permission to reproduce or cite will generally be granted, the Association expects that written requests for permission to reproduce will be submitted in advance, in the usual publication request format.

2. Proceedings

The North American Nursing Diagnosis Association plans to continue the pattern of publishing Proceedings of each Conference held. The Proceedings are intended to provide attendees and other interested parties

    Complete texts of invited papers and panel presentations
    Texts or summaries of scheduled presentations including research papers, poster presentations, etc.
    Summary materials from discussion sessions
    Current accepted diagnostic terminology and taxonomy
    Bibliographic materials used at the conference

3. Editing of Proceedings

NANDA will employ an individual with established editorial skills to prepare the Proceedings manuscript for publication. Selection will be based on materials submitted to the Publications Committee regarding

    Prior publication experience
    Samples of editorial work
    Time commitment

NANDA will negotiate the publication contract with the selected editor and publishing firm. Copyright will be held by the publisher and by NANDA.

4. Other publications

From time to time the Publications Committee may identify materials which should be made available to nurses through special publications. These might include discussions of individual diagnoses, "how to use diagnoses" guidebooks, or works

related to taxonomy development. Decisions will be made on a case by case basis regarding copyright, editorial control, and method of publication.
  Work plan: Publications of Proceedings
         Other publications

Report of the Membership Committee

MEMBERS

Ann Becker, Chairperson
Andrea Bircher
Mary Lee Kirkland
Peggy McComb
Christine Miaskowski
Winnifred Mills

The Committee has not met but has been in contact through the mail. The first meeting will be held during the Sixth Conference.
  The following goals have been established:
  1. Explore mechanisms for increasing membership throughout North America (working with Public Relations committee)
  2. Identify appropriate information to be obtained from members (i.e., area of specialization, nursing diagnosis interest, etc.) that can be stored in and easily retrieved from a computer
  3. Determine whether the cost of the newsletter subscription should be included in the membership fee (working with Publications committee)

Report of the Public Relations Committee

MEMBERS

Derry Ann Moritz, Chairperson
Kristine Gebbie
Barbara McGuire
Dee-J Putzier
Marylouise Welch

RESPONSIBILITIES OF THE PUBLIC RELATIONS COMMITTEE, ACCORDING TO BYLAWS

. . . shall promote the relationship with other nursing and health professionals and keep the association abreast of their trend and pertinent activities. The Committee shall serve as the advocate/spokesman for general affairs to the Association.

ACTIVITIES TO DATE

Conference call 2/22/84 to establish goals for immediate future (including individual tasks)
Promote NANDA Conference through national professional media

Meeting 4/4/84 to establish long-term goals:
  Determine budgetary needs
  Identify primary targets for P.R. efforts
    Specialty groups: ANA Committee on Specialty Organizations, Council of Specialty Groups
    ANA/American Nurse
    Journals: *American Journal of Nursing, Nursing, RN, Canadian Nurse*
  Send representatives of NANDA to state, national, and Canadian conferences
  Forward press releases of NANDA activities to appropriate specialty organizations
  Collect data on cost and effectiveness of displays at state and regional association meetings; publicize NANDA at health-related organizations
  Have material on NANDA in each formally organized nursing group by October 1985
  Get logo professionally produced by July 1984
  Continue efforts at news coverage beyond professional media, get one major cover article during next 6 months

Report of the Nominating Committee

The Nominating Committee has not yet met; however, an attempt will be made to meet during the time we are in St. Louis. Objectives to be accomplished immediately are:
  1. To examine the process used for the 1983 elections and recommend changes to the Board if appropriate.
  2. To establish a time frame for the nomination process.
  3. To establish a budget to include the nomination and election process.
Offices to be elected effective July, 1985, are as follows:
  President
  Secretary
  3 Board Members
  1 member of the nominating committee
According to the bylaws, the ballot must be prepared by December 1, 1984. Individuals interested in seeking office are invited to submit their names to the Chair of the Nominating Committee.

Report of the Research Committee

MEMBERS

  Gertrude K. McFarland, Chairperson
  Phyllis Jones
  Mi Ja Kim
  Elizabeth A. McFarlane
  Chris Tanner
  Phyllis Kritek

DESCRIPTION OF RESEARCH COMMITTEE FROM NANDA BYLAWS

The Research Committee shall promote conducting research studies and review research papers for the publications of the Association.

TENTATIVE GOALS

1. To stimulate networking/collaboration among nurses interested in and/or conducting research relevant to the development and application of nursing diagnoses by
   a. Developing a data bank containing such information as researchers involved in nursing diagnoses research; nature of research being conducted; methodology used; and tools utilized
   b. Developing a method of information storage and distribution of data
   c. Identifying and developing appropriate relationships with organizations of importance to or with interest in nursing diagnoses research
2. To stimulate the conducting of nursing diagnoses research by
   a. Exploring the feasibility of and (based upon the assessed need) planning and implementing a Regional or National Conference on Nursing Diagnoses Research that focuses on issues, concerns, and research completed/in progress that is of interest to nurse researchers.
   b. Exploring the feasibility of and (based upon findings) initiating a journal focusing on nursing diagnoses research and related scholarly activities.
   c. Developing position papers on critical issues relevant to nursing diagnoses research.

PROPOSED COMMITTEE STRUCTURE

Subcommittees will be composed of three to four members, chaired by a Research Committee member, and focusing on one of the major areas of concentration identified above.

The committee will meet several times during the Conference.

Report of the Taxonomy Committee

MEMBERSHIP

Phyllis Kritek, Chairperson
Lois Hoskins
Mary Kerr
Susan Onopa
Barbara Rottkamp
Judy Warren
Board Advisors: Mary Hurley, Winifred Mills

NANDA BYLAWS REQUIREMENTS: TAXONOMY COMMITTEE

1. Shall develop and regularly review a taxonomic system for the diagnoses
2. Shall promote the taxonomy for use
3. Shall promote collaboration with groups supporting other established health-related taxonomies

ACTIVITIES WHICH THE COMMITTEE WILL COMPLETE

1. Review of work to date on taxonomy:
   a. Review of previous conference work on taxonomies
   b. Review of Theorist Group work
   c. Review of uses/advantages/disadvantages of alphabetic list
   d. Review of work of Fifth Conference Taxonomy Group
2. Establish a taxonomic system for current and new diagnoses
3. Establish a system for inclusion, in the taxonomy, of new and changed diagnoses
4. Identify mechanisms for promoting the taxonomy
5. Target groups of health-related professionals with whom to collaborate on taxonomies, and generate appropriate networks and goals

Consider for review a NANDA taxonomic system at the Seventh Conference.

Report of the Diagnosis Review Committee

MEMBERSHIP

Phyllis Kritek, Chairperson
Lynda Hall Carpenito
Cynthia Dougherty
Dorothea Fox Jakob
Julie Rovtar
Maureen Shekleton
Board Advisors: Kristie Gebbie, Derry Moritz

NANDA BYLAWS REQUIREMENTS: DIAGNOSIS REVIEW COMMITTEE

1. Shall review proposed diagnoses and recommend acceptance/modification/rejection to the Board
2. Shall appoint specialized clinical/technical review task forces in specific clinical areas to review diagnoses prior to Committee action
3. Shall designate the format for submission of proposed diagnoses or changes to existing diagnoses
4. Shall prepare proposed diagnoses in final form as recommended for membership voting

ASSUMPTIONS FOR COMMITTEE ACTIVITIES

1. Creating a review process for the approval of new diagnoses will precede creating a review process for changes to existing diagnoses.
2. Creating functional mechanisms for all phases and eventualities of the review process will be a priority.
3. The review process will be cyclic in character, with a theoretically endless series of progressions.
4. The *NANDA Newsletter* will be the initial vehicle for regular communication with the membership on all phases of the development, implementation, and refinement of the review process.
5. The established rules of public domain apply to all diagnoses which are approved by the membership.

ACTIVITIES WHICH THE COMMITTEE WILL COMPLETE

1. Delineation of all phases of the review process
2. Creation of appropriate forms for documentation, voting, etc.
3. Development of guidelines for submission of diagnoses
4. Identification of specific decision points in a cyclic review timeline
5. Appointment of specialized clinical/technical review task forces
6. Utilization of NANDA Newsletter for communication with the membership on developments/actions of the Committee
7. Implementation of the review process
8. Clarification of public status of work of individual proposers of tentative new diagnoses
9. Exploration of publication procedures with the Publication Committee
10. Refinement and revisions of procedures as necessary or appropriate

General Assembly "review and comment on proposed diagnoses" (Bylaws, Art, VIII, Sec. 2) will occur for the first time at the Seventh Conference.

Report of the Financial Committee

Fiscal year 1984 (from July 1983 to February 1984 and future projections). Balance carried over from fiscal year 1983 = $17,838.47.

Month	Income	Expenses	Balance
July	514.00	314.48	18,037.99
August	834.00	365.02	18,506.97
September	622.00	4,206.47	14,922.50
October	5,592.61	2,035.10	18,480.01
November	553.00	2,152.35	16,880.66
December	2,247.00	1,524.22	17,603.44
January	12,025.00	2,230.81	27,397.63
February	11,042.00	2,304.97	36,134.66
Projections for March and April:			
	$42,850.00	$16,453.00	$62,531.66

Explanation for projections: The large income would be due from Conference fees which have not been deposited, and the expenses would be the estimated expenses for the Sixth Conference, using 400 participants as a base figure.

• • •

Six-month totals for income and expense categories (7/1/83 to 1/1/84):

Income

Dues	$ 2,790.00
Newletter	2,215.00
Bibliography	28.00
Royalties	4,714.61
Conference fees	450.00
Miscellaneous	165.00
TOTAL	$10,362.61

Expenses

Salaries	$4,971.27
FICA/Work. Comp.	338.63
Telephone	3.28
Postage	325.87
Newsletter	666.84
Board reimbursements	3,773.79
Copy center	103.21
Supplies	30.99
MC/Visa	2.00
Conferences	266.10
Computer expenses	115.66
Miscellaneous	0
TOTAL	$10,597.64

Expected estimated balance after conference $62,531.66

Awards ceremony

ANN BECKER, M.S.N., R.N.

At this the first conference sponsored by the North American Nursing Diagnosis Association, it is appropriate that we recognize individuals who have contributed their ideas, talent, and support to the national effort to identify and classify nursing diagnoses.

Prior to the early 1970s minimal information about nursing diagnosis was available to nurses. Since 1973 when the First National Conference on Classification of Nursing Diagnosis was sponsored by the Saint Louis University School of Nursing and Allied Health Professions, there has been a proliferation of activities and literature related to nursing diagnosis. During these years the National Group for the Classification of Nursing Diagnosis continued the effort begun in 1973, until the present association was established in 1982.

To honor these individuals each will receive a plaque which states "For Outstanding Contributions to Nursing Diagnosis," her name, and 1984. In addition each person will have her name placed on a plaque which will remain in the NANDA office. It is a pleasure to introduce the awardees:

Kristine M. Gebbie was one of the faculty members at St. Louis University who conceived the idea of calling together 100 outstanding nurses to initiate "the clear articulation of those health problems that comprise the domain of nursing and the classification of the problems into a taxonomic system." She subsequently coordinated the nursing diagnosis clearinghouse until she left the university. Kristine edited the proceedings of the first and second national conferences and has written many articles about nursing diagnosis. She has made numerous presentations throughout the United States and Canada. Currently she is treasurer of the association and chairperson of the Publications committee.

It is a pleasure to recognize Kristine M. Gebbie for her numerous contributions to nursing diagnosis and thank her for making it possible for us to be here today.

Mary Ann Lavin (Sister Mary Frances, CP) was one of the faculty members at St. Louis University who conceived the idea of calling together one hundred outstanding nurses to initiate "the clear articulation of those health problems that comprise the domain of nursing and the classification of the problems into a taxonomic system." She continued to be active in the national effort and assisted with activities at the clearinghouse. Mary Ann coedited the proceedings of the first national conference and coauthored an article on nursing diagnosis. In 1978 she joined the Passionist nuns and her formal activities with nursing came to an end.

It is a pleasure to recognize Mary Ann Lavin for her contributions to nursing diagnosis and to thank her mother, Mrs. Frances Neudeck, for joining us today to accept the award.

Sister Mary Teresa Noth, S.S.M., was dean of the St. Louis University School of Nursing and Allied Health Professions when the idea of a national conference on nursing diagnosis was conceived. When approached by the faculty, she provided support from the school and her own personal encouragement. Throughout her tenure as dean, she continued this support by making available facilities and staff for the clearinghouse which is still housed at the School of Nursing. Sister Teresa is an advocate for nursing and, through her willingness to encourage a new idea, the movement to identify and classify nursing diagnoses has expanded nationally and internationally.

It is a pleasure to recognize Sister Mary Teresa Noth for her contributions to nursing diagnosis and thank her for making it possible for us to be here today.

Marjory Gordon had completed a study of nursing diagnosis for her doctoral dissertation prior to her participation in the first national conference. After the conference, she became chairperson of the task force of the national group. Under her leadership the task force stimulated implementation and research of nursing diagnosis and organized four national conferences. During this time the formal structure of the North American Nursing Diagnosis Association was established. Marjory has spoken on nursing diagnosis with many groups in the United States and other countries. She has authored numerous articles, edited a symposium on the implementation of nursing diagnosis, and has published the book, *Nursing Diagnosis: Process and Application.* Currently she is the first president of the association.

It is a pleasure to recognize Marjory Gordon for her numerous contributions to nursing diagnosis and thank her for making it possible for us to be here today.

Sister Callista Roy was a participant at the first national conference and has continued to be involved in the activities of the association. When the need for an organizing principle for nursing diagnoses was discussed, she assumed leadership of a group of nurse theorists. As chairperson of this group, she brought together theorists with differeing views of nursing and nursing diagnosis. These individuals subsequently presented to the national group their conceptual schema and patterns of unitary man. It was Sister Callista's "belief in the values of theoretical frameworks for organizing all aspects of clinical practice" that led her to initiate this group and encourage its activities. Sister has also authored a number of articles and spoken with various groups about nursing diagnosis.

It is a pleasure to recognize Sister Callista Roy for her contributions to nursing diagnosis and thank her for her ideas and support.

Summary and recommendations

AUDREY M. McLANE, Ph.D., R.N.

The North American Nursing Diagnosis Association, known by its members as NANDA, met for the first time as a formal organization during the Sixth Conference on Classification of Nursing Diagnoses. NANDA supercedes the National Task Force on Classification of Nursing Diagnosis, a loose association of persons interested in the development of a taxonomy of nursing diagnoses, which directed the activities of the national conferences from 1973 until 1982, when by-laws were formally adopted for NANDA.

While nurses attended the early conferences by invitation, based on their knowledge and expertise in the field of nursing diagnosis, more recently, 1982 and 1984, invitations were extended to the general nursing community. Some 460 nurses attended the Sixth Conference, which is more than twice the number who attended any other national conference. The increase probably resulted from the combined effects of a more structured organization with standing committees and the growing perception of nurses that nursing diagnoses have relevance for research, practice, and education.

From my own observations and from my discussions with participants, the program of the Sixth Conference met the objectives set forth by the Program Committee, i.e., it provided a Janus View of nursing diagnoses—a look back, an appreciation of our origins, and a look forward to glimpse the future. Some of the invited papers presented during the general sessions and the methodologic papers presented during the scientific sessions incorporated suggestions for the future of NANDA, the work of its committees, and for nursing diagnosis research. Highlights from the invited and scientific papers have been selected to provide background for this summary and recommendations.

Since NANDA's *raison d'être* is the development of a taxonomy, Kritek's paper which evolved from the work of the Taxonomy Committee at the 1982 conference (Kim, McFarland, and McLane, 1984) merits special attention. The work of the Taxonomy Committee consisted of categorizing the diagnostic labels at four levels of abstraction, with Level I as the most abstract and Level IV as the least. According to Kritek, Level I looks more like category sets and Level III looks more like the things we write care plans about. Examples of Level I are: fear, comfort, and coping. Examples of Level III are: self-care deficit, constipation, and grieving. After categorizing each label at a level of abstraction, nine taxonomic trees were developed using the patterns of unitary man, i.e., a taxonomy was developed using the patterns of unitary man as the principle of classification. It is imperative that conference participants study and determine the relevance of the taxonomy for a variety of purposes in practice, research, and education. In addition, nurses working on new phenomena are encouraged to look for placement of new diagnoses within the taxonomic trees.

During the period of 1982 to 1984, a total of 25 suggestions for new diagnostic labels were received. The review process and criteria for acceptance were not in place prior to this meeting, so no formal action was taken on any new diagnoses. In the future, information about new diagnoses will be printed in the Nursing Diagnosis Newsletter which members receive as part of their membership in NANDA. The names of new proposed diagnostic labels and the names of the persons working on them will be reported in the Newsletter to provide for more networking during the diagnostic review process.

Another major paper related to the developing taxonomy was presented by Kirk (1984), who elaborated and expanded the patterns of unitary man. Since the nurse theorists who developed the Unitary Man Framework no longer meet as a group, it was exciting to find that theoretical work on the framework is continuing. Using Kuhn's (1970) notion of normal science, one could say that scientific work on the taxonomy may become part of normal science in the discipline of nursing during the current decade.

Gordon (1984) presented a major paper on the structure of the 62 diagnostic categories; i.e., she examined them from a structural perspective. She pointed out that 43 of the categories lack a definition (although the category name reflects the operational definition) and 49 have no "critical indicators," i.e., an indicator which must be present in order to make a diagnosis. Since the defining characteristics provide the structure for the cognitive processes involved in making a diagnosis, it is not surprising that Gordon and other speakers urged participants to contribute to the scientific work needed to validate the diagnoses.

The validation of diagnostic labels must be given a high priority. Clinical validation models must supplant or at least supplement the nurse validation models which are usually based on variations of the Delphi technique. Validation studies could be done by graduate students in master's and doctoral programs in research studies for theses/dissertations and in practicums designed to develop clinical research skills. As the number of scientific papers related to a single diagnostic category increases substantially, expert clinicians, graduate students, and researchers could meet for the express purpose of refining a diagnostic category. These meetings could be held in conjunction with Regional Nursing Diagnoses Conferences or annual meetings of regional research societies.

Clinton's methodological presentation on IDEA, an interactive computer program, merits careful study for use in diagnostic validation studies. IDEA stands for Inductive Data Exploration and Analysis (Rogers and Shure, 1971). As Clinton pointed out, IDEA is different from the classical techniques in many ways. First, they (the classical techniques) require that all variables be scaled at least at an interval level of measurement. "IDEA is free of the assumption concerning level of measurement and distribution shape" (Clinton,

1984). When confronted with nominal data, researchers usually use dummy coding which makes interpretation of results extremely difficult. In IDEA, Clinton pointed out, any characteristic of a variable which can be made explicit can be accounted for in a unique inductive routine. Not only is IDEA able to handle nominal level data, but it is also not an additive model. That is say, if a variable does not contribute significantly to the dependent variable in certain subjects, it is not calculated into the model for those subjects. This is a key feature for diagnostic validation studies, since it provides a means for discovering which indicators are significant in contributing to nursing diagnoses in different subjects. A third important feature of IDEA is that it provides for human control in the procedure. IDEA will follow the researchers' direction to search for a pattern in the data set; it will rank-order all indicators in terms of their chi-square significance values and suggest to the researcher the next step in building a tree or a model. The investigator decides at decision points how the analysis should continue. Although these are just a few highlights of Clinton's presentation, it is clear that the application of IDEA would "serve to refine nursing diagnoses in a scientifically lawful and clinically relevant fashion" (Clinton, 1984).

Two other methodological papers with implications for diagnostic validation studies were presented. Fehring suggested two practical methods for gathering quantifiable evidence for the validation of nursing diagnoses. The approaches he described produce numerical ratios that reflect standardized diagnostic confidence. Lackey also emphasized the need to validate and standardize the diagnostic labels and presented three studies which demonstrated the use of the Q Methodology to validate the defining characteristics of diagnoses.

Lang, chairperson of the ANA Steering Committee on Classification of Nursing Practice Phenomena, shared the goals of that Committee as they relate to (1) policy regarding classification systems; (2) development of a blueprint for identifying and classifying nursing practice phenomena; (3) the relationship between ANA and NANDA; (4) monitoring the state of the art of classification systems; and (5) promoting an understanding of the state of the art of classifications of nursing practice phenomena (Lang, 1984). Lang's suggestions will be used to guide the organization's activities with respect to ANA during the coming biennium. A meeting between ANA and NANDA representatives was held during the conference to initiate discussion about joint sponsorship of consensus conferences for specific diagnostic categories.

In response to the call for abstracts for this conference, 104 abstracts of research and scholarly papers were submitted to NANDA's Program Committee. Of these, 39 were selected via a two-tier blind review process. Eighteen were selected for poster and 21 for paper presentations. Using a suggestion made by Lang (1984), both paper and poster presentations were evaluated for

TABLE 1   **Paper and poster presentations: relevance to ANA social policy statement centerfold**

	Paper	Poster
Epidemiological	0	6
Phenomena/nursing diagnoses	6	9
Theory application	2	0
Intervention	0	1
Outcome	2	0
Documentation	2	1
Diagnostic reasoning	2	1
Methodological	3	0
Implementation	4	0

their relationship to the centerfold of the Social Policy Statement (Table 1). Of 15 presentations which focused on the phenomena itself, 9 were posters and 6 were paper presentations. This breakdown could be interpreted in many ways, but the most obvious explanation is that researchers need to increase the rigor of the methodologies used for indentifying and validating diagnostic labels. The methodological papers presented at this meeting should influence the future direction of nursing diagnosis research and have a major impact on the quality of future studies.

Other conference activities which have implications for the future include: the formal recognition of five persons who were critical to the development of the organization; networking for Special Interest Groups; and facilitating the work of the Regional Nursing Diagnosis Groups. The five persons honored were Kristine Gebbie, Mary Ann Lavin, Sister Mary Teresa Noth, Marjory Gordon, and Sister Callista Roy. An ad hoc committee has been established to determine whether or not to continue such recognition and, if so, to develop a more formal process.

Ten Special Interest Groups met for the first time at this Sixth Conference and have begun networking in the following areas:

Clinical implementation
Computerization
Critical care
Curriculum
Long-term care
Mental health
Reimbursement/DRGs
Research
Taxonomy
Wellness

News from these groups will be carried in the Nursing Diagnosis Newsletter and plans are underway to provide for more meeting time at the next conference. It is anticipated that meeting space will be provided for Special Interest Groups the afternoon before the beginning of the next conference. Mary Ann Kelly, a member of the program committee, has agreed to coordinate the activities of these groups.

In addition to the special interest groups, representatives of sixteen regional groups met at the Conference to discuss regional needs and goals. Some of the groups also had a regional meeting at the conference. News from the regions will be carried in future Newsletters. Provisions will be made for these groups to meet at the Seventh Conference on Classification of Nursing Diagnoses, which will be held in St. Louis, March 9 to 12, 1986. Laura Rossi, a member of the Program Committee, has agreed to coordinate the activities of the Regional Groups.

Many of the perennial dilemmas which faced participants attending earlier conferences still remain. Health/wellness-oriented clinicians and researchers continue to express concern about the problem focus of the current diagnostic labels. Other dilemmas center around the absence of an agreed-upon definition of a nursing diagnosis; continued use of the alphabet as the organizing principle for the diagnostic labels; the question of etiology; and the difficulties arising from computerization of nursing diagnoses. Resolution of the dilemmas must come from theoretical and scientific work, not from some arbitrary process, regardless of how democratic.

Since no new diagnoses were formally processed during the Fifth and Sixth Conferences, the development of procedures for refinement of the diagnostic review process has the highest priority during the coming biennium. What constitutes adequate research support for provisional summary descriptions of new phenomena must be decided so that rules developed from a research base can be used with confidence to guide the differentiation of one phenomenon from another. The Board of Directors of NANDA looks with confidence to its standing committees and its membership to meet the challenges set forth in this conference during the next biennium.

REFERENCES

American Nurses' Association: Nursing: a social policy statement, Kansas City, Mo., 1980, The Association.

Clinton, J.: Nursing diagnosis research methodologies. Paper presented at the Sixth Conference on Classification of Nursing Diagnoses, St. Louis, 1984.

Fehring, R.J.: Validating diagnostic labels: Standardized methodology. Paper presented at the Sixth Conference on Classification of Nursing Diagnoses, St. Louis, 1984.

Gordon, M.: Structure of diagnostic categories. Paper presented at the Sixth Conference on Classification of Nursing Diagnoses, St. Louis, 1984.

Kim, M.J., McFarland, G.K., and McLane, A.M., editors: Classification of nursing diagnoses—Proceedings of the Fifth National Conference, St. Louis, 1984, The C.V. Mosby Co.

Kirk, L.: The design for relevance, revisited: an elaboration of the conceptual framework for nursing diagnoses. Paper presented at the Sixth Conference on Classification of Nursing Diagnoses, St. Louis, 1984.

Kritek, P.B.: Report of the group work on taxonomies. In Kim, M.J., McFarland G.K., and McLane, A.M., editors: Classification of nursing diagnoses—Proceedings of the Fifth National Conference, St. Louis, 1984, The C.V. Mosby Co.

Kuhn, T.S.: The structure of scientific revolutions, ed. 2, Chicago, 1970, The University of Chicago Press.

Lackey, N.R.: Use of the Q methodology in validating defining characteristics of specified nursing diagnoses. Paper presented at the Sixth Conference on Classification of Nursing Diagnoses, St. Louis, 1984.

Lang, N.: ANA Steering Committee on Classification of Nursing Practice Phenomena: Current and future directions. Paper presented at the Sixth Conference on Classification of Nursing Diagnoses, St. Louis, 1984.

Rogers, M.S., and Shure, G.H.: A user's guide to IDEA in the CCBS system. Los Angeles, 1971, U.C.L.A. Center for Computer-Based Behavioral Studies.

Appendix D # North American Nursing Diagnosis Association

OFFICERS

President: Marjory Gordon
Vice-President: Phyllis Kritek
Secretary: Jane Lancour
Treasurer: Kristine Gebbie

BOARD OF DIRECTORS

Ann Becker
Mary Hurley
Gertrude McFarland
Audrey McLane
Winnifred Mills
Derry Moritz
Joyce Shoemaker

COMMITTEE CHAIRPERSONS

Program	Audrey McLane
Publication	Kristine Gebbie
Membership	Ann Becker
Diagnosis Review	Phyllis Kritek
Research	Gertrude McFarland
Public Relations	Derry Moritz
Taxonomy	Phyllis Kritek
Master Plan Ad Hoc	Marjory Gordon
Nominations	Joyce Shoemaker

PROGRAM COMMITTEE

Audrey M. McLane, Chairperson
Ann Becker
Mi Ja Kim
Richard J. Fehring

ABSTRACT REVIEW PANEL

The Program Committee would like to thank the following persons who assisted them in reviewing abstracts. The abstracts were sent for a blind review to three reviewers, and then given final review by the Program Committee. There were a total of 104 abstracts submitted.

Dr. Janet Awtrey
Dr. Kenneth Cianfrani
Dr. Richard Fehring
Dr. Frances Fickess
Dr. Marjory Gordon
Dr. June Gray
Dr. Edward Halloran

Dr. Mary Ann Kelly
Dr. Nancy Lackey
Dr. Joanne McCloskey
Dr. Gertrude McFarland
Dr. Elizabeth McFarlane
Ms. Judith Fitzgerald Miller
Dr. Helen Niskala
Dr. Myrna Pickard
Dr. Sue Ellen Pinkerton
Dr. Sue Popkess-Vawter
Dr. Evelyn Redding
Dr. Barbara Rottkamp
Dr. Virginia Saba
Dr. Joyce Shoemaker
Dr. Ruth Stolenwerk
Dr. Rosemary Wang
Dr. Helen Yura
Dr. Shirley Ziegler

SPECIAL INTEREST GROUPS

The purposes of the Special Interest Groups (SIGs) were to provide opportunities for:
1. Informal sharing of nursing diagnoses activities, e.g., research in progress, demonstration projects, implementation, etc.
2. Networking with nurses interested in common areas of concern relative to nursing diagnoses.

Group	Group Title	Leader	Recorder
1	Clinical implementation	Ann McCourt	Joan Duslak
2	Computerization	Joan Norris	Linda Grilley
3	Critical care	Cynthia Dougherty	Naomi Yoshimoto
4	Curriculum	Lynne Kreutzer	Ken Cianfrani
5	Long term care	Terry Mullen	Barbara Hammer
6	Mental health	Barbara Krainovich	Nona Lemieux
7	Reimbursement/DRG	Luette Lutjens	Donna Hartweg
8	Research	Elizabeth McFarlane	Nancy Lackey
9	Taxonomy	Phyllis Kritek	Sr. Regina Maibusch
10	Wellness	Dorothea Jakob	Pat deSilva

Participants of the Sixth Conference on the Classification of Nursing Diagnoses*

Marilyn Abraham, **1**
Tucson, AZ

Frenita Agbayani, **8**
Matteson, IL

Dianna Aideuis, **1**
Saxapahaw, NC

Margaret Alexander, **10**
Milwaukee, WI

Janice Allen, **7**
Denver, CO

Patricia Allen, **8**
Philadelphia, PA

Solita Amoranto, **3**
Chicago, IL

Jackie A. Anderson, **2**
Renton, WA

Karen Anderson, **7**
Plainwell, MI

Denise Antle, **3**
Davenport, IA

Jacquelyn Armitage, **1**
Middleton, MA

Janet Awtrey, **10**
Cottondale, AL

Mary Axelrod, **1**
Chicago, IL

Carol Baer, **2**
Medfield, MA

Patricia Bailey, **4**
Scranton, PA

Betty Baines, **5**
Clemson, S.C.

Sue Baird, **8**
Milwaukee, WI

Kathleen Baldwin, **7**
Peoria Heights, IL

Linda Banks, **8**
Des Moines, IA

Bonnie Barndt-Maglio, **8**
Huber Heights, OH

Margaret Barry, **1**
Vacaville, CA

Vivian Barry, **10**
Chicago, IL

Beverly Bartlett, **4**
Granby, MA

Susan Bash, **10**
Beavercreek, OH

Linda Baas, **8**
Cincinnati, OH

Phyllis Bastone
Cape Elizabeth, ME

Karen Batty, **1**
Oak Park, IL

Billie Baughman, **4**
Bowling Green, KY

Patricia Beach, **4**
Toledo, OH

Margaret Beard
Denton, TX

Ann Becker
St. Louis, MO

Ruth Becker
Detroit, MI

Nancy Beckman, **8**
Detroit, MI

Gloria Belling, **4**
Wauwatosa, WI

Gwenthalyn Bello, **3**
Ann Arbor, MI

JoAnne Bennett, **10**
New York, NY

Debra Berry, **7**
Carson City, MI

Andrea Bircher
Oklahoma City, OK

Virginia Blackmer, **1**
Franklin, NH

Carol Blankenship, **1**
Johnson City, TN

Virginia Blom, **1**
Sioux City, IA

Kathleen Bloom, **4**
Jacksonville, FL

Lynn Bobel, **3**
St. Clair Shores, MI

Lenore Boles, **6**
Norwalk, CT

Margaret Boone, **9**
Thunder Bay, Ont.

Carol Booth, **6**
Kansas City, KS

Eleanor Borkowski, **3**
Redlands, CA

Lucy Brand, **2**
Thompsonville, MI

Ruth Braulick, **1**
San Antonio, TX

Kathleen Breunig, **7**
Wauwatosa, WI

Margaret Briody, **9**
Rochester, N.Y.

Ann L. Brodt, **7**
Galesburg, IL

Sharon Brown, **1**
Willmar, MN

Sandra Brus, **3**
Wheaton, IL

Vivian Brzezicki
St. Clair Shores, MI

Betty Buckwalter, **1**
Indianapolis, IN

Gloria Bulechek, **8**
Solon, IA

Sandra Burgener
Fisber, IL

Barbara Burke, **10**
Dearborn, MI

Joseph T. Burley, **1**
Ocean Springs, NJ

Lucy Callaghan
Overland Park, KS

Maggie Campbell, **6**
Kansas City, MO

Janice Cantrall, **1**
Burlington, KY

---

*The number listed behind the name indicates which special interest group the person attended.

Kathleen Canty-Rowe, 7
Duxbury, MA

Glee Carreon, 1
Ann Arbor, MI

Sue Carroll
Seattle, WA

Linda Carpenito, 4
Mickleton, NJ

Janet Carstens, 4
Cape Girardeau, MO

Mildred Case, 4
Berrien Springs, MI

Suzanne Cascino, 3
Chicago, IL

Vicki Chambers, 1
Biloxi, MS

Betty Chang
Los Angeles, CA

Sheron Chisholm, 9
Petoskey, MI

Dianne Christopherson, 3
Melrose, MA

Kenneth L. Cianfrani
Moline, IL

Cynthia Clapp, 1
Cabery, IL

Rene Clark
Fairway, KS

Jacqueline Clinton
Milwaukee, WI

Jeanette Clough, 8
Wakefield, MA

Pat Cole, 1
Des Moines, IA

Marga Coler, 8
Amherst, MA

Luna Collado, 8
Orland Park, IL

Evelyn Cook, 5
Topeka, KS

Rodney Copley
Oklahoma City, OK

Cynthia Coviak, 8
Ada, MI

Carol Craft
St. Louis, MO

Jennifer Craig, 8
West Vancouver, BC

Laraine Crane, 7
Milwaukee, WI

Susan Creager, 5
Mattawan, MI

Nancy Creason, 8
Champaign, IL

Patricia Creuims
Milton, MA

Betty Croonquist, 4
Kandiyohi, MN

Joan Crosley, 9
Babylon, NY

Phyllis Curtis, 5
Kalamazoo, MI

Kathy Czurylo, 1
Des Plaines, IL

Marlas Daerr, 2
Whitefish Bay, MI

Joyce Dains, 8
Houston, TX

Carol Daisy, 4, 10
Glastonbury, CT

Joanne Dalton, 8
Duxbury, MA

Jeanette Daly, 4
Moline, IL

Barbara Damvelt
Kalamazoo, MI

Constance D'Argenio, 1
Greenwich, CT

Kay Davis, 1
Iowa City, IA

Malessa Dean, 2
Memphis, TN

Joan Deming, 3
Philadelphia, PA

Patricia deSilva, 10
Milwaukee, WI

Carol Dickel, 7
Davenport, IA

Geri L. Dickson, 10
Milwaukee, WI

Jacquelyn Dietz, 10
Chicago, IL

Ann Dillon, 4
New Lenox, IL

Ellen Dillon, 3
Cedar Rapids, IA

Kathy Dillon, 1
Olivia, MN

Joan T. Dolan, 1
Great River, NY

JoAnne Donhan, 3
Olathe, KS

Cynthia Dougherty, 3
Coralville, IA

Therese Dowd, 8
Lincoln, NE

Kathleen Dracup
Santa Monica, CA

Diane Drevs, 2
Moville, IA

Dorothy Dunn, 10
Kalamazoo, MI

Joan Dunn, 10
Grand Island, NY

Joan Duslak
Downers Grove, IL

Brenda Dutil, 5
Jonquière, Quebec

Patricia Eagan, 2
Pine Bluff, AR

Jennifer Early, 6
Des Plaines, IA

Pat Ebright, 7
Cincinnati, OH

Kathryn Eckerle, 1
Dayton, OH

Tommie Edwards, 6
Ypsilanti, MI

Judith Effken, 2
West Simsbury, CT

Kathleen Ennen, 1
Champaign, IL

Pam Erekson, 2
Oxford, OH

Virginia Erickson, 3
Saco, ME

Linda Erlich
Philadelphia, PA

Teresa Fadden, 8
Milwaukee, WI

Jill Fargo
Milwaukee, WI

Richard Fehring, 8
Wauwatosa, WI

Donna Fellinger, **2**
Williston, VT

Luanne Fendrich, **1**
Peoria, IL

Frances Fickess, **8**
Loma Linda, CA

Anita Fisher, **1**
Toronto, Ont.

James Flaherty, **7**
Smithtown, NY

Karen Fondry, **1**
East Montpelier, VT

Catherine Foster, **8**
Kansas City, MO

Jane Fraher, **2**
San Antonio, TX

Marilyn Frenn, **10**
Milwaukee, WI

Margaret Freundl, **9**
Johnson City, TN

Ellen Garneau, **7**
Meredith, NH

Elizabeth Gale, **8**
Richmond, KY

Christine Galante
Temple Hills, MD

Gramatice Garofallou, **1**
Bronx, NY

Kathrine Garthe, **4**
Northport, MI

Kay Gatkins, **4**
Macon, GA

Kristine Gebbie
Portland, OR

Kathleen Gettrust, **9**
Dousman, WI

Annette Gillis, **8**
Calgary, Alberta

Brian Golden, **2**
Cape Girardeau, MO

Lorraine Goodwin, **1**
Chicago, IL

Marjory Gordon
Brighton, MA

Pamela Gotch, **3**
Franklin, WI

Marie Gould, **8**
Hillside, IL

Angelynn Grabau, **2**
Lincoln, NE

Pauline Green
Edmonston, MD

Faye Gregory, **4**
Garden Grove, CA

Elizabeth Gren, **4**
Plainwell, MI

Linda Grilley, **2**
Wausau, WI

Pauline Guay, **4**
No. Andover, MA

Meg Gulanick, **3**
Wheaton, IL

Linda Guyton, **2**
Olathe, KS

Teresa Gyldenvand, **8**
West Des Moines, IA

Barbara Haas
Yarmouth, ME

Iora Haglund, **3**
Farmington, MI

Carolyn Hall, **7**
Cincinnati, OH

Barbara Hammer, **5**
Marshalltown, IA

Donna Hartweg, **7**
Bloomington, IL

Carol Hayes-Christiansen, **4**
Gainesville, FL

Karen Heaphy, **1**
Jackson Heights, NY

Patricia Hearns, **3**
Lawton, MI

Barbara Heater
Florissant, MO

Ann Henrick, **7**
Northlake, IL

Mary K. Hermann, **9**
Evansville, IN

Katharyne Higgins, **1**
Masury, OH

Doris Hill, **1**
Chicago, IL

Ida Hilliard, **5**
Butler, PA

Sharon Hilton, **7**
Santa Ana, CA

Elizabeth Hiltunen, **8**
Ipswich, MA

Eloise Hippensteel, **4**
Bloomsburg, PA

Rosemarie C. Hogan, **4**
Cleveland, OH

Nancy Hnat
Elmsford, NY

Beth Holstein, **3**
Forest Park, IL

Barbara Hoshiko, **2**
University Heights, OH

Lois Hoskins, **9**
Silver Spring, MD

Don Hudson, **1**
San Francisco, CA

Ann Hunt, **4**
West Lafayette, IN

Mary Hurley, **3**
Saddle Brook, NJ

Nancy Rae Ignatowicz, **3**
Bourbonnais, IL

Mary Ingersoll, **2**
St. Louis, MI

Carol Jacobs, **10**
Racine, WI

Dorothea Jakob, **10**
Toronto, Ont.

Carolyn Jarvis
Bloomington, IL

Jean Jenny, **4**
Nepean, Ont.

Lucille Joel
Newark, NJ

Nancy Johncola
Johnstown, PA

Betty Johnsen, **2**
Oak Park, IL

Brenda Johnson, **2**
Ashkam, IL

Lois Johnson, **5**
St. Louis, MI

Dorothy Jones, **10**
Boston, MA

Eileen Jones, **8**
Oshkosh, WI

Katherine Jones, **1**
Ypsilanti, MI

Mildred Jones, **1**
Fairfax, VA

Phyllis Jones
Toronto, Ont.

Kathleen Justice, **1**
North Glenn, CO

Dorothy Kavalhuna
Richland, MI

Lisa Kelley, **4**
Marshalltown, IA

Mary Ann Kelly
Seneca, SC

Patricia Kelly, **4**
Harleysville, PA

Donna Kennedy, **2**
Granby, MA

Patricia Kenyon, **2**
Yuma, AZ

Mary Kerr, **9**
Gibsonia, PA

Remedios Kho, **1**
Chicago, IL

Judy Kieffer, **4**
Louisville, KY

Mary Lou Kiley, **8**
South Euclid, OH

Mi Ja Kim
Des Plaines, IL

Jacquelin Kinsman, **2**
Berrien Spring, MI

Lark Kirk
Cleveland, OH

Terrie Kirkpatrick, **6**
Greenville, SC

Eleanore Kirsch, **3**
Milwaukee, WI

Mary Klingersmith, **1**
Chicago, IL

Mary Klinzing, **1**
West Des Moines, IA

Geraldine Knapp, **1**
Kalamazoo, MI

Mary Kolbe, **1**
Lincoln, NE

Mary Kontz, **1**
Miami, FL

Sue Kovats
Kalamazoo, MI

Barbara Krainovich
Garden City, NY

Vicki Kraus, **7**
Iowa City, IA

Lynne Kreutzer
Oak Park, IL

Phyllis Kritek
Whitefish Bay, WI

Patricia Kucharski, **8**
Norwell, MA

Joan Kulpa, **1**
Peoria, IL

Susan Labarthe, **7**
Worcester, VT

Nancy Lackey
Overland Park, KS

Jane Lancour
Wauwatosa, WI

Norma Lang
Milwaukee, WI

Dorothy Larson
Topeka, KS

Karen Lawson, **8**
Columbus, KS

Carla Lee, **7**
Wichita, KS

Helena Lee, **10**
Milwaukee, WI

Deborah Lekan-Rutledge, **4**
Chapel Hill, NC

Susan Lembright, **2**
Xenia, OH

Nona Lemieux
Grand Forks, ND

Patricia Lemon, **1**
Bellevue, NE

Ruth Leo, **10**
Grove City, PA

Rona Levin, **8**
Westbury, NY

Anna Lieske, **8**
Milwaukee, WI

Margaret Lindsay, **1**
Hesperia, CA

Chi-Hui Lo
Chicago, IL

Frances Logan, **3**
Ottawa, Ont.

Margaret Logan, **9**
Rockford, IL

Kay Lopez
New Orleans, LA

Annette Lueckenotte, **10**
Normal, IL

Roberta Luedke, **1**
Kent, WA

Margaret Lunney, **7**
Staten Island, NY

Marilyn Luther, **10**
Kalamazoo, MI

Louette Lutjens, **7**
Plainwell, MI

Anita Lymburner, **7**
Nashau, NH

Meridean Maas, **5**
Iowa City, IA

Suzanne MacAvoy, **8**
Ridgefield, CT

Marianne MacNeil
Teaneck, VT

Eunice Madsen, **1**
Murfreesboro, TN

Lou Ann Madson, **2**
Shorewood, WI

Kathleen Mahoney, **8**
Corpus Christi, TX

Regina Maibusch
Milwaukee, WI

Jo Ann Maklebust
Livonia, MI

Carol Mandle, **8**
Lexington, MA

Anne Manton, **8**
Westwood, MA

Patricia Martin, **8**
Beaver Creek, OH

Jean Marie Martinson, **4**
Minneapolis, MN

Sandra Matthews, **4**
Toronto, Ont.

Mary McAuliffe, **8**
Pac Palisades, CA

Donna McCarthy, **3**
Ann Arbor, MI

JoAnne McCloskey
Iowa City, IA

Margaret McComb, **6**
Portland, OR

Kathryn McCormack, **1**
Cape Girardeau, MO

Ann McCourt
North Easton, MA

Kyra McCoy, **4**
Madison, WI

Diane McDaniel, **1**
Marietta, GA

Adrienne McDermott
Chicago, IL

Sandra McDonald, **4**
Marion, IA

Mary McDowell, **4**
Richmond, KY

Mary McElroy, **3**
Columbus, OH

Elizabeth McFarlane, **8**
Burke, VA

Gertrude McFarland, **8**
Oakton, VA

Anne McGuire
St. Louis, MO

Barbara McGuire
Vancouver, BC

Janet McKnight, **10**
Hamilton, Ont.

Audrey McLane
Milwaukee, WI

Ruth McShane
Cudhay, WI

Marie McQueen, **6**
Philadelphia, PA

Peg Mehmert, **2**
Davenport, IA

Bonnie Meyer, **4**
Cincinnati, OH

Lorenza Meza, **5**
APO Miami, FL

Emmy Miller
Richmond, VA

Judith Miller, **8**
Wauwatosa, WI

Karen Miller, **10**
Milwaukee, WI

Mary Ann Miller, **10**
Pittsburgh, PA

Winnifred Mills, **4**
Vancouver, BC

Mary Moberg, **4**
St. Paul, MN

Martha Montgomery, **7**
Detroit, MI

Sue Moorhead, **4**
Davenport, IA

Derry Moritz
New Haven, CT

Carol Morris, **8**
Miami, FL

Susan Moseley, **1**
Nashville, TN

Sharon Moudry, **2**
Minneapolis, MN

Terry Mullen, **5**
Palmer, MA

Dawneane Munn, **4**
Lincoln, NE

Dianne Munns, **6**
Melcher, IA

Judith Myers, **7**
St. Louis, MO

Deborah Nadzam
Cleveland Heights, OH

Charlotte Naschinski
Silver Spring, MD

Lois Newman, **1**
Wichita, KS

Angela Nicoletti, **8**
Newton, MA

Mary Niemeyer, **7**
Ann Arbor, MI

Lucy Anne Nolan, **10**
Augusta, GA

Mary Nordtvedt, **10**
Pierre, SD

Margaret Noreuil
Springfield, IL

Joan Norris
Omaha, NE

Linda O'Brien, **7**
Toronto, Ont.

Syble Oldaker
Denton, TX

Sandra Owens-Jones
Great Lakes, IL

Rhonda Panfilli, **2**
Taylor, MI

Linda Parenteau, **1**
Arlington, VA

Ruth Parker, **8**
Baltimore, MD

Elinor Parsons, **2**
West Chicago, IL

Roselle Partridge, **1**
Indianapolis, IN

Ann Paterson, **1**
Nashville, TN

Carol Pavlish, **4**
Prior Lake, MN

Marilyn Peasley, **1**
Marshalltown, IA

Luella Penner, **5**
Hudson, WI

Harriet Pfotenhauer, **4**
Richmond, KY

Marguerite Pike, **10**
Clarendon Hills, IL

Norma Pinnell
Godfrey, IL

Nancy Pogue, **2**
St. Joseph, IL

Barbara Pokorny, **10**
Bowie, MD

Sue Popkess-Vawter, **8**
Prairie Village, KS

Beverly Post, **10**
Oak Park, IL

Patricia Potter, **7**
Overland, MO

Cynthia Poznanski, **8**
Silver Spring, MD

Marie Price, **4**
Bruce Mines, Ont.

Marilyn Price, **4**
Seattle, WA

Pricilla Quillen, **7**
Oxford, OH

Michelle Quinn, **7**
Chicago, IL

Marilyn Rantz, **5**
Delavan, WI

Marilynn Rathbun, **8**
Kalamazoo, MI

Ellen Reichenbach
O'Fallon, IL

Ann Reilly
Bridgewater, MA

Agatha Reiners, 3
Clara City, MN

Sally Remus, 3
Toronto, Ont.

Charla Renner, 2
Bloomington, IL

Marion Resler, 2
St. Louis, MO

Paula Rich, 7
Philadelphia, PA

Marilyn Richardson, 2
Oxford, OH

Martha Roark, 1
Prairie Village, KS

Paul Roland, 4
Oxford, MA

Beverly Ross, 4
Indianapolis, IN

Jo Ellen Ross, 1
Iowa City, IA

Laura Rossi, 3
Medway, MA

Phyllis Roth, 8
Danville, IL

Barbara Rottkamp, 9
Westbury, NY

Julie Rovtar, 2
Chicago, IL

Frances Rowley, 2
Greenfield, WI

Laurie Rufolo, 8
Staten Island, NY

Lavonne Russell, 4, 10
Grand Forks, ND

Polly Ryan, 3
Wauwatosa, WI

Susan Ryan, 9
Wauwatosa, WI

Marge Rydlewski, 9
Charlottesville, VA

Vivianne Saba, 4
Montreal, Quebec

Karen Sadowski, 8
Birmingham, MI

Fusako Sato, 3
Chicago, IL

Mary E. Schaertl, 3
Bourbonnais, IL

Amella Schechinger, 7
Philadelphia, PA

Cynthia Schneider, 4
Oklahoma City, OK

Lorraine Schweidenbach, 10
Kalamazoo, MI

Vivki Schreckengost, 3
Hermitage, PA

Pam Schroeder, 8
Milwaukee, WI

Patricia Schultz, 8
Chicago, IL

Leann Scroggins, 1
Rochester, MN

Frank Shaffer
New York, NY

Evangeline R. Shank, 3
Sterling, IL

Kathleen Sheppard
Katy, TX

Joyce K. Shoemaker
Philadelphia, PA

Suzanne Sikma, 7
Seattle, WA

DeLanne A. Simmons
Omaha, NE

Margie Sipe, 4
Wellesley, MA

Diann Smith
Indianapolis, IN

Janet Smith, 6
Philadelphia, PA

Linda Smith, 4
Franksville, WI

Catherine Spearing, 7
Baltimore, MD

Martha Spies, 9
St. Louis, MO

Valerie Sproule, 4
Surrey, BC

Margaret Stafford, 3
Northlake, IL

Roberta Standafer, 4
Cedar Rapids, IA

Richard Stavale, 1
Omaha, NE

Paula Stopjik, 1
Wheeler, MI

Marsal Stoll, 4
Getzville, NY

Claudia Storhoff, 1
Vacaville, CA

Kathy Strong, 4
West Bend, WI

Janet Studer, 1
Topeka, KS

Rosemarie Suhayda
Woodridge, IL

Alice Swan, 7
Roseville, MN

Linda Sweigart, 2
New Castle, IN

Judith Sylvester, 6
Greenville, SC

Barbara Tacinelli, 2
New York, NY

Susan Taylor, 8
Columbia, MO

Juanita Theile, 8
Shawano, WI

Mildred Thieleman, 1
Paducah, KY

Roberta Thiry
Pittsburg, KS

Kathie Thomas
Kansas City, MO

June Thompson, 3
Houston, TX

Carol Tippe, 10
Coralville, IA

Marita Titler
Alburnett, IA

Lavon Titus, 5
Marshalltown, IA

Debra Tribett, 3
Bethesda, MD

Sally Tripp, 10
Amherst, MA

Sue Truex, 8
Urbana, IL

Janice Twiss, 7
Gretha, NE

Joyce Ulrich, **7**
Kalamazoo, MI

Danielle Valois, **4**
Belleville, Quebec

Barbara Vassallo, **2**
Willingboro, NJ

Carol Viamontes, **1**
Bridgewater, NJ

Karen Vincent, **8**
Brookline, MA

Anne Voith, **8**
Glendale, WI

Peggy Wagner, **3**
Brookfield, WI

Jane Wall, **8**
Milwaukee, WI

Rosemary Wang, **4**
Barrington, NH

Christine Ward, **7**
Honolulu, HI

Judith Warren, **8**
Mililani, HI

Kathy Watson, **1**
Livonia, MI

Judith Weatherall, **8**
Champaign, IL

Carolyn Weber, **8**
Wichita, KS

Susan Weitekamp, **4**
Rantoul, IL

Mary Lou Welch, **10**
W. Hartford, CT

Constance Welzel, **7**
Seaford, NY

Kathleen Wendt, **2**
Farmington, MI

Harriet Werley, **8**
Milwaukee, WI

Una Westfall, **8**
Portland, OR

Georgia Whitley, **4**
Plainfield, IL

Joie Whitney, **7**
Seattle, WA

Paul Wibbenmeyer, **7**
Chicago, IL

Ellen Wilson, **3**
Libertyville, IL

William Windels, **6**
Underhill, VT

Marina Wolfe, **1**
Terre Haute, IN

Sue Woolsey, **3**
Evansville, IN

Jackie Wylie, **8**
Kalamazoo, MI

Karen York, **3**
Dayton, OH

Naomi Yoshimoto, **3**
Honolulu, HI

Pamela Youngbauer, **1**
Milwaukee, WI

Dorothy Zelenski
Johnstown, PA

Natalie Zimmerman, **1**
Brookfield, WI

Karin Zuehls, **4**
West Burlington, IA

Appendix F Regional group meeting

LAURA ROSSI, M.S.N., R.N.

There was much excitement at this conference, where nineteen representatives from fifteen regional groups met to discuss common issues and concerns. Although no formal relationship between NANDA and these groups exists at the present time, there was a genuine interest in maintaining open channels of communication supporting the development of new regional groups. Each group currently functions to meet the specific needs of its area. Dissemination of up-to-date conference news is a primary focus; however, other needs range from educational programming to research consultation. Groups are financially supported locally by individual state nurses associations or independent dues-paying membership structures.

Regional group representatives were encouraged to utilize the NANDA newsletter as a mechanism for networking between conferences. Plans to establish a regular meeting time for regional groups at each conference are currently underway.

Representatives and regions

Beverly J. Bartlett
Western Mass Nursing Diagnosis Group

Joanne Bennett
American Journal of Nursing

Lenore Boles
Connecticut Nursing Diagnosis Group

Eleanor H. Borkowski
Western Regional Nursing Diagnosis Group

Lynda Juall Carpenito
Mid-Atlantic Nursing Diagnosis Group

Kenneth L. Cianfrani
Midwest Nursing Diagnosis Task Force

Rodney Copley
Cindy Schneider
Central Oklahoma Nursing Diagnosis Group

Richard J. Fehring
Linda F. Gulley
Wisconsin Nursing Diagnosis Interest Group

Mary Ann Kelly
Southern Regional

Pat Kucharski
Laura Rossi
Mass Conference Group for Classification of Nursing Diagnosis

Anita Lymburner
New Hampshire Nursing Diagnosis Group

Audrey McLane
NANDA—Program Committee Chairperson

Peggy McComb
Northwest Nursing Diagnosis Committee
Oregon

Roselle Partridge
Indiana Nursing Diagnosis Interest Group

Marion Resler
Mid-America Regional Nursing Diagnosis Group

Kathy Sheppard
Texas Nursing Diagnosis Interest Group

Index